CRITICAL PERSPECTIVES ON RACIAL AND ETHNIC DIFFERENCES IN HEALTH IN LATE LIFE

Norman B. Anderson, Rodolfo A. Bulatao, and
Barney Cohen, Editors

Panel on Race, Ethnicity, and Health in Later Life

Committee on Population

Division of Behavioral and Social Sciences and Education

NATIONAL RESEARCH COUNCIL
OF THE NATIONAL ACADEMIES

THE NATIONAL ACADEMIES PRESS
Washington, D.C.
www.nap.edu

THE NATIONAL ACADEMIES PRESS • 500 Fifth Street, N.W. • Washington, D.C. 20001

NOTICE: The project that is the subject of this report was approved by the Governing Board of the National Research Council, whose members are drawn from the councils of the National Academy of Sciences, the National Academy of Engineering, and the Institute of Medicine. The members of the committee responsible for the report were chosen for their special competences and with regard for appropriate balance.

This study was supported by Contract No. N01-OD-4-2139, TO #78 between the National Academy of Sciences and the National Institute on Aging and a grant from the Andrew W. Mellon Foundation. Any opinions, findings, conclusions, or recommendations expressed in this publication are those of the authors and do not necessarily reflect the views of the organizations or agencies that provided support for the project.

Library of Congress Cataloging-in-Publication Data

Critical perspectives on racial and ethnic differences in health in late life / Norman B. Anderson, Rodolfo A. Bulatao, and Barney Cohen, editors ; Panel on Race, Ethnicity, and Health in Later Life, Committee on Population, Division of Behavioral and Social Sciences and Education.
   p. ; cm.
Includes bibliographical references.
ISBN 0-309-09211-6 (pbk.)
1. Minority older people—Health and hygiene—United States. 2. Older people—Health and hygiene—United States—Cross-cultural studies. 3. Discrimination in medical care—United States. 4. Health status indicators.
[DNLM: 1. Health Status—Aged. 2. Ethnic Groups. 3. Health Behavior—Aged. 4. Socioeconomic Factors. WB 141.4 C934 2004] I. Anderson, Norman B. II. Bulatao, Rodolfo A., 1944- III. Cohen, Barney, 1959- IV. National Research Council (U.S.). Panel on Race, Ethnicity, and Health in Later Life.
  RA564.8.C75 2004
  362.198'97'00973—dc22

                 2004017317

Additional copies of this report are available from the National Academies Press, 500 Fifth Street, N.W., Lockbox 285, Washington, D.C. 20055; (800) 624-6242 or (202) 334-3313 (in the Washington metropolitan area); http://www.nap.edu.

Printed in the United States of America

Suggested citation: National Research Council. (2004). *Critical Perspectives on Racial and Ethnic Differences in Health in Late Life*. N.B. Anderson, R.A. Bulatao, and B. Cohen, Editors. Panel on Race, Ethnicity, and Health in Later Life. Committee on Population, Division of Behavioral and Social Sciences and Education. Washington, DC: The National Academies Press.

THE NATIONAL ACADEMIES
Advisers to the Nation on Science, Engineering, and Medicine

The **National Academy of Sciences** is a private, nonprofit, self-perpetuating society of distinguished scholars engaged in scientific and engineering research, dedicated to the furtherance of science and technology and to their use for the general welfare. Upon the authority of the charter granted to it by the Congress in 1863, the Academy has a mandate that requires it to advise the federal government on scientific and technical matters. Dr. Bruce M. Alberts is president of the National Academy of Sciences.

The **National Academy of Engineering** was established in 1964, under the charter of the National Academy of Sciences, as a parallel organization of outstanding engineers. It is autonomous in its administration and in the selection of its members, sharing with the National Academy of Sciences the responsibility for advising the federal government. The National Academy of Engineering also sponsors engineering programs aimed at meeting national needs, encourages education and research, and recognizes the superior achievements of engineers. Dr. Wm. A. Wulf is president of the National Academy of Engineering.

The **Institute of Medicine** was established in 1970 by the National Academy of Sciences to secure the services of eminent members of appropriate professions in the examination of policy matters pertaining to the health of the public. The Institute acts under the responsibility given to the National Academy of Sciences by its congressional charter to be an adviser to the federal government and, upon its own initiative, to identify issues of medical care, research, and education. Dr. Harvey V. Fineberg is president of the Institute of Medicine.

The **National Research Council** was organized by the National Academy of Sciences in 1916 to associate the broad community of science and technology with the Academy's purposes of furthering knowledge and advising the federal government. Functioning in accordance with general policies determined by the Academy, the Council has become the principal operating agency of both the National Academy of Sciences and the National Academy of Engineering in providing services to the government, the public, and the scientific and engineering communities. The Council is administered jointly by both Academies and the Institute of Medicine. Dr. Bruce M. Alberts and Dr. Wm. A. Wulf are chair and vice chair, respectively, of the National Research Council.

www.national-academies.org

Contributors

MAUREEN R. BENJAMINS, School of Public Health, University of Illinois, Chicago

DEBBIE BRADSHAW, Burden of Disease Research Unit, Medical Research Council, Tygerberg, South Africa

MARY E. CAMPBELL, Department of Sociology, University of Wisconsin-Madison

AMITABH CHANDRA, Department of Economics, Dartmouth College, Hanover, NH

RODNEY CLARK, Department of Psychology, Wayne State University, Detroit, MI

BARNEY COHEN, The National Academies, Washington, DC

RICHARD S. COOPER, Department of Preventive Medicine and Epidemiology, Loyola University Stritch School of Medicine, Maywood, IL

EILEEN M. CRIMMINS, Andrus Gerontology Center, University of Southern California

CATHERINE CUBBIN, Stanford Prevention Research Center, Stanford University School of Medicine

DAVID M. CUTLER, Department of Economics, Harvard University

JENNIFER L. EGGERLING-BOECK, Department of Sociology, University of Wisconsin-Madison

DOUGLAS EWBANK, Sociology Department, University of Pennsylvania

BRUCE H. FRIEDMAN, Department of Psychology, Virginia Polytechnic Institute and State University

THOMAS A. GLASS, Department of Epidemiology, Johns Hopkins Bloomberg School of Public Health

MARK D. HAYWARD, Department of Sociology, Pennsylvania State University

CLYDE HERTZMAN, Center for Health Services and Policy Research, University of British Columbia, Vancouver, Canada

ROBERT A. HUMMER, Population Research Center and Department of Sociology, University of Texas at Austin

WEI-CHIN HWANG, Department of Psychology, University of Utah

GUILLERMINA JASSO, Department of Sociology, New York University

RIA LAUBSCHER, Burden of Disease Research Unit, Medical Research Council, Tygerberg, South Africa

JOHN W. LYNCH, Department of Epidemiology, University of Michigan

JENNIFER J. MANLY, GH Sergievsky Center and Taub Institute for Research on Alzheimer's Disease and the Aging Brain, Columbia University

DOUGLAS S. MASSEY, Department of Sociology and Woodrow Wilson School of Public and International Affairs, Princeton University

RICHARD MAYEUX, GH Sergievsky Center and Taub Institute for Research on Alzheimer's Disease and the Aging Brain, Columbia University

NOLWAZI MBANANGA, Burden of Disease Research Unit, Medical Research Council, Tygerberg, South Africa

CARLOS F. MENDES DE LEON, Department of Internal Medicine, Rush Presbyterian St. Luke's Medical Center, Chicago, IL

JEFFREY D. MORENOFF, Department of Sociology, University of Michigan

HECTOR F. MYERS, Department of Psychology, University of California, Los Angeles

JAMES Y. NAZROO, Department of Epidemiology and Public Health, University College London, England

ROSANA NORMAN, Burden of Disease Research Unit, Medical Research Council, Tygerberg, South Africa

ALBERTO PALLONI, Department of Sociology, University of Wisconsin-Madison

RICHARD G. ROGERS, Population Program and Department of Sociology, University of Colorado at Boulder

MARK R. ROSENZWEIG, John F. Kennedy School of Government, Harvard University

GARY D. SANDEFUR, Department of Sociology, University of Wisconsin-Madison

MICHELLE SCHNEIDER, Burden of Disease Research Unit, Medical Research Council, Tygerberg, South Africa

TERESA E. SEEMAN, School of Medicine, University of California, Los Angeles

JONATHAN S. SKINNER, Department of Economics, Dartmouth College, Hanover, NH

JAMES P. SMITH, RAND Corporation, Santa Monica, CA

KRISELA STEYN, Burden of Disease Research Unit, Medical Research Council, Tygerberg, South Africa

JULIAN F. THAYER, Gerontology Research Center, National Institute on Aging, Baltimore, MD

MARILYN A. WINKLEBY, Stanford Prevention Research Center, Stanford University School of Medicine

Preface

The Panel on Race, Ethnicity, and Health in Later Life was established in 2001 under the auspices of the Committee on Population of the National Research Council. The panel's task was to inform the National Institute on Aging about recent research findings on racial and ethnic differences in health in late life and to help in developing a future research agenda for reducing them. This project was a follow-up to a 1994 Committee on Population workshop, which resulted in a volume of papers published by the National Academy Press, *Racial and Ethnic Differences in the Health of Older Americans*.

The panel was asked to organize a 2-day workshop, bringing together leading researchers from a variety of disciplines and professional orientations to summarize current research and to identify research priorities. That workshop was held in March 2002 in Washington, D.C. The panel also was asked to produce a summary of the state of knowledge incorporating this information and to provide recommendations for further work. The initial plan called for the papers and the panel report to be published in a single volume, but it was decided to publish the papers and the panel report separately. The papers are presented in this volume. The panel's final report is available in a companion volume, *Understanding Racial and Ethnic Differences in Health in Late Life: A Research Agenda*.

The papers in this volume have been reviewed in draft form by individuals chosen for their diverse perspectives and technical expertise, in accordance with procedures approved by the Report Review Committee of the National Research Council. The purpose of this independent review is to provide candid and critical comments that will assist the institution in making its published volume as sound as possible and to ensure that the volume meets institutional standards for objectivity, evidence, and responsiveness to the charge. The review comments remain confidential to protect the integrity of the process.

We thank the following individuals for their review of one or more papers in this volume: Dolores Acevedo-Garcia, Department of Society, Human Development, and Health, Harvard School of Public Health; Norman B. Anderson, American Psychological Association, Washington, DC; Eileen M. Crimmins, Andrus Gerontology Center, University of Southern California; Angus S. Deaton, Woodrow Wilson School of Public and International Affairs, Princeton University; Troy Duster, Department of Sociology, University of California at Berkeley; Irma T. Elo, Department of Sociology, University of Pennsylvania; David V. Espino, Department of Family and Community Medicine, University of Texas Health Science Center at San Antonio; Maria Evandrou, Age Concern Institute of Gerontology, King's College London, England; W. Reynolds Farley, Population Studies Center, University of Michigan; Vicki A. Freedman, Polisher Research Institute, Abramson Center for Jewish Life, North Wales, PA; W. Parker Frisbie, Population Research Center, University of Texas at Austin; Lucy Gilson, Centre for Health Policy, University of Witwatersrand, Johannesburg, South Africa; Jules Harrell, Psychology Department, Howard University; James S. House, Institute of Gerontology, University of Michigan; James S. Jackson, Research Centre for Group Dynamics, University of Michigan; John Jemmott, Annenberg School for Communication, University of Pennsylvania; Christopher Jencks, John F. Kennedy School of Government, Harvard University; Elizabeth A. Klonoff, Department of Psychology, San Diego State University, California; Neal M. Krause, Institute of Gerontology, University of Michigan; Diana J. L. Kuh, Department of Epidemiology and Public Health, University College London, England; Nancy S. Landale, Department of Sociology, Pennsylvania State University; Gerald E. McClearn, Department of Biobehavioral Health, Pennsylvania State University; Alberto Palloni, Department of Sociology, University of Wisconsin-Madison; Lynda Powell, Department of Preventive Medicine, Rush University Medical Center, Chicago, IL; Thomas C. Ricketts, III, School of Public Health, University of North Carolina at Chapel Hill; Teresa E. Seeman, School of Medicine, University of California, Los Angeles; James P. Smith, RAND Corporation, Santa Monica, CA; Keith E. Whitfield, Department of Health and Human Development, Pennsylvania State University; and David R. Williams, Department of Sociology, University of Michigan, Ann Arbor.

Although the reviewers listed above provided many constructive comments and suggestions, they were not asked to endorse the content of any of the papers nor did they see the final version of any paper before this publication. The review of this volume was overseen by Charles B. Keely, Georgetown University. Appointed by the National Research Council, he was responsible for making certain that an independent examination of the papers was carried out in accordance with institutional procedures and that all review comments were carefully considered. Responsibility for the final content of this volume rests entirely with the authors.

Contents

ACCESS TO HEALTH CARE

SECTION IV: THE CHALLENGE OF IDENTIFYING EFFECTIVE INTERVENTIONS

SECTION V: TWO INTERNATIONAL COMPARISONS

1

Introduction

Barney Cohen

Life expectancy at birth in the United States has improved dramatically over the past century—from about 46.3 years for men and 48.3 years for women in 1900 to about 74.1 years for men and 79.5 years for women in 2000 (National Center for Health Statistics [NCHS], 2003). But the story behind this piece of good news is a story in two parts. During the first half of the century, life expectancy at birth rose largely because of improvements in nutrition, housing, hygiene, and medical care, as well as the prevention and control of major childhood infectious diseases (NCHS, 2003). But throughout the second half of the century, advances in medicine—particularly in relation to the treatment of heart disease and stroke—along with healthier lifestyles, improvements in access to health care, and better general overall health before reaching age 65 combined to result in continued improvements in life expectancy (Fried, 2000). As a result, in the first half of the 20th century, life expectancy at birth rose dramatically while gains in life expectancy above age 65 were relatively modest. Between 1900 and 1950, life expectancy at birth rose 42 percent for men and 47 percent for women, while life expectancy at 65 only rose 11 percent for men and 23 percent for women. But between 1950 and 2000, the pattern was completely different. In the second half of the century, demographers recorded small gains in life expectancy at birth and large gains in life expectancy above age 65. Life expectancy at birth over this latter period rose 13 percent for men and 12 percent for women, while life expectancy at age 65 rose 31 percent for men and 28 percent for women.

Although universally lauded as a great success story, the increase in life expectancy at older ages over the second half of the century has renewed important concerns about the existence of significant racial and ethnic differences in health. This country's progress on race-related issues is often measured by trends in major indicators of economic and social well-being, such as income or percentage of people in poverty, but few indicators offer more dramatic social commentary than the existence of large racial and ethnic differences in life expectancy. Blacks continue to experience much poorer health than whites, both before and after age 65, even though the black-white gap has narrowed over much of the century. The most recent data available from death certificates indicate that age-adjusted death rates for blacks are 33 percent higher than for whites (NCHS, 2003). On the other hand, age-adjusted death rates for other racial and ethnic minority groups are often lower than the comparable rate for whites, although there is much misunderstanding and misreporting on this point. Age-adjusted death rates for Hispanics (to the extent that they can be considered a discrete and identifiable segment of American society) are 22 percent lower than for non-Hispanic whites (NCHS, 2003), a surprise to many given their far lower average socioeconomic position and their generally poor level of health care coverage. Furthermore, the available data from death certificates suggest that, if taken at face value, both the American Indian and Alaskan Native populations and the Asian and Pacific Islander populations enjoy relatively lower age-adjusted death rates than non-Hispanic whites.

Undoubtedly some fraction of the minority advantage is attributable to measurement errors because death rates for both these minority groups are known to be underestimated (Rosenberg et al., 1999). Even so, when re-searchers have attempted to adjust the data or reestimate rates using other data sources, the relative ranking described rarely changes (Chapter 3, this volume). Within these various groups, there is much heterogeneity. Among Hispanics, Puerto Ricans generally experience relatively poorer health out-comes than Cubans and Mexican Americans, while among Asians and Pacific Islanders, Samoans and Native Hawaiians generally have worse health than other Asians. Further complicating the picture of relative health is the fact that, although it is generally true that blacks fare worse than other groups, the relative ordering of the other groups is inconsistent. For example, while most studies find that Hispanics fare worse with respect to such health outcomes as diabetes, infectious diseases, and chronic liver disease, they also find a Hispanic advantage for cardiovascular disease, cancer, and pulmonary diseases (Palloni and Arias, 2003).

To date, little research on racial and ethnic differences in health has been directed specifically toward the elderly, and there is still a need for great concern about broad health disadvantages of certain subpopulations, but particularly with regard to the situation of elderly blacks relative to whites. In 1950, there was no survival advantage of white men over black men above age 65. For women, it was only 0.2 of a year (NCHS, 2003). By 1970, it was 0.6 of a year for men and 1.4 years for women, and by 2000, the survival advantage of whites over blacks above age 65 was 2 years for men and 1.9 years for women (NCHS, 2003). This situation changed little over the 1990s.

A further reason for concern over racial and ethnic differences in health is that as a nation, the United States is becoming increasingly diverse. Currently, Hispanics, non-Hispanic blacks, Asians, and American Indians constitute 27 percent of the population, with blacks being the largest ethnic minority group. In 2003, Hispanics overtook non-Hispanic blacks and became the largest minority group. By 2050, half of the U.S. population will be either Hispanic, non-Hispanic black, Asian, or American Indian. In terms of the population aged 65 and over, the changes will be even more dramatic. Current projections suggest that by 2050, the total number of whites aged 65 and over will double. But, over the same period, the number of elderly blacks will more than triple and the number of elderly Hispanic and "other race" populations will increase 11-fold.

Responding to all these concerns, the National Institute on Aging (NIA) requested the National Research Council (NRC) to help guide its efforts to eliminate racial and ethnic differences in the health of older Americans. Specifically, the NIA asked the NRC to review research in this area and to identify research priorities that it might fund. Given that the debate about racial disparities in health has become highly political (see Vedantam, 2004), the case for clear and dispassionate scientific research could hardly be greater.

In addressing its charge, the NRC was forced to confront a large and burgeoning theoretical and empirical literature involving researchers in public health, medicine, and virtually all of the social and behavioral sciences. To make sense of this rapidly growing field, the NRC appointed an ad hoc panel, chaired by Norman Anderson, to prepare a report summarizing the main research lessons learned and offering recommendations to NIA for future directions for policy research and data collection in this important area. To help guide the panel, a series of background papers was commissioned. Revised versions of these papers are included as chapters in this volume.

THE SIGNIFICANCE OF THE CHAPTERS IN THIS VOLUME

Taken collectively, the chapters map out many of the major themes of interest to researchers and policy-makers concerned with racial and ethnic inequalities in health. The authors, all people at the forefront of research in their particular field, provide state-of-the-art assessments of the research in their area and identify major gaps in data, theory, and research design.

The papers represent a broad diversity of scholarly perspectives. Many different disciplines have made theoretical and empirical contributions to the study of health and the current collection is, to some extent, an amalgamation of concepts and insights—both new and old—obtained from various disciplines, each with its own domain of interest and style of analyzing and presenting data. Inevitably, the empirical basis for certain conclusions is stronger than for others. For example, while enough large high-quality longitudinal data sets are now available to be able to link socioeconomic resources confidently to observed racial and ethnic differences in health, few data have been collected on the cumulative effects over time of perceived racism on health (Chapter 9, this volume, Chapter 13, this volume). Thus, while some authors review research fields that employ mature methodologies and standard approaches, others report on new avenues of research that are still very much in their infancy. In these latter cases, concepts, methods, and measures still need to be refined. Nevertheless, each paper conveys important ideas that merit careful consideration.

SECTION I: THE NATURE OF RACIAL AND ETHNIC DIFFERENCES

Complicating our ability to study racial and ethnic differences is the fluid nature of the social construct of race, which needs to be understood in a particular social and historical context. Race is not a very meaningful biological categorization. Although it can be defined as phenotypic differences in skin color, hair texture, and other physical attributes, these are not (as often wrongly perceived) the surface manifestations of deeper underlying differences in attributes such as intelligence, temperament, or physical stature. Nevertheless, as we all know, race remains an extremely powerful predictor of life chances as well as social, psychological, and behavioral group differences.

In Chapter 2, Gary D. Sandefur, Mary E. Campbell, and Jennifer Eggerling-Boeck discuss some of the problems of defining and measuring racial and ethnic groups in the United States, how information on racial and ethnic composition has been collected at different points in time in some of the major health data sources, and how this has had important implications for our understanding of racial and ethnic differences in health among the elderly.

There are numerous examples in the study of race in the United States of racial categories and/or data collection efforts changing over time. For example, consider the case of the American Indian population. Since 1960, this population has grown principally as a result of the increased numbers of persons choosing to claim American Indian as their racial identity, as opposed to choosing white or some other race (Eschbach, 1993; Harris,

1994; Passel, 1976; Passel and Berman, 1986). A large proportion of those changing their reported identity from one Census to the next have tended to be of mixed race, which with high rates of intermarriage among American Indians, is likely to be an increasingly frequent occurrence. Interestingly, intermarriage has not only affected how people identify themselves, but in some cases it has led to tribes reconsidering how they define themselves (Thornton, 1996). These factors make it more problematic to compare results over time and across studies for American Indians than for other groups.

Perhaps the one recent policy change that is likely to have the greatest long-run implications is the recent directive of the Office of Management and Budget that allowed individuals to choose more than one racial category in the 2000 Census. Up until then, Americans could choose only one racial category to describe their race. Sandefur et al. examine the impact of this change. They conclude that allowing multiple responses to the "race" question in the 2000 Census has had only a modest impact on the measured racial composition of the U.S. population (see also Hirschman et al., 2000). However, this could easily change over time because it is quite possible that many blacks of mixed racial descent did not identify themselves as such in the 2000 Census because they never had the option to do so in the past (Korgen, 1999).

With these caveats in mind, Robert A. Hummer, Maureen R. Benjamins, and Richard G. Rogers (Chapter 3) summarize what is known about racial and ethnic differences in older health and mortality from large nationally representative data sets, and they discuss the extent to which the observed health differences correspond with differences in sociodemographic factors across population groups. Not surprisingly, the authors document that racial and ethnic differences in health, activity limitation, and active life persist well into later life, despite overall improvements in the general health of the U.S. population. The basic pattern is remarkably consistent over time and across data sources. Blacks have worse overall health across a number of indicators than white elders, while Hispanics and Asian American elders tend to fare better than whites. A major question revolves around the reliability of data on the health of Native American elderly. Note, however, that there is a great deal of heterogeneity in health outcomes within racial and ethnic categories, particularly among Hispanics (e.g., consider Puerto Ricans versus Cubans or Mexican Americans), Asian Americans, and American Indians. Hummer et al. also find that excess black mortality, relative to whites, is concentrated among the younger elderly population, with negligible differences beyond age 80. The authors show that education and income differences across groups continue to play an important role, explaining the overall worse health of non-Hispanic blacks, Native Americans, and, to a lesser degree, Hispanics in old age.

An ongoing debate remains about whether a true black-white crossover in mortality occurs among the oldest old. For many years analysis of mortality data has suggested that the black mortality curve crosses over the white mortality curve in later life so that, at the oldest ages, blacks have an advantage (see, e.g., Manton and Stallard, 1997; Nam et al., 1978). However, racial differences in death rates at older ages are especially vulnerable to distortion both because age misreporting is unusually common at these ages and because any distortions that occur are amplified by the severe slope of the age distribution itself (Coale and Kisker, 1986; Preston et al., 1996). And recent analysis by Preston and colleagues suggests that if there is a crossover, it is postponed to very high ages where data quality is most suspect (Preston et al., 2003).

Hummer et al. also compare the racial and ethnic differences among the elderly with those exhibited by younger age groups, and they find similar relative differences over the entire life course. For example, despite the fact that infant mortality rates have declined for all racial and ethnic groups over the past 50 years, large racial and ethnic differences remain. For a variety of reasons, including differences in underlying health status, socioeconomic circumstances, and the availability and use of health care, infant, neonatal, and postneonatal mortality rates for blacks are more than twice as high as for whites. Infant mortality for Hispanics is quite similar to whites, although under the Hispanic banner there is a degree of heterogeneity, with infant mortality rates being highest for Puerto Rican mothers and lowest for Cuban mothers. Similarly, although mortality rates among children and young adults also have declined over the past 50 years, large differences remain. Homicide and suicide rates, for example, vary by age, sex, and race. In 2000, homicide rates for black males aged 15 to 24 were 18 times as great as for non-Hispanic white males the same age (NCHS, 2003).

The second overview paper, by Jennifer J. Manly and Richard Mayeux (Chapter 4), examines in depth the ethnic differences in dementia and Alzheimer's disease. The major findings are that blacks and Hispanics have higher prevalence and incidence of cognitive impairment, dementia, and Alzheimer's disease than whites. American Indians have a lower rate of Alzheimer's disease than whites, but equivalent rates of overall cognitive impairment and dementia. The authors argue that because no research has been able to convincingly overcome the overwhelming influence of cultural and educational experience on cognitive test performance, the true extent of cross-cultural differences in cognitive impairment, dementia, or Alzheimer's remains an open question. Not surprisingly, therefore, researchers are still a long way from understanding how, controlling for education, observed differences can be explained by biological risk factors such as cerebrovascular disease, differential exposure to environmental risk factors, or genetic risk factors (Chapter 4, this volume). Some intriguing recent cross-national evidence suggests that racial and ethnic differences in rates of dementia may be the result of complex gene-environmental interactions. It remains to be seen, however, whether researchers will be able to disentangle biological and genetic risk factors from their sociocultural or environment context (Chapter 4, this volume).

SECTION II: TWO KEY CONCEPTUAL AND METHODOLOGICAL CHALLENGES

The papers by Clyde Hertzman (Chapter 5), Alberto Palloni and Douglas C. Ewbank (Chapter 6), and Guillermina Jasso and colleagues (Chapter 7) highlight important analytical and methodological insights that have emerged from research in this area over the past couple of decades.

In Chapter 5, Hertzman argues the need for a life-course approach to the study of health. Events over one's life can have a long-run and cumulative impact on one's health, affecting a diverse range of outcomes from general well-being to physical functioning and chronic disease. For example, studies have linked fetal and early child nutrition to a wide range of disease outcomes in later life, including heart disease, diabetes, obesity, high blood pressure, age-related memory loss, and schizophrenia (see Barker, 1998). Similarly, findings related to the nature of racial and ethnic differences in health and mortality in older ages need to be interpreted within a life-course framework. Hertzman sets out various mechanisms through which early experiences can affect adult health status, distinguishing among latency, pathway, and cumulative effects. Hertzman's chapter implies an urgent need for much better data in order to understand how various life-course factors (e.g., socioeconomic position over the life cycle, family history, migration history, work history, cumulative stress, child and early adult health experience) exhibit different general patterns across racial and ethnic groups, thereby contributing to differential impacts on older adult health by race or ethnic group.

The next papers, by Palloni and Ewbank (Chapter 6) and Jasso et al. (Chapter 7), focus on the conceptual and methodological challenges that arise in the study of observed racial and ethnic differences in health from the potential existence of certain types of selection processes. Generally speaking, standard regression coefficients that are obtained from data drawn from nonrandom samples are not of direct interest because they may exaggerate or attenuate estimates of effects of membership in a particular race or ethnic group that occur due to the existence of other mechanisms. For example, in the classic case of sample selection bias, standard regression coefficients confound meaningful structural parameters with the parameters of a function that determines the probability that the observation makes its way into the nonrandom sample (Heckman, 1979). Perhaps the best known and simplest example of a problem analogous to that identified by Heckman operating in demography relates to the issue of differential survival among population subgroups, which can produce mortality cross-overs. If one subgroup is disadvantaged at an early age, then heterogeneity implies that its members will appear to be less disadvantaged or even advantaged at older ages (Vaupel et al., 1979). Palloni and Ewbank demonstrate that selection effects can, in some cases at least, be quite large, and if ignored could lead to misinterpretation of observable data and to erroneous policy prescriptions.

Palloni and Ewbank's general conclusions regarding the value of controlling for selection are generally reinforced by the paper by Jasso et al., who use the particularly salient example of immigrant health to discuss the dangers of using censored (i.e., nonrandomly selected) samples to estimate behavioral relationships. With immigration a driving force in accounting for the future growth of the American population, scholarly and policy-related interest in immigration and health, and how the two are related, is perhaps greater today than ever before. A recurrent finding in the immigrant health literature is that Mexican and non-Mexican Hispanics experience better health, lower adult mortality rates, and lower infant mortality than African Americans and non-Hispanic whites and that the health of immigrants appears to deteriorate with duration of stay in the United States (Chapter 6, this volume). Various explanations have been put forward as to why this might be the case. These include the possibility that migrants come from a cultural milieu that promotes more favorable behavioral profiles in terms of diet, smoking, and alcohol consumption, and more cohesive social networks and social support mechanisms (see Chapter 6, this volume). However, it is also possible that immigrants are healthier because of positive selection of migration for health (or for other endowments or traits that are correlated with health). In other words, their initially superior health status preceded and facilitated their immigration.

Drawing on their survey of legal immigrants who obtained their green cards in 1996, Jasso et al. discuss the problems of using cross-sectional data to investigate these issues. The authors provide strong empirical support to Palloni and Ewbank's concerns regarding the importance of accounting for selectivity bias in interpreting data on racial and ethnic differences in health. They argue persuasively that controlling for health selection (i.e., the propensity of immigrants to be healthier than a representative person in the sending country) is critical to understanding patterns of immigrant health. The authors also develop a theoretical model that attempts to explain the diversity in health selection among immigrants. This work provides a sounder theoretical grounding for research on immigration and health than has previously been available.

SECTION III: THE SEARCH FOR CAUSAL PATHWAYS

Over the past 20 years, papers on racial and ethnic differences in health have shifted away from straightforward descriptive studies toward more analytical studies that attempt to explain the underlying causes and mechanisms behind these differences. The next nine papers in the volume attempt to summarize scientific knowledge about the main factors that contribute to the existence of racial and ethnic differences in health in later life, as described earlier. As many of the authors point out in their chapters, the search for evidence on causal factors has been a stubborn problem, fraught with methodological and conceptual difficulties.

Each of the nine chapters in this section of the volume focuses on a particular factor or set of factors, which often parallel the interest(s) of a particular scientific discipline. Group differences in health are the product of both biology and individual choice, the former modified in some cases by environmentally sensitive gene expression and the latter strongly influenced by economic, social, and cultural conditions. While the volume itself aspires to be comprehensive in its coverage of the major health risks, individual papers introduce concepts and insights from quite different disciplines, not all of which have been fully integrated. Thus, individual chapters can only provide a general treatment of a particular set of relationships, detailing the research evidence in one particular area without attempting to integrate these observations into a comprehensive theory or framework, which, in any event, is still far beyond the current capacities of the field (National Research Council, 2004).

Genetic Factors

Probably no aspect of the debate about the causes of racial differences in health is potentially more sensitive than the discussion about the extent to which genetic factors are in any way responsible. There are numerous historical examples of scientific mischief in the support of racism. The discovery in 1851 of drapetomania (a mental disease that caused slaves to run away from plantations) is only one of a series of misguided attempts over the 19th and early 20th centuries to distinguish biological differences between the races. Yet recent research on genetic variation within human populations has reopened the debate over the validity of race as a sensible research variable (Sankar and Cho, 2002). Proponents of using race assert that there is a useful degree of association between genetic differences and racial classifications, so that the use of race as a research variable is warranted. Critics, on the other hand, argue that bundling the population into four or five broad groups according to skin color and other physical traits is not a useful way of summarizing genetic variation when we know now that there are at least 15 million genetic polymorphisms in humans, of which an unknown number underlie variation in (normal and) disease traits (Burchard et al., 2003). Hence critics argue that there is as much or more genetic variation within the major population groups than between them.

The gene pools of different racial or ethnic groups may contain different frequencies of alleles at different loci that are pertinent to health status or to disease processes. In Chapter 8, Richard S. Cooper explains that there are two ways that genes may be relevant to the study of health differences. First, genetic differences in disease among racial and ethnic groups are particularly relevant for simple genetic disorders caused by a single gene mutation in populations that descend from a relatively small number of founders and that remain endogamous for a large part of their history. An example is the prevalence of Tay-Sachs disease among Ashkenazi Jews. However, such single-gene disorders are generally rare and scientists are only just beginning to confront the challenge of understanding the genetic basis of complex genetic disorders such as asthma, cancer, and diabetes, which likely involve multiple, potentially interacting, genes and environmental factors (see also Burchard et al., 2003).

This leads to the second way that genes may be relevant to the study of health differences, namely through environmental factors, which may vary by ethnic group, and which might interact with genotype to produce difference outcomes. (Note that environment in this context is defined as all influences not coded in DNA.) Significant resources are now being devoted to elucidating further the importance of gene-environment interactions in a wide range of diseases. Although the volume of research in this area is growing rapidly, it is still in the early stages. Cooper is perhaps more pessimistic than some about the prospect of disentangling the role of genetic factors in explaining racial differences in health in the near future. But, given that most of the major diseases differing in frequency among the standard racial classifications appear to be diseases of complex etiology, involving a complex genetic basis and a strong environmental component influencing how this inherited susceptibility is expressed, and given that the environmental milieu of different racial and ethnic groups is quite different in many important respects, the challenge of disentangling the role of genetic factors from other possible explanatory variables appears hard to overstate (Neel, 1997). Nevertheless, the potential for further study is increasing greatly, with growing numbers of large population-based social and behavioral studies also collecting clinical and genetic data (Kington and Nickens, 2001).

Economic and Social Risk Factors

Chapters 9, 10, and 11 review the extent to which racial and ethnic differences in economic, social, and personal resources contribute to racial and ethnic differences in the health and well-being of older adults.

In Chapter 9, Eileen M. Crimmins, Mark D. Hayward, and Teresa E. Seeman review the complex interactions linking race, socioeconomic status, and health. The United States ranks first among industrialized countries with respect to measures of inequality of both income and wealth (Wilkinson, 1996; Wolff, 1996). This is important not only from a social justice perspective, but also because studies in recent decades have demonstrated a strong and persistent inverse gradient between mortality and socioeconomic status, even among those near the top of the socioeconomic distribution (Marmot et al., 1991).

Controlling for socioeconomic status eliminates a significant proportion—but not all—of the observed racial differences in chronic health between blacks and non-Hispanic whites, but not between Hispanics and non-Hispanic whites (Hayward et al., 2000). Nevertheless, for a number of reasons, it is extremely difficult to quantify succinctly the nature of the relationship between socioeconomic resources and health outcomes. First, the meaning and measurement of socioeconomic status has varied a fair amount across studies, and findings from different studies are not always directly comparable. Second, some authors have found the relationship between socioeconomic status and health to be decidedly nonlinear, while others have observed an essentially linear relationship. Third, no data set has truly come to grips with the cumulative and dynamic nature of the relationship over the entire lifecycle. Furthermore, there is growing evidence that conditions in early life or even in utero can profoundly influence one's risk for certain chronic conditions much later in life (Barker, 1998; Elo and Preston, 1992). Finally, although it has been well established that variations in socioeconomic status produce health differences, there is now an increasing appreciation of the need to recognize the alternative casual pathway, namely that among the elderly poor health can also lead to significantly reduced wealth (Smith, 1999). Recognizing the bidirectional nature of the relationship makes it difficult to interpret results from cross-sectional data. Finally, there is still a great deal of ambiguity surrounding the exact mechanisms by which socioeconomic inequality influences health (Deaton, 2001).

Using data from a number of major health surveys of the U.S. population, Crimmins et al. investigate how socioeconomic status—as indicated by educational attainment, family income, and wealth—varies across race and ethnicity. The authors find that the prevalence of diseases, functioning loss, and disability are all negatively related to socioeconomic status (i.e., lower socioeconomic status implies more health problems). The authors also examined the variability in disease and disability prevalence by socioeconomic status within racial and ethnic groups to determine whether the relationships were the same for all ethnic groups. They found that the strongest socioeconomic effects are within the white group.

Undoubtedly, the effects of economic resources on health and well-being are determined to some extent by the sociocultural environment. Building on the chapter by Crimmins et al., Carlos Mendes de Leon and Thomas A. Glass (Chapter 10) review the evidence on the effects of social and other personal resources on health and well-being. Evidence is accumulating to suggest that social and personal resources also play an important role in understanding differences in health and well-being among older adults. Social resources—which can include factors such as the strength of social and community networks, the level of social engagement, and the degree of participation in formal and informal organizations—have been linked with prolonged survival and decreased risk of age-related physical and cognitive disabilities (Chapter 10, this volume). But there is little evidence to suggest that there are substantial differences by race and ethnicity in either social or personal resources among the elderly. While older blacks tend to have similarly sized or slightly smaller social networks than older whites, these networks are more likely to include extended family members (Chapter 10, this volume). Similarly, older whites tend to be more engaged than older blacks with volunteer activities through formal and informal organizations, while older blacks tend to be more involved than older whites in faith-based organizations. Hence the authors conclude that there is little evidence to suggest that differences in social resources play a major role in producing the observed racial and ethnic differences in health in later life. The authors speculate that there may be more important racial and ethnic differences in community networks, given the stark differences in neighborhood characteristics in which different racial and ethnic groups live.

The challenge of reviewing the literature on the effects of neighborhoods and residential contexts on health among the elderly is taken up in Chapter 11 by Jeffrey D. Morenoff and John W. Lynch. Communities and neighborhoods are potentially important levels of aggregation for designing interventions aimed at improving health, yet few studies exist that focus specifically on the linkages between neighborhoods and elderly health. Consequently, the authors are forced to extend their review far beyond direct consideration of the effects of neighborhood influences on the elderly. A considerable body of research on the neighborhood context of health now exists and shows that context matters. Multilevel studies consistently show that poor neighborhoods with concentrated poverty are associated with significantly elevated risks of poor health and overall mortality, even after controlling for individual differences in household income. Unfortunately, however, different investigators have operationalized the concept of neighborhood in different ways, making it difficult to reach definite conclusions about the magnitude and importance of these kinds of effects (Chapter 11, this volume). Studies on neighborhood effects now need to move away from the descriptive to focus more on the question of why context matters for health. With this in mind, Morenoff and Lynch advance the notion of a life-course perspective that emphasizes the importance of cumulative effects. This implies that cross-sectional data would likely underestimate the true strength of neighborhood effects and that more attention needs to be focused on a multilevel longitudinal approach that can incorporate information on neighborhood characteristics over a protracted period.

Behavioral Risk Factors

An enormous amount of research over the past 20 years or so has confirmed the link between certain diseases and health outcomes and various health-damaging and health-promoting behaviors. Smoking, for example, is now known to be a major risk factor for several forms of cancer, chronic bronchitis, emphysema, and cardiovascular disease, while alcoholism is an important risk factor for numerous health outcomes, including cirrhosis of the liver and pancreatitis (U.S. Department of Health and Human Services, 1991). Alcohol is also a factor in approximately half of all homicides, suicides, and motor vehicle fatalities. Similarly, regular physical activity and correct nutrition have been shown to lower one's overall risk of mortality as well as being linked to the risk of certain diseases such as cardiovascular disease, non-insulin-dependent diabetes, osteoarthritis, and depression (U.S. Department of Health and Human Services, 1991).

The paper by Marilyn A. Winkleby and Catherine Cubbin (Chapter 12) explores the extent to which these and other health-damaging or health-promoting behaviors vary by racial and ethnic group. Few studies have examined racial and ethnic differences in health behavior among the elderly, especially using large-scale, nationally representative samples. Drawing on data from the 2000 Behavioral Risk Factor Surveillance System, the authors compare rates of smoking, obesity, leisure-time physical activity, diet, alcohol consumption, and cancer screening practices by racial and ethnic group, age, sex, and sociodemographic status. The differences between racial and ethnic groups are far from consistent. By some indicators, non-Hispanic whites behave in a more healthy manner than non-Hispanic blacks and/or Hispanics, but for other indicators, the opposite it true. For example, for women aged 65 to 74, non-Hispanic whites tend to smoke more than blacks or Hispanics. But for comparably aged men, blacks are the heaviest smokers. Similarly, elderly black women are less likely to engage in leisure-time physical activity and more likely to be obese than non-Hispanic whites or Hispanics, while elderly Hispanic men report significantly lower rates of leisure-time physical activity than non-Hispanic whites or blacks. Significantly, the authors find that these and similar differences in health-promoting or health-damaging behavior exist within each racial and ethnic group by important sociodemographic indicators, including age, sex, educational attainment, household income, and, for Mexican Americans, country of birth and language spoken. These differences clearly have important implications for prevention and public health (see Chapter 17, this volume).

Biobehavioral Factors

The next three chapters, by Hector F. Myers and Wei-Chin Hwang (Chapter 13), Rodney Clark (Chapter 14), and Julian F. Thayer and Bruce H. Friedman (Chapter 15), all explore various aspects of the relationships among stress, psychosocial risk and resilience, and racial and ethnic differences in health. Recent conceptual advances in health research have stressed the importance of an integrative approach that incorporates the interplay among genetic, behavioral, psychosocial, and environment factors over time (National Research Council, 2001). For many years, the study of stress has been considered a potentially important pathway connecting a person's experience, living and working conditions, interpersonal relations, and other behavioral variables to biological factors that more directly influence health. Stress is a known risk factor for hypertension, and the significantly higher prevalence of hypertension in blacks has led some researchers to theorize that there may be an important link between a negative psychological environment, cumulative stress, and hypertension and some of the observed racial differences in health.

Important new attempts to understand the relationship between environmental and behavioral challenges and stressors, health, and disease have introduced the concepts of allostasis and allostatic load (see Chapter 13, this volume). Stress is actually just part of the body's normal regulatory system. Stress causes and modulates a diversity of physiological effects that can either directly enhance resistance to disease or cause damage, thereby making the body more susceptible to disease (Institute of Medicine, 2001). But it is the repeated wear and tear on the body as a function of repeated insults that can lead to negative health effects and which is referred to as a body's allostatic load. This concept has received a lot of attention in medical circles (see, e.g., McEwen, 1998). In Chapter 13, Myers and Hwang outline a biopsychosocial model of cumulative psychological and physical vulnerability and resilience in later life, in which chronic stress burden and psychosocial resources for coping are hypothesized as playing a significant role in accounting for ethnic differences in mental health.

The central hypothesis in these biobehavioral models is that the differential burden of lifetime stress contributes to ethnic differences in health. Chapters 13 and 14 review some of the major potential sources of stress, including race, social class, immigrant acculturation, and age. Other researchers have emphasized the importance of looking at other potential sources of stress such as the degree of job control in the workplace (see, e.g., Marmot et al., 1997). These chapters are necessarily somewhat speculative because very little research has attempted to model or estimate the cumulative effects of various sources of stress. This is partly because of problems of measurement, concepts, and definition that need to be overcome. It is also partly because modeling and estimating dynamic processes over time are extremely complex and data-hungry endeavors. One of the methodological challenges of the work in this area is that much of it is based on subjective measures of stress (i.e., respondents reporting that they are feeling or felt stressed) rather than on measuring objective stressors such as particular life events (e.g., job loss, divorce). In addition, there is always the possibility that the causality runs in the other direction, namely that poor health status leads to higher perceived stress (Kington and Nickens, 2001).

Recently, researchers have turned their attention to investigating the impact of repeated encounters with racism or discrimination on physiologic activity (see, e.g., February 2003 special issue of the *American Journal of Public Health* as well as Chapter 14, this volume). Studies that attempt to relate physical health status to self-reported encounters with racism have been inconsistent (Chapter 14, this volume), but there is a growing body of research from community studies that discrimination is associated with multiple indicators of poorer physical and, especially, mental health status (Williams et al., 2003). Nevertheless, research on the health impact of racism and discrimination is still very much in its infancy, and difficult methodological challenges and controversies need to be overcome (Krieger, 1999). Racism and discrimination are subjective measures that are arguably far harder to measure than, say, socioeconomic status. The problem is even more complex once one accepts that the effects of discrimination can accumulate over a lifetime and even spill over into subsequent generations (National Research Council, 1989). Furthermore, racism and discrimination are not measured directly in large social and economic surveys. Hence data tend to come from laboratory research in controlled clinical settings. Clark (Chapter 14) suggests several ways to strengthen research in this area.

Another important avenue of research in this area revolves around the observation that people differ widely in their ability to deal with particular situations, including overcoming adversity. A growing body of research indicates that a number of psychosocial factors, including personality, resilience, coping style, early life experience, availability of social supports, and religiosity can serve to moderate the stress-health relationship in adults, including the elderly (Chapter 13, this volume). But, although some researchers have proposed that there may be important racial and ethnic differences in coping styles that relate to health outcomes (see, e.g., James, 1994, on John Henryism), few high-quality studies in this area have been conducted (Chapter 13, this volume).

In the next chapter, Thayer and Friedman collect recent findings that relate psychosocial factors such as stress and perceived racism to the functioning of the autonomic nervous system, which regulates all aspects of cardiovascular function. Our understanding of the multilevel and bidirectional relationships between behavioral and biologic processes has been enriched in recent years by advances in technology and by conceptual advances in the behavioral, biological, and medical sciences (Institute of Medicine, 2001). Recent research has uncovered many previously unknown links among the central nervous system, the endocrine system, and the immune system (Institute of Medicine, 2001). Thayer and Friedman's chapter reemphasizes the need for multilevel studies that address the interplay among physiological, behavioral, affective, cognitive, and social processes and their shared impact on health.

Access to Health Care

The chapter by Amitabh Chandra and Jonathan S. Skinner (Chapter 16) examines the extent to which the spatial distribution of health care and health outcomes across the United States varies by hospital referral region. Differential health care access and quality is a major public policy challenge. The United States is the only developed country in the world that does not have national health coverage, and 40 million Americans do not have any form of health care coverage (Institute of Medicine, 2001). Hispanics in particular are relatively underserved with respect to health coverage, partly because of their relatively low socioeconomic status and partly due to other contributing factors related to their degree of acculturation, language barriers, immigration status, and types of jobs in which they are engaged (Suárez, 2000). How much differential coverage contributes to racial and ethnic differences in health outcomes is unclear, however, because Hispanics do not appear to fare any worse than non-Hispanic whites with respect to a number of health outcomes. Infant mortality rates for Hispanics, for example, are essentially identical to non-Hispanic whites and have been for more than a decade (NCHS, 2003).

Chandra and Skinner argue that the correlation between minority status and health outcomes is confounded by differential access to medical services, specifically by substantial geographic variation in treatment and outcome patterns. Minorities tend to seek care from different hospitals and from different physicians than non-Hispanic whites, in large part a reflection of the general spatial distribution of the United States population with concentrations of minorities in certain hospital referral regions. Chandra and Skinner demonstrate that regional variation in the utilization of health care, and in outcomes, potentially can account for a substantial part of the observed racial and ethnic disparities in health. This implies a different set of policy prescriptions than if the underlying source of racial differences in health were primarily due to differences in treatment within hospitals or communities or differences in the self-management of disease (Goldman and Smith, 2002; Institute of Medicine, 2003).

SECTION IV: THE CHALLENGE OF IDENTIFYING EFFECTIVE INTERVENTIONS

What can be done about the existence of large and persistent differences in health outcomes by racial and ethnic group that essentially cannot be fully explained by traditional arguments? One starting point is the observation that approximately half of all deaths in the United States can be traced to various health-damaging behaviors, especially tobacco use, poor diet, low activity patterns, and excessive alcohol consumption (McGinnis and Foege, 1993). To the extent that racial differences in health can be attributed to differences in group behavior (see Chapter 12, this volume), then it may be possible to develop programs that can educate and encourage people to modify their behavior. Although there are numerous examples of successful public awareness campaigns, the real challenge has always been to get people to convert new knowledge into sustained behavioral change. Most people, for example, know that if they change certain behaviors (e.g., exercise more, eat and drink more responsibly, avoid cigarettes), they would reduce their risk of certain diseases. But the $30 to $50 billion spent annually on various types of diet products testifies to the self-control problems that many people face (Cutler et al., 2003). In Chapter 17, David M. Cutler reviews the evidence on the effectiveness of large-scale behavioral health interventions that have been implemented at the individual, community, and national levels. Behavioral change is notoriously difficult to achieve and overall there is not very compelling evidence that large-scale interventions have worked. Although there have been studies that show that effective change is possible, by and large interventions have had smaller effects than were originally anticipated (Chapter 17, this volume). There are, however, some important exceptions to this generalization, including the 1964 report of the Surgeon General on the harmful effects of smoking and the Mothers Against Drunk Driving campaign that began in the early 1980s. Cutler notes that in both of these cases, the interventions occurred at the national level, the message conveyed was simple and straightforward, and the behavioral change required was clear. In general, however, more research is needed on why some health interventions succeed while others fail (Chapter 17, this volume).

SECTION V: TWO INTERNATIONAL COMPARISONS

The United States is not the only country in the world concerned about racial equity in health. In the final two papers in the volume, James Y. Nazroo (Chapter 18) and Debbie Bradshaw and colleagues (Chapter 19) offer international comparative perspectives on these issues from the United Kingdom and South Africa, respectively. Although both papers document slightly different patterns of racial and ethnic disparities in health than occur in the United States, they both suggest the centrality of particular casual factors including socioeconomic status, culture, racism, and, for immigrants, generation (i.e., first versus second or third) and period of migration (i.e., length of stay in country).

In Chapter 18, Nazroo investigates the relationship between age and ethnic inequalities in health in the United Kingdom, in relation to socioeconomic circumstances, migration status, extent of racial harassment, duration of stay, and cohort. Given the complexity of factors involved, the author finds it difficult to come to any firm conclusions. A particularly vexing problem is that although most minorities in the United Kingdom have arrived since the Second World War, different ethnic subgroups have tended to enter the country in waves, making it extremely difficult to untangle the effects of age, period, and cohort on health. As Nazroo points out, this underscores the utility of collecting and analyzing these issues using longitudinal panel data.

In Chapter 19, Bradshaw and colleagues review recent data and analyses on the nature of racial disparities in health in South Africa, a country that has witnessed extraordinary political and social change over the past 10 to 15 years as the government has attempted to overcome the legacy of apartheid. Again the complexity of the issues and the lack of long-term data prevent the authors drawing firm conclusions about how these profound economic and social changes are affecting racial differences in health by age. Nevertheless, the available evidence suggests that socioeconomic and cultural factors as well as health behaviors are important determinants of health in South Africa.

The Way Ahead

The purpose of this chapter is not to outline an agenda for future research in this area. That task has already been undertaken by the NRC's Panel on Race, Ethnicity, and Health in Later Life. Their conclusions and recommendations are presented in a companion volume (see National Research Council, 2004). Nevertheless, taken together, the chapters in this volume highlight both the strengths and weaknesses of the existing knowledge base. Perhaps the main message is that after decades of research in this area, there are still large and persistent differences in health by racial and ethnic groups that cannot be explained fully by traditional arguments such as differences in socioeconomic status, access to health care, or health behaviors.

Clearly, then, there is still a need to continue to monitor changes in the health status of different racial and ethnic groups and to understand the causal factors underlying these differences. Even if there is no way to weigh their relative importance, there is fairly broad agreement among the disciplines that the list of major causes is fairly self-contained: socioeconomic status, education, health risk behavior, psychosocial factors including stress, access to and quality of health care, culture, genetic factors, and environmental and occupational risk factors (Kington and Nickens, 2001). Because of the interaction and the multiple causal pathways between these various factors (e.g., low socioeconomic status leads to poor health, but poor health can also lead to less wealth), the exact contribution that each factor contributes to the observed health differences by race remains unknown. Further research, particularly with emphasis on the integration of data from various disciplines, is therefore essential.

A full understanding and complete consensus on the reasons underlying these observed differences will likely continue to elude us for some time. Nevertheless, the papers in this volume indicate that high-quality research is under way in many disciplines. Increasingly, this research points to the need for a more integrative approach to health that accounts for the interactions among genetic, behavioral, psychosocial, and environmental factors over time. The chapters in this volume represent a useful step forward, but it is only one among many that will ultimately need to be undertaken before sustainable progress in our understanding of the causes of racial and ethnic differences in health in later life can be made. My hope is that these papers will be useful to those charged with making and implementing public policy as well as to scholars from different disciplines wishing to build on this foundation.

ACKNOWLEDGMENTS

I am grateful to Richard S. Cooper, Eileen M. Crimmins, Clyde Hertzman, Charles B. Keely, Faith Mitchell, Alberto Palloni, Jane Ross, James P. Smith, and Marilyn A. Winkleby for their comments on an earlier draft.

REFERENCES

Barker, D.J.P. (1998). *Mothers, babies and health in later life* (2nd ed.). Edinburgh, Scotland: Churchill Livingstone.

Burchard, E.G., Ziv, E., Coyle, N., Gomez, S.L., Tang, H., Karter, A.J., Mountain, J.L., Pérez-Stable, E.J., Sheppard, D., and Risch, N. (2003). The importance of race and ethnic background in biomedical research and clinical practice. *New England Journal of Medicine, 348*(12), 1170-1175.

Coale, A.J., and Kisker, E.E. (1986). Mortality crossovers. Reality or bad data? *Population Studies, 40*(3), 389-401.

Cutler, D.M., Glaeser, E.L., and Shapiro, J.M. (2003). *Why have Americans become more obese?* (NBER Working Paper No. 9446). Cambridge, MA: National Bureau of Economic Research.

Deaton, A. (2001). *Health, inequality, and economic development.* (NBER Working Paper No. 8318). Cambridge, MA: National Bureau of Economic Research.

Elo, I.T., and Preston, S.H. (1992). Effects of early-life conditions on adult mortality: A review. *Population Index, 58*(2), 186-212.

Eschbach, K. (1993). Changing identification among American Indians and Alaska Natives. *Demography, 30*(4), 635-652.

Fried, L.P. (2000). Epidemiology of aging. *Epidemiologic Reviews, 22*(1), 95-106.

Goldman, D.P., and Smith, J.P. (2002). Can patient self-management help explain the SES health gradient? *Proceedings of the National Academy of Sciences, 99*(16), 10929-10934.

Harris, D. (1994). The 1990 census count of American Indians: What do the numbers really mean? *Social Science Quarterly, 75*(3), 580-593.

Hayward, M.D., Crimmins, E.M., Miles, T.P., and Yu, Y. (2000). The significance of socio-economic status in explaining the racial gap in chronic health conditions. *American Sociological Reviews, 65*(6), 910-930.

Heckman, J.J. (1979). Sample selection bias as a specification error. *Econometrica, 47*(1), 153-161.

Hirschman, C., Alba, R., and Farley, R. (2000). The meaning and measurement of race in the U.S. Census: Glimpses into the future. *Demography, 37*(3), 381-393.

Institute of Medicine. (2001). *Coverage matters: Insurance and health care.* Committee on the Consequences of Uninsurance. Washington, DC: National Academy Press.

Institute of Medicine. (2003). *Unequal treatment: Confronting racial and ethnic disparities in health care.* Committee on Understanding and Eliminating Racial and Ethnic Disparities in Health Care. B.D. Smedley, A.Y. Stith, and A.R. Nelson (Eds.). Washington, DC: The National Academies Press.

James, S.A. (1994). John Henryism and the health of African Americans. *Culture, Medicine, and Psychiatry, 18*(2), 163-182.

Kington, R.S., and Nickens, H.W. (2001). Racial and ethnic differences in health: Recent trends, current patterns, and future directions. In N.J. Smelser, W.J. Wilson, and F. Mitchell (Eds.), *America becoming: Racial trends and their consequences* (vol. II, pp. 253-310). Washington, DC: National Academy Press.

Korgen, K.O. (1999). *From black to biracial: Transforming racial identity among Americans.* Westport, CT: Praeger.

Krieger, N. (1999). Embodying inequality: A review of concepts, measures, and methods for studying health consequences of discrimination. *International Journal of Health Services, 29*(2), 295-352.

Manton, K.G., and Stallard, E. (1997). Health and disability differences among racial and ethnic groups. In L.G. Martin and B.J. Soldo (Eds.), *Racial and ethnic differences in the health of older Americans* (pp. 43-105). Committee on Population, Commission on Behavioral and Social Sciences and Education, National Research Council. Washington, DC: National Academy Press.

Marmot, M.G., Davey-Smith, G., Stansfeld, S., Patel, C., North, F., Head, J., White, I., Brunner, E., and Feeny, A. (1991). Health inequalities among British civil servants: The Whitehall II Study. *Lancet, 337*, 1387-1393.

Marmot, M.G., Bosma, H., Hemingway, H., Brunner, E., and Stansfeld, S.A. (1997). Contribution of job control and other risk factors to social variations in coronary heart disease incidence. *Lancet, 350*, 235-239.

McEwen, B.S. (1998). Protective and damaging effects of stress mediators. *New England Journal of Medicine, 338*(3), 171-179.

McGinnis, J.M., and Foege, W.H. (1993). Actual causes of death in the United States. *Journal of American Medical Association, 270*(18), 2207-2212.

Nam, C.B., Weatherby, N.L., and Ockay, K.A. (1978). Causes of death which contribute to the mortality crossover effect. *Social Biology, 25*, 306-314.

National Center for Health Statistics. (2003). *Health, United States, 2003*. Hyattsville, MD: Author.

National Research Council. (1989). *A common destiny: Blacks and American society*. Committee on the Status of Black Americans. G.D. Jaynes and R.M. Williams (Eds.). Washington DC: National Academy Press.

National Research Council. (2001). *New horizons in health: An integrative approach*. Committee on Future Directions for Behavioral and Social Sciences Research at the National Institutes of Health. B.H. Singer and C.D. Ruff (Eds.). Washington, DC: National Academy Press.

National Research Council. (2004). *Understanding racial and ethnic differences in health in late life: A research agenda*. Panel on Race, Ethnicity, and Health in Later Life. R.A. Bulatao and N.B. Anderson (Eds.). Committee on Population, Division of Behavioral and Social Sciences and Education. Washington, DC: The National Academies Press.

Neel, J.V. (1997). Are genetic factors involved in racial and ethnic differences in late-life health? In L.G. Martin and B.J. Soldo (Eds.), *Racial and ethnic differences in the health of older Americans* (pp. 210-232). Committee on Population, Commission on Behavioral and Social Sciences and Education, National Research Council. Washington, DC: National Academy Press.

Palloni, A., and Arias, E. (2003). *A re-examination of the Hispanic mortality paradox*. Paper presented at the meeting of the Population Association of America, Minneapolis, Minnesota, May 1-3.

Passel, J.S. (1976). Provisional evaluation of the 1970 Census count of American Indians. *Demography, 13*(3), 397-409.

Passel, J.S., and Berman, P.A. (1986). Quality of 1980 Census data for American Indians. *Social Biology, 33*, 163-182.

Preston, S.H., Elo, I.T., Rosenwaike, I., and Hill, M. (1996). African American mortality at older ages: Results of a matching study. *Demography, 33*(2), 193-209.

Preston, S.H., Elo, I.T., Hill. M.E., and Rosenwaike, I. (2003). *The demography of African Americans, 1930-1990*. Dordrecht, The Netherlands: Kluwer Academic.

Rosenberg, H.M., Maurer, J.D., Sorlie, P.D., Johnson, N.J., MacDorman, M.F., Hoyert, D.L., Spitler, J.F., and Scott, C. (1999). *Quality of death rates by race and Hispanic origin: A summary of current research*. (Vital Health Statistics, Series 2. Data Evaluation and Methods Research. No. 128). Hyattsville, MD: U.S. Department of Health and Human Services.

Sankar, P., and Cho, M.K. (2002). Towards a new vocabulary of human genetic variation. *Science, 298*, 1337-1338.

Smith, J.P. (1999). Healthy bodies and thick wallets: The dual relation between health and economic status. *Journal of Economic Perspectives, 13*(2), 145-166.

Suárez, Z.E. (2000). Hispanics and health care. In P.S.J. Cafferty and D.W. Engstrom (Eds.), *Hispanics in the United States* (pp. 195-235). New Brunswick, NJ: Transaction.

Thornton, R. (1996). Tribal membership requirements and the demography of 'old' and 'new' Native Americans. In G.D. Sandefur, R.R. Rindfuss, and B. Cohen (Eds.), *Changing numbers, changing needs: American Indian demography and public health* (pp. 103-112). Washington, DC: National Academy Press.

U.S. Department of Health and Human Services. (1991). *Healthy people 2000: National health promotion and disease prevention objectives*. Washington, DC: Author.

Vaupel, J.W., Manton, K.G., and Stallard, E. (1979). The impact of heterogeneity in individual frailty on the dynamics of mortality. *Demography, 16*(3), 439-454.

Vedantam, S. (2004). Racial disparities played down. *The Washington Post*, January 14, p. A17.

Wilkinson, R.G. (1996). *Unhealthy societies: The afflictions of inequality*. New York: Routledge.

Williams, D.R., Neighbors, H.W., and Jackson, J.S. (2003). Racial/ethnic discrimination and health: Findings from community studies. *American Journal of Public Health, 93*(2), 200-208.

Wolff, E.N. (1996). *Top heavy: The increasing inequality of wealth in America and what can be done about it*. New York: New Press.

Section I

The Nature of Racial and Ethnic Differences

2

Racial and Ethnic Identification, Official Classifications, and Health Disparities

Gary D. Sandefur, Mary E. Campbell,
and Jennifer Eggerling-Boeck

Our picture of racial and ethnic disparities in the health of older Americans is strongly influenced by the methods of collecting data on race and ethnicity. At one level there is a good deal of consistency in data collection. Most Americans and most researchers have in mind a general categorical scheme that includes whites, blacks, Asians, Hispanics, and American Indians. Most Americans and nearly all researchers are also aware that these general categories disguise significant heterogeneity within each of these major groups. To the extent possible, recent research has attempted to identify and compare subgroups within each of the major racial and ethnic groups, making distinctions by country of origin, nativity, and generation within the United States. Most researchers generally agree that these categories are primarily social constructions that have changed and will continue to change over time.

Once we begin to explore more deeply the ways in which data on the elderly population are collected, however, we discover inconsistency across data sets and time. Part of this variation is from inconsistency in the way that Americans think and talk about race and ethnicity. Race and ethnicity are words that carry heavy intellectual and political baggage, and issues surrounding racial and ethnic identities are often contested within and across groups. The debate over racial and ethnic categories prior to the 2000 Census is one of the most recent, but by no means the only, example of these contests. Several advocacy groups pressured the Office of Management and Budget (OMB) to revise its racial and ethnic categories and data collection schemes (see Farley, 2001, and Rodriguez, 2000, for discussions of the controversies). This resulted in several significant changes, including the most well-known change, which allowed individuals to choose more than one racial category in the 2000 Census. Although most national and many local data collection efforts follow the federal guidelines, they vary in the way in which questions are constructed and in the order in which they appear in the questionnaire or interview schedule. Such seemingly trivial differences in measurement lead to different distributions of responses about racial and ethnic identity (Hirschman, Alba, and Farley, 2000).

Another inconsistency that has troubled health researchers is the collection of racial and ethnic data using different criteria across data sources. A good example of this is the mismatch between self-selected race (which is used in most data sets) and the observer-selected race that is often used for death certificates. Comparisons between next-of-kin racial identifications and death certificates have shown that a large proportion of, for example, black Hispanics are misidentified on death certificates. This leads to a significant overestimate of their life expectancy because the race-specific mortality rates are inaccurate (Swallen and Guend, 2001).

The purpose of this chapter is to examine the implications of how we measure racial and ethnic identity for our understanding of racial and ethnic disparities in health, especially among the elderly.[1] We focus on the official classifications used to produce statistics on the health status of the elderly, and because self-identification is the fundamental tool used to assign individuals to the official categories, we explore factors associated with self-identification.[2] Although we emphasize identification and classification involving the elderly, much of what we have to say applies to other age groups as well. We first look at what the social science literature has to say about the ways in which individuals and society construct racial and ethnic identities. Second, we examine how information on race and ethnicity is recorded in some of the major federal data sets used to study health disparities among the elderly. We then discuss some of the major problems in our national system of collecting and reporting on health disparities. We conclude with some recommendations for achieving greater consistency in the collection and reporting of racial and ethnic information.

RACIAL AND ETHNIC IDENTITY

Historical Understandings of Racial and Ethnic Identity

Over time, academic and popular understandings of racial and ethnic identities have changed dramatically. Prior to the 20th century, racial and ethnic groups were perceived as permanent, biological types. Scholars of race and ethnicity turned to Biblical passages and, later, theories of natural history to explain the origins of differences among ethnic and racial groups

(Banton, 1998). They concluded that these group differences were natural and immutable. Cornell and Hartmann (1998) explain that the paradigms popular among social scientists in the late 19th and early 20th centuries "conceived ethnic and racial groups as biologically distinct entities and gave to biology the larger part of the responsibility for differences in the cultures and the political and economic fortunes of these groups" (Cornell and Hartmann, 1998, p. 42).

The work of Franz Boas shifted the model describing racial and ethnic differences from one stressing biology to one that focused on cultural differences (Cornell and Hartmann, 1998). This shift implied that racial and ethnic groups were dynamic rather than static. These paradigmatic changes influenced the work on race in the emerging Chicago School of Sociology, which led to an assimilationist model of racial and ethnic identities (Cornell and Hartmann, 1998). In this model, the inherent flexibility of racial and ethnic identities would eventually lead to the assimilation of distinctive racial and ethnic minority groups into the mainstream culture. However, developments in the middle of the 20th century, such as strengthening ethnic and racial conflicts, forced social scientists to reconsider the question of racial and ethnic identities.

Two paradigms, primordialism and circumstantialism, emerged in the post-assimilationist era (Cornell and Hartmann, 1998). Proponents of primordialism asserted that for each individual "ethnicity is fixed, fundamental, and rooted in the unchangeable circumstances of birth" (Cornell and Hartmann, 1998, p. 48). Those favoring circumstantialism claimed that individuals and groups claim ethnic or racial identities when these identities are in some way advantageous. As more and more social scientific research investigated racial and ethnic identities, it became clear that neither model was able to fully explain the complexities of these phenomena. The most prevalent current view on racial and ethnic identities is a social constructionist model (Banton, 1998; Cornell and Hartmann, 1998; Nagel, 1996). Within this system, "the construction of ethnicity is an ongoing process that combines the past and the present into building material for new or revitalized identities and groups" (Nagel, 1996, p. 19).[3]

As views of racial and ethnic identities have changed over time, so have official categories and measurement procedures. The U.S. Census has classified people into racial groups since its origin in 1790. However, the list of categories and the method of measuring race or ethnicity has changed many times in the intervening decades, as the political and economic forces shaping the collection of racial data have changed. In early Censuses, enumerators answered the race question based on their perception of the individual. The earliest Censuses used slave status as a proxy for a racial category, the only race options being "free White persons, slaves, or all other free persons" (Sandefur, Martin, Eggerling-Boeck, Mannon, and Meier, 2001; U.S.

Bureau of the Census, 1973). In later years more specific categories for those of mixed African American and white descent, such as mulatto, quadroon, and octoroon, were used (Lee, 1993). Asian groups have been listed on the form since the late 1800s. Chinese, Japanese, and Filipino were the first Asian groups to appear on the Census; later Korean, Vietnamese, Asian Indian, and other Asian groups were added to the list. American Indians were included as a separate group beginning in 1870. The Census question measuring the Hispanic population has also varied over time. Enumerators have used a Spanish surname, the use of the Spanish language in the home, and the birthplace of the respondent or parents to indicate Hispanic ethnicity.

In 1970, racial classification on the Census changed from enumerator identification to self-identification. This change had a relatively minor impact on the count of racial and ethnic groups in 1970 compared to 1960. However, it created a situation that led to significant changes in counts during subsequent years. This methodological shift proved to be especially influential for American Indians. During the period between 1960 and the end of the 20th century, the size of the American Indian population as measured by the Census increased much more than could be accounted for by migration or births (Eschbach, 1993; Nagel, 1996). This increase was because persons whom enumerators had previously identified as being of another race began self-identifying as American Indian and, after 1970, there was increased self-identification as American Indian by those who earlier self-identified or were identified by their parents as being in some other group (Nagel, 1996).

In 1997 OMB announced new standards for federal data on race and ethnicity (OMB, 1999). Following the OMB standards, the 2000 Census used the five suggested racial categories: White, black/African American, American Indian/Alaska Native, Asian, and Native Hawaiian/other Pacific Islander. The Census Bureau also added a sixth category, "some other race." The Native Hawaiian/other Pacific Islander was separated from the Asian category for the first time. A second and even more influential change allowed respondents to choose more than one racial category.[4] Prior to the 2000 Census, the U.S. Bureau of the Census conducted several tests—including the 1996 Race and Ethnic Targeted Test—to consider the implications of changing the way in which data were collected for the counts of racial and ethnic groups in the United States.[5] The major conclusion that came out of this test was that allowing individuals to choose more than one racial group had a very small impact on the measured racial composition of the population (Hirschman et al., 2000; U.S. Bureau of the Census, 1997).

Based on these results, Hirschman and colleagues (2000) predicted that 1 to 2 percent of whites and blacks in the 2000 Census would identify with more than one race and that the numbers of respondents who identified solely as American Indian or Asian would not be significantly different from what one would find if people were constrained to pick only one race. On the other hand, they predicted that some who in the past had recorded their race as white or "some other race" would report more than one race. Their predictions turned out to be correct. In Census 2000, 97.6 percent of the U.S. population reported only one race. Of the 2.4 percent, or 6.8 million, who reported more than one race, 32 percent reported white and "some other race," 16 percent reported white and American Indian/Alaska Native, 13 percent reported white and Asian, and 11 percent reported white and black or African American (U.S. Bureau of the Census, 2001c). Another way to look at these figures, however, is to note that the size of the population reporting two or more races is larger than the American Indian or Pacific Islander populations and about half the size of the Asian population.

The Social Constructionist Paradigm of Racial and Ethnic Identity

Changes in the U.S. Census categories over time reflect changes in the ways in which Americans think about race and ethnicity as well as political conflicts over these views. Changes in official classifications in turn helped shape the discussion of race and ethnicity in subsequent decades. Within the paradigm of social constructionism, racial and ethnic groups are understood as socially created, rather than biologically given, realities. Relatively trivial (and even overlapping) phenotypical differences or group customs are used to categorize groups, and then society proceeds to attach a socially constructed meaning to these differences. The socially constructed meaning of racial/ethnic groups most often takes an evaluative tone.[6] Given their social origins, racial and ethnic identities continually change over time and with varying circumstances. Changes are a result of forces from both outside and within the racial/ethnic group. Cornell and Hartmann employ the terms *assertion* and *assignment* to illustrate this interaction of forces shaping identities. They conclude that racial and ethnic identities "involve not only circumstances but active responses to circumstances by individuals and groups" (Cornell and Hartmann, 1998, p. 77). Nagel (1996, p. 21) agrees, stating, "ethnic identity is, then, a dialectic between internal identification and external ascription." Of course, the relative influence of assignment and assertion varies by group. Waters (1990) demonstrates that white ethnics have a great degree of choice about their ethnic identity. They can choose a particular identity to highlight, and this choice can fluctuate across time and situations. However, she notes that many members of racial and ethnic minority groups do not have this degree of choice. For these individuals, identity is heavily ascribed by society. This is especially the case for individuals who have "markers" that associate them with a particular racial and/or ethnic group. These markers can be physical such as skin color, or they can involve surnames or accents.

Changes in a racial or ethnic identity can occur at both the group and individual levels. In other words, the racial/ethnic categories a society accepts and utilizes can change over a period of time; in addition, the racial/ethnic label an individual chooses can change over time.[7] Nagel (1996) described the extensive changes in American Indian identity in the second half of the 20th century. Social factors such as the civil rights movement, World War II, and federal Indian policy led to an "ethnic renewal" among American Indians. This, in turn, led to a revised understanding of the American Indian category; it also led many individuals who previously identified as some other race to change their ethnic identity from some other category to American Indian. In this case, ethnic identity changed at both the group and individual levels. Espiritu (1992) outlines the ways in which the meaning of the Asian American category has changed over time and with varying social and political circumstances.[8]

Although all racial and ethnic identities are socially constructed, some categories are more prone to change than others. Waters (1990) notes that the ethnic options employed by white Americans are generally not available to African Americans, Asian Americans, Native Americans, or Hispanics. Nagel notes that some racial and ethnic identities appear more rigid than others (1996, p. 26). In the United States, the racial category African American has been a relatively closed and static category. The common identity rule for this group is the rule of hypodescent, under which any amount of black ancestry, no matter how small, makes one African American.[9] Individuals in this group have much less opportunity to claim varied identities and to have these identities socially recognized. In many cases even those biracial (African American and white) individuals with a white parent have difficulty claiming a non-black identity (Korgen, 1998; Rockquemore and Brunsma, 2002).

Another reason for varying levels of change in racial categories over time is the varying extent of racial intermarriage for different groups. Intermarriage, however, has less of an impact on the self-identification of older Americans than on younger Americans. Native Americans have historically had high intermarriage rates, leading to a large group of persons with both white and Native American ancestry. The intermarriage rates for Asian Americans and Hispanics have been increasing and are now at significant levels. For all these groups, the most common racial group to intermarry with is white. Therefore, there are significant numbers of persons whose ancestry is partially white and partially Native American, Asian American, or Hispanic. These individuals are faced with a choice of how to identify racially or ethnically. Many factors can lead to a particular identity choice. In their study of children with one Asian and one non-Asian parent, Xie and Goyette (1997) show that factors such as the gender, national ancestry, and language patterns of the Asian parent affect the racial identity of the child. The race of the non-Asian parent also has an effect. Given these differences in racial and ethnic options across groups, it is important to examine the specific circumstances (historical and current) for each group and examine the ways in which these circumstances have affected the racial/ethnic identity processes for the group.

African Americans

As mentioned, the African American racial category has relatively rigid boundaries in U.S. society. Inclusion in the black category is guided by the rule of hypodescent. Davis (1991) provides a thorough outline of the ways in which this system of racial categorization evolved in U.S. society. Both African Americans and whites have largely accepted this system of racial classification. Therefore, most persons with African American ancestry have a strong socially imposed identity. If they were to choose another identity, they would likely receive little social support for this identity. The findings of Waters (1991) support these ideas. She found that although more than half of her interview respondents were aware of non-black ancestors, none of the respondents reported that they would identify with this part of their ancestry. She concludes "the 'one-drop rule' operates to keep non-black ancestors from mattering to black individuals' present day identifications" (Waters, 1991, p. 68).

However, there is some evidence that this situation is changing, or at least becoming more complex, due to increased interracial marriage among African Americans and increased immigration of persons of African descent. Intermarriage rates for African Americans, though still much smaller than rates for other groups, have been increasing significantly over the past few decades. This has created a sizable population of biracial (black-white) persons. Korgen (1998) studied the experiences of this group and found important generational differences. Biracial individuals born after the civil rights movement were much more likely to identify as biracial; those born before the movement were less likely to identify in this manner, primarily because they believed this identity would not have been socially supported or recognized. Rockquemore and Brunsma (2002) found a number of different identification strategies among their sample of young biracial (black-white) respondents: Monoracial identity (as either white or black), biracial identity, situationally shifting identity, and racially transcendent identity. This wide variation in racial identity among those with the same racial parentage indicates that the one-drop rule of racial identity for African Americans may be slowly weakening.

The increased immigration of individuals of African descent (primarily from Africa and the Caribbean) further complicates the social construction of African American identity. Second-generation black immigrants face an inherent tension: Their parents, in general, hold negative stereotypes of black Americans, and yet these second-generation persons are often identified as American blacks by others because they lack the ethnic markers of their parents (e.g., accent) (Waters, 1994, 1999). As with biracial individuals, this group shows evidence of a variety of racial identities. Among Waters' respondents, some black immigrants adopted a black American identity, others had a strong ethnic identity (e.g., Jamaican, Trinidadian), and still others embraced an immigrant identity. These recent studies suggest that although African American historically has been an extremely rigid racial category, the situation may be slowly changing.

Asian Americans

Any examination of racial identity among Asian Americans must be informed by an awareness of important subgroup differences. Several subgroups, such as Chinese, Japanese, Filipino, and Asian Indian, are usually included in the Asian racial category. In 2000, Chinese Americans continued to be the largest Asian American group, with more than 2.7 million individuals reporting Chinese alone or in combination with other racial groups. More than 2 million recorded Filipino as one of their racial identities. The groups with more than 1 million included, in order of size, Asian Indian, Korean, Vietnamese, and Japanese. These subgroups differ widely with respect to language, culture, education, income levels, and immigration history. Furthermore, many Asian Americans identify more closely with their particular subgroup than with the panethnic identity. In many cases, using the panethnic label Asian can mask important variations among subgroups.

Members of Asian subgroups arrived in America with no perception of the Asian racial category. This is true for all of the umbrella groups used in the United States. Most Europeans entered the United States with little idea of a common European identity. The same can be said for African Americans, Hispanics, and Native Americans. *National* identities (e.g., Chinese, Japanese, Filipino) were much more relevant to members of these Asian subgroups, influencing many aspects of everyday life. Cornell and Hartmann (1998), for example, describe the Asian racial identity of recent Vietnamese and Cambodian immigrants as assigned and thin. The identity is assigned because although Vietnamese or Cambodian identity is much more salient to these immigrants, U.S. society for the most part ignores subgroup differences and groups all these individuals under the racial category Asian. The Asian identity is thin because it does not organize much of the social life and activities of these individuals. Furthermore, unlike the case for Hispanics, there is no factor such as language that unifies the Asian population as a whole.

Writing about the evolution of the Asian American panethnic label, Espiritu (1992, p. 6) notes, "the term Asian American arose out of the racist discourse that constructs Asians as a homogeneous group." More recently, however, Asian American panethnicity has also been constructed from within the group. Specifically, Espiritu (1992) focuses on the ways in which organizations have drawn on and extended the panethnic label as a way of claiming resources and gaining political influence. In her research, Kibria (1997) found that Chinese- and Korean-American respondents did have a sense of belonging to an "Asian race." They understood that Asian groups were perceived by the dominant society as physically similar, they felt a common history of experiences resulting from being labeled Asian, and they had a sense of an Asian American culture. However, for most respondents the Chinese- or Korean-American identity was more important than Asian American identity (Kibria, 1997).

Intermarriage has a large impact on the racial identity of Asian Americans. This group has relatively high rates of outmarriage. In the 1990s, 24.2 percent of Asian American wives and 12.3 percent of Asian American husbands were married to someone in a different racial group (Sandefur et al., 2001). The children of these intermarried couples face choices about their racial self-identification. Saenz, Hwang, Aguirre, and Anderson (1995) and Xie and Goyette (1997) examined the factors that affect the racial self-identification of children with one Asian and one non-Asian parent. Saenz et al. (1995) used data from the 1980 Public Use Microdata Sample (PUMS) from California and restricted their analyses to children of Asian-Anglo marriages. They found that the probability of the child identifying as Asian was increased for children whose Asian parent is the father as opposed to the mother, who speak a language other than English, who are first generation, who live in areas with higher concentrations of the Asian parent's ethnic group, who live in areas with less ethnic heterogeneity, and whose Asian parent is Asian Indian, Korean, Filipino, or Japanese (Saenz et al., 1995).

Xie and Goyette (1997) had similar findings using the 1990 PUMS for children with one Asian and one non-Asian parent. Their results show that children are more likely to be identified as Asian if they are of the first or third generation, their father (as opposed to mother) is Asian, or their Asian parent speaks a non-English language. Their results on ancestry of the Asian parent, however, contradict those of Saenz et al. (1995). Xie and Goyette (1997) found that those whose Asian parent is Chinese or Japanese were more likely to identify as Asian than those whose parent was Indian, Korean, or Filipino. Finally, they found that children whose non-Asian parent was African American or Hispanic were significantly less likely to identify as Asian.

Hispanic Americans

Similar to Asian Americans, there is wide variation among Hispanic subgroups. The three largest Hispanic subgroups in the United States are Mexicans, Puerto Ricans, and Cubans. The case for Hispanics is further complicated by the fact that "Hispanic" is usually considered an ethnic identity, rather than a racial one. Therefore, in the Census and most survey data, the Hispanic ethnicity and race questions are separate. Hispanics, then, can be racially identified as white, black, Asian, or Native American.[10]

Differences among the Hispanic subgroups include median age, immigration history, geographic distribution, fertility and family patterns, health status and mortality rates, income and education levels, and occupational distribution (Maldonado, 1991; Sandefur et al., 2001). Survey data that do not separate these subgroups run the risk of masking important variations among the groups.

Hispanics also have significant rates of intermarriage. In the 1990s, 16.1 percent of Hispanic wives and 13.1 percent of Hispanic husbands were married to non-Hispanics (Sandefur et al., 2001). As with Asian Americans, this means that the children of these unions can potentially make choices about their self-identification. However, this is complicated by the fact that in most cases the Hispanic question is asked separately from the race question. This fact makes it much easier for children with one Hispanic and one non-Hispanic parent to identify with the race/ethnicity of both parents on a survey.

Several authors have investigated factors that lead adolescents with Hispanic ancestry to make particular racial/ethnic identity choices. Eschbach and Gomez (1998) investigate what factors led particular Hispanic adolescents to switch their self-identity (as measured on surveys 2 years apart) from Hispanic to non-Hispanic. Factors such as speaking Spanish, having a higher concentration of Hispanic students in the school, living in a Census tract with a concentration of co-ethnics, and having a lower socioeconomic status were related to a reduced likelihood of switching to a non-Hispanic identity. Those who spoke only English were more likely to shift to a non-Hispanic identity.[11] The authors conclude that the results identify "linguistic assimilation and spatial deconcentration as the structural mechanisms through which experience in the United States leads to uncertainty about ethnic identification as a Hispanic" (Eschbach and Gomez, 1998, p. 86).

Portes and MacLeod (1996) examined the use of the Hispanic panethnic label by second-generation children whose parents were born in Latin

America. National origin had the strongest effects on use of the Hispanic label. Cubans were least likely to use the panethnic label, followed by Colombians, and then Mexicans. Dominicans and Nicaraguans were most likely to identify as Hispanic. Greater acculturation and greater parental status were related to a lower likelihood of adopting the panethnic identity.

This complex set of factors affecting the Hispanic population creates an uncertain future for the racial identity of Hispanics. Because Hispanic status is usually asked separately from racial group membership, Hispanic Americans can usually choose a racial identity as well. However, many Hispanics believe that they do not fit into any of the other available racial groups. The studies reviewed indicate that Hispanic identity may become less salient as structural assimilation occurs for the group. Furthermore, many Hispanics reject the panethnic label in favor of their particular national identity (e.g., Mexican or Puerto Rican).

Native Americans

Racial identity is also a complex issue for Native Americans. However, it is complex for different reasons. The history of tribal membership, Native American relations with the U.S. government, and interracial marriage are the primary factors affecting issues of racial identity for American Indians. Cornell (1990) outlines the macrolevel historical factors affecting Native American identity. The treaty system and the removal of tribes to geographically remote areas reinforced tribal identities rather than racial identities (e.g., Navajo rather than American Indian). Nagel (1996) describes the more recent emergence of a Native American panethnic identity. Factors such as experiences in World War II, the civil rights movement, and certain federal Indian policies led to the intensification and increased saliency of a racial identity as Native American.

This situation is further complicated by the many ways in which Native American identity can be defined.[12] Nagel (1996, p. 234) concludes that in the post-Red Power era, "Indian individual and collective identities have become increasingly problematic and contested. There are widespread ambiguities and disputes about who is an Indian, how many American Indians there are in the United States, who should be permitted to assert Indian ethnicity, and who has the right to represent Indian interests." Unlike other racial and ethnic groups, the federal government has outlined specific methods to classify Native Americans. These definitions can be at odds with state, tribal, and individual definitions of who qualifies as Native American. In order to receive federal services, Indian tribes must be federally recognized. Lack of tribal recognition denies tribal members official Native American status in the view of the federal government. Tribal definitions of Native American identity vary widely in their required blood quantum.

Some tribes require a particular percentage of ancestry or "blood quantum" in order for individuals to be considered tribal members. Of course, the Census and most surveys measure race by self-identification, so individuals not considered Native American in the previous cases would be counted as Native American in these surveys.

American Indians have racially intermarried at even greater rates than Asian Americans and Hispanic Americans. In the 1990s, 60.2 percent of Native American wives and 58.8 percent of Native American husbands were married to someone of another racial group.[13] As with the previous groups, these high levels of intermarriage have produced a group of individuals who face choices about their racial identity. Nagel (1996) describes the ethnic renewal of American Indians in the latter half of the 20th century. Part of this renewal was the shifting of racial identities of multiracial persons with American Indian ancestry from a racial identification with their other ancestry group (usually white) to a racial identification as Native American. As the social and political atmosphere of the United States made American Indian identity more attractive, the numbers of those choosing this identity grew. Eschbach, Supple, and Snipp (1998) found that more highly educated persons living in cities were more likely to shift to a Native American identity in the Census. Self-identification shifts such as these can initially create apparent improvements in the demographic characteristics of Native Americans as a group. When analyzing longitudinal data on outcomes such as income, education, and health, researchers should consider possible identity shifts.

Summary

Existing evidence on racial and ethnic identity suggests that the early 21st century is a time of changing notions of racial and ethnic identity as immigration continues to fuel the growth of the Asian and Hispanic populations, as intermarriage rates continue to increase, and as the federal government begins to take into account the implications of mixed racial heritage or origins. As the previous discussion shows, the way in which Americans have seen themselves and one another has been influenced by the federal racial and ethnic classification schemes. At the same time, these classification schemes have responded to changes in how people identify themselves and others. The changes between the 1990 and 2000 Censuses are only the more recent examples of these shifts.

Next we review the racial and ethnic classification schemes employed by some of the largest federal data sets used to study racial and ethnic disparities in the health of the aging population. Although we discuss only a few of the major data sets, this will help us to understand the limitations of the available data for the study of these complex racial and ethnic identities.

RACIAL AND ETHNIC IDENTIFICATION IN EXISTING DATA USED TO STUDY HEALTH DISPARITIES

What we know about racial and ethnic differences in health is, of course, largely driven by the kind of racial and ethnic data available. There are many sources of information about health, so it would be impossible to discuss all the intricacies of how racial and ethnic data are collected for health surveys. However, a few major federal data collection efforts are very important in their own right, and have a significant impact on how other surveys collect racial and ethnic data. For this reason, it is important to examine how the largest federal data sets measure race and ethnicity. In this section, we will discuss the measurement of race and ethnicity in the Census, National Health and Nutrition Examination Survey, Hispanic Health and Nutrition Examination Survey, National Health Interview Survey, and vital statistics.

The Decennial Census

Despite its limited measures of health and aging, changes in the Census will affect our understanding of health for two reasons. First, the Census provides one of the largest data sets available to researchers, which allows panethnic groups to be broken down into subgroups, such as nationality groups. Thus, we must rely on the Census for our information about some of the smallest groups. Second, many other large surveys look to the Census and the guidelines set by OMB to decide how to frame their own race and ethnicity items, so changes in the Census often affect many other surveys.

As noted earlier, the 2000 Census permitted individuals to identify with more than one racial group. This change could have a significant effect on health statistics for some groups because it is clear from early results that some groups have a much higher percentage of multiracial individuals than others. In other words, groups such as American Indians and Asian Americans are likely to have a much higher percentage of their population switch to a multiracial identity than African Americans or whites. This will change our understanding of racial differences in health to the degree that these multiracial individuals differ from the monoracial groups they were selecting before.

Older people were less likely than younger people to be affected by this change. Table 2-1 contains some information on the racial composition of the population of different ages from Census 2000. These figures illustrate

TABLE 2-1 Percentage Distribution into Racial Categories by Age Group, 2000

Age Group	White Only, Including Hispanic	Black Only	American Indian Only	Asian Only	Pacific Islander Only	Other Race Only	Two or More Races	Hispanic (of any race)
Total	75	12	0.8	4	0.1	5.0	2.0	13
Under 5	67	15	1.0	3	0.2	8.0	5.0	19
Under 18	69	15	1.0	4	0.1	8.0	4.0	17
18–64	76	12	0.8	4	0.1	5.0	2.0	12
65–69	84	9	0.5	3	0.1	2.0	1.0	6
75–79	88	8	0.4	2	0.04	1.0	0.9	4
85+	90	7	0.2	1	0.05	0.8	0.8	4

SOURCE: U.S. Bureau of the Census (2000).

the well-known fact that the population of individuals 65 and older is less diverse than the younger population. More importantly for our purposes, the results show that the percentage of people who report (or are reported as) being of two or more races declines consistently as we move upward through the age groups.

Hispanic identity has been and continues to be measured in a question separate from racial identification. Individuals were constrained to choose only one Hispanic group in the Hispanic identification question (although they could include multiple identities in the question about ancestry) (U.S. Bureau of the Census, 2001b). The question about Hispanic origins was placed before the race question because research indicated that individuals who were asked about their Hispanic origins first were more likely to answer the race question and less likely to choose "other race" as a response than if the order of the questions was reversed (Hirschman et al., 2000). Hirschman and colleagues (2000) argue convincingly that there is little reason to keep the Hispanic origin and race questions separate. In fact, there are good reasons for putting them together. The results from the 1996 Race and Ethnic Targeted Test (RAETT) laid out by Hirschman and colleagues showed that the percentage of individuals who did not respond to the question about race declined significantly when the Hispanic and race questions were combined into an origins question and people were allowed to select more than one group. They argue that the concept of origins seems to be closer to how most Americans think about diversity than the old concepts of race and ethnicity.

One issue raised by combining the race and Hispanic questions is whether this affects our ability to identify and study black Hispanics. Many Americans regard substantial numbers of Cubans, Puerto Ricans, and Hispanics from other countries of origin in Central and South America as black. Black Hispanics are of interest to social scientists and to those who are interested in monitoring health because they represent an interesting combination of ascribed statuses. We do not know to what extent those who are seen as black Hispanics by Americans and thus by social scientists necessarily see themselves in the same way; they may identify more as black or more as Hispanic. Consequently, all we can do is compare the results of various forms of self-identification, including the old way of forcing a choice of race followed by a choice of Hispanic origin, the 2000 Census way of forcing a choice of Hispanic origin followed by allowing people to choose more than one racial category, or the Hirschman and colleagues proposal to combine the two questions and allow individuals to choose more than one. Table 2-2 shows the percentage of individuals who identified as both black and Hispanic in the 1990 Census, the 2000 Census, and in the combined panel (with the option of choosing more than one response) in the RAETT. In 1990, 3.4 percent of the Hispanic population self-identified or were identified by the householder as black, while 42.7 percent were identified as "other race" (McKenney and Bennett, 1994). In the 2000 Census, 2 percent of the Hispanic population was recorded as black, 42.2 percent as "other race," and 6.3 percent as two or more races (U.S. Bureau of the Census, 2001a). In the combined question used in the 1996 RAETT, approximately 75 percent of Hispanics identified themselves as Hispanic only, while 0.9 percent identified as black and only 0.6 percent identified as "other race." This suggests that most Hispanics see themselves as Hispanics only. The next most common category was white and Hispanic. Most importantly, the percentage of individuals who do not respond to the race question is reduced dramatically by using a combined question,

TABLE 2-2 Racial Distribution of the Hispanic Population (percentage)

	Data Source		
Racial Category	1990 Census	2000 Census	1996 Race and Ethnic Targeted Test: Combined
White	51.7	47.9	22.6
Black	3.4	2.0	0.9
American Indian	0.7	1.2	0.5
Asian	1.4	0.3	—
Pacific Islander	—	0.1	—
Other	42.7	42.2	0.6
Two or more races	—	6.3	0.1
Hispanic only	—	—	75.0

NOTES: The Asian and Pacific Islander categories were separate in the 2000 Census; the RAETT results are from Panel F (combined question; mark all that apply).
SOURCES: U.S. Bureau of the Census (1997, 2001a); U.S. Bureau of the Census Website, data from the 1990 Census.

especially among Hispanics. A combined question would reduce the count of black Hispanics, but given the choice of "other" in the 2000 Census, it is not clear that we have ever had a good count of the population that would be regarded as black and Hispanic by other Americans. The best we can hope for, and what we should try for, is a count that represents how people see themselves.

National Health and Nutrition Examination Survey and Hispanic Health and Nutrition Examination Survey

The National Health and Nutrition Examination Survey (NHANES) is a national survey of the health and nutritional characteristics of the U.S. civilian, noninstitutionalized population (excluding those who live on American Indian reservations). The Centers for Disease Control and Prevention's (CDC's) National Center for Health Statistics conducts the surveys. Since 1999, the NHANES has been an annual survey; before that, the NHANES was a multiyear survey that was done three times (NHANES I covered 1971-1974, NHANES II covered 1976-1980, and NHANES III covered 1988-94). The NHANES is a useful data set for health researchers because it includes both a home interview with basic demographic information and health tests that are administered by medical personnel in a "mobile examination center."

Information on the racial and ethnic characteristics of the respondents comes from the home interview. Since the NHANES III, African Americans and Mexican Americans have been oversampled in the NHANES (along with adolescents, older individuals, and pregnant women) to allow for better estimation of the health characteristics of these populations. The most recent NHANES first asks respondents to indicate whether they identify with a Hispanic subgroup. Then respondents are asked to self-identify with one of the major racial categories. For most estimates by race and ethnicity, the researcher needs 3 years of NHANES to obtain an adequate sample size. Many of the results of the NHANES that are reported are still limited to reports of only whites, blacks, and Mexican Americans because of constraints of the sample size.

The Hispanic Health and Nutrition Examination Survey (HHANES) is a national probability sample from 1982 to 1984 that provides health and demographic information for Hispanic adults and youth. The goal of this survey was to provide a sample large enough (about 16,000) to allow estimation of the health of Hispanics in general, as well as of specific groups such as Mexican Americans, Cuban Americans, and Puerto Ricans. To do this, the NHANES instrument was adapted in small ways (such as the addition of an acculturation scale) and translated into Spanish so respondents could choose to participate in Spanish or English.

To accomplish the goal of a large sample of Mexican Americans, Cuban Americans, and Puerto Ricans, the HHANES sampled three localized areas with high concentrations of the three groups. The Cuban-American sample comes from the Miami (Dade County) area, with a sample size of 2,244. The Mexican-American sample comes from selected counties in five southwestern states[14] with a sample size of 9,894. The Puerto Rican sample was selected from the New York City area, with a sample size of 3,786. In all areas, all Hispanics were asked to complete the survey, so there are small numbers of Hispanic respondents from other groups.

This geographical selection means, however, that the HHANES is really a survey of Hispanics in the most concentrated locations in the United States. The health outcomes of Hispanics might be different in areas where they are much less concentrated, an issue that cannot be addressed with HHANES data. The HHANES is also not designed to give a representative sample of any other Hispanic subgroups, so it does not inform us about, for example, the health experiences of Central and South American Hispanics in the United States.

National Health Interview Survey (NHIS)

The National Health Interview Survey (NHIS) is another representative sample of the civilian noninstitu-tionalized population of the United States. The survey, also run by the National Center for Health Statistics, is designed to cover basic health and demographic items, with supplements for specific health topics. The NHIS has been interviewing households since 1957, and is a continuous cross-sectional survey. In addition to these data, the Longitudinal Study of Aging (LSOA) is based on the 1984 NHIS sample, with baseline information drawn from the NHIS Supplement on Aging administered in that year.

The NHIS covers Hispanics, non-Hispanic whites, non-Hispanic African Americans, and Asian Americans. In 1985, the NHIS began oversampling African Americans. In 1995, the NHIS expanded its oversample to include Hispanics. An important change for researchers interested in racial and ethnic differences was the addition in 1992 of a detailed breakdown for Asian American groups. Since 1992, information has been available for nine Asian subgroups, and this information can be used to study these groups if the data are pooled over years to achieve a sample of sufficient size. The NHIS also collected the "observed race" of respondents, as recorded by the interviewers, in the past, but this practice ended in 1997. Once OMB released its new guidelines for collecting racial and ethnic data in federal surveys, the NHIS race and ethnicity questions were revised.

Since 2000, the NHIS has asked four questions about race and ethnicity. Respondents are asked if they identify as Hispanic, and those who do are asked to select a specific Hispanic origin group. Then respondents are asked to self-identify with a racial group, and those who select more than one race are asked a follow-up question to determine which single race "best represents" the respondent's race (see Division of Health Interview Statistics, 2002, for details). This format is particularly useful to researchers because it allows multiracial identification and provides a simple way to bridge past and current data. To create racial groups that are comparable to past data, the researcher can allocate multiracial individuals to the single race they select.

Vital Statistics Data

States are required to keep track of vital statistics for their populations, and the federal government compiles this information into national vital statistics. These data include information on births, marriages, divorces, deaths, and fetal deaths. These data are used to create fundamental statistics such as the average life expectancy in the United States and infant mortality information. This information is often broken down by race and ethnicity, providing a wealth of information about basic health inequalities. The data are especially useful because they are available for small geographical units and available over a long period of time.

Because the states are the first collectors of vital statistics, there is variation in how these records are kept. However, national standards provide a guideline that states are encouraged to follow. For example, a national standard death certificate can be used or adapted by states, so most states have similar forms. These forms usually have separate Hispanic ethnicity and race questions, similar to the Census.

Although vital statistics are essential to understanding health in the United States, they also suffer from one of the most well-known problems with respect to racial and ethnic identification. Documentation has clearly shown that mortality rates, especially for smaller groups, are flawed partly because of the way in which race and ethnicity are recorded on death certificates. This means that births, where the race of the child is usually identified by the parent, do not match with deaths, where the race of the deceased may be identified by a stranger.

The National Mortality Follow-Back Surveys (NMFS) of 1986 and 1993 provided some opportunities to investigate the implications of the misreporting of racial and ethnic group membership on the death certificates (Hahn, 1992; Swallen and Guend, 2001). Each NMFS was based on a national sample of death certificates. The NMFS contacted next of kin and hospital personnel to verify information on the death certificates. This created the opportunity for researchers to compare the racial and ethnic identification on the death certificate provided by whoever completed the death certificate at the time of death with the information provided by next of kin. The results show, for example, that while 86 percent of white Hispanics were classified correctly on the death certificates, only 54 percent of black Hispanics were classified correctly. Swallen and Guend (2001) adjust the life expectancies at birth (e_0) for black and white Hispanics for these misclassifications. The life expectancies for black Hispanic males drops from 77.28 to 65.01 and for black Hispanic females from 89.15 to 74.47. The reasons for these drops are clear: The current method of identifying race and ethnicity on the death certificates undercounts black Hispanic deaths, leading to an overestimation of life expectancy for this group. Swallen and Guend also find that these adjustments are more important for Hispanics than for non-Hispanics, but also more important for black Hispanics than for white Hispanics. The unadjusted life expectancy at birth for white Hispanic men is 65.65, while the adjusted life expectancy is 63.15. The black advantage among Hispanic men goes from nearly 12 years in the unadjusted rates to less than 2 years in the adjusted rates. It is also important to note that other data quality problems can significantly affect our understanding of racial and ethnic differences in health. Elo and Preston (1994), for example, note that racial differences in age misreporting significantly affect comparisons of white and black mortality at older ages.

THE LIMITATIONS OF EXISTING DATA SOURCES

The types of data we have reviewed here have several limitations for the study of racial and ethnic differences in health. Williams, Lavizzo-Mourey, and Warren (1994) review a number of these limitations. The first obvious weakness is that most of the large national surveys do not allow the researcher to examine subgroups within the major racial and ethnic groups. With the exception of surveys such as the HHANES, most data sources regularly used to examine the health characteristics of Americans are national samples with sample sizes too small to allow the specification of subgroups. The major panethnic categories used by researchers, however, contain such significant variation within them that it is difficult to draw useful conclusions about the population. We generally lack data on specific nationality groups for Asian Americans, for example, and yet we can be fairly sure that Japanese Americans and Vietnamese Americans will have significant differences in their health outcomes because there are such sizable differences in their class status. Similarly, Hispanics come from a wide range of ethnic backgrounds, and it is unreasonable to assume that early Cuban-American immigrants will have the same health characteristics as recent Mexican-American arrivals. Asian Americans and Hispanics are therefore most difficult to study using national data sources because their groups are both numerically small and very diverse. Therefore, most of the studies of the health of these subgroups

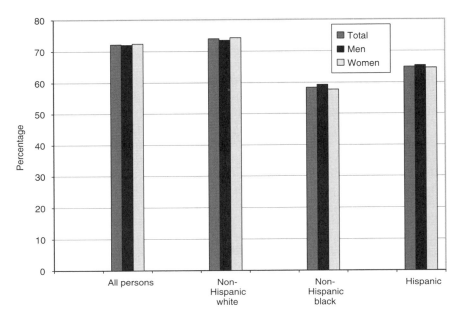

FIGURE 2-1 Percentage of persons aged 65 or older who reported good to excellent health, 1994 to 1996.
SOURCE: Federal Interagency Forum on Aging Related Statistics (2000).

do not come from these national data sets, but from state health surveys in states such as Hawaii, California, and Florida.

Figure 2-1 illustrates the type of information that is generally available in government publications (Federal Interagency Forum on Aging Related Statistics, 2000). This information is based on averaging over 3 years of data from the NHIS for the population aged 65 and older. An advantage of these data is that the numerator and the denominator are calculated using the same individuals. These data show that during the 1994-1996 period, 74 percent of non-Hispanic whites, 58.4 percent of non-Hispanic blacks, and 64.9 percent of Hispanics 65 and older reported they were in good to excellent health. These differences reveal continuing health disparities among the elderly for blacks, whites, and Hispanics. Unfortunately, they also disguise a good deal of heterogeneity within these groups. The Hispanic group consists of more than 25 national origin groups with wide variation in health status (Sorlie, Backlund, Johnson, and Rogot, 1993; Vega and Amaro, 1994; Williams, 2001). African American health status also varies with socioeconomic status, region of birth within the United

States, generation in the United States, and country of origin for recent immigrants from the Caribbean (Williams, 2001).

Many surveys force respondents to choose one race/ethnicity, which will become an increasingly significant problem as the multiracial population of the United States continues to grow. There are exceptions to this, of course, including the current NHIS and 2000 Census, so these sources need to be studied to see how multiracial identification might change our understanding of racial and ethnic health disparities. Currently, however, the multiracial population of the United States is overwhelmingly a young one, so this limitation should have a limited impact on studies of the health of the elderly (see, for example, Root, 1996).

Finally, death certificates greatly undercount the number of deaths for some racial and ethnic groups, and overcount deaths for other racial groups, because the observers identifying the race and ethnicity of the deceased identify them differently than they were identified in the Census. This draws our attention to the important fact that racial and ethnic identification can depend on *who* is identifying the individual. This is an important idea to bear in mind, especially when the source of the identification is different across data sets.

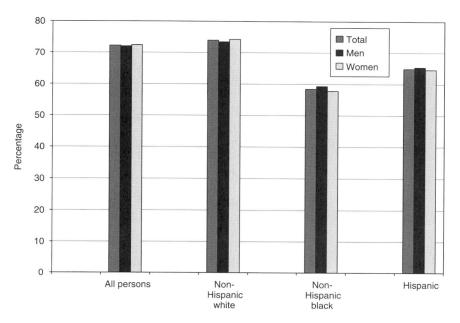

FIGURE 2-2 Age-adjusted death rates due to stroke by race and Hispanic origin. SOURCE: Keppel et al. (2002).

We give one final illustration of the problems created by our current data collection and health surveillance systems. Figure 2-2 contains information on the 1990 and 1998 age-adjusted death rates due to stroke that come from Keppel, Pearcy, and Wagener (2002). According to these statistics, the highest death rate due to stroke is among blacks and the lowest is among Hispanics. However, as the authors of the report note, these death rates make no adjustments for the poor reporting of race and ethnicity on the death certificates. The Hispanic death rate due to stroke is undoubtedly higher than that reported in Figure 2-2. Furthermore, the nature of the Hispanic population changed considerably between 1990 and 1998 due to immigration, and these statistics do not provide information separately by nativity or year of arrival. The Hispanic figures also disguise a good deal of heterogeneity across the different countries of origin of individuals within this category.

SUMMARY, CONCLUSIONS, AND RECOMMENDATIONS

Summary of Racial Identification and Data Challenges

Our review of how we collect data on racial and ethnic groups suggests that in some ways an accurate picture of racial and ethnic disparities in health will remain elusive. This is because societal definitions of racial and ethnic group membership as well as individuals' perceptions of their own racial and ethnic identities change over time. Furthermore there is a great deal of heterogeneity within racial and ethnic categories, including nationality subgroups, generation, language usage, and socioeconomic status. Only recently—1970 in the U.S. Census—have we permitted individuals to select their own race and ethnicity. Only in the 2000 Census were individuals permitted to select more than one racial identity. Research suggests that this change will have different effects on the elderly and young populations; for example, many older blacks of mixed racial descent do not identify themselves as such now because they never had the option in the past (Korgen, 1998).

Our review revealed that a major problem with the available official statistics is the relative paucity of data at the national level for people who do not identify as "black" or "white." Only fairly recently have data been available for Hispanics or Asians (and these are often problematic, as already mentioned). Information on mortality for Native Americans has generally been confined to Indian Health Service reports, not nationally representative data. This greatly restricts our understanding of historical trends in morbidity disparities. We know from some analyses of morbidity and mortality that statistics for these umbrella groups are misleading and disguise a good deal of variability within the groups. Health disparities vary with socioeconomic status within all of these umbrella groups. The picture would be more understandable if we looked at more detailed subgroups, including those differentiated by national origin, generation in the United States, and socioeconomic status. However, such differentiation is not always feasible with population-based survey data that sample enough cases to analyze Asians and Hispanics but not enough to examine specific origin groups or distinguish between the native born and the foreign born.

Implications for Health Outcomes

The ways in which we measure racial and ethnic identity have important implications for our understanding of racial and ethnic disparities in health among the elderly. Health outcomes might be influenced by both the racial and ethnic self-identification of individuals, and the discriminatory actions of others. The effects of discrimination on health occur because of how other people view an individual, which may or may not correspond with how an individual sees himself or herself. Nonetheless, it is clear that self-identification is the best way for gathering information about racial and ethnic identity. It gives people the opportunity to express how they see themselves, and it allows for greater consistency across data sources because most surveys use some form of self-identification. The Centers for Disease Control (now the Centers for Disease Control and Prevention) endorsed self-identification as the most desirable method for using race and ethnicity in public health surveillance (Centers for Disease Control, 1993). In addition, observer identification of race and ethnicity is heavily influenced by characteristics of the observer and context (Harris, 2002), so there is no consistent way to evaluate an individual's observed race in survey settings.

There are also good reasons to believe that self-identified race and ethnicity would have significant impacts on health outcomes. First, self-identification has an important influence on the self-selected peer group and community, which can in turn have meaningful effects on the availability of health services and an individual's tendency to utilize those services. Second, self-identification is related to the choice of media and cultural outlets, and these sources may contain messages about health behaviors such as smoking, eating habits, or visiting doctors. Finally, self-identification is often influenced by observer identifications, and so can also serve as a proximate measure of how others racially classify an individual.

The results of Census 2000 suggested that at this point in time a small minority of Americans took advantage of an opportunity to identify themselves as members of more than one racial or ethnic group (U.S. Bureau of the Census, 2001a). As the social science work on racial and ethnic identification and the biological work showing little evidence of biological racial groups become more widely disseminated, Americans may move to what Hirschman and colleagues (2000) refer to as an origins-based self-identification system. However, as these authors and other authors point out, Americans still see African Americans as somehow different from other racial and ethnic groups (Cornell and Hartmann, 1998; Waters, 1991). African Americans have the fewest ethnic options of any group in the United States. Changes in measurement over time, therefore, will have a greater impact on some groups than others.

The battles that led up to the 2000 Census illustrate the political problems that arise over efforts to modify racial and ethnic classification schemes. The fact that there is no scientific basis for preferring a particular set of categories makes the political issues even more intractable. One can compare this to the issue of adjusting results based on sampling. Here there are statistical theoretical reasons for arguing that such adjustments are appropriate. These become influential, although not conclusive, in the political debate. When we are looking at racial and ethnic classification schemes, there is no established theoretical perspective that suggests some schemes are better than others, and the scientific debates are largely confined to comparability issues (wanting to study trends over time, compare groups across studies, or ensure that the denominator includes all of the people in the numerator when computing rates based on two different data sets). Nonetheless, what we have learned up to this point suggests the following:

- Self-identification should be the standard method of collecting racial and ethnic information. In the case of death certificates, race and ethnicity should always be determined by asking the next of kin or someone familiar with the individual. This would bring data collection efforts into line with what most other federal agencies do in this area.

- People should not be constrained to choose only one group; they should be permitted to choose as many as they wish. This again is in the spirit of the CDC recommendation of relying on self-identification, and would bring other data collection efforts in line with the 2000 Census and the NHIS. Researchers would then have the option of collapsing more detailed categories in various ways.

- The race and Hispanic questions should be combined into an origins question. The question might be phrased as "What are this person's racial or Hispanic origins? Mark one or more origins to indicate what this person considers himself/herself to be." This goes beyond what federal policy currently specifies, but it would substantially reduce nonresponse to the race question and lessen the need to allocate individuals into racial categories.

- Sampling designs that attempt to oversample specific Asian or Hispanic subgroups are better than those that attempt to oversample the generic Asian or Hispanic categories. Nonetheless, statistics on "Hispanics" and "Asians" are more useful than no statistics at all, especially if people recognize the heterogeneity of the categories they are using.

ACKNOWLEDGMENTS

Work on this chapter was supported by funds provided to the Wisconsin Center for the Demography of Health and Aging by the National Institute of Aging. We thank Rodolfo Bulatao, Christopher Jencks, Ann Meier, Molly Martin, members of the Committee on Ethnic Disparities in Aging Health, and two anonymous reviewers for their comments and suggestions.

ENDNOTES

1. A number of related issues are outside the scope of this chapter. We do not, for example, look at how the strength and saliency of racial/ethnic identities in people's lives are associated with their health and well-being. Furthermore, we do not look at the roles of prejudice and discrimination in the differential treatment of individuals by the health care system.

2. The major exception to the use of self-identification in classifying individuals is the death certificate, in which someone who is generally not a member of the deceased's family, often a funeral home director, assigns racial and ethnic identity, sometimes without any consultation with family members.

3. The social constructionist model will be described further in this chapter.

4. Race questions employed by the Census will be discussed further in this chapter.

5. The results of this test should be regarded as suggestive rather than definitive because it was a simple, inexpensive mail out/mail back design with very low response rates. Nonetheless, it provides intriguing information about how people respond to alternative questions about racial and Hispanic identity.

6. For a detailed discussion of the ways in which the social construction of racial and ethnic groups takes place, see Cornell and Hartmann (1998).

7. An example of the former would be the use of Hindu and quadroon as common racial terms earlier in U.S. history and their disuse at this point in time. An example of the latter would be someone with some Asian and some white ancestry changing their racial identification from white to Asian or biracial.

8. Waters (1990) and Cornell and Hartmann (1998) provide further examples of the ways in which racial/ethnic identities can change at both the group and individual levels over time.

9. However, Davis (1991) and Nagel (1996) show that, indeed, there have been changes over time in the meanings associated with the "black" racial category.

10. However, many Hispanics choose "other" as their preferred racial identity, rejecting a racial identity in any of these groups. Rodriguez (2000) examines the reasons that 40 percent of Hispanics racially identified as "other race" in the 1980 and 1990 Censuses.

11. However, the results do vary somewhat by subgroup.

12. Snipp (1997) provides a helpful summary of the history of Native American classification.

13. However, some of those included in this statistic are possibly multiracial themselves.

14. The states are Texas, Colorado, New Mexico, Arizona, and California.

REFERENCES

Banton, M. (1998). *Racial theories*. Cambridge, England: Cambridge University Press.

Centers for Disease Control. (1993). Use of race and ethnicity in public health surveillance. Summary of the CDC/ATSDR Workshop. *Morbidity and Mortality Weekly Report, 42*(RR-10), 1-17.

Cornell, S. (1990). Land, labour and group formation: Blacks and Indians in the United States. *Ethnic and Racial Studies, 13*, 368-388.

Cornell, S., and Hartmann, D. (1998). *Ethnicity and race: Making identities in a changing world*. Thousand Oaks, CA: Pine Forge Press.

Davis, F.J. (1991). *Who is black? One nation's definition*. University Park: Pennsylvania State University Press.

Division of Health Interview Statistics. (2000). *NHIS Survey description*. Available: ftp://ftp.cdc.gov/pub/Health_Statistics/NCHS/Dataset_Documentation/NHIS/2000/srvydesc.pdf [Accessed July 2, 2003].

Elo, I.T., and Preston, S.H. (1994). Mortality, race, and the family: Estimating African-American mortality from inaccurate data. *Demography, 31*, 427-458.

Eschbach, K. (1993). Changing identification among American Indians and Alaska Natives. *Demography, 30*, 635-652.

Eschbach, K., and Gomez, C. (1998). Choosing Hispanic identity: Ethnic identity switching among respondents to high school and beyond. *Social Science Quarterly, 79*, 74-90.

Eschbach, K., Supple, K., and Snipp, C.M. (1998). Changes in racial identification and the educational attainment of American Indians, 1970-1990. *Demography, 35*, 35-43.

Espiritu, Y.L. (1992). *Asian American panethnicity: Bridging institutions and identities*. Philadelphia: Temple University Press.

Farley, R. (2001). *Identifying with multiple races: A social movement that succeeded but failed?* (PSC Research Report No. 01-491). Ann Arbor: University of Michigan, Population Studies Center at the Institute for Social Research.

Federal Interagency Forum on Aging Related Statistics. (2000). *Older Americans 2000: Key indicators of well-being*. Washington, DC: Author.

Hahn, R.A. (1992). The state of federal health statistics on racial and ethnic groups. *Journal of the American Medical Association, 267*(2), 268-271.

Harris, D.R. (2002). *In the eye of the beholder: Observed race and observer characteristics* (PSC Research Report No. 02-522). Ann Arbor: University of Michigan, Population Studies Center at the Institute for Social Research.

Hirschman, C., Alba, R., and Farley, R. (2000). The meaning and measurement of race in the U.S. Census: Glimpses into the future. *Demography, 37*, 381-394.

Keppel, K.G., Pearcy, J.N., and Wagener, D.K. (2002). *Trends in racial and ethnic specific rates for the health status indicators, 1990-98*. (Healthy People Statistical Notes, No. 23). Hyattsville, MD: National Center for Health Statistics.

Kibria, N. (1997). The construction of "Asian American": Reflections on intermarriage and ethnic identity among second generation Chinese and Korean Americans. *Ethnic and Racial Studies, 20*, 523-544.

Korgen, K.O. (1998). *From black to biracial: Transforming racial identity among Americans*. Westport, CT: Praeger.

Lee, S.M. (1993). Racial classifications in the U.S. Census: 1890-1990. *Ethnic and Racial Studies, 16*, 75-94.

Maldonado, L. (1991). Latino ethnicity: Increasing diversity. *Latino Studies Journal, 2*, 49-57.

McKenney, N., and Bennett, C. (1994). Issues regarding data on race and ethnicity: The Census Bureau experience. *Public Health Reports, 109*(1), 16-25.

Nagel, J. (1996). *American Indian ethnic renewal: Red power and the resurgence of identity and culture.* New York: Oxford University Press.

Office of Management and Budget. (1999). *Provisional guidance on the implementation of the 1997 standards for federal data on race and ethnicity.* Available: http://www.whitehouse.gov/omb/inforeg/race.pdf [Accessed July 2, 2003].

Portes, A., and MacLeod, D. (1996). What shall I call myself? Hispanic identity formation in the second generation. *Ethnic and Racial Studies, 19,* 523-547.

Rockquemore, K.A., and Brunsma, D.L. (2002). *Beyond black: Biracial identity in America.* Thousand Oaks, CA: Sage.

Rodriguez, C.E. (2000). *Changing race: Latinos, the census, and the history of ethnicity in the United States.* New York: New York University Press.

Root, M.P.P. (1996). *The multiracial experience: Racial borders as the new frontier.* Thousand Oaks, CA: Sage.

Saenz, R., Hwang, S.S., Aguirre, B.E., and Anderson, R.N. (1995). Persistence and change in Asian identity among children of intermarried couples. *Sociological Perspectives, 38,* 175-194.

Sandefur, G.D., Martin, M.A., Eggerling-Boeck, J., Mannon, S., and Meier, A. (2001). An overview of racial and ethnic demographic trends. In N.J. Smelser, W.J. Wilson, and F. Mitchell (Eds.), *America becoming: Racial trends and their consequences* (pp. 40-102). Washington, DC: National Academy Press.

Snipp, M.C. (1997). Some observations about racial boundaries and the experiences of American Indians. *Ethnic and Racial Studies, 20,* 667-689.

Sorlie, P.D., Backlund, E., Johnson, N.J., and Rogot, E. (1993). Mortality by Hispanic status in the United States. *Journal of the American Medical Association, 270*(20), 2464-2468.

Swallen, K., and Guend, A. (2001). *Data quality and adjusted Hispanic mortality in the United States, 1989-1991.* Unpublished manuscript, University of Wisconsin-Madison.

U.S. Bureau of the Census. (1973). *Population and housing inquiries in the U.S. Decennial Censuses, 1790-1970.* (Working Paper 39). Washington, DC: Author.

U.S. Bureau of the Census. (1997). *Results of the 1996 race and ethnic targeted test. (Population Division,* Working Paper 18). Washington, DC: Author.

U.S. Bureau of the Census. (2000). *Population by age, sex, race, and Hispanic or Latino origin for the United States.* Washington, DC: Author.

U.S. Bureau of the Census. (2001a). *Overview of race and Hispanic origin: Census 2000 brief.* Washington, DC: Author.

U.S. Bureau of the Census. (2001b). *The Hispanic population: Census 2000 brief.* Washington, DC: Author.

U.S. Bureau of the Census. (2001c). *The two or more races population: 2000.* Washington, DC: Author.

Vega, W., and Amaro, H. (1994). Latino outlook: Good health, uncertain prognosis. *Annual Review of Public Health, 15,* 39-67.

Waters, M. (1990). *Ethnic options: Choosing identities in America.* Berkeley: University of California Press.

Waters, M. (1991). The role of lineage in identity formation among black Americans. *Qualitative Sociology, 14,* 57-76.

Waters, M. (1994). Ethnic and racial identities of second-generation black immigrants in New York City. *The International Migration Review, 28,* 795-820.

Waters, M. (1999). *Black identities: West Indian immigrant dreams and American realities.* New York: Russell Sage Foundation.

Williams, D.R. (2001). Racial variations in adult health status: Patterns, paradoxes, and prospects. In N.J. Smelser, W.J. Wilson, and F. Mitchell (Eds.), *America becoming: Racial trends and their consequences* (vol. II). Washington, DC: National Academy Press.

Williams, D.R., Lavizzo-Mourey, R., and Warren, R.C. (1994). The concept of race and health status in America. *Public Health Reports, 109,* 26-41.

Xie, Y., and Goyette, K. (1997). The racial identification of biracial children with one Asian parent: Evidence from the 1990 Census. *Social Forces, 76,* 547-570.

REFERENCES FOR DATA SETS

(text order)

1990 and 2000 Census: http://www.Census.gov/population/www/socdemo/race.html

NHANES: http://www.cdc.gov/nchs/nhanes.htm

HHANES: http://www.cdc.gov/nchs/about/major/nhanes/hhanes.htm

NHIS: http://www.cdc.gov/nchs/nhis.htm

LSOA: http://www.cdc.gov/nchs/about/otheract/aging/lsoa.htm

Vital Statistics: http://www.cdc.gov/nchs/nvss.htm

3

Racial and Ethnic Disparities in Health and Mortality Among the U.S. Elderly Population

Robert A. Hummer, Maureen R. Benjamins,
and Richard G. Rogers

Racial/ethnic differences in health and mortality stand at the heart of the public health agenda of the United States (Kington and Nickens, 2001; Martin and Soldo, 1997; Williams, 2001; Williams and Collins, 1995). One of the three main goals of the *Healthy People 2000* initiative was to reduce health disparities among Americans (U.S. Department of Health and Human Services [DHHS], 1991). Now, one of the two primary goals of *Healthy People 2010* is to eliminate health disparities (DHHS, 2000). Although racial/ethnic health disparities have been the focus of much previous research, the rapidly changing age, racial/ethnic, and health landscape of the country makes it critical to continually update and assess such disparities.

The goals of this chapter are to document racial/ethnic health and mortality disparities among the elderly population of the United States and to examine some simple models of health and mortality that take into account basic demographic and socioeconomic factors. We focus on the five major racial/ethnic subpopulations in the United States: non-Hispanic blacks, non-Hispanic whites, the Hispanic origin population, Asian and Pacific Islanders (APIs), and Native Americans. In several portions of the chapter, the health and mortality patterns of Mexican Americans, the nation's largest Hispanic subpopulation, are discussed. We recognize there is substantial ethnic, cultural, geographic, and socioeconomic heterogeneity within the five main racial/ethnic categories here. Nevertheless, key limitations with population-based data sets, particularly for the elderly, limit the comparative analyses that are possible even across these five broad groups.

The chapter is organized into six sections. First, we outline overall mortality and cause-specific mortality disparities by race/ethnicity among the elderly population (ages 65+) in the United States. Second, we describe racial/ethnic disparities across general indicators of health for the U.S. elderly population. Third, we briefly compare current racial/ethnic health and mortality disparities among the elderly with those observed for younger age groups. Fourth, we examine whether health and mortality disparities among the elderly correspond with racial/ethnic differences in some key sociodemographic characteristics. Fifth, we present some simple models of health and mortality disparities among the elderly to assess the impact of those sociodemographic factors on the observed differentials. Our concluding section summarizes the findings from the chapter, notes some important data limitations in understanding the national picture of racial/ethnic health disparities among the elderly, and briefly notes future research needs.

RACIAL/ETHNIC MORTALITY DISPARITIES AMONG THE ELDERLY

Overall Mortality Disparities Using Vital Statistics and Census Data

We begin by examining racial/ethnic disparities in older adult mortality. The National Center for Health Statistics (NCHS) constructs official mortality rates based on U.S. Vital Statistics (numerator) and Census (denominator) data. The advantages of these data sources are that they are large and cover the entire population, including individuals in nursing homes, long-term care institutions, and prisons. Although important and informative, there are some well-known limitations with the quality and reliability of the official death rates by race/ethnicity, especially among the elderly (Coale and Kisker, 1986; Elo and Preston, 1997; Kestenbaum, 1992; Lauderdale and Kestenbaum, 2002; Preston, Elo, Rosenwaike, and Hill, 1996; Rosenberg et al., 1999; Rosenwaike and Hill, 1996). One problem is reporting disparities between the two data sources. Disparities may occur because racial/ethnic identification on the Census is completed most often by a household member, while identification at the time of death is assigned most often by a funeral director (Rosenberg et al., 1999). Another problem is that a number of recent studies have shown significant levels of age misreporting among the elderly, which can seriously bias old-age mortality estimates (e.g., Preston et al., 1996). Third, Census undercount, particularly of racial and ethnic minority populations, can artificially bias mortality estimates for these groups upward, although adjustments can be made for the estimated undercount (Rosenberg et al., 1999). Despite these limitations, these official data remain a key source for describing racial/ethnic mortality disparities by age, sex, and geographic area.

Panel A of Table 3-1 presents official death rates per 100,000 by race/ethnicity and sex for 5-year age groups among the U.S. elderly population in 1999 (Hoyert, Arias, Smith, Murphy, and Kochanek, 2001); Panel B presents rate ratios for the specific racial/ethnic, age, and sex groups vis-à-vis non-Hispanic white elders. As the ratios in Panel B demonstrate, the reported mortality rates of most of the racial/ethnic minority groups (e.g., persons of Hispanic, API, and Native American origin) are lower than or roughly equal to those of non-Hispanic whites at ages 65 to 69 and tend to become comparatively more advantaged at the advanced ages. Among non-Hispanic blacks, the mortality rates are 30 to 50 percent higher than non-Hispanic whites at ages 65 to 79, converge quite rapidly at ages 80 to 84, and eventually cross over among persons ages 85+. Although levels of mortality are higher among men than women for each racial/ethnic and age group, the relative disparities by race/ethnicity vary little by sex. Thus, these official rates depict non-Hispanic blacks to have the highest mortality among most of the elderly age groups, while rates for APIs, Hispanics, and Native Americans are generally lower than non-Hispanic whites.

Recent demographic work has been undertaken to evaluate and reestimate black, white, and Asian-American mortality estimates among the elderly for the various sources of bias mentioned (e.g., Elo, 2001; Hill, Preston, and Rosenwaike, 2000; Lauderdale and Kestenbaum, 2002; Preston et al., 1996). The reestimates suggest that the *general* mortality patterns for these three population groups described remain consistent; that is, black mortality remains significantly higher than that of whites for most elderly age groups, with the greatest disparities occurring among the young-old (ages 65-74), and then convergence and crossover at the oldest ages (Hill et al., 2000). Likewise, new estimates of Asian-American older adult mortality were shown to be lower than whites, although the advantage may not be as great as demonstrated in the official data (Lauderdale and Kestenbaum, 2002).

However, a debate continues about whether a real black-white mortality crossover occurs among the oldest-old (Nam, 1995). Although researchers for many years have documented such a mortality crossover using a number of different data sets and have concluded that it appears to be real (Johnson, 2000; Kestenbaum, 1992, 1997; Manton, Poss, and Wing, 1979; Manton and Stallard, 1997; Nam, Weatherby, and Ockay, 1978; Parnell and Owens, 1999), others have been more skeptical because of the data quality concerns (Coale and Kisker, 1986; Preston et al., 1996). The most recent, carefully produced evidence by a research team from the latter group continues to find a racial mortality crossover occurring at ages 90 to 94 for females and 95+ for males (Hill et al., 2000). Although the crossover is identified at an older age than a number of other researchers have found, the weight of the evidence, using a number of nationally based U.S. data sources, is strong that a black-white crossover exists. Probably more important, the evidence from

TABLE 3-1 Death Rates per 100,000 by Race/Ethnicity and Death Rate Ratios Compared with Non-Hispanic Whites for the Elderly Population of the United States, Official U.S. Mortality Data, 1999

Sex and Age Group	Non-Hispanic Black	Hispanic Origin	Asian/Pacific Islander	Native American	Non-Hispanic White
Panel A: Death Rates					
Females					
65-69	2,231.3	1,125.8	862.7	1,743.5	1,515.0
70-74	3,516.5	1,662.1	1,403.9	2,410.1	2,372.3
75-79	5,123.2	2,591.2	2,273.1	3,145.7	3,802.6
80-84	7,714.4	4,300.9	4,261.6	4,502.8	6,492.2
85+	14,474.3	8,838.7	8,396.6	6,395.1	15,284.6
Males					
65-69	3,567.2	1,841.1	1,358.4	2,471.2	2,433.4
70-74	5,236.8	2,704.7	2,394.6	3,246.0	3,780.8
75-79	7,455.4	3,913.0	3,828.0	4,358.5	5,712.0
80-84	10,546.4	5,696.6	5,957.6	5,165.3	9,286.8
85+	16,321.0	9,842.3	11,343.5	6,946.2	17,539.1
Panel B: Death Rate Ratios vis-à-vis Non-Hispanic Whites					
Females					
65-69	1.47	0.74	0.57	1.15	1.00
70-74	1.48	0.70	0.59	1.02	1.00
75-79	1.35	0.68	0.60	0.83	1.00
80-84	1.19	0.66	0.66	0.69	1.00
85+	0.95	0.58	0.55	0.42	1.00
Males					
65-69	1.47	0.76	0.56	1.02	1.00
70-74	1.39	0.72	0.63	0.86	1.00
75-79	1.31	0.69	0.67	0.76	1.00
80-84	1.14	0.61	0.64	0.56	1.00
85+	0.93	0.56	0.65	0.40	1.00

SOURCE: Derived from Hoyert et al. (2001).

Hill et al. (2000) shows that mortality rates among aged 80+ U.S. whites (and, given their similarity to white rates, black rates as well) are lower than reports in other low-mortality countries with good data, as originally documented for the U.S. white population by Manton and Vaupel (1995).

Notably, and in contrast to the in-depth work devoted to investigating data quality and refining old-age black and white mortality estimates, relatively few researchers have examined data quality or corrected for age misreports among other racial/ethnic groups (see Lauderdale and Kestenbaum, 2002, for an excellent exception that examines Asian-American mortality). Among the studies that have examined death rates across the life course, Rosenberg et al. (1999, p. 9) find that for population groups other than non-Hispanic whites and blacks, "levels of mortality are seriously biased from mis-reporting in the numerator and under-coverage in the denominator of the death rates." Their findings suggest that officially reported death rates for Native Americans may be more than 20 percent too low, while those reported for APIs and Hispanics may be about 11 percent and 2 percent too low, respectively. On the other hand, Rosenberg et al. (1999) found that officially reported rates for non-Hispanic whites and non-Hispanic blacks were most likely 1 percent and 5 percent too high, respectively. Their refined estimates of age-adjusted death rates across the life course suggest that API and Hispanic death rates still remain the lowest (in that order), while Native American adjusted rates are higher than those of non-Hispanic whites but lower than those of non-Hispanic blacks. How these adjustments for known sources of error specifically influence elderly adult death rates is unknown, although one recent report found that Native American adult decedents were most likely to be misclassified at older adult ages (Stehr-Green, Bettles, and Robertson, 2002). Thus, the officially reported mortality disparities shown in Table 3-1 should be interpreted with great caution, with the low mortality levels for Native Americans, especially at the oldest ages, particularly suspect. We will present alternative estimates of racial/ethnic mortality disparities among the elderly, based on survey data linked to mortality follow-up information below.

Cause-Specific Mortality Disparities Using Vital Statistics and Census Data

Following up on the documentation of overall mortality by race/ethnicity, Table 3-2 (also see Figure 3-1) presents cause-specific mortality rates (per 100,000 population) by race/ethnicity for the leading causes of death among the elderly population by gender. These rates are standardized to the gender-specific age distributions of the non-Hispanic white population. Similar to the overall mortality rates, substantial caution is warranted again, particularly for Hispanics, APIs, and Native Americans, because of problems of racial/ethnic misclassification of decedents, age misreporting, and Census undercount (Rosenberg et al., 1999).

For women (Panel A, Table 3-2), diseases of the heart, malignant neoplasms, and cerebrovascular diseases are the three leading causes of death for most racial/ethnic groups and account for 61 to 66 percent of deaths among all groups except Native Americans. For the two leading causes, non-Hispanic black rates are roughly twice as high as those reported for

TABLE 3-2 Racial/Ethnic Disparities in Cause-Specific Mortality Rates (per 100,000 population) for the Top 10 Causes of Death Among the U.S. Elderly Population, 1999

Underlying Cause of Death	Non-Hispanic Black	Hispanic Origin	Asian/Pacific Islander	Native American	Non-Hispanic White
Panel A: Females					
Heart diseases	1,861.9	974.7	735.4	894.7	1,715.2
Malignant neoplasms	1,029.3	513.9	513.9	547.3	955.4
Cerebrovascular diseases	506.3	233.4	278.1	248.4	481.1
Chronic lower respiratory diseases	140.9	99.6	75.5	169.9	294.9
Influenza and pneumonia	140.1	90.6	72.5	133.3	173.3
Alzheimer's disease	95.7	61.3	*	65.6	167.4
Diabetes mellitus	298.6	200.0	109.6	292.5	129.0
Accidents	*	41.6	40.6	82.8	85.3
Nephritis, nephrotic syndrome, and nephrosis	160.3	54.3	49.0	92.5	72.8
Septicemia	140.0	42.7	31.9	52.7	67.5
Residual (all other causes)	984.2	508.0	399.6	628.0	903.0
TOTAL	5,357.4	2,820.1	2,306.0	3,207.7	5,044.8
Panel B: Males					
Heart diseases	2,045.5	1,178.6	1,114.3	1,164.7	1,929.9
Malignant neoplasms	1,797.1	816.9	840.7	831.5	1,428.9
Cerebrovascular diseases	473.7	247.8	333.9	244.0	380.4
Chronic lower respiratory diseases	295.7	165.2	186.4	223.6	403.5
Influenza and pneumonia	172.0	103.6	119.6	133.0	172.2
Alzheimer's disease	*	*	*	*	99.8
Diabetes mellitus	247.2	191.4	111.6	241.1	142.4
Accidents	123.1	75.9	68.6	131.5	112.2
Nephritis, nephrotic syndrome, and nephrosis	177.5	70.2	69.4	62.8	92.6
Septicemia	149.6	46.6	43.6	57.0	65.6
Residual (all other causes)	1,048.9	622.6	552.0	686.8	902.9
TOTAL	6,530.3	3,518.7	3,440.1	3,776.0	5,730.3

*This cause of death was not listed in the top 10 for this particular racial/ethnic group and therefore is included in the residual category.

SOURCE: Anderson (2001).

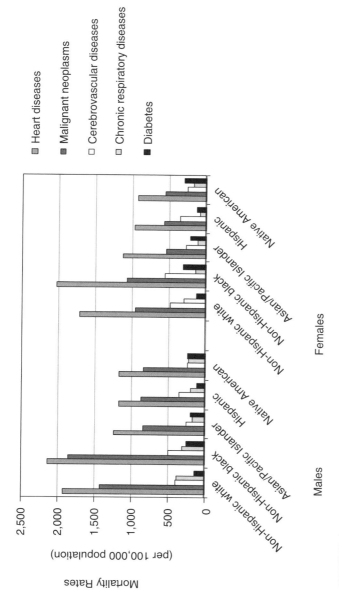

FIGURE 3-1 Cause-specific age-standardized mortality rates by race/ethnicity for the five leading causes of death among the elderly, U.S. population, 1999.

Hispanics, APIs, and Native Americans. For Native Americans, diabetes is the third leading cause of death and the three aforementioned causes account for just 53 percent of all deaths. High cause-specific rates of respiratory disease and Alzheimer's disease stand out among non-Hispanic whites, while non-Hispanic blacks have the highest rates for diseases of the heart, malignant neoplasms, cerebrovascular diseases, influenza/pneumonia, diabetes mellitus, nephritis, septicemia, and the residual category. API women stand out for having the lowest rate for several of the causes, exhibiting especially low rates of respiratory diseases, influenza/pneumonia, Alzheimer's disease, diabetes mellitus, and septicemia. For example, the age-standardized rate of respiratory disease mortality for API women (75.5) is roughly 69 percent lower than among non-Hispanic white women (294.9), and the rate of septicemia mortality for API women (31.9) is about 85 percent lower than exhibited by non-Hispanic black women (140.0).

For elderly men (Panel B, Table 3-2), non-Hispanic blacks and non-Hispanic whites, in that order, also exhibit by far the highest rates of heart disease and malignant neoplasm mortality. For all groups except non-Hispanic whites, cerebrovascular disease is the third leading cause, while for non-Hispanic whites, respiratory disease is the third leading cause. Indeed, similar to the rates for women, non-Hispanic white elderly men exhibit, by far, the highest reported mortality rate for chronic lower respiratory diseases. Non-Hispanic white men (like their counterpart women) are also characterized by the highest reported rates of Alzheimer's disease mortality. For most causes, however, rates are highest among non-Hispanic black male elders. For example, death rates for nephritis and related causes, septicemia, and diabetes mellitus are highest, by far, among non-Hispanic black men in comparison to all other groups. Relatively high rates of diabetes mellitus also stand out for Native American and Hispanic males, while accident mortality is the highest among Native American male elders. As with women, the API male population is characterized by the lowest overall rates of mortality and lowest rates for several specific causes of death

Overall Mortality Disparities Using a Survey-Based Data Set

Large, population-based survey data sets, with links to follow-up mortality information, provide another important source of information regarding mortality disparities among the elderly. Using survey-based data sets linked to follow-up death records (i.e., the National Death Index) to analyze adult mortality patterns in the United States offers some important advantages and disadvantages. Key advantages include the fact that the racial/ethnic identifying information is provided by the individual or a coresident of the individual, while, in contrast, official U.S. mortality data are based on reports of race/ethnicity provided by the funeral director that may or may not match the individual's own racial/ethnic identity reported in the Census (Rosenberg et al., 1999). Second, and perhaps most important, survey-based data sets provide an array of covariates measured at the time of the survey from which the racial/ethnic patterns of mortality can be understood more thoroughly (e.g., Rogers, Hummer, and Nam, 2000), an enormous advantage over the more limited vital statistics-based data.

On the other hand, the survey-based data sets do not cover the complete population: They are samples of the U.S. population and most often exclude the noninstitutionalized population (i.e., persons in nursing homes and prisons) by design. The matched data sets are also believed to miss between 2 and 5 percent of decedents during the mortality follow-up period (e.g., NCHS, 2000). This may particularly influence the findings for racial/ethnic groups that have high percentages of immigrants. Because the identification of deaths is heavily influenced by matching Social Security numbers from the death file to the original survey report, the quality of matches has been shown to be lesser among heavily immigrant populations (Hummer, Rogers, Amir, Forbes, and Frisbie, 2000; Liao et al., 1998). Third, again for some racial/ethnic groups composed of a large percentage of immigrants (e.g., Mexican Americans), return migration to the country of origin, after their original inclusion in the survey, may also bias survey-based follow-up estimates of mortality downward, although one recent study suggests that return migration effects cannot account for the relatively low adult mortality rates that have been demonstrated for the U.S. Hispanic population (Abraido-Lanza, Dohrenwend, Ng-Mak, and Turner, 1999). However, this hypothesis has never been tested directly using mortality records from out-migration countries such as Mexico. Finally, sample sizes among the oldest-old population in most nationally based survey data sets tend to be quite small, particularly for mortality follow-up purposes, thus providing unstable estimates at the oldest ages and making detailed cause-specific and sex-specific analyses for relatively small racial/ethnic populations unstable.

The National Health Interview Survey—Multiple Cause of Death (NHIS-MCD) linked data set (NCHS, 2000) is perhaps the finest of this kind for the study of mortality patterns within the U.S. population. The National Health Interview Survey (NHIS) conducted by the National Center for Health Statistics is an annual health interview of a nationally representative sample of individuals. It is the primary source of information on the health of individuals in the United States. The annual survey includes information from approximately 100,000 people (encompassing nearly 40,000 households annually) regarding central items such as age, sex, race/ethnicity, nativity, income, education, and self-reported health and activity limitation status. Moreover, its link to the National Death Index provides a unique opportunity to examine mortality patterns among racial/ethnic groups with a large prospective data set.

TABLE 3-3 Predicted Racial/Ethnic Mortality Disparities by Age for the Elderly Population of the United States, NHIS-MCD, 1989-1997

Age	Non-Hispanic Black[a]	Mexican Origin[a,b]	Other Hispanic[a,b]	Asian/ Pacific Islander[a]	Native American	Non-Hispanic White[a]
65	1.40	0.84	0.87	0.36	1.19	1.00
70	1.27	0.84	0.87	0.46	1.13	1.00
75	1.15	0.84	0.87	0.59	1.07	1.00
80	1.04	0.84	0.87	0.76	1.02	1.00
85	0.94	0.84	0.87	0.97	0.97	1.00

[a]Main effect of race/ethnicity was statistically different (p < .05) from non-Hispanic whites.
[b]Race/ethnicity by age interaction term was not statistically significant. Thus, disparities vis-à-vis non-Hispanic whites are constant across ages.
SOURCE: Derived from NCHS (2000).

Table 3-3 and Figure 3-2 show estimated racial/ethnic disparities in older adult (65+) mortality for men and women combined at several specific ages. Non-Hispanic whites are specified as the reference group, as is the case in most studies of U.S. mortality. The disparities are estimated using results from a proportional hazards model of mortality risk applied to the NHIS-MCD linked data set (NCHS, 2000). The equations specified mortality risk as a function of race/ethnicity, sex, age, and race/ethnicity by age interaction terms (which account for the possible widening or narrowing of mortality disparities vis-à-vis non-Hispanic whites with increasing age). The race/ethnicity by age interaction effects proved to be statistically significant for non-Hispanic blacks, APIs, and Native Americans and, thus, the racial/ethnic disparities in comparison to non-Hispanic whites for these groups are shown to vary by age. Data in Table 3-3 include 82,868 individuals aged 65 and older at the time of the baseline interviews, which were conducted in six different NHIS survey years, 1989 through 1994. Mortality follow-up was assessed through the end of 1997, which resulted in 20,145 deaths.

These survey-based, follow-up mortality results show non-Hispanic black mortality to be 40 percent higher than non-Hispanic white mortality at age 65, with convergence and eventual crossover at the oldest ages. This disparity is modestly smaller than what was shown in Table 3-1, where for adults aged 65 to 69, non-Hispanic black females and males were each shown to exhibit 47 percent higher mortality than their non-Hispanic white counterparts. The results in Table 3-3 also show 19 percent higher Native American mortality compared to non-Hispanic whites at age 65 (although the small number of Native American deaths yielded a statistically nonsignificant overall difference in comparison to non-Hispanic whites). Perhaps more important, the survey-based results in Table 3-3 for Native Americans do *not* show substantially lower mortality among Native Americans at the oldest ages, as exhibited in the official mortality data in Table 3-1. The survey-based data in Table

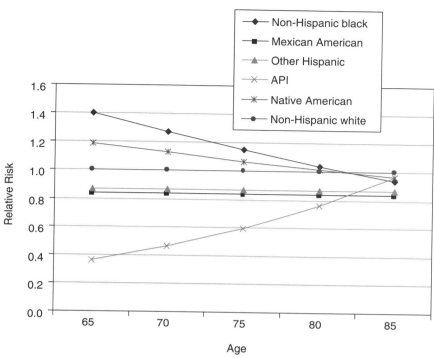

FIGURE 3-2 Predicted racial/ethnic mortality disparities by age, United States, 1989-1997.

3-3 continue to demonstrate lower Hispanic than non-Hispanic white mortality among the elderly. However, the Hispanic mortality advantage using these data is not nearly as wide as evidenced in the officially reported data seen in Table 3-1. Finally, API elderly mortality is significantly lower than non-Hispanic whites throughout the age range, with evidence of convergence to non-Hispanic white levels among the oldest-old. These disparities are quite similar to those reported by Elo and Preston (1997), who used survey-based (Current Population Surveys) follow-up mortality data from the 1979-1985 National Longitudinal Mortality Study data set. Perhaps the only difference of note is that the Hispanic groups presented in Table 3-3 exhibit only moderately (e.g., 13 to 16 percent) lower mortality than non-Hispanic whites, as opposed to the larger advantages (e.g., 21 to 37 percent) reported by Elo and Preston from the earlier time period.

In sum, the mortality results show that racial/ethnic disparities remain relatively unchanged in comparison to the results of Elo and Preston (1997), who used data from approximately a decade earlier. Non-Hispanic black mortality is roughly 40 percent higher at age 65 than non-Hispanic whites, with this disparity decreasing and crossing over at the very old ages. The mortality advantage for Hispanic elders compared to non-Hispanic whites is probably closer to 15 percent, as seen in the survey-based data set findings, rather than the officially reported 25 to 50 percent, although selective out-migration and poorer quality death matches may still be important, and unaccounted for, biasing factors, particularly for Mexican Americans. This Hispanic advantage also has been reported by a number of others at the national level (Hummer et al., 2000; Liao et al., 1998; Sorlie, Backlund, Johnson, and Rogot, 1993). API elderly mortality appears to be the most favorable of all, as consistently found now across several data sources (also see Elo and Preston, 1997; Lauderdale and Kestenbaum, 2002; Rogers, Hummer, Nam, and Peters, 1996), although some subpopulations (e.g., Native Hawaiians, Samoans) may experience higher mortality (Hoyert and Kung, 1997). A major question revolves around Native American elder mortality compared to non-Hispanic whites. Although officially reported data show large advantages for Native American elders, data quality issues are believed to be of greatest concern for this racial/ethnic group (Rosenberg et al., 1999; Stehr-Green et al., 2002). The survey-based results suggest that, at the very least, Native American older adult mortality is not lower than non-Hispanic whites. Nonetheless, data quality issues for Native Americans, as well as for Hispanics and APIs, should be kept in mind. Furthermore, note that these racial/ethnic groups are both internally very heterogeneous (e.g., by level of socioeconomic status, geographic dispersion, history of discrimination, cultural background) and, for Hispanics and APIs in particular, composed of a large percentage of immigrants. This heterogeneity is discussed in several chapters throughout this volume.

RACIAL/ETHNIC DISPARITIES IN HEALTH AND ACTIVITY LIMITATIONS AMONG THE ELDERLY

Disability and Active Life Expectancy

While mortality studies provide one set of evidence regarding racial/ethnic patterns of health, a number of other outcome variables help to round out the general picture of health disparities among the U.S. elderly population. As with a great deal of research on mortality disparities, much work in the health and activity limitations area has compared the black and white populations, with some attention in recent work given to Hispanics (for excellent recent examples using nationally representative data, see Hayward, Crimmins, Miles, and Yang, 2000; Manton and Gu, 2001; Manton and Stallard, 1997; Smith and Kington, 1997a, 1997b). An important exception is the recent work of Hayward and Heron (1999), who utilized life table models with Public Use Microdata Sample data from the 1990 U.S. Census (to obtain disability estimates) and U.S. Vital Statistics data (to obtain mortality estimates) to compare patterns of disability and active life expectancy across five racial/ethnic populations. Measures of *active life expectancy* gauge "the number of years individuals can expect to live without a limitation of activity resulting from chronic disease or impairment" (Hayward and Heron, 1999, p. 77). Thus, although this particular measure is bounded by life expectancy for all racial/ethnic groups, it can fluctuate quite extensively based on the relative health and disability levels of a population group throughout the life course.

A subset of the Hayward and Heron (1999) findings is summarized in Table 3-4 (also see Figure 3-3). These results show substantial differences in

TABLE 3-4 Disability Prevalence Rates and Estimates of Active Life Expectancy by Race/Ethnicity, Age, and Sex, United States, 1990

Indicator and Age Group	Non-Hispanic White	Non-Hispanic Black	Hispanic	Asian/Pacific Islander	Native American
Panel A: Males					
Disability prevalence (%):					
Ages 60-64	23.7	32.5	22.9	13.9	40.8
Ages 70-74	32.2	41.7	30.3	22.1	49.5
Ages 80-84	44.0	52.7	40.5	35.5	55.4
Average years of active life remaining:					
Age 60	12.8	9.8	12.0	16.5	10.8
Age 70	7.5	5.9	7.1	10.0	6.9
Age 80	3.8	3.2	3.5	5.4	4.0
Expected remaining active life (%):					
Age 60	66.9	58.6	69.9	74.3	49.8
Age 70	60.4	51.4	65.0	67.3	45.4
Age 80	50.6	42.6	54.5	57.3	40.0
Panel B: Females					
Disability prevalence (%):					
Age 60-64	19.0	33.4	21.0	13.6	36.0
Age 70-74	28.6	43.6	29.6	24.3	42.6
Age 80-84	47.3	58.7	48.7	41.8	58.4
Average years of active life remaining:					
Age 60	15.4	11.6	14.2	18.2	13.9
Age 70	9.0	6.9	8.2	10.9	9.0
Age 80	4.1	3.5	3.6	5.3	5.2
Expected remaining active life (%):					
Age 60	65.5	53.4	66.2	68.9	50.9
Age 70	56.4	45.3	57.7	59.9	44.7
Age 80	42.3	34.7	44.7	47.4	37.1

SOURCE: Hayward and Heron (1999).

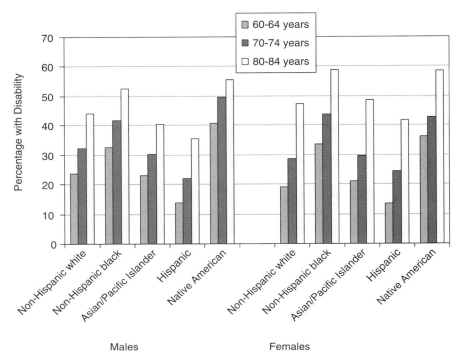

FIGURE 3-3 Racial/ethnic disparities in disability prevalence by age group, U.S. elderly population, 1990.

disability prevalence and active life for U.S. elders by race/ethnicity. Panel A of Table 3-4, which shows the findings for men, demonstrates that Native Americans and blacks have the highest disability prevalence at each age group. Furthermore, these two groups have the fewest years of active life remaining (with the exception of Native Americans at age 80) and the lowest percentage of remaining active life at each specific age. On the other hand, API elderly men have the lowest disability prevalence at each age group and the highest level and percentage of active life remaining at each specific age. Finally, Hispanic males exhibit slightly lower levels of disability and higher percentages of remaining active life than non-Hispanic whites.

While disability prevalence for women (Panel B, Table 3-4; also see Figure 3-3) tends to be somewhat lower than men at age group 60 to 64 and higher than men at age group 80 to 84, racial/ethnic patterns are similar to men. That is, Native Americans and blacks exhibit the highest levels of disability at each age group among the elderly, and API rates are the lowest. Again, Hispanic and white patterns are quite similar. In all, however, the findings emphasize the relative good health of the API elderly population and the high levels of disability and inactive elder life among the black and

Native American populations. Notably, the relatively low mortality rates documented for the Native American population, as reported in official mortality data, are contrasted with their very high levels of disability and inactive life among the elderly (Hayward and Heron, 1999, p. 88). However, the survey-based mortality results from Native Americans (from Table 3-3) correspond much more closely to these disability results. The high levels of disability among the black population corresponds with their high levels of mortality, although it is important to note that one study recently documented a sharper decline in black disability compared to nonblacks between 1994 and 1999 (Manton and Gu, 2001).

Self-Reported Health and Activity Limitations

Table 3-5 presents data on *self-reported health status* and *activity limitations* by race/ethnicity, drawn from 1989 to 1994 pooled National Health Interview Surveys, allowing for the specification of patterns across relatively small racial/ethnic populations. Self-reported health status is a five-point (excellent, very good, good, fair, poor), easily collected, and frequently utilized measure of general health status. Self-reported health has been demonstrated to have a powerful influence on subsequent mortality risk for the U.S. elderly population (Idler and Benyamini, 1997; Rogers et al., 2000) and for a number of racial/ethnic groups (McGee, Liao, Cao, and Cooper, 1999), although the predictive effect for subsequent mortality risk among Hispanic immigrants is much weaker (Finch, Hummer, Reindl, and Vega, 2002). Ratings of "poor" and "fair" are particularly risky categories when gauged with subsequent probabilities of survival (Rogers et al., 2000).

At the descriptive level, Panel A of Table 3-5 shows wide variation in male self-reported health status by race/ethnicity. While just 18.2 percent of API adults aged 65 to 74 report fair or poor health, 35.4 percent of Native Americans and 41.3 percent of non-Hispanic blacks do so. Mexican American elders aged 75 to 84 and 85+ also exhibit quite high levels of poor and fair self-reports, although this may be due, at least in part, to the generally lower levels of health reported among the Hispanic immigrant population (Angel and Guarnaccia, 1989; Cho, Frisbie, Hummer, and Rogers, in press; Shetterly, Baxter, Mason, and Hamman, 1996). It is clear that API and non-Hispanic white individuals exhibit the most favorable levels of self-reported health, while non-Hispanic blacks, Native Americans, and Mexican Americans display the least favorable results. Female patterns of self-reported health status by race/ethnicity (Panel B, Table 3-5) do not differ appreciably from the male patterns.

For activity limitations, the measure utilized in Table 3-5 groups together individuals who reported one of the following: (1) they were unable to perform their major activity, (2) they were limited in their major activity,

TABLE 3-5 Self-Reported Health and Activity Limitations by Race/
Ethnicity, Sex, and Age Group, United States, 1989-1994[a]

Indicator and Age Group	Non-Hispanic White	Non-Hispanic Black	Mexican American	Other Hispanic	Asian/ Pacific Islander	Native American
Panel A: Males						
Self-rated health:						
% fair or poor						
65-74 years	24.5	41.3	34.1	30.0	18.2	35.4
75-84 years	30.8	47.3	45.3	34.6	17.4	51.0
85+ years	32.0	51.4	56.6	40.3	—[b]	—
Activity limitations:						
% with limitations						
65-74 years	35.0	41.6	39.3	36.3	22.1	44.6
75-84 years	39.5	48.1	38.4	35.2	32.2	36.4
85+ years	49.6	59.5	70.8	51.6	30.8	—
N	28,508	3,544	588	601	432	148
Panel B: Females						
Self-rated health:						
% fair or poor						
65-74 years	23.0	41.0	36.0	32.0	20.9	34.2
75-84 years	29.1	45.8	44.7	41.7	35.0	40.5
85+ years	34.0	46.2	48.1	44.9	—	—
Activity limitations:						
% with limitations						
65-74 years	32.8	43.2	39.9	34.3	20.0	42.9
75-84 years	41.0	51.1	41.4	47.3	33.5	66.5
85+ years	60.8	65.7	57.2	68.6	43.5	63.2
N	40,749	5,753	783	973	561	228

[a]Weighted data.
[b]Dashes denote inadequate cell sizes.
SOURCE: Pooled National Health Interview Surveys, 1989-1994.

or (3) they were limited in other activities. Each of these categories has been linked to higher subsequent mortality risk in a recent follow-up study, with the "limited in other activities" category displaying the most modest mortality effects (Rogers et al., 2000, pp. 190-191). Nevertheless, we group them together here in order to provide estimates of racial/ethnic disparities in activity limitation for the five population subgroups under consideration, by specific age group. Recall, too, that these data are nationally representative of the noninstitutionalized U.S. elderly population.

Similar to the Hayward and Heron (1999) disability findings abstracted in Table 3-4, the NHIS findings from Table 3-5 show that, for both men and women, non-Hispanic blacks and Native Americans are most apt to report limitations at ages 65 to 74, while API individuals are least likely to report limitations. Both male and female non-Hispanic blacks continue to display relatively unfavorable patterns among the oldest age groups as well, with the percentage of activity-limited persons being the highest or next-to-highest when compared to the other racial/ethnic groups. Aside from the API population, non-Hispanic whites generally exhibit the most favorable patterns across each of the age groups considered. The activity limitation patterns of Mexican Americans and other Hispanics are more favorable than those of Native Americans and blacks at ages 65 to 74, but less favorable at ages 85+. However, the Mexican American and other Hispanic figures for the oldest-old, as well as those for Native Americans and the API population, must be considered with great caution because of the very small sample sizes of these groups in the NHIS, even when using 6 years of pooled data.

In sum, several sources of health and activity limitation data point to the relatively favorable profiles of API and non-Hispanic white elders, respectively, in comparison to the other racial/ethnic groups. For non-Hispanic black, Native American, and, to a lesser degree, Hispanic elders, the portrait is much less favorable. These summary health and activity limitation results by race/ethnicity are not entirely consistent with those shown for mortality earlier, where Hispanics exhibited favorable patterns compared to non-Hispanic whites, and Native Americans, depending on the data source, displayed either lower or modestly higher levels of mortality compared to elderly non-Hispanic whites. Such inconsistencies between the mortality and health/activity limitation findings could be due to a number of data quality and reliability issues, including the mortality data limitations already discussed. The possible selective nature of the migration process, both in terms of immigration and emigration, may also have strong impacts on the patterns of health and mortality for elderly Hispanics and APIs. Furthermore, cultural and language differences in the interpretation and responses to the health questions in survey data may influence those findings as well. Despite these ambiguities, the weight of the evidence strongly suggests that black and Native American elders are the least well off in terms of health *and* mortality, while API elders tend to be the most advantaged across most of the outcomes examined. Hispanics, while displaying modestly lower elder mortality than non-Hispanic whites, exhibited higher levels of poor and fair health, slightly lower levels of active life expectancy, and a higher level of activity limitations than non-Hispanic whites.

COMPARING RACIAL/ETHNIC DISPARITIES AMONG THE ELDERLY WITH THOSE EXHIBITED BY YOUNGER AGE GROUPS

Mortality

The mortality and health disparities described previously focus on the elderly (aged 65+, or in some cases, aged 60+) population, based on findings from several nationally representative data sets. One important question that emerges is how these relative disparities compare with those exhibited during earlier parts of the life course. We first turn to officially reported mortality rates for different age groups, shown in Table 3-6. Mortality rates for 1999 are shown for U.S. infants, and for younger adults aged 20 to 24, 40 to 44, and 60 to 64, with the older adult rates for those aged 70 to 74 and 80 to 84 displayed for context. Males and females are combined in this table for the sake of parsimony.

Rates for blacks are more than twice as high as whites during infancy and young adulthood, narrow but are still nearly twice as high during middle-aged adulthood, and then converge in older adulthood to near equity among persons aged 80 and over. These results are consistent with

TABLE 3-6   A Comparison of Racial/Ethnic Disparities in Mortality for Different U.S. Age Groups, 1999

	Non-Hispanic White	Non-Hispanic Black	Hispanic	Asian/Pacific Islander	Native American
Infant Mortality					
Infant mortality rate (per 1,000 live births)	5.8	14.1	5.7	4.8	9.3
Rate ratio versus non-Hispanic whites	—	2.43	0.98	0.83	1.60
Younger Adult Mortality					
Rate (per 100,000) for ages 20-24	78.8	163.0	97.9	48.1	151.8
Rate ratio versus non-Hispanic whites	—	2.07	1.24	0.61	1.93
Rate (per 100,000) for ages 40-44	208.0	466.2	192.8	101.7	331.9
Rate ratio versus non-Hispanic whites	—	2.24	0.93	0.49	1.60
Rate (per 100,000) for ages 60-64	1,225.8	2,060.8	913.8	706.2	1,379.3
Rate ratio versus non-Hispanic whites	—	1.68	0.75	0.58	1.13
Older Adult Mortality					
Rate (per 100,000) for ages 70-74	2,997.8	4,227.5	2,115.3	1,812.5	2,785.7
Rate ratio versus non-Hispanic whites	—	1.41	0.71	0.60	0.93
Rate (per 100,000) for ages 80-84	7,546.4	8,702.5	4,838.3	4,979.3	4,770.9
Rate ratio versus non-Hispanic whites	—	1.15	0.64	0.66	0.63

SOURCES: Hoyert et al. (2001); Mathews, MacDorman, and Menacker (2002).

numerous NCHS publications over the years, and with other data sources in a number of major mortality studies over the last 30 years (Kitagawa and Hauser, 1973; Rogers et al., 2000; Sorlie, Backlund, and Keller, 1995). Major cause of death contributors for the especially high levels of black mortality during younger adulthood include elevated levels of homicide and infectious disease mortality relative to whites (Anderson, 2001; Rogers, 1992). Earlier-age major onsets of diabetes-, heart disease-, and cancer-related mortality among middle-aged blacks relative to whites are even more important in understanding this pattern. For example, non-Hispanic black adults aged 55 to 64 suffered from 3.11 times higher mortality due to diabetes, 1.96 times higher heart disease mortality, and 1.44 times higher cancer mortality compared to non-Hispanic whites aged 55 to 64 in 1999; these relative cause of death differences were 2.16, 1.23, and 1.22, respectively, at ages 75 to 84 (Anderson, 2001).

Officially reported Hispanic mortality is equal to or lower than that of non-Hispanic whites across the life course, with the exception of young adulthood (Table 3-6). As with non-Hispanic blacks, elevated risks of homicide and infectious disease mortality help to account for this excess young adult Hispanic mortality (Anderson, 2001; Hummer et al., 2000; Rosenwaike, 1991). Native American infant and younger adult mortality is also significantly higher than non-Hispanic whites, a pattern that is divergent from that shown for older adults vis-à-vis non-Hispanic whites. The exceptionally favorable pattern for the Native American elderly population, again, must be viewed as highly suspect; clearly, our survey-based results for older adult mortality do not show this same pattern. API mortality rates are the lowest of these racial/ethnic groups at each age group. Although data quality issues are at least partially accountable for the reported low mortality rates for the API population (Rosenberg et al., 1999), low API infant mortality provides additional evidence of this group's overall healthy profile. Indeed, racial/ethnic patterns of infant mortality are less subject to misreports of race/ethnicity in comparison to patterns of adult mortality because infant death statistics are based on maternal race/ethnicity, which is reported on the infant's birth certificate in the mother's presence at the time of birth (Hummer et al., 1999a). Infant mortality rate equity between Hispanics and non-Hispanic whites, likewise, is strong evidence for the relatively favorable overall mortality experience of Hispanics at the national level.

Health and Activity Limitations

Table 3-7 turns to health and activity limitation disparities at different ages, using pooled data from the 1989-1994 National Health Interview Surveys. Panel A, which focuses on self-reported health, demonstrates that non-Hispanic whites report the most favorable health for most age groups exam-

TABLE 3-7 A Comparison of Racial/Ethnic Disparities in Self-Reported Health and Activity Limitations for Different Age Groups, United States, 1989-1994

Age Group and Indicator	Non-Hispanic White	Non-Hispanic Black	Mexican American	Other Hispanic	Asian/Pacific Islander	Native American
Panel A: Self-Reported Health						
20-24						
% fair or poor self-rated health	3.7	7.3	6.5	6.0	4.0	7.1
Ratio versus non-Hispanic whites	—	1.9	1.8	1.6	1.1	1.9
40-44						
% fair or poor self-rated health	7.5	17.1	15.1	12.9	7.9	20.2
Ratio versus non-Hispanic whites	—	2.3	2.0	1.7	1.1	2.7
60-64						
% fair or poor self-rated health	20.5	39.3	33.9	31.0	25.0	36.0
Ratio versus non-Hispanic whites	—	1.9	1.7	1.5	1.2	1.8
70-74						
% fair or poor self-rated health	25.3	41.0	33.7	34.3	19.4	35.1
Ratio versus non-Hispanic whites	—	1.6	1.3	1.4	0.8	1.4
80-84						
% fair or poor self-rated health	31.3	50.6	48.9	45.0	36.2	53.0
Ratio versus non-Hispanic whites	—	1.6	1.6	1.4	1.2	1.7

Panel B: Activity Limitations

20-24						
% with activity limitations	6.9	6.8	4.8	6.6	3.9	6.6
Ratio versus non-Hispanic whites	—	1.0	0.7	1.0	0.6	1.0
40-44						
% with activity limitations	14.1	17.7	13.1	14.9	7.1	27.8
Ratio versus non-Hispanic whites	—	1.3	0.9	1.1	0.5	2.0
60-64						
% with activity limitations	30.8	42.3	34.7	34.2	20.4	37.8
Ratio versus non-Hispanic whites	—	1.4	1.1	1.1	0.7	1.2
70-74						
% with activity limitations	31.5	38.5	36.0	31.8	16.9	38.3
Ratio versus non-Hispanic whites	—	1.2	1.1	1.0	0.5	1.2
80-84						
% with activity limitations	45.2	46.2	46.2	55.1	35.5	57.9
Ratio versus non-Hispanic whites	—	1.0	1.0	1.2	0.8	1.3

NOTE: Weighted data.
SOURCE: National Health Interview Surveys, 1989-1994.

ined. For example, for adults aged 60 to 64, non-Hispanics blacks are 1.9 times as likely to report fair or poor health as non-Hispanic whites, Mexican Americans are 1.7 times as likely, other Hispanics are 1.5 times as likely, and Native Americans are 1.8 times as likely. Differences between the API and non-Hispanic white populations are modest at most ages, although the API population tends to report slightly worse health when compared to non-Hispanic whites. As is the case with mortality by age, the racial/ethnic disparities in self-reported health are largest during young adulthood and are narrower among the elderly, although unlike the mortality rates shown earlier, non-Hispanic whites demonstrate the most favorable self-reported health, even in old age.

For most age groups, non-Hispanic blacks and Native Americans tend to report the poorest health. Mexican Americans and other Hispanics are not very different from one another or from Native Americans on this measure, reporting relatively poor health in comparison to non-Hispanic whites at every age (Markides, Rudkin, Angel, and Espino, 1997). The subjectivity involved in measures of self-reported health, particularly across racial/ethnic and highly concentrated immigrant populations (Angel and Guarnaccia, 1989; Finch et al., 2002), should temper any strong conclusions being made from such direct comparisons. Nevertheless, self-reported health has been demonstrated to be a strong predictor of subsequent mortality risk for each of these racial/ethnic groups at the national level, even net of socioeconomic and other health controls (McGee et al., 1999). Therefore, this measure must be considered yet another important indicator of the overall health of these populations.

Panel B of Table 3-7 turns to age-related racial/ethnic disparities in activity limitations. As with ratings of self-reported health, these assessments tend to be much less favorable when considering the older age groups, as might be expected. However, racial/ethnic disparities for this measure are much narrower than those exhibited for self-reported health and, like the mortality disparities shown in Table 3-6, favor APIs at each age group (see Hayward and Heron, 1999, for a similar comparison across younger and older age groups that also shows favorable rates of activity limitation among Asian Americans). Interestingly, Mexican Americans are characterized by their most favorable level of activity limitations compared to non-Hispanic whites at ages 20 to 24, when their mortality rates are highest compared to non-Hispanic whites. At ages 60 to 64 and 70 to 74, reports of activity limitations are modestly higher among Mexican Americans compared to non-Hispanic whites (Markides et al., 1997). Finally, for most age groups, non-Hispanic blacks and Native Americans again exhibit the least favorable results, with differentials reduced somewhat among the elderly groups, but remaining moderate in size.

HOW DO HEALTH AND MORTALITY DISPARITIES AMONG THE ELDERLY CORRESPOND WITH DIFFERENTIALS IN SOCIODEMOGRAPHIC FACTORS?

Another aim of this chapter is to compare the extent to which the observed racial/ethnic health and mortality disparities among the elderly correspond with differentials in sociodemographic factors across these population groups. Table 3-8 and Figures 3-4 through 3-6 summarize this endeavor by using pooled NHIS data from 1989 to 1994 to examine four key factors that have been linked to the health and mortality patterns of U.S. adults: gender, nativity/duration of residence in the United States, educational level, and family income. NHIS data are used to correspond with the health and mortality models that are estimated in the next section of this chapter. Thus, it should be kept in mind that these data are representative of the noninstitutionalized older adult population and do not reflect the total population of U.S. elders. The sociodemographic factors are examined for the elderly population as a whole (ages 65+, labeled "overall" in the table), as well as for the 65 to 74 and 75+ subgroups.

As might be expected, each racial/ethnic population includes more females than males, with this gender disparity larger among the oldest old. The descriptive tabulations demonstrate much greater heterogeneity in nativity/duration patterns by race/ethnicity (Figure 3-4). Consistent with recent immigration patterns, API (65.4 percent), other Hispanic (67.8 percent), and Mexican American (39.3 percent) elders are far more likely to be foreign born in comparison to the other groups. Interestingly, though, there is wide variation when comparing Mexican-Americans, other Hispanics, and APIs. Indeed, other Hispanic and API elders are the least likely to be U.S. born, and API individuals are most likely to be of short duration in the United States (e.g., 23.3 percent have resided in the United States less than 10 years). Thus, the health and socioeconomic characteristics of recent elderly migrants from Asia have vast demographic potential to make a major impact on this group's health and mortality patterns. On the other hand, a majority of Mexican American elders are U.S. born and less than 3 percent of this elderly group have resided in the United States for less than 10 years. Indeed, an overwhelming majority of Mexican American and other Hispanic foreign-born elderly residents report residing in the United States for 10 or more years. Among the predominantly U.S.-born racial/ethnic groups, non-Hispanic white (6.1 percent) elders are more likely to be foreign born than non-Hispanic blacks (3.2 percent) or Native Americans (4.2 percent), with most non-Hispanic white foreign-born elders residing in the United States for 10 or more years. Note that for Native Americans, foreign-born individuals are presumably those who have migrated from Canada or Latin America.

TABLE 3-8 Percentage Distributions for Selected Demographic and Socioeconomic Variables by Race/Ethnicity for Individuals 65 Years and Above, 1989-1994

	Non Hispanic White	Non-Hispanic Black	Mexican American	Other Hispanic	Asian/ Pacific Islander	Native American
Male						
Overall	41.7	40.1	44.3	39.4	44.1	39.0
65-74 years	44.8	42.5	45.2	41.1	43.2	41.9
75+ years	37.1	36.0	42.0	36.4	45.8	33.7
Nativity/duration						
U.S. born						
Overall	93.9	96.8	60.7	32.2	34.6	95.8
65-74 years	94.9	96.5	67.8	33.7	35.7	96.3
75+ years	92.5	97.3	46.6	29.7	32.2	94.8
Foreign born < 10 years						
Overall	0.3	0.6	2.2	7.7	23.3	0.7
65-74 years	0.3	0.7	2.0	7.1	23.5	0.4
75+ years	0.2	0.5	2.8	8.9	23.1	1.3
Foreign born 10+ years						
Overall	5.8	2.6	37.1	60.0	42.1	3.6
65-74 years	4.8	2.8	30.3	59.3	40.8	3.3
75+ years	7.3	2.2	50.6	61.4	44.7	4.0
Education						
Lowest (0-8 years)						
Overall	35.1	56.3	71.6	50.0	44.8	53.5
65-74 years	30.3	50.5	67.9	46.0	42.3	46.4
75+ years	42.2	66.1	79.1	57.3	50.0	66.0
Low (9-11 years)						
Overall	12.9	16.2	9.1	10.9	8.5	15.2
65-74 years	12.7	18.1	10.3	11.2	7.8	16.1
75+ years	13.3	12.9	6.7	10.3	10.2	13.8
Medium (12 years)						
Overall	29.8	17.4	12.3	21.6	24.0	16.7
65-74 years	33.0	20.3	13.8	23.7	25.1	19.5
75+ years	25.0	12.4	9.2	17.6	21.7	11.7
High (13-15 years)						
Overall	11.3	5.2	3.9	7.1	8.5	10.8
65-74 years	12.2	5.8	4.5	8.1	9.9	13.6
75+ years	10.1	4.1	2.8	5.3	5.4	5.9
Highest (16+ years)						
Overall	10.9	5.0	3.1	10.5	14.2	3.8
65-74 years	11.9	5.3	3.6	11.0	14.9	4.4
75+ years	9.4	4.5	2.3	9.5	12.7	2.7
Income[a]						
Low ($0-$15,999)						
Overall	39.5	66.5	59.1	51.3	23.7	59.0
65-74 years	32.8	62.1	57.4	48.6	21.0	56.9
75+ years	50.4	74.0	62.3	53.2	29.8	62.4

TABLE 3-8 Continued

	Non Hispanic White	Non-Hispanic Black	Mexican American	Other Hispanic	Asian/Pacific Islander	Native American
Medium ($16,000-$29,999)						
Overall	33.1	21.6	25.5	26.9	25.2	29.6
65-74 years	35.5	24.7	25.6	28.5	27.2	33.1
75+ years	29.4	16.3	25.1	24.1	20.7	23.6
High ($30,000-$44,999)						
Overall	14.2	7.1	10.4	9.9	19.9	7.6
65-74 years	16.4	7.7	12.0	11.0	20.1	7.3
75+ years	10.7	5.9	7.3	7.9	19.6	8.0
Highest ($45,000+)						
Overall	13.2	4.9	5.1	11.9	31.2	3.9
65-74 years	15.3	5.5	5.0	11.9	31.7	2.6
75+ years	9.9	3.8	5.3	11.8	30.0	6.0
N	69,257	9,297	1,371	1,574	993	376

aPercentages based on individuals who answered the question. Individuals with missing data were excluded.

NOTE: Weighted data.

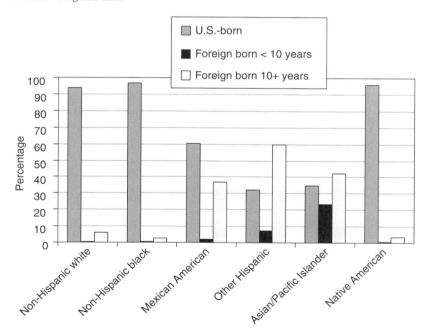

FIGURE 3-4 Nativity and duration by race/ethnicity for individuals 65 and older, U.S. noninstitutionalized population, 1989-1994.

Nativity/duration has been shown to be associated with adult health (Cho et al., in press; Frisbie, Cho, and Hummer, 2001) and mortality risks (Elo and Preston, 1997; Hummer et al., 1999b; Kestenbaum, 1986; Rogers et al., 2000; Singh and Siahpush, 2001) within a variety of racial/ethnic populations at the national level. For the most part, immigrants to the United States have been shown to exhibit favorable levels of adult health and mortality in comparison to the native-born population (with cause-specific mortality exceptions; see, e.g., Singh and Siahpush, 2001; Toussaint and Hummer, 1999), with foreign-native born disparities usually reported to be wider for health outcomes than for mortality risk. Explanations for favorable immigrant health and mortality include the selectivity of healthy individuals migrating to the United States, the selectivity of unhealthy individuals emigrating from the United States, the protective effects of the culture of origin from various sending countries, and the negative influences of U.S. culture, particularly for health behaviors such as cigarette smoking and dietary intake. The favorable levels of health and mortality for immigrants may also wear away with increasing time spent in the United States (Cho et al., in press; Frisbie et al., 2001), although few studies have had the necessary longitudinal data at the national level to directly test this proposition. Chapter 7 in this volume deals with the issue of immigrant health in much greater detail.

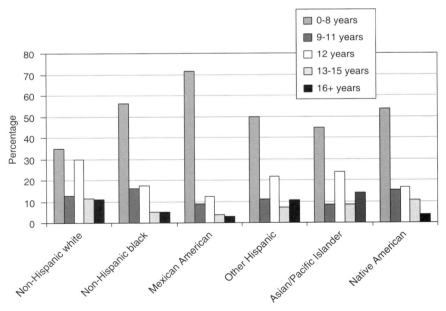

FIGURE 3-5 Years of education by race/ethnicity for individuals 65 and older, U.S. noninstitutionalized population, 1989-1994.

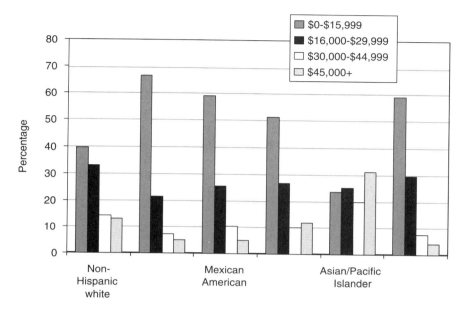

FIGURE 3-6 Income level by race/ethnicity for individuals 65 and older, U.S. non-institutionalized population, 1989-1994.

Differences in education (Figure 3-5) and family income (Figure 3-6) across these racial/ethnic groups are also substantial and, most notably in terms of education, do not always correspond with the health and mortality disparities outlined previously. Mexican American elders have the lowest educational levels of any of these groups: 71.6 percent attended 8 or fewer years of school, with the percentage even higher among Mexican American individuals aged 75 and older. More than half of Native American, non-Hispanic black, and other Hispanic elders also have fewer than 9 years of schooling, although again, age group differences within the elderly are substantial given generally increasing levels of schooling throughout the 20th century for all racial/ethnic groups. Corresponding more closely with their relative health and mortality profiles, non-Hispanic white elders (52 percent), followed by APIs (46.7 percent), are most likely to have completed at least 12 years of schooling, with this pattern consistent both for the 65 to 74 and 75+ groups. API elders (12.7 percent) exhibit the highest percentage of 16+ years of education.

Levels of family income by race/ethnicity correspond quite well with the health and mortality patterns of the elderly. Non-Hispanic black and Native American elders are characterized by very high percentages of individuals who live in the lowest family income category ($0-15,999), both overall and for the 65 to 74 and 75+ subgroups. Correspondingly, individuals in these two groups are also least likely to live in families in the highest income category. Mexican American elders also exhibit a highly unfavorable income distribution compared to non-Hispanic whites and APIs. Indeed, API individuals report living in the most favorable income situation of any racial/ethnic group, with just 23.7 percent reporting living in the low category and 31.2 percent reporting living in the highest ($45,000+) category. For all racial/ethnic groups, income levels are more favorable among individuals ages 65 to 74 compared to those 75+.

In sum, the descriptive data show especially wide nativity/duration and socioeconomic differences across racial/ethnic groups. The educational and income variables clearly show the socioeconomically advantaged position of the non-Hispanic white and API populations, with the income advantage for non-Hispanic whites and APIs particularly striking in comparison to non-Hispanic blacks, Hispanics, and Native Americans. On the other hand, non-Hispanic black, Native American, and Mexican American elders exhibit much worse off socioeconomic profiles that, at least for blacks and Native Americans, correspond with their health outcomes. Widely differing nativity/duration profiles, even among the heavily immigrant populations, also point to the substantial complexity of understanding health and mortality patterns across these groups.

BASIC RACIAL/ETHNIC MODELS OF OLDER ADULT HEALTH, ACTIVITY LIMITATIONS, AND MORTALITY

The last major section of this chapter presents basic models of racial/ethnic disparities in older adult health, activity limitations, and mortality, using data taken from pooled samples of the National Health Interview Survey from 1989 to 1994. Because of its size and the ability to pool multiple years together, this is one of the only nationally representative data sets that allow for modeling of health outcomes for the elderly population across the racial/ethnic groups under consideration here. Indeed, Preston and Taubman (1994, p. 291) described the NHIS as the "most authoritative source of national data on socioeconomic differences in health status." We note that the same is true for examining racial/ethnic health disparities at the national level. Here, we focus on the influences of basic demographic and socioeconomic factors on the racial/ethnic disparities, and particularly how controlling for such factors in a progressive manner (e.g., Mirowsky, 1999) influences the baseline differences.

Table 3-9 focuses on racial/ethnic disparities in self-reported health status among the elderly, using logistic regression models that contrast those individuals with poor/fair self-reported health versus those with good/very good/excellent health. Model 1 shows the baseline racial/ethnic disparities in comparison to non-Hispanic whites, controlling only for age and sex. Non-Hispanic blacks, Native Americans, Mexican Americans, and other Hispanics all exhibit higher odds of poor/fair self-reported health compared to non-Hispanic whites, while the API population demonstrates lower odds. Interestingly, these disparities are largely unaffected with the addition of a race/ethnicity by age interaction term (Model 2), although it is the case that the non-Hispanic black-white disparity is largest at age 65 and decreases with age. The inclusion of nativity/duration (Model 3) also has a limited impact on the racial/ethnic health differences. In this case, the foreign born of less than 10 years in the United States are moderately (43 percent) more likely to report poor/fair health compared to the U.S.-born elderly, which may be due to the interpretation of, and response categories for, the self-reported health question (Angel and Guarnaccia, 1989; Finch et al., 2002).

Model 4 adds educational level. Education is an especially important indicator of socioeconomic status for the elderly because it is usually determined early in life, can be assessed quite easily for all individuals, influences health behavior and the use of health services, and is very important in influencing occupational position and the generation of wealth throughout the life course (Preston and Taubman, 1994). Thus, a great deal of research has assessed educational differences in the health and mortality of U.S. adults and has continued to find sizable, graded differences (Christenson and Johnson, 1995; Elo and Preston, 1996; Feldman, Makuc, Kleinman, and Cornoni-Huntley, 1989; Freedman and Martin, 1999; Rogers et al., 2000; Ross and Mirowsky, 1999; Smith and Kington, 1997a, 1997b), with some studies even pointing to growing inequalities since 1960 (Pappas, Queen, Hadden, and Fisher, 1993; Preston and Elo, 1995). For the elderly population considered in Table 3-9, the educational differences in self-reported health are graded and wide; for example, individuals with 0-8 years of education are 2.6 times as likely to indicate poor/fair self-reported health compared to individuals with 16+ years of education. Furthermore, the addition of education results in a measurable reduction in the racial/ethnic disparities in self-reported health, particularly for non-Hispanic blacks, Mexican Americans, and Native Americans compared to non-Hispanic whites. However, even with the addition of this powerful socioeconomic variable, sizable racial/ethnic disparities remain in self-reported health, particularly between non-Hispanic blacks and whites.

Model 5 additionally considers family income. While recent studies on the health of the elderly have justifiably criticized reliance on household income as *the* proxy for the availability of household economic resources (Smith and Kington, 1997a, 1997b), the yearly NHIS contains no consistent measure of household assets, liabilities, or overall net worth. Thus,

TABLE 3-9 Odds Ratios of Racial/Ethnic Differences in Elderly Self-Reported Health, United States, 1989-1994

| | Odds Ratios for Fair/Poor Self-Rated Health[a] | | | | |
	Model 1	Model 2	Model 3	Model 4	Model 5
Race/ethnicity [NH white][b]					
Non-Hispanic black	2.14***	2.34***	2.34***	2.02***	1.82***
Mexican American	1.83***	1.77***	1.76***	1.42***	1.30**
Other Hispanic	1.49***	1.38**	1.35**	1.27**	1.18
Asian/Pacific Islander	0.81*	0.82	0.75*	0.74*	0.81
Native American	1.68***	1.65*	1.65*	1.47	1.33
Gender [female]					
Male	1.06***	1.06***	1.06***	1.07***	1.13***
Age, continuous in years	1.03***	1.03***	1.03***	1.02***	1.02***
Age * race/ethnicity					
Age * non-Hispanic black		0.99**	0.99**	0.99*	0.99
Age * Mexican American		1.00	1.00	1.01	1.01
Age * other Hispanic		1.01	1.01	1.01	1.01
Age * Asian/Pacific Islander		1.00	1.00	1.00	1.00
Age * Native American		1.00	1.00	1.00	1.01
Nativity/duration [U.S. born]					
Foreign born, <10 years in U.S.			1.43**	1.39*	1.45**
Foreign born, 10+ years in U.S.			0.98	0.97	0.98

Education [16+ years]					
0-8 years				2.59***	2.10***
9-11 years				2.41***	1.94***
12 years				1.64***	1.41***
13-15 years				1.27***	1.16***
Income [$45,000+]					
Low ($0-$15,999)					2.18***
Medium ($16,000-$29,999)					1.43***
High ($30,000-$44,999)					1.22***
Missing					1.77***
−2 * log-likelihood	95,938.1	95,928.1	95,912.6	94,351.0	93,493.1
Degrees of freedom	7	12	14	18	22
N	82,040	82,040	82,040	82,040	82,040

[a]Weighted data.
[b]Reference categories are in brackets.

SOURCE: Pooled National Health Interview Surveys, 1989-1994.

NOTE: *** = $p < 0.001$, ** = $p < 0.01$, * = $p < 0.05$.

there remain important, unmeasured components of socioeconomic inequality in this set of models (also see Kaufman, Cooper, and McGee, 1997, for a critique of socioeconomic measurement in studies of racial/ethnic health disparities). Furthermore, caution is warranted in interpreting the effects of income as fully causal; indeed, substantial literature points to the effects of health status on income as well as income on health (e.g., Mulatu and Schooler, 2002; Smith and Kington, 1997b).

The results for income are consistent with those for education in that a strong, graded association is evident, with individuals in the lowest family income category more than twice as likely to be in poor/fair health compared to individuals in the highest income category. Racial/ethnic disparities in self-reported health are further reduced with the addition of income, although significant differences remain between non-Hispanic blacks and non-Hispanic whites and between Mexican Americans and non-Hispanic whites. Nevertheless, it is clear that socioeconomic factors are instrumental in helping to account for the relatively poor self-reported health for non-Hispanic black, Mexican American, other Hispanic, and Native American elders in comparison to non-Hispanic whites. In contrast, API elders display marginally favorable self-reported health compared to non-Hispanic white elders, with education and family income differences between the API and non-Hispanic white groups having little impact.

Table 3-10 turns to racial/ethnic disparities in activity limitations for the elderly. Model 1 shows that API adults exhibit the most favorable patterns, with more than 40 percent lower odds of limitation compared with non-Hispanic whites. This baseline advantage is relatively unaffected by controls for nativity/duration and socioeconomic factors. On the other hand, Native Americans, non-Hispanic blacks, and Mexican Americans exhibit significantly higher levels of activity limitations than non-Hispanic whites that are, again, largely unaffected by controlling for nativity/duration, but substantially reduced with controls for education and income. In fact, the Mexican American difference with non-Hispanic whites is reduced to nonsignificance after controlling for education and income differences across groups, while the higher odds for non-Hispanic blacks and Native Americans are substantially reduced. Again, the important role of socioeconomic variables for poorer health outcomes among elderly Native Americans, non-Hispanic blacks, and Mexican Americans is demonstrated.

Finally, Table 3-11 displays results from proportional hazard models of racial/ethnic disparities in elder mortality risk. As exhibited in the descriptive portion of this chapter earlier, mortality disparities display somewhat different patterns than health disparities among the elderly. Model 1, for example, shows that non-Hispanic blacks exhibit just a 13 percent higher overall risk of mortality than non-Hispanic whites, controlling for age and sex, while Mexican Americans, other Hispanics, and, especially, APIs ex-

TABLE 3-10 Odds Ratios for Racial/Ethnic Differences in Elderly
Activity Limitations, United States, 1989-1994

	Odds Ratios for Activity Limitations[a]			
	Model 1	Model 2	Model 3	Model 4
Race/ethnicity [non-Hispanic white][b]				
Non-Hispanic black	1.44***	1.44***	1.32***	1.24***
Mexican American	1.22**	1.27***	1.13*	1.08
Other Hispanic	1.09	1.17*	1.13	1.09
Asian/Pacific Islander	0.56***	0.58***	0.57***	0.61***
Native American	1.54**	1.53**	1.42*	1.36*
Gender [female]				
Male	0.99	0.99	0.99	1.03
Age, continuous in years	1.04***	1.04***	1.04***	1.03***
Nativity/duration [U.S. born]				
Foreign born, <10 years in U.S.		1.10	1.07	1.10
Foreign born, 10+ years in U.S.		0.87** *	0.86***	0.86***
Education [16+ years]				
0-8 years			1.58***	1.34***
9-11 years			1.44***	1.21***
12 years			1.15***	1.02
13-15 years			1.14***	1.06
Income [$45,000+]				
Low ($0-$15,999)				1.81***
Medium ($16,000-$29,999)				1.30***
High ($30,000-$44,999)				1.15***
Missing				1.35***
−2 * log-likelihood	107,766.1	107,740.6	107,222.5	106,597.9
Degrees of freedom	7	9	13	17
N	82,040	82,040	82,040	82,040

[a]Weighted data.
[b]Reference categories are in brackets.
NOTE: *** = p < 0.001, ** = p < 0.01, * = p < 0.05.
SOURCE: Pooled National Health Interview Surveys, 1989-1994.

hibit lower elderly mortality than non-Hispanic whites. The age by racial/
ethnicity interactions shown in Model 2 reconfirm the converging black-
white and API-white mortality disparities with age and demonstrate the
substantial mortality disadvantage for blacks and mortality advantage for
APIs, relative to non-Hispanic whites, at age 65. For example, at age 65,
Model 2 demonstrates that non-Hispanic blacks exhibit a 41 percent higher
risk of mortality compared to non-Hispanic whites. The nativity/duration
association with mortality risk, exhibited in Model 3, is moderately strong
and maintains that strength through the complete set of models. The foreign born of less than 10 years of duration in the United States exhibit a 26
percent lower risk of mortality compared to the native born, while the
foreign born of 10 or more years of duration display an 18 percent lower
risk compared to the native born. Again, the interpretation of these differ-

TABLE 3-11 Hazard Ratios for Racial/Ethnic Differences in Elderly Mortality Risk, United States, 1989-1997

	Hazard Ratios of Mortality[a]				
	Model 1	Model 2	Model 3	Model 4	Model 5
Race/ethnicity [non-Hispanic white][b]					
Non-Hispanic black	1.13***	1.41***	1.41***	1.34***	1.30***
Mexican American	0.83**	0.85	0.88	0.83	0.80
Other Hispanic	0.85***	0.87	0.97	0.96	0.93
Asian/Pacific Islander	0.63***	0.36***	0.41***	0.41***	0.43***
Native American	1.00	1.19	1.19	1.15	1.11
Gender [female]					
Male	1.72***	1.72***	1.72***	1.73***	1.76***
Age, continuous in years	1.09***	1.09***	1.09***	1.09***	1.09***
Age * race/ethnicity					
Age * non-Hispanic black		0.98***	0.98***	0.98***	0.98***
Age * Mexican American		1.00	1.00	1.00	1.00
Age * other Hispanic		1.00	1.00	1.00	1.00
Age * Asian/Pacific Islander		1.05***	1.05***	1.05***	1.05***

Age * Native American	0.99	0.99	0.99	0.98	0.99
Nativity/duration [U.S. born]					
Foreign born, <10 years in U.S.			0.74*	0.73**	0.74*
Foreign born, 10+ years in U.S.			0.82***	0.82***	0.82***
Education [16+ years]					
0-8 years				1.35***	1.24***
9-11 years				1.29***	1.18***
12 years				1.20***	1.13***
13-15 years				1.10*	1.05
Income [$45,000+]					
Low ($0-$15,999)					1.36***
Medium ($16,000-$29,999)					1.18***
High ($30,000-$44,999)					1.11*
Missing					1.17***
-2 * log-likelihood	727,370.4	727,315.6	727,263.8	727,092.5	726,941.7
Degrees of freedom	7	12	14	18	22
N	82,040	82,040	82,040	82,040	82,040

[a]Weighted data.

[b]Reference categories are in brackets.

NOTES: *** = $p < 0.001$, ** = $p < 0.01$, * = $p < 0.05$.

SOURCE: National Health Interview Survey—Multiple Cause of Death linked file (NCHS, 2000).

entials is difficult because of immigrant and emigrant migration selectivity as well as the generally higher quality of death matches among the native-born population in comparison to the foreign born. Interestingly, though, the racial/ethnic disparities are only modestly influenced with the control for nativity/duration, demonstrating that the observed, rather favorable, elder mortality patterns for Mexican Americans, other Hispanics, and APIs are not solely due to the substantial foreign-born composition of these groups.

Models 4 and 5 further include education and family income, respectively. Although each of these factors exhibits a graded association with mortality risk in the expected direction, the socioeconomic differences are moderate in size and of weaker magnitude than for the health outcomes examined earlier. The somewhat weaker association of socioeconomic factors with older adult mortality has been noted in a number of national studies (e.g., Kitagawa and Hauser, 1973; Rogers et al., 2000), although the explanation for this phenomenon remains elusive. Moreover, although controlling for education and income in Models 4 and 5 works to help reduce the black-white mortality gap, differences between these two groups remain. Moreover, the relative mortality disparities between the other racial/ethnic populations and whites change only slightly with the introduction of the socioeconomic factors.

CONCLUSION

Despite the national-level priority on understanding and eliminating health disparities, we know far less about racial/ethnic differences in older adult health, activity limitations, and mortality than is the case among infants, children, and younger adults. It is imperative that the research community push for a greater understanding of these disparities, particularly given the continuing documentation of disparities across groups, the changing racial/ethnic composition of the nation, and an aging population. This chapter set out to document racial/ethnic disparities in older adult health and mortality using large, recent, nationally based data sets; to compare the disparities to earlier portions of the life course; to document how the health and mortality disparities correspond with racial/ethnic differences in sociodemographic factors; and to demonstrate how health and mortality disparities are influenced by controlling for those basic demographic and social factors.

To briefly summarize the findings, we have documented continuing racial/ethnic disparities in health, activity limitations, and active life among U.S. elders. Non-Hispanic black, Native American, and, to a lesser degree, Mexican American and other Hispanic elders were shown to have overall worse health across a number of indicators compared to non-Hispanic whites, while API elders displayed more favorable patterns across a number of the indicators. Mortality disparities were found to be less pronounced than health disparities among the elderly, although non-Hispanic blacks were clearly found to have the highest mortality risks using several different data sources. Excess black mortality, in comparison to whites, is concentrated among the younger elderly population, with negligible differences beyond age 80. Nevertheless, a comparison of the present mortality differentials with those of Elo and Preston (1997) from roughly a decade previous show no evidence of closure of the black-white mortality gap among the younger elderly population, even in the recent context of declining mortality for all groups. Racial/ethnic disparities in elderly health and mortality were also found to be generally of smaller magnitude than the disparities shown for younger U.S. adults, although levels of poor health, activity limitations, and mortality risks increase for all racial/ethnic groups with age.

This chapter also documented wide socioeconomic differences between racial/ethnic groups in old age. Our models also showed that education and income differences across groups continue to play an important part in the overall worse health of non-Hispanic blacks, Native Americans, and to a lesser degree, Hispanics in comparison to non-Hispanic whites and the API population. Other demographic and social factors were shown to differ quite markedly across groups. The widely varying immigration experiences across racial/ethnic groups will continue to differentiate Hispanic and API elders from blacks, whites, and Native Americans. Further nativity/duration differences were noted even within the highly concentrated immigrant populations; for example, API foreign-born elders are much more likely to have recently migrated to the United States in comparison to Hispanic foreign-born elders.

In our discussion and analyses, we have focused on the associations between sociodemographic factors, including age, sex, nativity, education, and income, and racial/ethnic disparities in health and mortality. But we must not overlook other important factors that may be associated with these disparities, such as health behaviors—tobacco use, alcohol consumption, diet, and exercise; health conditions—such as obesity and diabetes; mental and addictive disorders—such as drug abuse; and environmental and neighborhood factors—including crime and safety (Rogers, Hummer, and Krueger, 2004). Thus, although we have identified some of the major social and demographic factors that influence racial/ethnic health and mortality patterns, there are surely other areas of research that can further clarify the mechanisms that contribute to these patterns. Importantly, untangling the causal associations between socioeconomic factors and health outcomes, and understanding these associations *within* each racial/ethnic subgroup, should be a major research priority in the coming years.

Important data availability and reliability issues continue to hinder the more complete understanding of racial/ethnic health and mortality disparities among the elderly at the national level. Indeed, much of what is known about mortality among the elderly is based on vital statistics data, which have well-known limitations (e.g., very limited range of covariates, some mismatches of racial/ethnic reports between numerator and denominator data, and undercounts of minority groups in the denominator data), particularly for understanding minority group mortality levels and patterns. Matches between large survey-based data sets and mortality follow-up records (e.g., the NHIS-MCD, the National Longitudinal Mortality Study) have vastly improved our understanding in this area, but even those data sources have limited sets of variables to allow for the full comprehension of mortality patterns across racial/ethnic groups, as well as coverage gaps and matching problems. Nevertheless, such large survey-based data sources currently present the greatest opportunities for most thoroughly documenting and modeling racial/ethnic patterns of mortality across a wide variety of racial/ethnic groups.

Longitudinal studies of health among the elderly have been limited, with a major recent improvement made by the Health and Retirement Study (HRS) data collection program. Still, even the HRS surveys offer very limited numbers of Hispanics, Asian Americans, and Native Americans, undermining their utility for understanding the full spectrum of racial/ethnic disparities in older adult health. Understanding Hispanic and API older adult health and mortality will be a substantial future challenge, particularly with continued large-scale migration and the possibility of circular and/or return migration to Mexico, other countries of Latin America, and Asia.

The diverse ethnic, cultural, and geographic factors that characterize all of these broad racial/ethnic groups, but perhaps especially the Hispanic and API populations, will pose a real challenge to the understanding of elderly health and mortality patterns in the United States. Racial/ethnic groups are characterized by internal variation by language, religion, geographic dispersion, immigration patterns, socioeconomic status, health behaviors, and other factors. Indeed, Hispanics include Mexican Americans, Cubans, Puerto Ricans, Central and South Americans, and other persons of Spanish descent. APIs include Chinese, Japanese, Filipinos, Indians and Pakistanis, Vietnamese, Koreans, Hawaiians, and many other individuals from varying backgrounds. Currently, we know relatively little about the health and mortality patterns of most of the component ethnic populations of the broad racial/ethnic groups, and documenting and understanding such patterns will be an important research challenge in the coming decades.

Perhaps most important, racial/ethnic disparities in health and mortality among U.S. elders cannot be fully understood without placing such patterns in a life-course context. The research community will need much better data to understand how life-course factors (e.g., migration experiences, socioeconomic fluctuations, childhood and early adult health and illness, family backgrounds, discriminatory histories) impact older adult health and mortality across various racial/ethnic groups. Disparate patterns of older adult health and mortality among racial/ethnic groups come about because of the varying demographic, social, economic, behavioral, and health and health care experiences of these groups over many years; thus, our more complete understanding of old-age health consequences relies on better tapping this differential accumulation of experiences.

In conclusion, the United States experienced a remarkable mortality decline and great improvements in health across the 20th century. All racial/ethnic groups participated in and contributed to these substantial changes, although some important health and mortality disparities remain. With further improvements in standards of living, safety and security, nutrition, and medicine, we can anticipate further health gains and longer lives among all racial/ethnic groups in the coming decades as well, and we can hope that *Healthy People 2010*'s goal of eliminating health disparities among racial/ethnic groups becomes a reality.

REFERENCES

Abraido-Lanza, A.F., Dohrenwend, B.P., Ng-Mak, D.S., and Turner, J.B. (1999). The Latino mortality paradox: A test of the "salmon bias" and healthy migrant hypotheses. *American Journal of Public Health, 89,* 1543-1548.

Anderson, R.N. (2001). Deaths: Leading causes for 1999. *National Vital Statistics Reports, 49*(11).

Angel, R., and Guarnaccia, P.J. (1989). Mind, body, and culture: Somatization among Hispanics. *Social Science and Medicine, 23,* 1229-1238.

Cho, Y., Frisbie, W.P., Hummer, R.A., and Rogers, R.G. (in press). Nativity, duration of residence, and the health of Hispanic adults in the United States. *International Migration Review.*

Christenson, B.A., and Johnson, N.E. (1995). Educational inequality in adult mortality: An assessment with death certificate data from Michigan. *Demography, 32,* 215-230.

Coale, A.J., and Kisker, E.E. (1986). Mortality crossover: Reality or bad data? *Population Studies, 40,* 389-401.

Elo, I.T. (2001). New African American life tables from 1935-1940 to 1985-1990. *Demography, 38,* 97-114.

Elo, I.T., and Preston, S.H. (1996). Educational differentials in mortality: United States, 1979-1985. *Social Science and Medicine, 42,* 47-57.

Elo, I.T., and Preston, S.H. (1997). Racial and ethnic differences in mortality at older ages. In L.G. Martin and B.J. Soldo (Eds.), *Racial and ethnic differences in the health of older Americans* (pp. 10-42). Committee on Population, Commission on Behavioral and Social Sciences and Education, National Research Council. Washington, DC: National Academy Press.

Feldman, J., Makuc, D., Kleinman, J., and Cornoni-Huntley, J. (1989). National trends in educational differences in mortality. *American Journal of Epidemiology, 129,* 919-933.

Finch, B.K., Hummer, R.A., Reindl, M., and Vega, W.A. (2002). Validity of self-rated health among Latino(a)s. *American Journal of Epidemiology, 155*(8), 755-759.

Freedman, V.A., and Martin, L.G. (1999). The role of education in explaining and forecasting trends in functional limitations among older Americans. *Demography, 36*, 461-473.

Frisbie, W.P., Cho, Y., and Hummer, R.A. (2001). Immigration and the health of Asian and Pacific Islander adults in the U.S. *American Journal of Epidemiology, 153*, 372-380.

Hayward, M.D., and Heron, M. (1999). Racial inequality in active life among adult Americans. *Demography, 36*, 77-91.

Hayward, M.D., Crimmins, E.M., Miles, T.P., and Yang, Y. (2000). The significance of socioeconomic status in explaining the racial gap in chronic health conditions. *American Sociological Review, 65*, 910-929.

Hill, M.E., Preston, S.H., and Rosenwaike, I. (2000). Age reporting among white Americans aged 85+: Results of a record linkage study. *Demography, 37*, 175-186.

Hoyert, D.L., and Kung, H. (1997). Asian or Pacific Islander mortality, selected states, 1992. *Monthly Vital Statistics Reports, 46*(1).

Hoyert, D.L., Arias, E., Smith, B.L., Murphy, S.L., and Kochanek, K.D. (2001). Deaths: Final data for 1999. *National Vital Statistics Reports, 49*(8).

Hummer, R.A., Biegler, M., DeTurk, P.B., Forbes, D., Frisbie, W.P., Hong, Y., and Pullum, S.G. (1999a). Race/ethnicity, nativity, and infant mortality in the United States. *Social Forces, 77*, 1083-1118.

Hummer, R.A., Rogers, R.G., Nam, C.B., and LeClere, F.B. (1999b). Race/ethnicity, nativity, and U.S. adult mortality. *Social Science Quarterly, 80*, 136-153.

Hummer, R.A., Rogers, R.G., Amir, S.H., Forbes, D., and Frisbie, W.P. (2000). Adult mortality differentials among Hispanic subgroups and non-Hispanic whites. *Social Science Quarterly, 81*, 459-476.

Idler, E., and Benyamini, Y. (1997). Self-rated health and mortality: A review of twenty-seven community studies. *Journal of Health and Social Behavior, 39*, 21-37.

Johnson, N.E. (2000). The racial crossover in comorbidity, disability, and mortality. *Demography, 37*, 267-283.

Kaufman, J., Cooper, R., and McGee, D. (1997). Socioeconomic status and health in blacks and whites: The problem of residual confounding and the resiliency of race. *Epidemiology, 8*, 621-628.

Kestenbaum, B. (1986). Mortality by nativity. *Demography, 23*, 87-90.

Kestenbaum, B. (1992). A description of the extreme aged population based on improved Medicare enrollment data. *Demography, 29*, 565-580.

Kestenbaum, B. (1997). *Recent mortality of the oldest old, from Medicare data.* Paper presented at the annual meeting of the Population Association of America, Washington, DC.

Kington, R.S., and Nickens, H.W. (2001). Racial and ethnic differences in health: Recent trends, current patterns, future directions. In N.J. Smelser, W.J. Wilson, and F. Mitchell (Eds.), *America becoming: Racial trends and their consequences* (vol. II, pp. 253-310). Commission on Behavioral and Social Sciences and Education, National Research Council. Washington, DC: National Academy Press.

Kitagawa, E.M., and Hauser, P.M. (1973). *Differential mortality in the United States: A study in socioeconomic epidemiology.* Cambridge, MA: Harvard University Press.

Lauderdale, D.S., and Kestenbaum, B. (2002). Mortality rates of elderly Asian American populations. *Demography, 39*(3), 529-540.

Liao, Y., Cooper, R.S., Cao, G., Durazo-Arvizu, R., Kaufman, J.S., Luke, A., and McGee, D.L. (1998). Mortality patterns among adult Hispanics: Findings from the NHIS, 1986-1990. *American Journal of Public Health, 88*, 227-232.

Manton, K.G., and Gu, S. (2001). Changes in the prevalence of chronic disability in the United States black and non-black population above age 65 from 1982 to 1999. *Proceedings of the National Academy of Sciences, 98*(11), 6354-6359.

Manton, K.G., and Stallard, E. (1997). Health and disability differences among racial and ethnic groups. In L.G. Martin and B.J. Soldo (Eds.), *Racial and ethnic differences in the health of older Americans* (pp. 43-104). Committee on Population, Commission on Behavioral and Social Sciences and Education, National Research Council. Washington, DC: National Academy Press.

Manton, K.G., and Vaupel, J.W. (1995). Survival after the age of 80 in the United States, Sweden, France, England, and Japan. *New England Journal of Medicine, 333,* 1232-1235.

Manton, K.G., Poss, S.S., and Wing, S. (1979). The black/white mortality crossover: Investigation from the perspective of the components of aging. *The Gerontologist, 19,* 291-300.

Markides, K.S., Rudkin, L., Angel, R.J., and Espino, D.V. (1997). Health status of Hispanic elderly. In L.G. Martin and B.J. Soldo (Eds.), *Racial and ethnic differences in the health of older Americans* (pp. 285-300). Committee on Population, Commission on Behavioral and Social Sciences and Education, National Research Council. Washington, DC: National Academy Press.

Martin, L.G., and Soldo, B.J. (1997). Introduction. In L.G. Martin and B.J. Soldo (Eds.), *Racial and ethnic differences in the health of older Americans* (pp. 1-9). Committee on Population, Commission on Behavioral and Social Sciences and Education, National Research Council. Washington, DC: National Academy Press.

Mathews, T.J., MacDorman, M.F., and Menacker, F. (2002). Infant mortality statistics from the 1999 period linked birth/infant death data set. *National Vital Statistics Reports, 50*(4).

McGee, D.L., Liao, Y., Cao, G., and Cooper, R. (1999). Self-reported health status and mortality in a multiethnic U.S. cohort. *American Journal of Epidemiology, 149,* 41-46.

Mirowsky, J. (1999). Analyzing the associations between mental health and social circumstances. In C.S. Aneshensel and J.C. Phelan (Eds.), *Handbook of the sociology of mental health* (pp. 105-123). New York: Kluwer Academic/Plenum.

Mulatu, M.S., and Schooler, C. (2002). Causal connections between SES and health: Reciprocal effects and mediating mechanisms. *Journal of Health and Social Behavior, 43*(1), 22-41.

Nam, C.B. (1995). Another look at mortality crossovers. *Social Biology, 42,* 133-142.

Nam, C.B., Weatherby, N.L., and Ockay, K.A. (1978). Causes of death which contribute to the mortality crossover effect. *Social Biology, 25,* 306-314.

National Center for Health Statistics. (2000). *National Health Interview Survey: Multiple cause of death public use data file, 1986-1994 survey years.* [Computer file and documentation.] Hyattsville, MD: Public Health Service.

Pappas, G., Queen, S., Hadden, W., and Fisher, G. (1993). The increasing disparity in mortality between socioeconomic groups in the United States, 1960 and 1986. *New England Journal of Medicine, 329,* 103-109.

Parnell, A.M., and Owens, C.R. (1999). *Evaluation of U.S. mortality patterns at old ages using the Medicare enrollment database.* Available: http://www.demographic-research. org /Volumes/Vol1/2 [Accessed July 2, 2003].

Preston, S.H., and Elo, I.T. (1995). Are educational differentials in adult mortality increasing in the United States? *Journal of Aging and Health, 7,* 476-496.

Preston, S.H., and Taubman, P. (1994). Socioeconomic differences in adult mortality and health status. In L.G. Martin and S.H. Preston (Eds.), *Demography of aging* (pp. 279-318). Committee on Population, Commission on Behavioral and Social Sciences and Education, National Research Council. Washington, DC: National Academy Press.

Preston, S.H., Elo, I.T., Rosenwaike, I., and Hill, M.E. (1996). African-American mortality at older ages: Results of a matching study. *Demography, 33,* 193-209.

Rogers, R.G. (1992). Living and dying in the USA: Sociodemographic determinants of death among blacks and whites. *Demography, 29,* 287-303.

Rogers, R.G., Hummer, R.A., Nam, C.B., and Peters, K. (1996). Demographic, socioeconomic, and behavioral factors affecting ethnic mortality by cause. *Social Forces, 74,* 1419-1438.

Rogers, R.G., Hummer, R.A., and Nam, C.B. (2000). *Living and dying in the USA: Behavioral, health, and social differentials of adult mortality.* San Diego, CA: Academic Press.

Rogers, R.G., Hummer, R.A., and Krueger, P.M. (2004). Adult mortality. In D.L. Poston, Jr., and M. Micklin (Eds.), *Handbook of population.* New York: Kluwer Academic/Plenum.

Rosenberg, H.M., Maurer, J.D., Sorlie, P.D., Johnson, N.J., MacDorman, M.F., Hoyert, D.L., Spitler, J.F., and Scott, C. (1999). Quality of death rates by race and Hispanic origin: A summary of current research. *Vital and Health Statistics, 2*(128).

Rosenwaike, I. (1991). *Mortality of Hispanic populations.* New York: Greenwood Press.

Rosenwaike, I., and Hill, M.E. (1996). The accuracy of age reporting among elderly African Americans: Evidence of a birth registration effect. *Research on Aging, 18,* 310-324.

Ross, C.E., and Mirowsky, J. (1999). Refining the association between education and health: The effects of quantity, credential, and selectivity. *Demography, 36,* 445-460.

Shetterly, S.M., Baxter, J., Mason, L.D., and Hamman, R.F. (1996). Self-rated health among Hispanic versus non-Hispanic white adults: The San Luis Valley Health and Aging Study. *American Journal of Public Health, 86,* 1798-1801.

Singh, G.K., and Siahpush, M. (2001). All-cause and cause-specific mortality of immigrants and natives born in the United States. *American Journal of Public Health, 91,* 392-399.

Smith, J.P., and Kington, R.S. (1997a). Demographic and economic correlates of health in old age. *Demography, 34,* 159-170.

Smith, J.P., and Kington, R.S. (1997b). Race, socioeconomic status, and health in late life. In L.G. Martin and B.J. Soldo (Eds.), *Racial and ethnic differences in the health of older Americans* (pp. 105-162). Committee on Population, Commission on Behavioral and Social Sciences and Education, National Research Council. Washington, DC: National Academy Press.

Sorlie, P.D., Backlund, E., Johnson, N.J., and Rogot, E. (1993). Mortality by Hispanic status in the United States. *Journal of the American Medical Association, 270,* 2464-2468.

Sorlie, P.D., Backlund, E., and Keller, J. (1995). U.S. mortality by economic, demographic, and social characteristics: The National Longitudinal Mortality Study. *American Journal of Public Health, 85,* 949-956.

Stehr-Green, P., Bettles, J., and Robertson, L.D. (2002). Effect of racial/ethnic misclassification of American Indians and Alaskan Natives on Washington state death certificates, 1989-1997. *American Journal of Public Health, 92,* 443-444.

Toussaint, D.W., and Hummer, R.A. (1999). Differential mortality risks from violent causes for foreign- and native-born residents of the United States. *Population Research and Policy Review, 18,* 607-620.

U.S. Department of Health and Human Services. (1991). *Healthy people 2000: National health promotion and disease prevention objectives.* Washington, DC: Public Health Service, Author.

U.S. Department of Health and Human Services. (2000). *Tracking healthy people 2010.* Washington, DC: Author.

Williams, D.R. (2001). Racial variations in adult health status: Patterns, paradoxes, and prospects. In N.J. Smelser, W.J. Wilson, and F. Mitchell (Eds.), *America becoming: Racial trends and their consequences* (vol. II, pp. 371-410). Commission on Behavioral and Social Sciences and Education, National Research Council. Washington, DC: National Academy Press.

Williams, D.R., and Collins, C. (1995). U.S. socioeconomic and racial differences in health: Patterns and explanations. *Annual Review of Sociology, 21,* 349-386.

4

Ethnic Differences in Dementia and Alzheimer's Disease

Jennifer J. Manly and Richard Mayeux

The proportion of ethnic minorities among the elderly in the United States is increasing. The U.S. Census Bureau estimates that the proportion of elders who are white and non-Hispanic will decline from 87 percent in 1990 to 67 percent in 2050. As compared to the 1990 Census, the population of Hispanic elders is expected to double in 2010, and will be 11 times greater by 2050. Of the 80.1 million elderly projected for 2050, 8.4 million (10.4 percent) will be black, as compared to 8 percent of elders in 1990. With these changes, ethnic minority populations will bear an increased share of the economic and social burden associated with diseases that predominantly affect the elderly, such as Alzheimer's disease (AD). This presents the potential for a major public health issue because ethnic minorities may be at higher risk for AD and dementia than non-Hispanic whites.

Investigations of ethnic populations that have migrated across several cultures offer the opportunity to study groups for which genetic factors essentially remain the same but environmental and cultural forces undergo dramatic change. At the same time, comparison of different racial groups residing in the same environment with similar socioeconomic status and equal exposure to risk factors may help to uncover genetic factors responsible for AD (Osuntokun et al., 1992).

The studies reviewed in this chapter examine ethnic differences in rates of broad categories such as "cognitive impairment" or "dementia" as well as specific neurodegenerative diseases such as Alzheimer's disease and vascular dementia. Cognitive impairment, a necessary prerequisite for diagnosis of any dementia, is determined using either screening tests, such as the

Mini-Mental State Exam (MMSE), or more sensitive and extensive neuropsychological test batteries incorporating individual measures such as Logical Memory from the Weschler Memory Scale. To meet clinical criteria for dementia, cognitive impairment must be of sufficient severity to interfere with activities of daily living. Cross-cultural research on dementia must contend with the fact that assessments of both cognitive impairment and daily functioning are susceptible to culturally dependent definitions and are quantified by measures that are sensitive to cultural and educational background.

There are many possible etiologies of progressive dementia, but the most frequent causes are Alzheimer's pathology and cerebrovascular disease. Although the exact etiology cannot be definitively determined before an autopsy, there are research criteria for AD and vascular dementia that have been shown to predict the specific pathological determination upon autopsy with up to 90 percent accuracy. However, the supporting research has involved almost exclusively white subjects. Few autopsy studies have been performed to confirm the accuracy of these diagnoses among ethnically diverse groups.

This chapter will first review the findings of epidemiological studies of dementia and AD among different ethnic groups within the United States and other countries. This review is not intended to be a comprehensive survey of AD epidemiology, which is available elsewhere (Chang, Miller, and Lin, 1993; Hendrie, 1998; Jorm, 1990; Larson and Imai, 1996; Yeo, Gallagher-Thompson, and Lieberman, 1996); rather, it is intended to highlight specific studies that emphasize the issues in research of ethnicity and AD. We will then explore some potential explanations for ethnic differences in rates of AD and dementia: (1) statistical limitations, (2) bias in measurement of cognitive functioning, (3) genetic factors, (4) nongenetic medical risk factors, and (5) social factors.

EPIDEMIOLOGY OF AD: CROSS-CULTURAL COMPARISONS

Ethnic Comparisons Within the United States

A number of studies have compared the rates of dementia and AD between ethnic groups residing in the United States. Despite differences in sampling methods and definitions of dementia as well as in definitions of race/ethnicity, the most frequent findings in reviewing this literature are that African Americans and Hispanics have higher prevalence and incidence of dementia and AD than whites. Native Americans appeared to have lower rates of AD in comparison to whites. Asian Americans had rates of dementia comparable to whites; however, whether there is the same proportion of AD compared to vascular dementia among Asian Americans and

Asian immigrants remains uncertain. Opinion differs on whether correction for education accounted for the different rates of dementia and AD found among these cultural groups.

Most U.S.-based studies have focused on comparing rates of dementia or AD among African Americans and Hispanics to rates among whites. These studies found higher rates of cognitive impairment, dementia, and AD among ethnic minorities than among whites (Folstein, Bassett, Anthony, Romanoski, and Nestadt, 1991; George, Landerman, Blazer, and Anthony, 1991; Gurland et al., 1998; Haerer, Anderson, and Schoenberg, 1987; Perkins et al., 1997; Prineas et al., 1995; Schoenberg, Anderson, and Haerer, 1985; Still, Jackson, Brandes, Abramson, and Macera, 1990; Teresi, Albert, Holmes, and Mayeux, 1999). One of the largest projects, a population-based, longitudinal study of 2,126 elderly residents of New York City, examined the incidence of AD among three ethnic/racial groups, self-defined according to U.S. Census criteria: Non-Hispanic whites, non-Hispanic blacks, and Hispanics (mostly Caribbean) (Tang et al., 2001). These individuals were identified as Medicare recipients residing in selected Census tracts of the neighborhoods of Washington Heights and Inwood. Using National Institute of Neurological and Communicative Disorders and Stroke and the Alzheimer's Disease and Related Disorders Associations (NINCDS-ADRDA) criteria, neurological examination, and results from an extensive neuropsychological test, the standardized incidence rate for non-Hispanic black elders (4.2 percent per person-year) and Caribbean Hispanics (3.8 percent per person-year) was significantly higher than that of the referent group, non-Hispanic whites, even after correcting for differences in years of education.

Another large study, the Duke Established Populations for Epidemiological Studies of the Elderly project, found no differences in frequency of dementia between African Americans and whites. This study described a sample of 4,136 participants (Fillenbaum et al., 1998), 55 percent of whom were African American. The sample was defined using multistage probability sampling with unequal probabilities of selection to sample community-dwelling residents age 65 and older within five adjacent counties, one urban and four rural. However, the way in which the racial groups were defined is unclear. The authors used the Consortium to Establish a Registry for Alzheimer's Disease (CERAD) Neuropsychological Test battery to assess cognitive functioning, and norms correcting for years of education (Unverzagt, Hall, Torke, and Rediger, 1996) were used for the determination of significant cognitive deficit and dementia. The prevalence of dementia among elders above age 67, as determined by clinical consensus, was 7 percent for African Americans and 7.2 percent for whites. There were also no differences in the 3-year incidence of dementia for African Americans (5.8 percent) versus whites (6.2 percent). The authors did not report incidence of dementia subtypes; therefore, it is possible that although the overall rates of dementia were similar among African Americans and whites, the frequencies of AD and vascular dementia may differ within the groups.

The rate of dementia on admission to nursing homes is higher among black residents than among white residents (Weintraub et al., 2000); however, findings from studies of long-term outcomes for African-American elders with dementia are not consistent. Mortality associated with dementia was found to be higher among blacks than non-Hispanic whites, especially among black males (Lanska, 1998). However, there were no statistically significant differences in survival from time of entry into the CERAD study of whites and African Americans after accounting for the effects of age, gender, and severity of dementia (Heyman, Peterson, Fillenbaum, and Pieper, 1996). However, for each of these studies, the exact way in which racial groups were defined was not stated.

The role of immigration and changes in environmental risk factors was examined in several epidemiological studies of elders with Japanese ancestry. The age-standardized prevalence of dementia (using Diagnostic and Statistical Manual of Mental Disorders—Third Edition [DSM-III] criteria) among Japanese-American men aged 71 to 93 living in Hawaii (White et al., 1996) was 7.6 percent. This rate was higher than Japanese men living in Japan (4 percent to 6 percent), and similar to prevalence rates in European populations. The age-standardized prevalence of AD (using NINCDS-ADRDA criteria) in this Japanese-American population was 4.7 percent. The authors suggested that environmental or cultural exposures associated with migration from Japan to Hawaii influenced the development of AD in these Japanese Americans. Similar results were reported in a study of 1,985 Japanese-American participants in the Kame project in King County, Washington (Graves et al., 1996). A cross-sectional study of dementia prevalence using the California Alzheimer's Disease and Diagnostic Treatment Centers found that, as compared to whites, Asian Americans had a greater proportion of vascular dementia and lower proportion of AD (Still et al., 1990), similar to studies of Asians in Asia (to be discussed).

Native Americans appear to have a lower rate of AD than whites, but equivalent rates of overall cognitive impairment or dementia. Hendrie et al. (1993) examined 192 Cree, aged 65 and older, living on two reserves in Manitoba, Canada, and an age-stratified sample of 241 English-speaking whites living in Winnipeg. Using the Community Screening Interview for Dementia (CSID) to screen for cognitive impairment, the authors found a significant difference between the age-adjusted prevalence of AD among the Cree Indians (0.5 percent) as compared to whites (3.5 percent), despite the two groups having an equivalent age-adjusted prevalence of dementia (4.2 percent in each population).

A study of Cherokee Indians living in northeastern Oklahoma (Rosenberg et al., 1996) used NINCDS-ADRDA criteria to identify 26 people aged 65 and older with AD, and then assessed an equal number of normal controls. The investigators found that as the genetic degree of Cherokee ancestry increased, the frequency of AD decreased. That is, after taking into account whether the ε4 allele of the apolipoprotein E (APOE) gene is present, elders with more than 50 percent genetic Cherokee ancestry were less likely to be in the AD group than the control group. Genetic degree of ancestry for each participant was calculated using genealogical records provided by the Cherokee Nation Tribal Registration Department. A limitation of this study is its case-control design; however, this study represents a unique method of examining the relationship of race/ethnicity to disease because the degree of ethnic ancestry was assessed (albeit not through formal genetic analysis), as opposed to classifying individuals into racial groups based on self-report or investigator observation.

South America

The racial, ethnic, cultural, and socioeconomic diversity found within South America provides an excellent opportunity to evaluate biological and environmental risk factors for cognitive impairment and Alzheimer's among elders; however, more work must be carried out in this area to equal the epidemiological information available in other regions. A study of dementia in Chile (Quiroga et al., 1999) found a prevalence of 5.98 percent for elders 65 years and older, with the majority of these cases meeting criteria for AD (60 percent). Dementia rates in Brazil appear to be equivalent to those found in Europe and among white Americans, and rates are highest among illiterates (Nitrini et al., 1995). Rates of dementia and cognitive impairment in other South American countries appear to be comparable to Europe and the United States (Mangone and Arizaga, 1999).

Africa

A number of studies lead Osuntokun and his colleagues to state that "No authentic case of AD has been reported in an indigenous black African" (Osuntokun, Ogunniyi, Lekwauwa, and Oyediran, 1991; Osuntokun et al., 1992). In a door-to-door survey of 1,122 individuals above the age of 40 (32 percent above the age of 65) in Ibadan, Nigeria, these investigators reported finding no cases of severe dementia. They found that 3.6 percent of the sample had cognitive impairment, but their functional activities were intact. The same research group found that in an autopsy series of 198 brains, none were found with AD-like pathological changes. Among elderly clinical patients in this area, a high frequency of vascular dementia was encountered.

Soon after these reports, Hendrie and his colleagues from the Indiana University School of Medicine and the University of Ibadan, Nigeria began investigating the epidemiology of dementia among community-dwelling African Americans living in Indianapolis and Yoruba living in Ibadan. This study hoped to take advantage of the fact that African Americans are predominantly of the lineage of West African blacks but reside in quite different environments than Nigerians, and are therefore likely to have different exposures to possible environmental risk factors. A total of 2,212 African-American elders and 2,494 Nigerians were assessed (Hendrie et al., 1995b). Door-to-door screening was performed in each population, but the exact way in which the American sample was defined as "African American" is unclear. Diagnoses were made under World Health Organization guidelines, using DSM-II-R and ICD-10 criteria for dementia and NINCDS-ADRDA criteria for AD. Age-adjusted prevalence rates for dementia (2.29 percent) and AD (1.41 percent) among community-dwelling Yoruba elders in Ibadan were significantly lower than rates of dementia (8.24 percent) and AD (6.24 percent) among African Americans. Age-standardized annual incidence rates of dementia (1.35 percent) and AD (1.15 percent) were significantly lower in Ibadan than rates of dementia (3.24 percent) and AD (2.52 percent) among African Americans in Indiana (Hendrie et al., 2001). Investigators in the Indianapolis-Ibadan study suggested several possible explanations for reduced rates among Nigerian elders, including differential mortality (those who would eventually develop AD may die at a younger age in Nigeria); the relatively younger age structure of the population; absence of environmental factors that might increase risk of AD; and disparate diagnostic criteria for functional decline. The authors also suggested that the Nigerians may have a lower rate of amyloid deposition as compared to African Americans; a recent study suggests that this is not the case among East Africans (Kalaria et al., 1997).

Asia

In general, it has been noted that although the overall rates of dementia are similar among Asian and European elders, the distribution of subtypes of dementia are different. Specifically, early studies indicate that Asian populations appear to have a larger proportion of vascular dementia (VAD), whereas in most European studies the relative proportion of AD is larger (Jorm, 1991; Yeo et al., 1996).

The Japanese were initially believed to have substantially lower prevalence of AD and higher prevalence of VAD (reviewed in Shadlen, Larson, and Yukawa, 2000). However, more recent studies have shown decreases in prevalence of VAD and increases in AD (Yamada et al., 1999). This changing pattern of dementia diagnosis could reflect changes in diagnostic accuracy, a decrease in VAD prevalence due to better control over cardiovascular risk factors, or an increase in AD prevalence due to Westernization of risk factors such as a diet rich in fat and cholesterol.

One interesting study estimated the prevalence of dementia among Japanese who immigrated to Brazil before World War II. The prevalence of dementia on the mainland of Japan was previously found to be approximately 8 percent (Ishii et al., 1999). Diagnosis of dementia was made using the DSM-IV criteria, and cognitive ability was assessed using the Cognitive Abilities Screening Instrument. Japanese immigrants were not found to differ from the mainland Japanese population or native Brazilians in the overall prevalence of dementia (7.8 percent) or distribution of dementia types (half of the cases were AD and half were VAD). This study argues against an effect of environmental factors (at least later in life) on dementia prevalence or subtype.

Zhang et al. (1990) found that among 5,055 older residents of Shanghai, China, the prevalence rate of dementia among those 65 years and older was 4.6 percent, with 65 percent of these individuals having clinical diagnosis of AD. Approximately 47 percent of the sample had no formal education, and another 29 percent had less than 7 years of education. Participants were screened with a Chinese version of the MMSE using specific cutoffs by educational level. Those below cutoffs were further administered Chinese versions of the Fuld Object Memory Test, a Verbal Fluency Test, and Digit Span and Block Design subtests from the Wechsler Adult Intelligence Scale-Revised (WAIS-R). The authors found that lack of education was a significant and independent risk factor for the prevalence of dementia.

Europe

Rocca et al. (1991) combined data from 23 population-based prevalence studies from several European countries (collected by the EURODEM Prevalence Research Group), all of which used DSM-III or similar criteria to diagnose dementia and NINCDS-ADRDA criteria for AD. Age-specific prevalence rates ranged from 0.3 percent in the 60 to 69 age group to 10.8 percent in the 80 to 89 age group. Another study of nondemented residents of Gothenburg, Sweden between the ages of 85 and 88 revealed an incidence of 36.3 per 1,000 per year for AD (Aevarsson and Skoog, 1997). The prevalence and incidence of vascular dementia (based on National Institute of Neurological Disorders and Stroke-Association Internationale pour la Recherche et l'Enseignement en Neurosciences criteria) among Swedish elders aged 85 and older appears to exceed that of AD (Aevarsson and Skoog, 1996, 1997; Skoog, Nilsson, Palmertz, Andreasson, and Svanborg, 1993).

The Liverpool Health and Ethnicity Project (McCracken et al., 1997) reported that the prevalence of dementia among a sample of 418 English-speaking elders with African, Caribbean, Chinese, Asian, and Middle Eastern backgrounds was comparable to that found among whites (2 to 9 percent). However, in this same study, the authors found that the prevalence of dementia among people who had the same ethnic backgrounds but were not English speaking was elevated (21 to 27 percent). The authors suggested that these higher rates were due to bias in the orientation test items. People who did not speak English were less likely to know their exact birth date, their address, or the name of the Prime Minister than were English speakers, but they did not differ on any other test items.

Israel

Treves et al. (1986) reported on a nationwide epidemiologic study of the incidence of AD among those aged 40 to 60 in Israel. Through examination of the Israeli National Neurologic Disease Register and clinical records of hospital patients, the authors found that the age- and sex-adjusted incidence of AD was higher among those who were born in Europe or America (2.9 per 100,000 population) than those born in Africa or Asia (1.4 per 100,000); however, there were no ethnic differences in survival.

A 5-point rating scale of cognitive and daily functioning and a short cognitive screening test that did not involve reading or writing were administered to 1,399 residents of Ashkelon, Israel, who were 75 and older (Korczyn, Kahana, and Galper, 1991). Half of the participants were born in Africa or Asia and half were born in Europe or America. Frequency of dementia increased with age, and rates were higher among those born in Africa or Asia, among women, and among those who could not read. The authors suggested that a low level of education was the likeliest explanation for these ethnic group and gender differences.

The prevalence of AD among the entire population of 823 elders aged 60 and older was also examined in the Arab community of Wadi-Ara in northeast Israel (Bowirrat, Treves, Friedland, and Korczyn, 1998). The majority of the participants were illiterate (42 percent of males and 96 percent of females). All participants were examined by an Arabic-speaking neurologist who used DSM-IV criteria to identify dementia and NINCDS-ADRDA criteria for AD. In that population, 20.5 percent had a diagnosis of AD, with the frequency of dementia increasing from 6 percent among those 70 years and younger to 49 percent among those 80 and older.

Similar to the Zhang et al. (1990) study, the authors found that illiteracy was a significant and independent risk factor for AD in this population.

India

The Indo-US Cross-National Dementia Epidemiology project has been established to compare rates of dementia among elderly residents of a rural area of northern India to elders living in Monongahela Valley in Pennsylvania (MoVIES project). The group initially reported an overall prevalence rate of 1.36 percent for all dementias and a prevalence rate of 1.07 percent for AD (meeting NINCDS-ADRDA criteria) among those aged 65 and older in a community survey of 5,126 residents of Ballabgarh, India (Chandra et al., 1998). A recent report (Chandra et al., 2001) found that AD incidence rates were among the lowest ever reported: 3.24 per 1,000 person-years for those aged 65 and older and 1.74 for those aged 55 and older. These rates were significantly lower than those among elders in the Monongahela Valley. As with the Indianapolis/Ibadan study, the authors suggested the possibility that lower life expectancy, short survival with AD, or short follow-up duration could help to explain low incidence rates. Notably, the group found that literacy level was not related to prevalence or incidence of dementia.

Autopsy Confirmation of AD Pathology

Neuropathological confirmation of the presence and severity of AD pathology among patients diagnosed with AD is the only way to confirm ethnic discrepancies in AD prevalence and incidence. However, African Americans and other ethnic minorities are less likely to consent to autopsy (Amaducci, Baldereschi, Doody, Chandra, and Gaines, 1997; Bonner, Darkwa, and Gorelick, 2000; Fillenbaum et al., 1996; Ganguli et al., 1991; Harrell, Callaway, and Powers, 1993). Therefore, there are few published studies comparing the rates of neuropathologically defined AD among different ethnic groups in the United States; most published neuropathological studies of AD have examined whites almost exclusively. The few studies with ethnically diverse samples have found, among those autopsied, no racial differences in frequency of AD pathology (de la Monte, Hutchins, and Moore, 1989), or that AD lesions are more prevalent among whites than among blacks (Miller, Hicks, D'Amato, and Landis, 1984). Small sample size is a problem for each of these studies, and because there is a much lower rate of consent for autopsy among African Americans, there may be a selection bias.

One study avoided selection bias by performing a survey of all autopsies on individuals ages 40 to 70 in the Maryland Chief Medical Examiner's office for an 8-year time period (Sandberg, Stewart, Smialek, and Troncoso, 2001). All died of "nonnatural" causes, mostly accidents and homicides. The researchers assessed the prevalence of senile plaques (SPs) and neurofibrillary tangles (NFTs) in three brain areas: the hippocampus, entorhinal cortex, and inferior temporal cortex. In their sample of 138 individuals, 42 percent were African American and 61 percent were younger than age 65. NFTs were most common after age 54 and were found mostly in the hippocampus and entorhinal cortex. SPs were less frequent overall, but were found mostly in people 75 years and older in the entorhinal cortex and inferior temporal cortex. Prevalence of neuritic plaques was consistently lower in African Americans than whites. Although the authors confirmed that prevalence of mixed SPs and NFTs was strongly correlated with age, there was no evidence that these pathological changes had any differences in frequency by race.

Imaging Evidence

Brain imaging studies, using both structural and functional methods, might provide an alternative line of evidence concerning AD pathology that could back up the epidemiological findings of ethnic discrepancies in AD. However, there are few studies of structural or functional brain imaging using diverse groups of elders. Studies of African-American elders with clinical diagnoses of AD have shown that magnetic resonance imaging (MRI)-determined measurements of hippocampal volume (Sencakova et al., 2001) and qualitative computerized tomography and MRI findings (Charletta, Gorelick, Dollear, Freels, and Harris, 1995) were similar to those reported in other imaging studies of primarily white patients. One study using MRI and Single Photon Emission Computed Tomography showed no major ethnic differences in degree of white-matter hyperintensities, ventricle-to-brain ratio, and uptake among 3,301 nondemented community-dwelling elders without a history of stroke or transient ischemic attack (Longstreth et al., 2000). Other research has found a higher prevalence of white-matter lesions among nondemented African-Americans elders, a predictable finding given that cardiovascular risk factors (e.g., hypertension, diabetes) are more common among African Americans (Lesser et al., 1996; Liao et al., 1997).

Summary

Within the United States, most studies found higher rates of dementia and AD among African Americans and Hispanics as compared to non-Hispanic whites; however, these findings have not yet been confirmed by autopsy or imaging studies. Native Americans appeared to have lower rates of dementia as compared to whites. The Indianapolis-Ibadan study showed that Nigerians had lower rates of AD as compared to African Americans; prevalence rates in Nigeria appeared to be significantly lower than those for whites and Hispanics in the United States as well. Studies of Japanese Americans indicated that they have lower rates of AD than American and European whites, higher than Japanese living in Japan. The prevalence of dementia and AD were also lower in China than in the United States and Europe. Within Israel, risk for dementia and AD appeared to be higher among those of African or Asian background than among those of American or European background. The prevalence of AD in rural India appeared to be very low, and comparable with the rates of dementia found in Ibadan, Nigeria. The Nigerian data cast doubt on the theory that there is something inherent in African ancestry that connotes higher risk of AD. Rates of AD among African-American, Caribbean Hispanic, and non-Hispanic white participants in the New York City study (Gurland et al., 1998; Tang et al., 2001) appear to be higher than other studies.

There are several possible explanations for these observed differences in rates of dementia across ethnic groups; we will discuss some of these factors in the following sections. These include statistical limitations, discrepancies in cognitive test performance, differential genetic factors, differences in prevalence of nongenetic medical risk factors, and differences in the social meaning and reaction to cognitive decline. Certainly, differential exposure to environmental risk factors may also help to explain ethnic group differences in frequency of AD; however, little work has been published addressing ethnic differences in these exposures.

STATISTICAL LIMITATIONS

A major problem in the studies reviewed here is that the concepts of ethnicity, race, and culture are often blurred, which can result in inconsistent and scientifically meaningless classification of people into groups (Lewontin, Rose, and Kamin, 1984; Wilkinson and King, 1987; Zuckerman, 1990). Because racial classifications are socially determined, changing over time and between geographical locations, different studies of "Hispanics" may yield incomparable findings because of the different populations gathered under that label. Although cross-national studies may offer powerful analyses of environmental and biological risk factors for cognitive impairment, it is important to remember that the meta-grouping of nationality is simply a proxy for the actual variables of interest, such as genetic makeup, cultural experience, or environmental exposure, and the conclusions that can be drawn from studies that do not measure these underlying factors are regrettably limited.

A number of basic socioeconomic variables are known to influence measures of cognitive and functional ability and to be associated with the risk of AD. Studies comparing ethnic groups within the United States, as well as comparing groups residing in different countries, face a challenge in proving that different rates of AD are due to racial or ethnic background and not simply a function of the vast disparities in socioeconomic factors that are almost always found between such groups.

The most common research strategy has been to attempt to correct for differences in socioeconomic status (SES) by using matching procedures, covariance, or other methods of statistical control. Several of the studies reviewed in the previous sections found that after correcting for years of education, there were "persisting" ethnic group differences in prevalence or incidence of AD. However, these methods depend on the assumption that there is no significant error in the measurement of SES indicators. This assumption is questionable in the extreme; large measurement error of SES variables such as educational attainment, occupation, and income is common because of their high vulnerability to differential unresponse, underreporting, and volatility over time (Elo, Preston, Rosenwaike, Hill, and Cheney, 1996). To conclude that biological or genetic factors drive differences in risk of AD between ethnic or cultural groups, researchers must deal with this problem of residual confounding.

Kaufman and colleagues have provided an excellent analysis of issues surrounding residual confounds in health outcome research (Kaufman and Cooper, 1995; Kaufman, Cooper, and McGee, 1997) that can also be directly applied to research on AD among ethnic and cultural groups. Sources of residual confounding include errors in categorization of the SES variable. Statistics such as income or education are often dichotomized, which introduces an assumption that individuals from each ethnic group within each category have equivalent social positions, or an equal distribution above and below the cutpoints. For example, if educational level is cut at 9 years, residual confounding will occur if the mean for African Americans below the cutpoint is 6 years and the mean for whites below the cutpoint is 8 years.

The use of aggregated SES measures can also inflate group effects; one simulation demonstrated that when SES was estimated for each ethnicity by using average income for that group, the effect of race as a predictor of outcome was inflated 38 percent as compared to a model where SES was estimated using individual values (Geronimus, Bound, and Neidert, 1996).

The final and most salient cause of residual confounding is incommensurability of SES variables. We use SES variables to "stand in" for unmeasured aspects of the cultural and social experience of ethnically diverse individuals. However, if the relationship between these unmeasured aspects and the SES variable differs systematically between ethnic or cultural groups, the variable is not commensurate. One example is years of education, in which the difference in payoff for any given level of educational attainment is vastly different between ethnic groups. In other words, matching on quantity of formal education does not necessarily mean that the quality of education received by each ethnic group is comparable, nor does it mean that the occupational or economic opportunities associated with that education are the same (Baker, Johnson, Velli, and Wiley, 1996; Loewenstein, Arguelles, Arguelles, and Linn-Fuentes, 1994).

Not only does the educational system of the United States differ from that of many other countries, but the quality of education within the United States is also variable. African Americans educated in the South before the Supreme Court's 1954 *Brown v. Board of Education* decision attended segregated schools, which were more poorly funded than white Southern schools and most integrated Northern schools (Anderson, 1988). Several researchers have demonstrated that school characteristics such as pupil expenditures, teacher quality, pupil-to-teacher ratios, presence of special facilities such as science laboratories, length of school year, and peer characteristics accounted for much of the difference in achievement and other outcomes (e.g., wage earnings) between African Americans and whites (Hanushek, 1989; Hedges, Laine, and Greenwald, 1994; Margo, 1985; O'Neill, 1990; Smith, 1984; Smith and Welch, 1977; Welch, 1966, 1973). African-American children were often employed or used as labor during the harvest, which reduced attendance during the year. This gap in "days attended" also contributes to differences in quality of education and literacy levels per "year" in school (Margo, 1990).

Despite this evidence that the number of years of education is an inconsistent estimate of educational experience when compared across ethnic groups, educational attainment remains the variable most commonly used by AD researchers to correct for differences in SES. The alternatives of income variables and occupational level are vulnerable to problems of incommensurability as well. Income level does not reflect standard value; that is, income is not equivalent to wealth because a certain level of income does not translate into the same resources, such as higher quality housing and health insurance, in minority communities.

Because of any one of these statistical factors, in a sufficiently large study race effects will always persist after adjustment, even if there is no true difference between groups. The problem is that effects that are actually from covariant factors are instead being attributed to race. When the concept of race is deconstructed into more meaningful variables (Kaufman and Cooper, 2001; Manly and Jacobs, 2001), the underlying reasons for racial or ethnic differences in rates of AD may be determined more definitively.

COGNITIVE TEST PERFORMANCE

Ethnic Differences and Cognitive Testing

The most commonly accepted research criteria for probable or possible AD (McKhann et al., 1984) require the diagnosis to be confirmed by neuropsychological tests demonstrating impairments of performance in memory and two other cognitive domains. However, few cognitive ability measures have been properly validated for use among ethnic minorities in the United States. Lack of such validation may account for the fact that, based on neuropsychological test performance, ethnic minorities are judged to be cognitively impaired more often than non-Hispanic whites. This section will review studies within and outside the United States that have compared the cognitive test performance of different ethnic groups, and describe constructs that might allow for more sophisticated investigations of ethnic differences in the future.

Use of the standard cutoff of 23 on the MMSE leads to overdiagnosis of dementia among African Americans, even after controlling for years of education (Bohnstedt, Fox, and Kohatsu, 1994). Racial, ethnic, and cultural differences have been found on MMSE performance and other screening measures before (Mast, Fitzgerald, Steinberg, MacNeill, and Lichtenberg, 2001; Unverzagt et al., 1996) and after adjusting for education (Escobar et al., 1986; Fillenbaum, Heyman, Williams, Prosnitz, and Burchett, 1990; Fillenbaum, Hughes, Heyman, George, and Blazer, 1988; Kuller et al., 1998; Salmon et al., 1989; Teresi, Albert, Holmes, and Mayeux, 1999; Welsh et al., 1995).

Difficulties in interpreting cognitive scores among ethnic minority elders are not limited to brief screening instruments; several studies have indicated that ethnic or cultural factors have a substantial effect on neuropsychological batteries (Adams, Boake, and Crain, 1982; Overall and Levin, 1978). Even when ethnic groups are matched on socioeconomic variables, discrepancies in neuropsychological test performance have remained (Jacobs et al., 1997; Kaufman, McLean, and Reynolds, 1988; Manly et al., 1998b; Reynolds, Chastain, Kaufman, and McLean, 1987). Roberts and Hamsher (1984) found that neurologically intact whites obtained significantly higher scores on a measure of visual naming ability than did neurologically intact African Americans, even after correcting for education level. Several other studies also reported ethnic differences in performance on tests of visual confrontation naming (Carlson, Brandt, Carson, and Kawas, 1998b; Lichtenberg, Ross, and Christensen, 1994; Ross, Lichtenberg, and Christensen, 1995; Welsh et al., 1995).

Ethnicity-related differences have been reported on measures of nonverbal abilities as well (Bernard, 1989; Brown et al., 1991; Campbell et al., 1996; Heverly, Ixaac, and Hynd, 1986; Miller, Bing, Selnes, Wesch, and Becker, 1993). Jacobs et al. (1997) found that Spanish-speaking elders scored significantly lower than age- and education-matched English-speaking elders on a measure of nonverbal abstraction (i.e., the Identities and Oddities subtest from the Mattis Dementia Rating Scale); multiple-choice matching and recognition formats of the Benton Visual Retention Test; and measures of category fluency and comprehension. In another study, healthy Spanish-speaking Mexicans and Mexican Americans who lived near a U.S.-Mexico border (n = 200) were compared with residents of Madrid, Spain (n = 218). After accounting for education, borderland residents obtained significantly lower scores on measures of recognition discriminability for stories and figures, learned fewer details from a story over five trials, and made more perseverative responses on the Wisconsin Card Sorting Task (Artiola i Fortuny, Heaton, and Hermosillo, 1998). There were some interactions between years of education and place of birth, suggesting that among those with high levels of education, borderland and Spanish participants performed similarly on several measures.

Unverzagt et al. (1996) gave the CERAD neuropsychological test battery to 83 normal, nondemented African-American elders who volunteered from the local community. Their study found significant effects of years of education on several test scores. Its African-American sample was older and less well educated, and scored significantly lower on every measure than a previously collected sample of primarily white elders (Morris et al., 1989). This study also found that well-established cutoffs for dementia (i.e., MMSE below 24 and standard CERAD cutoffs) (Welsh, Butters, Hughes, Mohs, and Heyman, 1992) would misclassify a large percentage of these normal African Americans as demented.

In another study using the CERAD, the performance of elderly African-American and white representative community residents in North Carolina was compared with that of African Americans in Indianapolis and with whites in the Monongahela Valley, Pennsylvania (Fillenbaum, Heyman, Huber, Ganguli, and Unverzagt, 2001). Although on average African Americans performed more poorly than whites after controlling for demographic characteristics, no significant racial differences were found in the North Carolina sample. Both African-American and white participants in North Carolina performed more poorly than their racial counterparts in the other two studies.

A study in rural Virginia (Marcopulos, McLain, and Giuliano, 1997) compared neuropsychological test performance between 69 African-American and 64 non-Hispanic white nondemented, community-dwelling elders, all of whom had less than 10 years of formal education. Although education accounted for a significant amount of variance in nearly every measure that was administered, race was an independent predictor of performance on WAIS-R Vocabulary and Block Design subtests, as well as Wechsler Memory Scale-Revised (WMS-R) Logical Memory Delay.

Manly et al. (1998a) found that after matching neurologically normal African-American and white groups on age and years of education, there were significant ethnic group differences on measures of figure memory, verbal abstraction, category fluency, and visuospatial skill. These discrepancies in test performance of education-matched African Americans and whites could not be accounted for by occupational attainment or history of medical conditions such as hypertension and diabetes.

In contrast, a number of studies have failed to find discrepancies in test performance among racial, ethnic, or cultural groups after participants were matched on years of education (Ford, Haley, Thrower, West, and Harrell, 1996; Marcopulos et al., 1997), after statistically adjusting for education (Loewenstein, Ardila, Rosselli, and Hayden, 1992; Marcopulos et al., 1997; Mungas, Marshall, Weldon, Haan, and Reed, 1996), or after cutscores were adjusted for those with low education (Murden, McRae, Kaner, and Bucknam, 1991). However, the statistical power to detect a significant difference in some of these studies was severely limited by their small sample sizes of nonwhite participants. For example, there were no significant ethnic differences among a small number of African Americans (n = 11) and whites (n = 32) with AD on measures of naming, picture vocabulary, verbal abstraction, verbal list learning, and pragmatic language use after controlling for MMSE score and years of education (Ripich, Carpenter, and Ziol, 1997). Another study found that among 18 black and 114 white participants who met NINCDS-ADRDA criteria for AD, there were no significant differences by race on decline in MMSE score over an average 2.5-year period, whereas left-handedness, more years of education, and family history of dementia were associated with more rapid decline (Rasmusson, Carson, Brookmeyer, Kawas, and Brandt, 1996).

A meta-analysis of studies published between 1973 and 1994, which conducted cross-cultural comparisons of cognitive test scores, revealed that cross-cultural differences were, as expected, greater in cross-national comparisons than intranational cross-ethnic comparisons. Cross-cultural differences in test performance increased with age and were most pronounced when the discrepancies in affluence between the groups were greatest. Differences in performance were also larger on tests developed in the West as compared to tests developed in non-Western areas. Differences were present across many cognitive domains, and were not limited to tasks that purported to assess abstract abilities (van de Vijver, 1997).

Taken together, most previous studies of ethnic group differences in performance on the MMSE and neuropsychological tests have shown that discrepancies between scores of different ethnic groups persist, despite equating groups on other demographics such as age, education, gender, and socioeconomic background. These discrepancies cause attenuated specificity of verbal and nonverbal neuropsychological tests, such that cognitively normal ethnic minorities are more likely to be misdiagnosed as impaired as compared to whites (Ford-Booker et al., 1993; Klusman, Moulton, Hornbostle, Picano, and Beattie, 1991; Manly et al., 1998b; Stern et al., 1992; Welsh et al., 1995). These findings indicate that not all tasks are functionally equivalent (Helms, 1992; Ratcliff et al., 1998). Although establishing test norms for each ethnic group may help with misdiagnosis (Miller, Heaton, Kirson, and Grant, 1997), there is variability of educational and cultural experiences within ethnicity that may decrease the accuracy of these norms. In the following sections, we will review research that has focused on the effects of within-group factors on cognitive test performance.

Years of Education/Quality of Education/Literacy

Extreme differences in educational level are often found between ethnic minorities and whites or between residents of developed and undeveloped countries. Illiteracy rates in the United States are highest among people aged 65 and over, but are especially elevated among ethnic minority elders (Kirsch, Jungeblut, Jenkins, and Kolstad, 1993). Cross-cultural researchers are therefore challenged to find measures that are sensitive to cognitive impairment across these broad educational backgrounds (Ratcliff et al., 1998). Although it is common for investigators to use covariance, matching procedures, or education-corrected norms in order to "equate" ethnic groups on years of education before interpreting neuropsychological test performance, as discussed earlier, these techniques ignore ethnic discrepancies in quality of education. Therefore, disparate school experiences could explain why many ethnic minorities obtain lower scores on cognitive measures even after controlling for years of education.

Presence of poor literacy skills among elders is a particularly relevant issue for neuropsychologists attempting to accurately detect dementia using cognitive measures. Reading level, as measured by a bilingual measure of reading comprehension, was found to be more related to MMSE score than were years of education, age, or ethnicity (Weiss, Reed, Kligman, and Abyad, 1995). These results suggest that interpretation of cognitive test performance is more dependent on knowledge of literacy or reading skills than years of education. Nevertheless, only a few studies have been conducted to identify ways to accurately assess literacy and reading level among elders that differ ethnically (Baker et al., 1996; Boekamp, Strauss, and Adams, 1995) and linguistically (Del Ser, Gonzalez-Montalvo, Martinez-Espinosa, Delgado-Villapalos, and Bermejo, 1997).

Our group recently reported a study that sought to determine if discrepancies in quality of education could explain differences in cognitive test scores between African-American and white elders matched on years of education. A comprehensive neuropsychological battery was administered to a sample of nondemented African-American and non-Hispanic white participants in an epidemiological study of normal aging and dementia in the Northern Manhattan community. The Reading Recognition subtest from the Wide Range Achievement Test-Version 3 (WRAT-3) was used as an estimate of quality of education. African-American elders obtained significantly lower scores than whites on measures of word list learning and memory, figure memory, abstract reasoning, fluency, and visuospatial skill even though the groups were matched on years of education. However, after adjusting the scores for WRAT-3 reading score, the overall effect of race was greatly reduced and racial differences on all tests (except category fluency and a drawing measure) became nonsignificant. Reading score also attenuated the effect of race after accounting for an estimate of test-wiseness, or familiarity with the testing situation. This finding suggests that years of education is an inadequate measure of the educational experience among multicultural elders, and that adjusting for quality of education may improve the specificity of certain neuropsychological measures across racial groups.

Despite the clear improvement in specificity that is provided by adjusting cognitive test scores for differences in educational experience across ethnic groups, some researchers caution against controlling for educational variables in studies of dementia because low education may itself be a risk factor for disease. The logic behind this argument will be discussed in the section on the nongenetic risk factor of cognitive reserve.

Acculturation

Most previous research on ethnicity has classified participants on the basis of physical appearance or self-identified racial/ethnic classification, rather than measuring the cultural variables that accompany ethnic group membership. However, as suggested by Helms (1992), specification of experiential, attitudinal, or behavioral variables that distinguish those belonging to different ethnic groups, and that also vary among individuals within an ethnic group, may allow investigators to understand better the underlying reasons for the relationship between ethnic background and cognitive test performance.

Level of acculturation is one way in which social scientists have operationalized within-group cultural variability. Acculturation is defined as the level at which an individual participates in the values, language, and practices of his or her own ethnic community versus those of the dominant culture (Landrine and Klonoff, 1996; Padilla, 1980). Previous studies have identified ideologies, beliefs, expectations, and attitudes as important components of acculturation, as well as cognitive and behavioral characteristics such as language and customs (Berry, 1976; Moyerman and Forman, 1992; Negy and Woods, 1992; Padilla, 1980).

Few studies have examined the relationship of cognitive test performance to within-group ethnic or cultural factors independent of those associated with SES. Arnold and colleagues (Arnold, Montgomery, Castenada, and Longoria, 1994) found a relationship between Hispanic acculturation and performance on selected tests of the Halstead-Reitan Battery among college students. Artiola i Fortuny et al. reported that among Mexican and Mexican-American residents of a U.S.-border region, percentage of life in which individuals lived in the United States was significantly and negatively related to number of words generated on a Spanish oral fluency measure, especially among those with fewer than 8 years of education. In addition, those who spent a larger percentage of their life in the United States made more perseverative errors on the Wisconsin Card Sorting Test, and bilingualism accounted for a significant amount of variance in performance on a Spanish Verbal Learning Test (Artiola i Fortuny et al., 1998).

Three studies have explored the relationship of African-American acculturation (as measured by the African American Acculturation Scale) (Landrine and Klonoff, 1994, 1995) to cognitive test performance. Manly et al. (1998c) found that among neurologically intact African Americans between the ages of 20 and 65, those who were less acculturated (more traditional) obtained lower scores on measures of general information and naming than more acculturated African Americans. Among elderly residents of Northern Manhattan (Manly et al., 1998b), acculturation accounted for a significant amount of variance in several neuropsychological measures assessing verbal and nonverbal abilities after accounting for age, education, and gender. Among elderly African Americans living in Jacksonville, Florida, acculturation accounted for a significant amount of variance in Verbal IQ (as measured by the Wechsler Adult Intelligence Scale), Boston Naming Test, and delayed recall of stories from the WMS-R (Lucas, 1998).

Taken together, investigations of acculturation level suggest that there are cultural differences within elders of the same ethnicity that relate to neuropsychological measures of verbal and nonverbal skills, and that accounting for acculturation may improve the accuracy of certain neuropsychological tests. Although previous research has focused on ethnic minority elders in the United States, it is likely that within-group cultural differences are also significant factors in the test performance of American elders who identify themselves as white or Caucasian, as well as ethnic groups outside the United States.

Racial Socialization

Level of comfort and confidence during the testing session may also vary among ethnic groups. The concept of stereotype threat has been described as a factor that may attenuate the performance of racial minorities on cognitive tests. Stereotype threat describes the effect of attention diverting from the task at hand to the concern that one's performance will confirm a negative stereotype about one's group. Steele and colleagues (Steele, 1997; Steele and Aronson, 1995) demonstrated that when a test consisting of difficult verbal GRE exam items was described as measuring intellectual ability, black undergraduates at Stanford University performed worse than SAT score-matched whites. However, when the same test was described as a "laboratory problem-solving task" or a "challenging test" that was unrelated to intellectual ability, scores of African Americans matched those of white students. Researchers have also shown that when gender differences in math ability were invoked, stereotype threat undermined performance of women on math tests (Spencer, Steele, and Quinn, 1999) and among white males (when comparisons to Asians were invoked) (Aronson et al., 1999). The role of stereotype threat in neuropsychological test performance of African Americans and Hispanics has not been investigated to date. In addition, it is likely that the salience of negative stereotypes differs among racial minorities, and therefore, stereotype threat will likely affect some test takers more than others. Investigation of the experiential, social, and cultural variables that affect vulnerability to stereotype threat should be examined.

Linguistic Issues

Translation of English-Language Tests

Clinicians and researchers sometimes erroneously assume that instruments are equivalent across populations as long as the test is administered in the native language of the individual. However, literal translation may not produce items with comparable word frequency and/or salience in each culture, resulting in different difficulty levels (Sano et al., 1997; Teng, 1996). In addition, idiosyncrasies of different languages may introduce problems in equating certain tests. For example, when asked to name as many animals as possible in a minute, Hispanics produce fewer exemplars than do Vietnamese. This discrepancy can be explained by the fact that most animal names in Spanish are multisyllabic, while most animal names in Vietnamese are monosyllabic (Kempler, Teng, Dick, Taussig, and Davis, 1998).

Translators of cognitive measures must use extreme caution and proper methods to adapt measures into another language. Artiola i Fortuny and Mullaney (1997) describe several examples of Spanish versions of tests that include syntactic, lexical, and spelling errors. These authors also suggest that investigators consult only those who possess native fluency and in-depth knowledge of the culture before attempting to translate a measure. The accuracy of translated and adapted instruments should be checked following established guidelines (Ardila, Rosselli, and Puente, 1994; Artiola i Fortuny and Mullaney, 1997; Brislin, 1970, 1980; Dick, Teng, Kempler, Davis, and Taussig, 2002; Fuld, Muramoto, Blau, Westbrook, and Katzman, 1988; Hall et al., 1996; LaCalle, 1987; Mungas, 1996; Ponton et al., 1996; Ritchie and Hallerman, 1989; Salmon, Jin, Zhang, Grant, and Yu, 1995; Teng et al., 1994; van de Vijver and Hambleton, 1996). Researchers and clinicians must also develop standards to determine in which language bilinguals should be assessed (Ponton et al., 1996).

Translation of measures is not simply a linguistic issue; measures must be culturally equivalent as well. That is, it must be determined whether the use of a particular test format to assess the cognitive skill of interest is equally valid within every culture in which the test will be administered (Teng, 1996; Teng et al., 1994).

Norms

Investigators must be aware that the published norms for tests administered in English are not necessarily valid when the tests are administered in another language. Furthermore, they should not assume that test norms can be applied to distinct populations simply because they share a language. For example, there is evidence that several instruments developed in Spanish-speaking countries may not be functionally or linguistically equivalent when used among Spanish speakers in the United States (Artiola i Fortuny et al., 1998). Similarly, tests and norms developed among a particular group of immigrants to the United States (e.g., Cuban Americans) may not be valid among other groups in the United States who share a language (e.g., Dominicans or Puerto Ricans) (Loewenstein et al., 1994).

Use of Interpreters

Misinterpretation is a serious threat to the reliability and validity of testing. Family members are often used as translators, but are not likely to be objective. Even translators who are reasonably fluent in both languages may not be familiar with many of the terms used in neuropsychological testing (Ardila et al., 1994; LaCalle, 1987). Increasing the linguistic diversity of testers and improving the availability of objective translators are thus worthwhile goals for investigators; when this is not feasible, the possibility of misinterpretation must be considered when interpreting results.

Development of Cross-Cultural Cognitive Tests

A number of measures have been adapted for use in different cultures and for multiple languages, and proven to be useful in distinguishing demented and nondemented elders in cross-cultural studies. The multiple sources of difficulty in linguistic and cultural test adaptation will often make it preferable to use a preexisting measure that has been validated; unfortunately, much work remains to be done in this area.

Fuld et al. (1988) compared a small number of [Japanese and white American] elders on the Fuld Object-Memory Test, a measure of memory for common objects. The Japanese and American groups were of similar educational and occupational attainment and were diagnosed as nondemented based on mental status exams. There were no differences in total recall between the two groups among elders aged 70 to 79. However, the 80- to 89-year-old Japanese group obtained slightly but significantly higher scores than both Americans (of all ages) and Japanese aged 70 to 79. The authors suggested that the manner in which participants were selected in Japan and the United States might have contributed to these findings; however, the results indicated that, for at least some groups, the Fuld Object Memory Test measured comparable cognitive functions in both cultures.

The Cognitive Abilities Screening Instrument (CASI) (Teng, 1996; Teng et al., 1994) was described as a family of similar tests designed for easy adaptability for cross-cultural research. The CASI has been adapted for use among elderly speakers of English, Japanese, Chinese, Vietnamese, and Spanish residing within a number of cultural and socioeconomic environments. The majority of the items were taken from the MMSE and the Hasegawa Dementia Screening Scale, and the measure has been shown to have acceptable sensitivity and specificity as a dementia screening instrument.

The Cross-Cultural Neuropsychological Battery (Dick et al., 2002) includes the CASI and 10 neuropsychological tests assessing memory for common objects, language, visuospatial skill, attention, reasoning, and psychomotor speed. Norms for the battery have been generated using 336 normal elders who identify as African American, white, Chinese, Hispanic, or Vietnamese. The authors found that years of education and ethnicity accounted for a significant amount of variance in performance on every measure except the learning, delayed recall, and recognition on the Common Objects Memory Test. These measures may be suitable for direct comparison between cultures, while for the rest of the battery, the use of norms may allow groups to be compared. However, further research is needed to determine the sensitivity and specificity of the Cross-Cultural Neuropsychological Battery to detect subtle cognitive impairment and early AD among ethnically diverse elders.

Salmon et al. (1995) reported the successful translation and adaptation of several neuropsychological measures (including the Fuld Object Memory Test, Boston Naming Tests, Category Fluency Tests, Wechsler Adult Intelligence Scale Vocabulary, Digit Span, and Digit Symbol subtests, Wechsler Intelligence Scale for Children-Revised Block Design subtest, Clock Drawing Tests, and Trail Making Test) for detection of dementia among Chinese elders participating in the Shanghai Dementia Survey. However, some items, especially tasks that required elders to draw, were influenced by both educational and cultural factors. Another cognitive screening instrument (the CSID) was developed and validated in a study comparing Cree Indians in Manitoba to European Manitobans (Hall et al., 1996), and was applied to a sample of African Americans in Indiana and Yorubans in Ibadan, Nigeria. Although there were significant ethnic group differences in individual items of the instrument and total score, these differences resolved after accounting for years of education. Ritchie and Hallerman (1989) found that among 78 elderly Israelis of diverse ethnic background (i.e., Russian, Moroccan, Polish, Argentine, and Iraqi), raw scores from the Iowa Screening Battery had acceptable sensitivity and specificity (82.2 percent and 80.6 percent, respectively) measured against the diagnosis of dementia based on a neurologist's and neuropsychologist's clinical examination.

Sano et al. (1997) used established translation and adaptation methods to test the validity of a number of global severity measures among 94 Spanish speakers and 306 English speakers. The MMSE, Clinical Dementia Rating Scale, Global Deterioration Scale, and Functional Assessment Staging proved able to discriminate participants with AD from controls and were all equally sensitive to disease severity. Mungas and colleagues also report the successful development of a neuropsychological test battery for English and Spanish speakers (Gonzalez, Mungas, Reed, Marshall, and Haan, 2001; Mungas, 1996; Mungas et al., 1996; Mungas, Reed, Marshall, and Gonzalez, 2000).

Although these findings are encouraging, more work is needed to be certain that the proposed cross-cultural measures are truly free of bias; many of these studies had a relatively limited number of subjects in each ethnic group studied, so it remains possible that the researchers were simply unable to detect the cultural biases that existed in their measures.

GENETICS

The APOE ε4 Story

Differences in genetic background could contribute to the disparate rates of dementia and AD among ethnic groups. Because of the identification of the APOE ε4 allele as a major risk factor for the development of AD (reviewed in Farrer et al., 1997; Kamboh, 1995; Roses, 1996), and an apparent protective effect of the ε2 allele among whites, several investigations (Corder et al., 1995) have focused on the role of APOE polymorphisms in the development of AD among other ethnic groups. Racial (Gerdes, Klausen, Sihm, and Faergeman, 1992; Kamboh, Sepehrnia, and Ferrell, 1989) and geographic (Lucotte, Loirat, and Hazout, 1997; Zekraoui et al., 1997) differences in the frequency of the APOE ε4 allele create opportunities to investigate the independent effects of genetics and environment on development of AD. It has also been suggested that racial differences affect the linkage between the ε4 allele and the density of SPs and number of NFTs found in the brain (Itoh and Yamada, 1996). Investigations of the risk associated with the APOE ε4 allele in different ethnic or cultural groups are currently taking place throughout the world.

Studies in the United States

A series of case-control studies (Maestre et al., 1995; Mayeux et al., 1993; Tang et al., 1996) comparing ethnic groups in the Washington Heights-Inwood Columbia Aging Project's (WHICAP's) community-based random sample found different degrees of association between AD risk and presence of the APOE ε4 allele. Among African Americans the association of the APOE ε4 allele to AD was weak or absent, but it was significant among white study participants. The ε4-associated risk among Hispanics in this project was intermediate to that of African Americans and whites.

The relationship between APOE genotype and ethnicity was investigated among elders with late-onset AD in Florida (Duara, Barker, Lopez-Alberola, and Loewenstein, 1996). Participants were classified into four ethnic groups: Ashkenazi Jewish (n = 100), Hispanic (n = 46), non-Hispanic white (n = 30), and African American (n = 19). Diagnosis of probable or possible AD was made using NINCDS-ADRDA criteria. The investigators found that age of onset was later in Ashkenazi Jewish elders than among African-American, Hispanic, and non-Hispanic non-Jewish whites. The ε4 allele frequency was 29 percent for the entire sample, which is significantly different from the 13.7 percent frequency reported among normal subjects aged 45 and over. These investigators found no ethnic differences in frequency of the ε4 allele (Ashkenazi Jewish = 30 percent; African American = 29 percent; Hispanic = 28 percent; and non-Hispanic non-Jewish white = 33 percent) or the ε2 allele. A later case-control study by the same group found that although the ε4 allele is a risk factor for AD among white non-Hispanics (392 AD patients, 202 normal subjects) and white Hispanics (188 AD patients, 84 normal controls) (Harwood et al., 1999), other risk factors such as low education and hypertension appear to be important only for white non-Hispanics.

A meta-analysis (Farrer et al., 1997) of raw data provided by 40 research teams, comprising 5,930 elders with AD and 8,607 normal controls, examined the association between APOE genotype and AD within four ethnic groups (whites, African Americans, Hispanics, and Japanese). Although there was an elevated frequency of APOE ε4 allele among elders with AD from every ethnic group, the ε4 allele's association with AD among whites was weaker than that of Japanese, but stronger than that of African Americans. The investigators found that among Hispanics, the ε3/ε4 genotype was associated with a significant risk for AD, but the ε4/ε4 genotype did not confer an increased risk, which they attributed to the small number of Hispanics who were homozygous for the ε4 allele.

All the studies described computed the risk associated with possession of an ε4 allele by using the ε3/ε3 genotype as a reference group. An incidence study by Tang et al. (1998) used a different approach by comparing participants in a longitudinal, random community cohort in Northern Manhattan (WHICAP) with and without the ε4 allele. African Americans and Hispanics with one or more ε4 allele were as likely to develop probable or possible AD as were whites; however, African Americans and Hispanics *without* an ε4 allele were two to four times more likely than whites to develop AD by age 90. Years of education did not account for these ethnic differences in AD incidence, and reclassifying elders who developed only mild disease (Clinical Dementia Rating Scale of 0.5) as normal did not alter the findings.

Indianapolis-Ibadan Study

In a pilot study, Hendrie and his colleagues (1995a) examined the APOE genotypes of the first 85 African-American participants in the Indianapolis study who were either normal (n = 54) or diagnosed with AD (n = 31) using NINCDS-ADRDA criteria. The frequency of the ε4 allele was 13.9 percent among normal African-American elders and 40.3 percent among African-American elders with AD. The investigators found that 22.6 percent of those with AD were homozygous for the ε4 allele, while only 3.7 percent of the normal controls were homozygous. The odds ratio (OR) associated with one copy of the ε4 allele was 4.14, while the OR associated with two copies of the ε4 allele was 17.16. This estimate of risk was at least as high as that found among white populations. The authors suggested that the overall frequency of the ε4 allele in their sample (13.9) was smaller than the reported frequency for the African-American population (26 percent) because of the general decrease in frequency of the ε4 allele with age (differential mortality). The risk associated with having an ε4 allele appeared to be independent of ethnic background.

At about the same time, these researchers reported an association between the presence of an ε4 allele and AD among Nigerians living in Ibadan (Osuntokun et al., 1995). Using NINCDS-ADRDA criteria, 12 elders with AD and 39 normal controls were identified from the community survey. There were no significant differences in the frequency of the ε4 allele between controls (20.5 percent) and elders with AD (16.7 percent). The authors noted that the frequency of the ε4 allele was higher among the Nigerian controls than among the African-American participants in Indianapolis, and concluded that differences in the expression of APOE ε4 allele or its receptors may explain its lack of association with AD. They also suggested the possibility that the presence of other genetic or environmental factors could intensify the effects of ε4 in those populations for which this genotype was a risk factor for AD.

In a follow-up to their pilot study (Sahota et al., 1997), the Indianapolis-Ibadan group examined a larger sample of 288 African-American participants, 60 of whom were diagnosed with AD using NINCDS-ADRDA criteria. They found that the OR was 4.83 for AD with the ε4/ε4 genotype, but did not reach significance for the ε3/ε4 genotype. The frequency of the ε4 allele among those with AD was significantly higher than it was among controls (34.17 percent versus 21.76 percent, respectively). It was also found that the ε2 allele was less frequent in the AD group than in the control group (4.17 percent versus 10.65 percent, respectively). These results did not change after the removal of elders who had cognitive impairment, but were not demented, from the control group. The investigators noted that their original findings were likely due to sampling bias, and concluded that the association between the APOE allele and AD among African Americans was weaker than that found among whites. Together with the Nigerian data, they suggested that other genetic or environmental factors reduced the ε4-associated risk for AD in populations of African origin.

Indo-U.S. Study

International differences in the APOE genotype risk of AD were also examined in the Indo-U.S. case-control study, which sampled individuals from two rural communities: Elders aged 55 or older in Ballabgarh, India (n = 4,450), and elders aged 70 or older in the Monongahela Valley region of Southwestern Pennsylvania (n = 886). Although frequency of APOE ε4 was significantly lower in Ballabgarh as compared to the Monongahela Valley, the association of the APOE ε4 allele with AD was the same across Indian and U.S. groups.

Cherokee Indians and AD

A small study performed among Cherokee Indians found no relationship between APOE genotype and AD diagnosis. However, there was a relationship of Cherokee ancestry with risk for AD: AD patients with a greater than 50 percent genetic degree of Cherokee ancestry constituted only 35 percent of the group with AD. In contrast, 17 (65 percent) of the control subjects were more than 50 percent Cherokee. Unfortunately, this remains the only research assessing the relationship between APOE genotype and AD risk among Native Americans.

Dominican Republic and the Caribbean

In contrast to sporadic AD, late-onset familial AD among Caribbean Hispanics is strongly associated with APOE ε4. A study of 203 Caribbean Hispanic families residing in the greater New York City area, the Dominican Republic, and Puerto Rico found that the presence of the APOE ε4 allele was strongly associated with AD. In addition, 8 of the 19 families with at least 1 family member with onset of dementia before age 55 showed an association with a previously unreported presenilin mutation. The same group found modest evidence of linkage to loci on chromosome 12p among 79 Caribbean Hispanic families with AD, which varied by age at onset of AD and by the presence or absence of the APOE-ε4 allele.

Summary

Taken together, the finding of ethnic variability in the association between AD and APOE ε4 could mean the following:

• The ε4 allele is in linkage disequilibrium with an AD susceptibility locus, rather than a direct cause of the disease. However, this possibility is unlikely because the APOE-AD association has been confirmed worldwide.
• African Americans and Hispanics may have genes modifying the expression of APOE. This is possible because regulatory sequences in enhancer/promoter regions of APOE are associated with modification in disease risk.
• Factors such as head injury or coronary artery disease may modify the biological effect of the ε4 allele.

Cross-national studies offer great promise in resolving these possibilities because they permit environmental risk factors for AD to be distinguished from genetic causes. However, they all suffer from the difficulty of accurately identifying parental populations for genetic studies that use admixed groups to map disease genes (Parra et al., 1998).

In addition, our ability to draw conclusions from these studies is hampered by many of the same issues that confound interpretation of studies of prevalence and incidence, such as small sample sizes and differences in identification of cases and controls; sampling strategies; definitions of race and ethnicity; and methods for measuring the risk associated with the possession of a particular APOE genotype (i.e., differences in reference group). When studies do not sufficiently address these problems, the generalizability of their results, as well as our ability to resolve discordant findings, is limited.

NONGENETIC RISK FACTORS

Stroke

Compared to non-Hispanic whites, African Americans have a 2.4-fold and Hispanics a twofold increase in stroke incidence (Sacco et al., 1998). Among patients with dementia, a higher proportion of African Americans and Asian/Pacific Islanders were found to have vascular dementia than whites and Hispanics (Gorelick et al., 1994). Therefore, cerebrovascular disease could partially explain higher rates of dementia among African Americans when all subtypes are considered together. It is also possible that vascular disease could help to explain higher incidence of AD among African Americans and Hispanics; among elders who meet the neuropathologic criteria for AD, those with concomitant lacunar infarcts are more likely to clinically express dementia (Snowdon et al., 1997). If this is the case, African Americans, who are at higher risk for stroke, may be at higher risk to develop the clinical signs of dementia even though they may be just as likely as whites to have AD pathology. One possible mechanism may be that silent infarcts decrease cognitive reserve and thus the brain's ability to compensate for AD pathology (Moroney et al., 1997).

Hypertension

The high prevalence of hypertension among African Americans is well known, and the frequency of hypertension is further increased among African Americans with Alzheimer's disease (Gorelick et al., 1994; Hargrave, Stoeklin, Haan, and Reed, 1998; Yeo et al., 1996). Hypertension places African Americans at higher risk for neurovascular pathology that is often found among people diagnosed with AD such as cerebral amyloid angiopathy, white-matter lesions, and vascular endothelial damage (Shadlen et al., 2000). However, the role this neurovascular pathology plays in AD and its significance remains uncertain.

Diabetes

Prevalence of diabetes is higher in African Americans and Hispanics; therefore, it is possible that this disorder, or the cardiovascular problems that go along with it, can help explain elevated rates of AD in these ethnic groups as compared to whites. The mechanisms underlying a possible association between diabetes and AD are unclear, but include the possibility that the production of glycation end products increase Alzheimer's pathology (Sasaki et al., 1998; Smith, Sayre, and Perry, 1996). However, elevated plasma levels of glucose and insulin are associated with reductions in plasma amyloid precursor protein (Boyt et al., 2000), and insulin decreases β-amyloid neurotoxicity in vitro (Takadera, Sakura, Mohri, and Hashimoto, 1993). A more tenable explanation is that the presence of diabetes increases the possibility that an individual will have a stroke or small-vessel disease, both of which increase the risk of AD and dementia diagnosis.

Studies of the relationship between diabetes mellitus and AD have produced conflicting results. Three longitudinal studies have reported an increased risk of dementia, including AD, among persons with diabetes (Brayne et al., 1998; Leibson et al., 1997; Ott et al., 1996, 1999). These studies had a limited ability to detect vascular dementia. If cases of stroke-associated dementia are misclassified as cases of AD, risk factors for stroke-associated dementia can appear to predict AD. One study found a relation of diabetes with vascular dementia (defined by criteria established by the California State Alzheimer's Disease Diagnostic and Treatment Centers) but not with AD (defined by NINCDS-ADRDA criteria; McKhann et al., 1984). A recent study (Luchsinger, Tang, Stern, Shea, and Mayeux, 2001) followed 1,262 ethnically diverse elders who were not demented at baseline for approximately 4.3 years. The adjusted relative risk for the composite outcome of Alzheimer's disease and cognitive impairment without dementia (or stroke) in subjects with diabetes was significant, at 1.6, whereas the adjusted relative risk of stroke-associated dementia in persons with diabetes was 3.4. Among blacks and Hispanics, one-third of the risk of stroke-associated dementia was attributable to diabetes as compared with 17 percent among whites. The risk for diabetes in relation to stroke-associated dementia varied by ethnic group; it was approximately twice as great in Hispanics and blacks as in whites.

Myocardial Infarction/Coronary Artery Disease

Coronary artery disease mortality is higher among African Americans and Hispanics than among whites (Williams, Massing, Rosamond, Sorlie, and Tyroler, 1999), and there is higher prevalence of risk factors for myocardial infarction, such as higher rates of diabetes among black and Mexican-American women and higher rates of hypertension among black men and women (Sundquist, Winkleby, and Pudaric, 2001). Because history of myocardial infarction and coronary artery disease have been associated with higher rates of dementia and presence of diffuse plaques in the brain, this health disparity may also contribute to epidemiologic observations of higher rates of AD among African Americans and Hispanics. It is possible that increased β-amyloid deposits in the neuropil and within neurons occur in the brains of nondemented individuals with heart disease (Aronson et al., 1990; Sparks et al., 1990). Individuals with two APOE ε4 alleles have higher plasma cholesterol, and are thus at higher risk for myocardial infarction (Sparks, Martin, Gross, and Hunsaker, 2000).

Head Injury

Head injury is a frequently reported risk factor for AD (reviewed in Kawas and Katzman, 1999). The most likely biological mechanism for an association between head injury and AD is that insult to the brain leads to increased production of β-amyloid containing diffuse plaques. One study found a 10-fold increase in the risk of AD with both an APOE ε4 allele and a history of traumatic head injury, but head injury in the absence of an APOE ε4 allele did not increase risk (Tang et al., 1996).

Given the evidence for this connection, the fact that an increased risk of traumatic brain injury has been reported among ethnic minority populations (Collins, 1990; Rosenthal and Ricker, 2000) might contribute to disparities in risk for AD. Supporting evidence comes from the finding that African-American patients with AD were more likely to have a history of head injury than African Americans with vascular dementia (Gorelick et al., 1994).

Exposure to Possible Protective Factors

Nonwhite and Hispanic women are less likely to receive counseling about estrogen replacement therapy from their physician and less aware of its health benefits (Gallagher, Geling, FitzGibbons, Aforismo, and Comite, 2000; Ganesan, Teklehaimanot, and Norris, 2000). Access to and utilization of health care is significantly lower among ethnic minorities than among whites in the United States. Therefore, there may be less exposure to possible protective factors for AD, including estrogen replacement therapy and antiinflammatory drugs. Ethnic differences in diet and vitamin intake may reduce exposure to antioxidants, which may also protect the brain from AD pathology.

Cognitive Reserve

Cognitive reserve is another possible explanation for ethnic differences in rates of dementia and AD. Studies of ethnically diverse samples indicate that lifetime experiences, reflected in years of education or occupational level, may be independent risk factors for incidence of dementia and cognitive impairment (Callahan et al., 1996; Stern, 2002; Stern et al., 1994). This has led to the proposal that educational and occupational experience provide a "cognitive reserve" against clinical manifestation of Alzheimer's neuropathology. In a recent review, Yaakov Stern conceptualized reserve as comprising both active and passive models (Stern, 2002). In the first model, the brain actively copes with AD pathology through compensation or more efficient use of brain networks. The passive model holds that innate ability or life experience determines the threshold of brain damage necessary to produce cognitive deficit. Operationalization of cognitive reserve includes measures of SES, such as years of education, income, or occupational attainment; anatomic measures such as brain size or synaptic count; or cognitive measures such as IQ.

Ethnic groups often have different levels of SES, and these SES variables may reflect either lack of educational or occupational experiences that contribute to cognitive reserve, or risk factors such as poor nutrition, toxic exposures, or poor health care that may diminish cognitive reserve. For example, cognitive decline appears to be faster (Stern, Albert, Tang, and Tsai, 1999; Unverzagt, Hui, Farlow, Hall, and Hendrie, 1998;) and associated with increased risk of mortality (Stern, Tang, Denaro, and Mayeux, 1995) among highly educated ethnic minorities. The cognitive reserve theory would explain this finding by stating that enriched educational experience produced an increased reserve in these individuals, delaying the onset of mental deterioration and thus reducing the interval between the initiation of memory loss and severe disability from dementia. In another study, childhood residence (rural versus urban) and educational level was evaluated in a random sample of 223 African-American elders, 180 of whom were neurologically normal and 43 of whom had AD (Hall, Gao, Unverzagt, and Hendrie, 2000). Childhood rural residence, combined with fewer than 7 years of school, was associated with an increased risk of AD. The authors hypothesized that low education by itself is not a major risk factor, but is a marker for other deleterious socioeconomic or environmental influences in childhood.

Operationalization of cognitive reserve is especially challenging among ethnic minorities. Variables such as years of education are often used as a proxy for an individual's degree of cognitive reserve. However, these variables may not necessarily represent native ability, especially among elders whose educational and occupational opportunities were limited because of institutionalized racism and poverty. When number of years of education is used to represent an experience that increased the brain's resistance to pathology or provided the brain with reserve, we cannot be sure that the same quantity of education provided the same quality of experience across ethnic groups. In addition, investigators must avoid confounding measures of reserve with outcome indicators. For example, IQ measures may be used to represent brain reserve, but the disease process itself may also affect such measures. Ideally, we would be able to use childhood measures of cognitive ability to predict development of dementia late in life. This was elegantly demonstrated in studies showing that low scores on measures of intelligence in childhood (Whalley et al., 2000) and low linguistic ability in the early 20s (Snowdon et al., 1997) were associated with low cognitive test scores and dementia late in life. This kind of research is limited among ethnic minorities, however, if the cognitive measure administered did not accurately reflect true cognitive ability due to cultural effects on test performance.

Discrepancies in quantity and quality of education, literacy, and the limitations placed on occupational attainment by institutionalized racism may help to explain the increased rates of dementia and AD among ethnic minorities and illiterate individuals. Nevertheless, a notable finding from the studies discussed earlier in this chapter is that the lowest incidence of dementia is found in rural India and West Africa, areas where elders have low levels of education and literacy. These disparate findings may be clarified in the future if longitudinal studies of cognitive reserve are conducted in both Western and non-Western countries.

CULTURAL BELIEFS ABOUT DEMENTIA AND COGNITIVE DECLINE

Social and cultural differences in the meaning of dementia and beliefs about cognitive decline among elders may play a part in the different rates of AD by ethnicity, and may also explain the lack of consensus on rates of AD across studies. Cultural values may include beliefs that dementia-related changes are part of the normal aging process rather than an abnormal process, such that in some groups and communities, cognitive decline may not elicit concern until symptoms are well beyond the early or mild stages (Hart, Gallagher-Thompson, Davies, Diminno, and Lessin, 1996). Differences in the meaning of cognitive decline highlight the need for community-based random samples and recruitment strategies that improve the rates of participation of ethnically diverse elders (Baker, 1996).

Individuals within some cultures may be more likely to view cognitive decline as disgraceful and something that should be kept within the family. A dementing illness may be difficult to accept when the ethnic elder may be the historian, mediator, and provider of emotional and financial support for many generations of family members living in the same home (Baker, 1992). Richards et al. (1998) found that although African-Caribbean elders living in London reported a larger number of family members living nearby and were more likely to live with at least one other family member, they received no more help from their families with activities of daily living, yet were more likely to have difficulties in this area.

One study found that black participants with AD evaluated at California Department of Health Alzheimer's Disease Diagnostic and Treatment Centers reported a shorter duration of illness at the time of initial diagnosis (Hargrave et al., 1998). However, after adjusting for years of education, blacks with AD had more advanced cognitive dysfunction (as assessed by the MMSE) and were more functionally impaired (as assessed by the Blessed Dementia Rating Scale) at the time of initial diagnosis. These findings may be due to reporting bias, testing bias, or both; it is also possible that cognitive decline is more rapid among African-American elders with AD.

Black elders evaluated at several dementia assessment centers were more likely than whites to be in poverty, living alone, and poorly educated (Cohen and Carlin, 1993). Blacks with dementia (both U.S.-born African Americans and African Caribbeans) were more likely to have psychotic symptoms, while whites were more likely to have depression (Cohen and Magai, 1999). The possible contribution of limited economic, educational, and health care resources throughout the lifespan must be considered when assessing all elders for dementia, but may be especially salient among ethnic minorities and immigrants. Access to basic resources may be restricted by institutionalized segregation or residence in poorly developed areas within or outside the United States, such that poor nutrition throughout the lifespan could be a risk factor for cognitive decline as an older adult (Artiola i Fortuny et al., 1998; Baker, 1992).

CONCLUSIONS AND FUTURE DIRECTIONS

We conclude that there are ethnic differences in the observed prevalence and incidence of cognitive impairment, dementia, and AD. Although studies conducted in the United States have differences in sampling methods, definitions of dementia, and definitions of race/ethnicity, it appears that African Americans and Hispanics have higher prevalence and incidence of dementia and AD than whites. These differences may be at least partially explained by discrepancies in the specificity of functional and neuropsychological instruments used to detect cognitive impairment across cultures. No research group has been able yet to overcome the strong influence of cultural and educational experience on cognitive test performance, the meaning of dementia, and the significance attributed to cognitive change in aging. However, even using the most accurate cognitive measures, cross-cultural differences in rates of cognitive impairment, dementia, and AD may still exist. These can be explained by differences in biological risk factors such as cerebrovascular disease, differential exposure to environmental risk factors, cognitive reserve, or genetic risk factors. Cross-national studies such as the Indianapolis-Ibadan study indicate that ethnic differences in rates of dementia may be a result of a complex gene-environment interaction. It remains to be seen whether such intricately entwined biological and genetic risk factors can be separated from their sociocultural or environmental context.

Cross-cultural researchers must be aware that racial and ethnic classifications are historically defined categories that are not direct reflections of genetic populations. There is also tremendous heterogeneity in cultural, linguistic, educational, and environmental exposures within traditionally defined racial and ethnic groups. Therefore, we believe that the highest priority for future cross-cultural research is to operationalize the behavioral, experiential, and biological factors that are assumed to differ between ethnic or racial groups. Without explicit measurement of one or more of these factors, the possible interpretations of differences between ethnic or racial groups are too varied and complex. For example, investigators of the genetics of AD could create comparison groups based on degree of shared ancestry using population-specific alleles, as opposed to self-reported racial or ethnic classifications.

Another crucial priority for cross-cultural investigations of cognitive impairment, dementia, and AD is to increase rates of autopsy among random samples of ethnic minority elders whose cognitive ability has been well characterized during life. Without neuropathological confirmation, we will never overcome the suspicion that our diagnoses are culturally biased, and without samples free of selection bias we can never determine if rates of AD pathology differ between ethnic groups. Improved pathological verification of dementia diagnoses will require large-scale education of communities about brain donation, as well as improved training of medical personnel on culturally sensitive discussion of autopsy. Another approach would be to refine anatomical and functional imaging techniques that can be used to accurately discriminate pathological changes associated with AD or vascular disease during life, and to detect these changes early in the course of the disorder.

The next priority is to improve the accuracy of cognitive tests used to detect impairment. Cultural experience has been hypothesized to correlate with specific cognitive variables such as problem-solving styles, speed versus accuracy tradeoffs, and salience or familiarity with items. Focus on these variables might guide research on cross-cultural differences in cognitive test performance and assist in the development of tests usable across cultures. Differences in quality of educational attainment within and between ethnic groups could be assessed with measures of reading level, and used in research on cognitive reserve. If cognitive reserve is a major factor in explaining ethnic differences in rates of dementia and AD, researchers should be able to demonstrate this using anatomic indicators of reserve such as brain size or brain network activity.

Despite the methodological difficulties cross-cultural dementia researchers must face, these investigations challenge our definitions of race and ethnicity, cognitive impairment, functional deficit, and the definition of dementia itself (Richards and Brayne, 1996). The ultimate validity check for constructs involving these concepts may be their ability to supersede cultural boundaries. The challenges are significant, but we expect that as we clarify the complex etiology of AD and move toward prevention, the struggle to deconstruct ethnicity, culture, and biology will inevitably enrich our understanding of the effect of culture on cognition, genetic and environmental influences on AD, as well as the normal aging process.

ACKNOWLEDGMENTS

Support was provided by federal grants AG07232, AG10963, AG08702, and RR00645, an Alzheimer's Association Grant (IIRG-98-020), the Taub Foundation, the Charles S. Robertson Memorial Gift for Alzheimer's Disease Research from the Banbury Fund, and the Blanchette Hooker Rockefeller Foundation. Tavis Allison provided editorial assistance for this chapter.

REFERENCES

Adams, R.L., Boake, C., and Crain, C. (1982). Bias in a neuropsychological test classification related to age, education and ethnicity. *Journal of Consulting and Clinical Psychology, 50,* 143-145.

Aevarsson, O., and Skoog, I. (1996). A population-based study on the incidence of dementia disorders between 85 and 88 years of age. *Journal of the American Geriatrics Society, 44,* 1455-1460.

Aevarsson, O., and Skoog, I. (1997). Dementia disorders in a birth cohort followed from age 85 to 88: The influence of mortality, refusal rate, and diagnostic change on prevalence. *International Psychogeriatrics, 9,* 11-23.

Amaducci, L., Baldereschi, M., Doody, R., Chandra, V., and Gaines, A.D. (1997). Cultural issues in the clinical diagnosis of Alzheimer's disease (position paper from the International Working Group on Harmonization of Dementia Drug Guidelines). *Alzheimer's Disease and Associated Disorders, 11*(Suppl. 3), 19-21.

Anderson, J.D. (1988). *The education of blacks in the South, 1860-1935.* Chapel Hill: University of North Carolina Press.

Ardila, A., Rosselli, M., and Puente, A.E. (1994). *Neuropsychological evaluation of the Spanish speaker.* New York: Plenum.

Arnold, B.R., Montgomery, G.T., Castaneda, I., and Longoria, R. (1994). Acculturation and performance of Hispanics on selected Halstead-Reitan neuropsychological tests. *Assessment, 1,* 239-248.

Aronson, M.K., Ooi, W.L., Morgenstern, H., Hafner, A., Masur, D., Crystal, H., et al. (1990). Women, myocardial infarction, and dementia in the very old. *Neurology, 40,* 1102-1106.

Aronson, J., Lustina, M.J., Good, C., Keough, K., Steele, C.M., and Brown, J. (1999). When white men can't do math: Necessary and sufficient factors in stereotype threat. *Journal of Experimental and Social Psychology, 35,* 29-46.

Artiola i Fortuny, L., and Mullaney, H. (1997). Neuropsychology with Spanish speakers: Language use and proficiency issues for test development. *Journal of Clinical and Experimental Neuropsychology, 19,* 615-622.

Artiola i Fortuny, L., Heaton, R.K., and Hermosillo, D. (1998). Neuropsychological comparisons of Spanish-speaking participants from the U.S.-Mexico border region versus Spain. *Journal of the International Neuropsychological Society, 4,* 363-379.

Baker, F.M. (1992). Ethnic minority elders: A mental health research agenda. *Hospital and Community Psychiatry, 43,* 337-338.

Baker, F.M. (1996). Issues in assessing dementia in African American elders. In G. Yeo and D. Gallagher-Thompson (Eds.), *Ethnicity and the dementias* (pp. 59-76). Washington, DC: Taylor and Francis.

Baker, F.M., Johnson, J.T., Velli, S.A., and Wiley, C. (1996). Congruence between education and reading levels of older persons. *Psychiatric Services, 47,* 194-196.

Bernard, L. (1989). Halstead-Reitan neuropsychological test performance of black, Hispanic, and white young adult males from poor academic backgrounds. *Archives of Clinical Neuropsychology, 4,* 267-274.

Berry, J.W. (1976). *Human ecology and cognitive style.* New York: Sage-Halstead.

Boekamp, J.R., Strauss, M.E., and Adams, N. (1995). Estimating premorbid intelligence in African-American and white elderly veterans using the American version of the National Adult Reading Test. *Journal of Clinical and Experimental Neuropsychology, 17,* 645-653.

Bohnstedt, M., Fox, P.J., and Kohatsu, N.D. (1994). Correlates of mini-mental status examination scores among elderly demented patients: The influence of race-ethnicity. *Journal of Clinical Epidemiology, 47,* 1381-1387.

Bonner, G.J., Darkwa, O.K., and Gorelick, P.B. (2000). Autopsy recruitment program for African Americans. *Alzheimer's Disease and Associated Disorders, 14,* 202-208.

Bowirrat, A., Treves, T., Friedland, R.P., and Korczyn, A.D. (1998). Illiteracy is a risk factor for Alzheimer's disease among Arab elderly in Israel. *Neurology, 50*(Suppl. 4), 229.

Boyt, A.A., Taddei, T.K., Hallmayer, J., Helmerhorst, E., Gandy, S.E., Craft, S., et al. (2000). The effect of insulin and glucose on the plasma concentration of Alzheimer's amyloid precursor protein. *Neuroscience, 95,* 727-734.

Brayne, C., Gill, C., Huppert, F.A., Barkley, C., Gehlhaar, E., Girling, D. M., et al. (1998). Vascular risks and incident dementia: Results from a cohort study of the very old. *Dementia and Geriatric Cognitive Disorders, 9,* 175-180.

Brislin, R.W. (1970). Back-translation for cross-cultural research. *Journal of Cross-Cultural Psychology, 1,* 185-216.

Brislin, R.W. (1980). Translation and content-analysis of oral and written material. In H.C. Triandis and J.W. Berry (Eds.), *Handbook of cross-cultural psychology, vol. 2: Methodology* (pp. 389-444). Boston: Allyn and Bacon.

Brown, A., Campbell, A., Wood, D., Hastings, A., Lewis-Jack, O., Dennis, G., et al. (1991). Neuropsychological studies of blacks with cerebrovascular disorders: A preliminary investigation. *Journal of the National Medical Association, 83,* 217-229.

Callahan, C.M., Hall, K.S., Hui, S.L., Musick, B.S., Unverzagt, F.W., and Hendrie, H.C. (1996). Relationship of age, education, and occupation with dementia among a community-based sample of African Americans. *Archives of Neurology, 53,* 134-140.

Campbell, A., Rorie, K., Dennis, G., Wood, D., Combs, S., Hearn, L., et al. (1996). Neuropsychological assessment of African Americans: Conceptual and methodological considerations. In R. Jones (Ed.), *Handbook of tests and measurement for black populations: Volume 2* (pp. 75-84). Berkeley, CA: Cobb and Henry.

Carlson, M.C., Brandt, J., Carson, K.A., and Kawas, C.H. (1998). Lack of relation between race and cognitive test performance in Alzheimer's disease. *Neurology, 50,* 1499-1501.

Chandra, V., Ganguli, M., Pandav, R., Johnston, J., Belle, S., and DeKosky, S. (1998). Prevalence of Alzheimer's disease and other dementias in rural India. *Neurology, 51,* 1000-1008.

Chandra, V., Pandav, R., Dodge, H.H., Johnston, J.M., Belle, S.H., DeKosky, S.T., et al. (2001). Incidence of Alzheimer's disease in a rural community in India: The Indo-U.S. study. *Neurology, 57,* 985-989.

Chang, L., Miller, B.L., and Lin, K.M. (1993). Clinical and epidemiologic studies of dementias: Cross-ethnic perspectives. In K.M. Lin, R.E. Poland, and G. Nakasaki (Eds.), *Psychopharmacology and psychobiology of ethnicity* (pp. 223-252). Washington, DC: American Psychiatric Press.

Charletta, D., Gorelick, P.B., Dollear, T.J., Freels, S., and Harris, Y. (1995). CT and MRI findings among African-Americans with Alzheimer's disease, vascular dementia, and stroke without dementia. *Neurology, 45,* 1456-1461.

Cohen, C.I., and Carlin, L. (1993). Racial differences in clinical and social variables among patients evaluated in a dementia assessment center. *Journal of the National Medical Association, 85,* 379-384.

Cohen, C.I, and Magai, C. (1999). Racial differences in neuropsychiatric symptoms among dementia outpatients. *American Journal of Geriatric Psychiatry, 7,* 57-63.

Collins, J.G. (1990). Types of injuries by selected characteristics. *Vital and Health Statistics, 175,* 1-68.

Corder, E.H., Saunders, A.M., Strittmatter, W.J., et al. (1995). Apolipoprotein E, survival in Alzheimer's disease patients, and competing risks of death and Alzheimer's disease. *Neurology, 45,* 1323-1328.

de la Monte, S.M., Hutchins, G.M., and Moore, G.W. (1989). Racial differences in the etiology of dementia and frequency of Alzheimer lesions in the brain. *Journal of the National Medical Association, 81,* 644-652.

Del Ser, T., Gonzalez-Montalvo, J.I., Martinez-Espinosa, S., Delgado-Villapalos, C., and Bermejo, F. (1997). Estimation of premorbid intelligence in Spanish people with the word accentuation test and its application to the diagnosis of dementia. *Brain and Cognition, 8,* 343-356.

Dick, M.B., Teng, E.L., Kempler, D., Davis, D.S., and Taussig, I.M. (2002). The Cross-Cultural Neuropsychological Test Battery (CCNB): Effects of age, education, ethnicity, and cognitive status on performance. In F.R. Ferraro (Ed.), *Minority and cross-cultural aspects of neuropsychological assessment* (pp. 17-41). Lisse, Netherlands: Swets and Zeitlinger.

Duara, R., Barker, W., Lopez-Alberola, R., and Loewenstein, D.A. (1996). Alzheimer's disease: Interaction of apolipoprotein E genotype, family history of dementia, gender, education, ethnicity, and age of onset. *Neurology, 46,* 1575-1579.

Elo, I.T., Preston, S.H., Rosenwaike, I., Hill, M., and Cheney, T.P. (1996). Consistency of age reporting on death certificates and Social Security records among elderly African Americans. *Social Science Research, 25,* 292-307.

Escobar, J.I., Burnam, A., Karno, M., Forsythe, A., Landsverk, J., and Golding, J.M. (1986). Use of the Mini-Mental State Examination (MMSE) in a community population of mixed ethnicity: Cultural and linguistic artifacts. *Journal of Nervous and Mental Disease, 174,* 607-614.

Farrer, L.A., Cupples, L.A., Haines, J.L., Hyman, B., Kukull, W.A., Mayeux, R., et al. (1997). Effects of age, sex, and ethnicity on the association between apolipoprotein E genotype and Alzheimer disease: A meta-analysis. APOE and Alzheimer Disease Meta Analysis Consortium. *Journal of the American Medical Association, 278,* 1349-1356.

Fillenbaum, G.G., Hughes, D.C., Heyman, A., George, L.K., and Blazer, D.G. (1988). Relationship of health and demographic characteristics to mini-mental state examination score among community residents. *Psychological Medicine, 18*, 719-726.

Fillenbaum, G.G., Huber, M.S., Beekly, D., Henderson, V.W., Mortimer, J., Morris, J.C., et al. (1996). The consortium to establish a registry for Alzheimer's Disease (CERAD). Part XIII: Obtaining autopsy in Alzheimer's disease. *Neurology, 46*, 142-145.

Fillenbaum, G.G., Heyman, A., Huber, M., Woodbury, M., Leiss, J., Schmader, K., Bohannon, A., and Trapp-Moen, B. (1998). The prevalence and 3-year incidence of dementia in older black and white community residents. *Journal of Clinical Epidemiology, 51*, 587-595.

Fillenbaum, G.G., Heyman, A., Huber, M.S., Ganguli, M., and Unverzagt, F.W. (2001). Performance of elderly African American and white community residents on the CERAD Neuropsychological Battery. *Journal of the International Neuropsychological Society, 7*, 502-509.

Folstein, M.F., Bassett, S.S., Anthony, J.C., Romanoski, A.J., and Nestadt, G.R. (1991). Dementia: Case ascertainment in a community survey. *Journal of Gerontology: Biological Sciences and Medical Sciences, 46*, 132-138.

Ford, G.R., Haley, W.E., Thrower, S.L., West, C.A.C., and Harrell, L.E. (1996). Utility of mini-mental state exam scores in predicting functional impairment among white and African American dementia patients. *Journals of Gerontology: Biological Sciences and Medical Sciences, 51*, 185-188.

Ford-Booker, P., Campbell, A., Combs, S., Lewis, S., Ocampo, C., Brown, A., Lewis-Jack, O., and Rorie, K. (1993). The predictive accuracy of neuropsychological tests in a normal population of African Americans. *Journal of Clinical and Experimental Neuropsychology, 15*, 64.

Fuld, P.A., Muramoto, O., Blau, A., Westbrook, L., and Katzman, R. (1988). Cross-cultural and multi-ethnic dementia evaluation by mental status and memory testing. *Cortex, 24*, 511-519.

Gallagher, T.C., Geling, O., FitzGibbons, J., Aforismo, J., and Comite, F. (2000). Are women being counseled about estrogen replacement therapy? *Medical Care Research and Review, 57*, 72-92.

Ganesan, K., Teklehaimanot, S., and Norris, K. (2000). Estrogen replacement therapy use in minority postmenopausal women. *Ethnicity and Disease, 10*, 257-261.

Ganguli, M., Ratcliff, G., Huff, F.J., Belle, S., Kancel, M.J., Fischer, L., et al. (1991). Effects of age, gender, and education on cognitive tests in a rural elderly community sample: Norms from the Monongahela Valley Independent Elders Survey. *Neuroepidemiology, 10*, 42-52.

George, L.K., Landerman, R., Blazer, D.G., and Anthony, J.C. (1991). Cognitive impairment. In L.N. Robins and D.A. Regier (Eds.), *Psychiatric disorders in America: The Epidemiologic Catchment Area Study* (pp. 291-327). New York: Free Press.

Gerdes, L.U., Klausen, I.C., Sihm, I., and Faergeman, O. (1992). Apolipoprotein E polymorphism in a Danish population compared to findings in 45 other study populations around the world. *Genetic Epidemiology, 9*, 155-167.

Geronimus, A.T., Bound, J., and Neidert, L.J. (1996). On the validity of using Census geocode characteristics to proxy individual socioeconomic characteristics. *Journal of the American Statistical Association, 91*, 529-537.

Gonzalez, H.M., Mungas, D., Reed, B.R., Marshall, S., and Haan, M.N. (2001). A new verbal learning and memory test for English- and Spanish-speaking older people. *Journal of the International Neuropsychological Society, 7*, 544-555.

Gorelick, P.B., Freels, S., Harris, Y., Dollear, T., Billingsley, M., and Brown, N. (1994). Epidemiology of vascular and Alzheimer's dementia among African Americans in Chicago, IL: Baseline frequency and comparison of risk factors. *Neurology, 44*, 1391-1396.

Graves, A.B., Larson, E.B., Edland, S.D., Bowen, J.D., McCormick, W.C., McCurry, S.M., et al. (1996). Prevalence of dementia and its subtypes in the Japanese American population of King County, Washington state: The Kame Project. *American Journal of Epidemiology, 144,* 760-771.

Gurland, B.J., Wilder, D., Lantigua, R., Stern, Y., Chen, J., Killeffer, E.H.P., et al. (1998). Rates of dementia in three ethnoracial groups. *International Journal of Geriatric Psychiatry, 14,* 481-493.

Haerer, A.F., Anderson, D.W., and Schoenberg, B.S. (1987). Survey of major neurologic disorders in a biracial United States population: The Copiah County Study. *Southern Medical Journal, 80,* 339-343.

Hall, K.S., Ogunniyi, A.O., Hendrie, H.C., Osuntokun, B.O., Hui, S., Musick, B., et al. (1996). A cross-cultural community based study of dementias: Methods and performance of the survey instrument in Indianapolis, U.S.A., and Ibadan, Nigeria. *International Journal of Methods in Psychiatric Research, 6,* 129-142.

Hall, K.S., Gao, S., Unverzagt, F.W., and Hendrie, H.C. (2000). Low education and childhood rural residence: Risk for Alzheimer's disease in African Americans. *Neurology, 54,* 95-99.

Hanushek, E. (1989). The impact of differential expenditures on school performance. *Educational Researcher, 18,* 45-51.

Hargrave, R., Stoeklin, M., Haan, M., and Reed, B. (1998). Clinical aspects of Alzheimer's disease in black and white patients. *Journal of the National Medical Association, 90,* 78-84.

Harrell, L.E., Callaway, R., and Powers, R. (1993). Autopsy in dementing illness: Who participates? *Alzheimer's Disease and Associated Disorders, 7,* 80-87.

Hart, V.R., Gallagher-Thompson, D., Davies, H.D., DiMinno, M., and Lessin, P.J. (1996). Strategies for increasing participation of ethnic minorities in Alzheimer's Disease Diagnostic Centers: A multifaceted approach in California. *Gerontologist, 36,* 259-262.

Harwood, D.G., Barker, W.W., Loewenstein, D.A., Ownby, R.L., St. George-Hyslop, P., Mullan, M., et al. (1999). A cross-ethnic analysis of risk factors for AD in white Hispanics and white non-Hispanics. *Neurology, 52,* 551-556.

Hedges, L.V., Laine, R.D., and Greenwald, R. (1994). Does money matter? A meta-analysis of studies of the effects of differential school inputs on student outcomes. *Educational Researcher, 23,* 5-14.

Helms, J.E. (1992). Why is there no study of cultural equivalence in standardized cognitive ability testing? *American Psychologist, 47,* 1083-1101.

Hendrie, H.C. (1998). Epidemiology of dementia and Alzheimer's disease. *American Journal of Geriatric Psychiatry, 6*(Suppl.), 3-18.

Hendrie, H.C., Hall, K.S., Pillay, N., Rodgers, D., Prince, C., Norton, J., et al. (1993). Alzheimer's disease is rare in Cree. *International Psychogeriatrics, 5,* 5-14.

Hendrie, H.C., Hall, K.S., Hui, S., Unverzagt, F.W., Yu, C.E., Lahiri, D.K., et al. (1995a). Apolipoprotein E genotypes and Alzheimer's disease in a community study of elderly African Americans. *Annals of Neurology, 37,* 118-120.

Hendrie, H.C., Osuntokun, B.O., Hall, K.S., Ogunniyi, A.O., Hui, S.L., Unverzagt, F.W., et al. (1995b). Prevalence of Alzheimer's disease and dementia in two communities: Nigerian Africans and African Americans. *American Journal of Psychiatry, 152,* 1485-1492.

Hendrie, H.C., Ogunniyi, A., Hall, K.S., Baiyewu, O., Unverzagt, F.W., Gureje, O., et al. (2001). Incidence of dementia and Alzheimer's disease in 2 communities: Yoruba residing in Ibadan, Nigeria, and African Americans residing in Indianapolis, Indiana. *Journal of the American Medical Association, 285,* 739-747.

Heverly, L.L., Isaac, W., and Hynd, G.W. (1986). Neurodevelopmental and racial differences in tactile-visual (cross-modal) discrimination in normal black and white children. *Archives of Clinical Neuropsychology, 1,* 139-145.

Heyman, A., Peterson, B., Fillenbaum, G., and Pieper, C. (1996). The consortium to establish a registry for Alzheimer's disease (CERAD): Part XIV: Demographic and clinical predictors of survival in patients with Alzheimer's disease. *Neurology, 46,* 656-660.

Ishii, H., Meguro, K., Ishizaki, J., Shimada, M., Yamaguchi, S., Sano, I., et al. (1999). Prevalence of senile dementia in a rural community in Japan: The Tajiri project. *Archives of Gerontology and Geriatrics, 29,* 249-265.

Itoh, Y., and Yamada, M. (1996). Apolipoprotein E and the neuropathology of dementia. *New England Journal of Medicine, 334,* 599-600.

Jacobs, D.M., Sano, M., Albert, S., Schofield, P., Dooneief, G., and Stern, Y. (1997). Cross-cultural neuropsychological assessment: A comparison of randomly selected, demographically matched cohorts of English- and Spanish-speaking older adults. *Journal of Clinical and Experimental Neuropsychology, 19,* 331-339.

Jorm, A.F. (1990). *The epidemiology of Alzheimer's disease and related disorders.* London and New York: Chapman and Hall.

Jorm, A.F. (1991). Cross-national comparison of the occurrence of Alzheimer's disease and vascular dementia. *European Archives of Psychiatry and Clinical Neuroscience, 240,* 218-222.

Kalaria, R.N., Ogeng'o, J.A., Patel, N.B., Sayi, J.G., Kitinya, J.N., Chande, H.M., et al. (1997). Evaluation of risk factors for Alzheimer's disease in elderly east Africans. *Brain Research Bulletin, 44,* 573-577.

Kamboh, M.I. (1995). Apolipoprotein E polymorphism and susceptibility to Alzheimer's disease. *Human Biology, 67,* 195-215.

Kamboh, M.I., Sepehrnia, B., and Ferrell, R.E. (1989). Genetic studies of human apolipoproteins: VI. Common polymorphism of apolipoprotein E in blacks. *Disease Markers, 7,* 49-55.

Kaufman, A.S., McLean, J.E., and Reynolds, C.R. (1988). Sex, race, residence, region, and education differences on the 11 WAIS-R subtests. *Journal of Clinical Psychology, 44,* 231-248.

Kaufman, J.S., and Cooper, R.S. (1995). Epidemiologic research on minority health: In search of the hypothesis. *Public Health Reports, 110,* 662-666.

Kaufman, J.S., and Cooper, R.S. (2001). Considerations of use of racial/ethnic classification in etiologic research. *American Journal of Epidemiology, 154,* 291-298.

Kaufman, J.S., Cooper, R.S., and McGee, D.L. (1997). Socioeconomic status and health in blacks and whites: The problem of residual confounding and the resilience of race. *Epidemiology, 8,* 621-628.

Kawas, C.H., and Katzman, R. (1999). Epidemiology of dementia and Alzheimer's disease. In R.D. Terry, R. Katzman, S.S. Sisodia, and K.L. Bick (Eds.), *Alzheimer's disease* (pp. 95-116). Philadelphia: Lippincott Williams and Wilkins.

Kempler, D., Teng, E.L., Dick, M., Taussig, I.M., and Davis, D.S. (1998). The effects of age, education, and ethnicity on verbal fluency. *Journal of the International Neuropsychological Society, 4,* 531-538.

Kirsch, I.S., Jungeblut, A., Jenkins, L., and Kolstad, A. (1993). *Adult literacy in America: The National Adult Literacy Survey.* Washington, DC: U.S. Department of Education, National Center for Education Statistics.

Klusman, L.E., Moulton, J.M., Hornbostle, L.K., Picano, J.J., and Beattie, M.T. (1991). Neuropsychological abnormalities in asymptomatic HIV seropositive military personnel. *Journal of Neuropsychological and Clinical Neurosciences, 3,* 422-428.

Korczyn, A.D., Kahana, E., and Galper, Y. (1991). Epidemiology of dementia in Ashkelon, Israel. *Neuroepidemiology, 10,* 100.

Kuller, L.H., Shemanski, L., Manolio, T., Haan, M., Fried, L., Bryan, N., et al. (1998). Relationship between ApoE, MRI findings, and cognitive function in the Cardiovascular Health Study. *Stroke, 29,* 388-398.

LaCalle, J.J. (1987). Forensic psychological evaluations through an interpreter: Legal and ethical issues. *American Journal of Forensic Psychology, 5,* 29-43.

Landrine, H., and Klonoff, E.A. (1994). The African American Acculturation Scale: Development, reliability, and validity. *Journal of Black Psychology, 20,* 104-127.

Landrine, H., and Klonoff, E.A. (1995). The African American Acculturation Scale II: Cross-validation and short form. *Journal of Black Psychology, 21,* 124-152.

Landrine, H., and Klonoff, E.A. (1996). *African American acculturation: Deconstructing race and reviving culture.* Thousand Oaks, CA: Sage.

Lanska, D.J. (1998). Dementia mortality in the United States: Results of the 1986 National Mortality Followback Survey. *Neurology, 50,* 362-367.

Larson, E.B., and Imai, Y. (1996). An overview of dementia and ethnicity with special emphasis on the epidemiology of dementia. In G. Yeo and D. Gallagher-Thompson (Eds.), *Ethnicity and the dementias* (pp. 9-20). Washington, DC: Taylor and Francis.

Leibson, C.L., Rocca, W.A., Hanson, V.A., Cha, R., Kokmen, E., O'Brien, P.C., et al. (1997). The risk of dementia among persons with diabetes mellitus: A population-based cohort study. *Annals of the New York Academy of Sciences, 826,* 422-427.

Lesser, I.M., Smith, M.W., Wohl, M., Mena, R.N., Mehringer, C.M., and Lin, K.M. (1996). Brain imaging, antidepressants, and ethnicity: Preliminary observations. *Psychopharmacology Bulletin, 32,* 235-242.

Lewontin, R., Rose, S., and Kamin, G. (1984). *Not in our genes: Biology, ideology, and human nature.* New York: Pantheon.

Liao, D., Cooper, L., Cai, J., Toole, J., Bryan, N., Burke, G., et al. (1997). The prevalence and severity of white matter lesions, their relationship with age, ethnicity, gender, and cardiovascular disease risk factors: The ARIC Study. *Neuroepidemiology, 16,* 149-162.

Lichtenberg, P.A., Ross, T., and Christensen, B. (1994). Preliminary normative data on the Boston Naming Test for an older urban population. *Clinical Neuropsychologist, 8,* 109-111.

Loewenstein, D.A., Ardila, A., Rosselli, M., and Hayden, S. (1992). A comparative analysis of functional status among Spanish- and English-speaking patients with dementia. *Journal of Gerontology, 47,* 389-394.

Loewenstein, D.A., Arguelles, T., Arguelles, S., and Linn-Fuentes, P. (1994). Potential cultural bias in the neuropsychological assessment of the older adult. *Journal of Clinical and Experimental Neuropsychology, 16,* 623-629.

Longstreth, W.T., Jr., Arnold, A.M., Manolio, T.A., Burke, G.L., Bryan, N., Jungreis, C.A., et al. (2000). Clinical correlates of ventricular and sulcal size on cranial magnetic resonance imaging of 3,301 elderly people: The Cardiovascular Health Study. Collaborative Research Group. *Neuroepidemiology, 19,* 30-42.

Lucas, J.A. (1998). Acculturation and neuropsychological test performance in elderly African Americans. *Journal of the International Neuropsychological Society, 4,* 77.

Luchsinger, J.A., Tang, M.X., Stern, Y., Shea, S., and Mayeux, R. (2001). Diabetes mellitus and risk of Alzheimer's disease and dementia with stroke in a multiethnic cohort. *American Journal of Epidemiology, 154,* 635-641.

Lucotte, G., Loirat, F., and Hazout, S. (1997). Pattern of gradient of apolipoprotein E allele *4 frequencies in western Europe. *Human Biology, 69,* 253-262.

Maestre, G., Ottman, R., Stern, Y., Gurland, B., Chun, M., Tang, M.-X., et al. (1995). Apolipoprotein E and Alzheimer's disease: Ethnic variation in genotypic risks. *Annals of Neurology, 37,* 254-259.

Mangone, C.A., and Arizaga, R.L. (1999). Dementia in Argentina and other Latin-American countries: An overview. *Neuroepidemiology, 18,* 231-235.

Manly, J.J., and Jacobs, D.M. (2001). Future directions in neuropsychological assessment with African Americans. In F.R. Ferraro (Ed.), *Minority and cross-cultural aspects of neuropsychological assessment*. Lisse, Netherlands: Swets and Zeitlinger.

Manly, J.J., Jacobs, D.M., Sano, M., Bell, K., Merchant, C.A., Small, S.A., et al. (1998a). Cognitive test performance among nondemented elderly African Americans and whites. *Neurology, 50,* 1238-1245.

Manly, J.J., Jacobs, D.M., Sano, M., Bell, K., Merchant, C.A., Small, S.A., and Stern, Y. (1998b). African American acculturation and neuropsychological test performance among nondemented community elders. *Journal of the International Neuropsychological Society, 4,* 77.

Manly, J.J., Miller, S.W., Heaton, R.K., Byrd, D., Reilly, J., Velasquez, R.J., et al. (1998c). The effect of African-American acculturation on neuropsychological test performance in normal and HIV positive individuals. *Journal of the International Neuropsychological Society, 4,* 291-302.

Marcopulos, B.A., McLain, C.A., and Giuliano, A.J. (1997). Cognitive impairment or inadequate norms: A study of healthy, rural, older adults with limited education. *Clinical Neuropsychologist, 11,* 111-131.

Margo, R.A. (1985). *Disenfranchisement, school finance, and the economics of segregated schools in the United States south, 1980-1910*. New York: Garland.

Margo, R.A. (1990). *Race and schooling in the South, 1880-1950: An economic history*. Chicago: University of Chicago Press.

Mast, B.T., Fitzgerald, J., Steinberg, J., MacNeill, S.E., and Lichtenberg, P.A. (2001). Effective screening for Alzheimer's disease among older African Americans. *Clinical Neuropsychologist, 15,* 196-202.

Mayeux, R., Stern, Y., Ottman, R., Tatemichi, T.K., Tang, M.-X., Maestre, G., et al. (1993). The apolipoprotein epsilon 4 allele in patients with Alzheimer's disease. *Annals of Neurology, 34,* 752-754.

McCracken, C.F., Boneham, M.A., Copeland, J.R., Williams, K.E., Wilson, K., Scott, A., et al. (1997). Prevalence of dementia and depression among elderly people in black and ethnic minorities. *British Journal of Psychiatry, 171,* 269-273.

McKhann, G., Drachman, D., Folstein, M., Katzman, R., Price, D., and Stadlan, E. (1984). Clinical diagnosis of Alzheimer's disease: Report of the NINCDS-ADRDA Work Group under the auspices of the Department of Health and Human Services Task Force on Alzheimer's disease. *Neurology, 34,* 939-944.

Miller, E.N., Bing, E.G., Selnes, O.A., Wesch, J., and Becker, J. (1993). The effects of sociodemographic factors on reaction time and speed of information processing. *Journal of Clinical and Experimental Neuropsychology, 15,* 66.

Miller, F.D., Hicks, S.P., D'Amato, C.J., and Landis, J.R. (1984). A descriptive study of neuritic plaques and neurofibrillary tangles in an autopsy population. *American Journal of Epidemiology, 120,* 331-341.

Miller, S.W., Heaton, R.K., Kirson, D., and Grant, I. (1997). Neuropsychological (NP) assessment of African Americans. *Journal of the International Neuropsychological Society, 3,* 49.

Moroney, J.T., Bagiella, E., Hachinski, V.C., Molsa, P.K., Gustafson, L., Brun, A., et al. (1997). Misclassification of dementia subtype using the Hachinski Ischemic Score: Results of a meta-analysis of patients with pathologically verified dementias. *Annals of the New York Academy of Sciences, 826,* 490-492.

Morris, J.C., Heyman, A., Mohs, R.C., Hughes, J.P., van Belle, G., Fillenbaum, G., et al. (1989). The Consortium to Establish a Registry for Alzheimer's Disease (CERAD): Part I. Clinical and neuropsychological assessment of Alzheimer's disease. *Neurology, 39,* 1159-1165.

Moyerman, D.R., and Forman, B.D. (1992). Acculturation and adjustment—a meta-analytic study. *Hispanic Journal of Behavioral Sciences, 14,* 163-200.

Mungas, D. (1996). The process of development of valid and reliable neuropsychological assessment measures for English- and Spanish-speaking elderly persons. In G. Yeo and D. Gallagher-Thompson (Eds.), *Ethnicity and the dementias* (pp. 33-46). Washington, DC: Taylor and Francis.

Mungas, D., Marshall, S.C., Weldon, M., Haan, M., and Reed, B.R. (1996). Age and education correction of mini-mental state examination for English and Spanish-speaking elderly. *Neurology, 46,* 700-706.

Mungas, D., Reed, B.R., Marshall, S.C., and Gonzalez, H.M. (2000). Development of psychometrically matched English and Spanish language neuropsychological tests for older persons. *Neuropsychology, 14,* 209-223.

Murden, R.A., McRae, T.D., Kaner, S., and Bucknam, M.E. (1991). Mini-mental state exam scores vary with education in blacks and whites. *Journal of the American Geriatrics Society, 39,* 149-155.

Negy, C., and Woods, D.J. (1992). The importance of acculturation in understanding research with Hispanic-Americans. *Hispanic Journal of Behavioral Sciences, 14,* 224-247.

Nitrini, R., Mathias, S.C., Caramelli, P., Carrilho, P.E., Lefevre, B.H., Porto, C.S., et al. (1995). Evaluation of 100 patients with dementia in Sao Paulo, Brazil: Correlation with socioeconomic status and education. *Alzheimer Disease and Associated Disorders, 9,* 146-151.

O'Neill, J. (1990). The role of human capital in earning differences between black and white men. *Journal of Economic Perspectives, 4,* 25-45.

Osuntokun, B.O., Ogunniyi, A.O., Lekwauwa, G.U., and Oyediran, A.B. (1991). Epidemiology of age-related dementias in the Third World and aetiological clues of Alzheimer's disease. *Tropical and Geographical Medicine, 43,* 345-351.

Osuntokun, B.O., Hendrie, H.C., Ogunniyi, A.O., Hall, K.S., Lekwauwa, U.G., Brittain, H.M., et al. (1992). Cross-cultural studies in Alzheimer's disease. *Ethnicity and Disease, 2,* 352-357.

Osuntokun, B.O., Sahota, A., Ogunniyi, A.O., Gureje, O., Baiyewu, O., Adeyinka, A., et al. (1995). Lack of an association between apolipoprotein E epsilon 4 and Alzheimer's disease in elderly Nigerians. *Annals of Neurology, 38,* 463-465.

Ott, A., Stolk, R.P., Hofman, A., van Harskamp, F., Grobbee, D.E., and Breteler, M.M. (1996). Association of diabetes mellitus and dementia: The Rotterdam Study. *Diabetologia, 39,* 1392-1397.

Ott, A., Stolk, R.P., van Harskamp, F., Pols, H.A., Hofman, A., and Breteler, M.M. (1999). Diabetes mellitus and the risk of dementia: The Rotterdam Study. *Neurology, 53,* 1937-1942.

Overall, J.E., and Levin, H.S. (1978). Correcting for cultural factors in evaluating intellectual deficit on the WAIS. *Journal of Clinical Psychology, 34,* 910-915.

Padilla, A.M. (1980). *Acculturation: Theory, models, and some new findings.* Boulder, CO: Westview Press.

Parra, E.J., Marcini, A., Akey, J., Martinson, J., Batzer, M.A., Cooper, R., et al. (1998). Estimating African American admixture proportions by use of population-specific alleles. *American Journal of Human Genetics, 63,* 1839-1851.

Perkins, P., Annegers, J.F., Doody, R.S., Cooke, N., Aday, L., and Vernon, S.W. (1997). Incidence and prevalence of dementia in a multiethnic cohort of municipal retirees. *Neurology, 49,* 44-50.

Ponton, M.O., Satz, P., Herrera, L., Ortiz, F., Urrutia, C.P., Young, R., et al. (1996). Normative data stratified by age and education for the Neuropsychological Screening Battery for Hispanics (NeSBHIS): Initial report. *Journal of the International Neuropsychological Society, 2,* 96-104.

Prineas, R.J., Demirovic, J., Bean, J.A., Duara, R., Gomez-Marin, O., Loewenstein, D.A., et al. (1995). South Florida Program on Aging and Health: Assessing the prevalence of Alzheimer's disease in three ethnic groups. *Journal of the Florida Medical Association, 82*, 805-810.

Quiroga, P., Calvo, C., Albala, C., Urquidi, J., Santos, J.L., Perez, H., et al. (1999). Apolipoprotein E polymorphism in elderly Chilean people with Alzheimer's disease. *Neuroepidemiology, 18*, 48-52.

Rasmusson, D.X., Carson, K.A., Brookmeyer, R., Kawas, C., and Brandt, J. (1996). Predicting rate of cognitive decline in probable Alzheimer's disease. *Brain and Cognition, 31*, 133-147.

Ratcliff, G., Ganguli, M., Chandra, V., Sharma, S., Belle, S., Seaberg, E., et al. (1998). Effects of literacy and education on measures of word fluency. *Brain and Language, 61*, 115-122.

Reynolds, C.R., Chastain, R.L., Kaufman, A.S., and McLean, J.E. (1987). Demographic characteristics and IQ among adults: Analysis of the WAIS-R standardization sample as a function of the stratification variables. *Journal of School Psychology, 23*, 323-342.

Richards, M., and Brayne, C. (1996). Cross-cultural research into cognitive impairment and dementia: Some practical experiences. *International Journal of Geriatric Psychiatry, 11*, 383-387.

Richards, M., Abas, M., Carter, J., Osagie, A., Levy, R., and Brayne, C. (1998). Social support and activities of daily living in older Afro-Caribbean and white UK residents. *Age and Ageing, 27*, 252-253.

Ripich, D.N., Carpenter, B., and Ziol, E. (1997). Comparison of African-American and white persons with Alzheimer's disease on language measures. *Neurology, 48*, 781-783.

Ritchie, K.A., and Hallerman, E.F. (1989). Cross-validation of a dementia screening test in a heterogeneous population. *International Journal of Epidemiology, 18*, 717-719.

Roberts, R.J., and Hamsher, K.D. (1984). Effects of minority status on facial recognition and naming performance. *Journal of Clinical Psychology, 40*, 539-545.

Rocca, W.A., Hofman, A., Brayne, C., Breteler, M.M., Clarke, M., Copeland, J.R., et al. (1991). Frequency and distribution of Alzheimer's disease in Europe: A collaborative study of 1980-1990 prevalence findings. The EURODEM-Prevalence Research Group. *Annals of Neurology, 30*, 381-390.

Rosenberg, R.N., Richter, R.W., Risser, R.C., Taubman, K., Prado-Farmer, I., Ebalo, E., et al. (1996). Genetic factors for the development of Alzheimer's disease in the Cherokee Indian. *Archives of Neurology, 53*, 997-1000.

Rosenthal, M., and Ricker, J.H. (2000). Traumatic brain injury. In R. Frank and T. Elliott (Eds.), *Handbook of rehabilitation psychology* (pp. 49-74). Washington, DC: American Psychological Association.

Roses, A.D. (1996). Apolipoprotein E alleles as risk factors in Alzheimer's disease. *Annual Review of Medicine, 47*, 387-400.

Ross, T.P., Lichtenberg, P.A., and Christensen, B.K. (1995). Normative data on the Boston Naming Test for elderly adults in a demographically diverse medical sample. *Clinical Neuropsychologist, 9*, 321-325.

Sacco, R.L., Boden-Albala, B., Gan, R., Chen, X., Kargman, D.E., Shea, S., et al. (1998). Stroke incidence among white, black, and Hispanic residents of an urban community: The Northern Manhattan Stroke Study. *American Journal of Epidemiology, 147*, 259-268.

Sahota, A., Yang, M., Gao, S., Hui, S.L., Baiyewu, O., Gureje, O., et al. (1997). Apolipoprotein E-associated risk for Alzheimer's disease in the African-American population is genotype dependent. *Annals of Neurology, 42*, 659-661.

Salmon, D., Jin, H., Zhang, M., Grant, I., and Yu, E. (1995). Neuropsychological assessment of Chinese elderly in the Shanghai Dementia Survey. *Clinical Neuropsychologist, 9,* 159-168.

Salmon, D.P., Riekkinen, P.J., Katzman, R., Zhang, M.Y., Jin, H., and Yu, E. (1989). Cross-cultural studies of dementia: A comparison of mini-mental state examination performance in Finland and China. *Archives of Neurology, 46,* 769-772.

Sandberg, G., Stewart, W., Smialek, J., and Troncoso, J.C. (2001). The prevalence of the neuropathological lesions of Alzheimer's disease is independent of race and gender. *Neurobiology of Aging, 22,* 169-175.

Sano, M., Mackell, J.A., Ponton, M., Ferreira, P., Wilson, J., Pawluczyk, S., et al. (1997). The Spanish Instrument Protocol: Design and implementation of a study to evaluate treatment efficacy instruments for Spanish-speaking patients with Alzheimer's disease: The Alzheimer's Disease Cooperative Study. *Alzheimer's Disease and Associated Disorders, 11*(Suppl. 2), 57-64.

Sasaki, N., Fukatsu, R., Tsuzuki, K., Hayashi, Y., Yoshida, T., Fujii, N., et al. (1998). Advanced glycation end products in Alzheimer's disease and other neurodegenerative diseases. *American Journal of Pathology, 153,* 1149-1155.

Schoenberg, B.S., Anderson, D.W., and Haerer, A.F. (1985). Severe dementia: Prevalence and clinical features in a biracial US population. *Archives of Neurology, 42,* 740-743.

Sencakova, D., Graff-Radford, N.R., Willis, F.B., Lucas, J.A., Parfitt, F., Cha, R.H., et al. (2001). Hippocampal atrophy correlates with clinical features of Alzheimer's disease in African Americans. *Archives of Neurology, 58,* 1593-1597.

Shadlen, M.F., Larson, E.B., and Yukawa, M. (2000). The epidemiology of Alzheimer's disease and vascular dementia in Japanese and African-American populations: The search for etiological clues. *Neurobiology of Aging, 21,* 171-181.

Skoog, I., Nilsson, L., Palmertz, B., Andreasson, L.A., and Svanborg, A. (1993). A population-based study of dementia in 85-year-olds. *New England Journal of Medicine, 328,* 153-158.

Smith, J.P. (1984). Race and human capital. *American Economic Review, 4,* 685-698.

Smith, J.P., and Welch, F. (1977). Black-white male wage ratios: 1960-1970. *American Economic Review, 67,* 323-328.

Smith, M.A., Sayre, L.M., and Perry, G. (1996). Diabetes mellitus and Alzheimer's disease: Glycation as a biochemical link. *Diabetologia, 39,* 247.

Snowdon, D.A., Greiner, L.H., Mortimer, J.A., Riley, K.P., Greiner, P.A., and Markesbery, W.R. (1997). Brain infarction and the clinical expression of Alzheimer's disease: The Nun Study. *Journal of the American Medical Association, 277,* 813-817.

Sparks, D.L., Hunsaker, J.C., III, Scheff, S.W., Kryscio, R.J., Henson, J.L., and Markesbery, W.R. (1990). Cortical senile plaques in coronary artery disease, aging and Alzheimer's disease. *Neurobiology of Aging, 11,* 601-607.

Sparks, D.L., Martin, T.A., Gross, D.R., and Hunsaker, J.C., III. (2000). Link between heart disease, cholesterol, and Alzheimer's disease: A review. *Microscopy Research and Technique, 50,* 287-290.

Spencer, S.J., Steele, C.M., and Quinn, D.M. (1999). Stereotype threat and women's math performance. *Journal of Experimental and Social Psychology, 35,* 4-28.

Steele, C.M. (1997). A threat in the air: How stereotypes shape intellectual identity and performance. *American Psychologist, 52,* 613-629.

Steele, C.M., and Aronson, J. (1995). Stereotype threat and the intellectual test performance of African Americans. *Journal of Personality and Social Psychology, 69,* 797-811.

Stern, Y. (2002). What is cognitive reserve? Theory and research application of the reserve concept. *Journal of the International Neuropsychological Association, 8,* 448-460.

Stern, Y., Andrews, H., Pittman, J., Sano, M., Tatemichi, T., Lantigua, R., et al. (1992). Diagnosis of dementia in a heterogeneous population: Development of a neuropsychological paradigm-based diagnosis of dementia and quantified correction for the effects of education. *Archives of Neurology, 49,* 453-460.

Stern, Y., Gurland, B., Tatemichi, T.K., Tang, M.-X., Wilder, D., and Mayeux, R. (1994). Influence of education and occupation on the incidence of Alzheimer's disease. *Journal of the American Medical Association, 271,* 1004-1010.

Stern, Y., Tang, M.-X., Denaro, J., and Mayeux, R. (1995). Increased risk of mortality in Alzheimer's disease patients with more advanced educational and occupational attainment. *Annals of Neurology, 37,* 590-595.

Stern, Y., Albert, S., Tang, M.-X., and Tsai, W.-Y. (1999). Rate of memory decline in AD is related to education and occupation: Cognitive reserve? *Neurology, 53,* 1942-1947.

Still, C.N., Jackson, K.L., Brandes, D.A., Abramson, R.K., and Macera, C.A. (1990). Distribution of major dementias by race and sex in South Carolina. *Journal of the South Carolina Medical Association, 86,* 453-456.

Sundquist, J., Winkleby, M.A., and Pudaric, S. (2001). Cardiovascular disease risk factors among older black, Mexican-American, and white women and men: An analysis of NHANES III, 1988-1994. Third National Health and Nutrition Examination Survey. *Journal of the American Geriatrics Society, 49,* 109-116.

Takadera, T., Sakura, N., Mohri, T., and Hashimoto, T. (1993). Toxic effect of a beta-amyloid peptide (beta 22-35) on the hippocampal neuron and its prevention. *Neuroscience Letters, 161,* 41-44.

Tang, M.-X., Maestre, G., Tsai, W.Y., Liu, X.H., Feng, L., Chung, W.Y., et al. (1996). Effect of age, ethnicity, and head injury on the association between APOE genotypes and Alzheimer's disease. *Annals of the New York Academy of Sciences, 802,* 6-15.

Tang, M.-X., Stern, Y., Marder, K., Bell, K., Gurland, B., Lantigua, R., et al. (1998). The APOE-ε4 allele and the risk of Alzheimer's disease among African Americans, whites, and Hispanics. *Journal of the American Medical Association, 279,* 751-755.

Tang, M.-X., Cross, P., Andrews, H., Jacobs, D.M., Small, S., Bell, K., et al. (2001). Incidence of AD in African-Americans, Caribbean Hispanics, and whites in northern Manhattan. *Neurology, 56,* 49-56.

Teng, E.L. (1996). Cross-cultural testing and the Cognitive Abilities Screening Instrument. In G. Yeo and D. Gallagher-Thompson (Eds.), *Ethnicity and the dementias* (pp. 77-85). Washington, DC: Taylor and Francis.

Teng, E.L., Hasegawa, K., Homma, A., Imai, Y., Larson, E., Graves, A., et al. (1994). The Cognitive Abilities Screening Instrument (CASI): A practical test for cross-cultural epidemiological studies of dementia. *International Psychogeriatrics, 6,* 45-58.

Teresi, J.A., Albert, S.M., Holmes, D., and Mayeux, R. (1999). Use of latent class analyses for the estimation of prevalence of cognitive impairment, and signs of stroke and Parkinson's disease among African-American elderly of central Harlem: Results of the Harlem Aging Project. *Neuroepidemiology, 18,* 309-321.

Treves, T., Korczyn, A.D., Zilber, N., Kahana, E., Leibowitz, Y., Alter, M., et al. (1986). Presenile dementia in Israel. *Archives of Neurology, 43,* 26-29.

Unverzagt, F.W., Hall, K.S., Torke, A.M., and Rediger, J.D. (1996). Effects of age, education and gender on CERAD neuropsychological test performance in an African American sample. *Clinical Neuropsychologist, 10,* 180-190.

Unverzagt, F.W., Hui, S.L., Farlow, M.R., Hall, K.S., and Hendrie, H.C. (1998). Cognitive decline and education in mild dementia. *Neurology, 50,* 181-185.

van de Vijver, F. (1997). Meta-analysis of cross-cultural comparisons of cognitive test performance. *Journal of Cross-Cultural Psychology, 28,* 678-709.

van de Vijver, F., and Hambleton, R.K. (1996). Translating tests: Some practical guidelines. *European Psychologist, 1,* 89-99.

Weintraub, D., Raskin, A., Ruskin, P.E., Gruber-Baldini, A.L., Zimmerman, S.I., Hebel, J.R., et al. (2000). Racial differences in the prevalence of dementia among patients admitted to nursing homes. *Psychiatric Services, 51,* 1259-1264.

Weiss, B.D., Reed, R., Kligman, E.W., and Abyad, A. (1995). Literacy and performance on the mini-mental state examination. *Journal of the American Geriatric Society, 43,* 807-810.

Welch, F. (1966). Measurement of the quality of education. *American Economic Review, 56,* 379-392.

Welch, F. (1973). Black-white differences in returns to schooling. *American Economic Review, 63,* 893-907.

Welsh, K.A., Butters, N., Hughes, J.P., Mohs, R.C., and Heyman, A. (1992). Detection and staging of dementia in Alzheimer's disease: Use of the neuropsychological measures developed for the Consortium to Establish a Registry for Alzheimer's Disease. *Archives of Neurology, 49,* 448-452.

Welsh, K.A., Fillenbaum, G., Wilkinson, W., Heyman, A., Mohs, R.C., Stern, Y., et al. (1995). Neuropsychological test performance in African-American and white patients with Alzheimer's disease. *Neurology, 45,* 2207-2211.

Whalley, L., Starr, J., Athawes, R., Hunter, D., Pattie, A., and Deary, I. (2000). Childhood mental ability and dementia. *Neurology, 55,* 1455-1459.

White, L., Petrovitch, H., Ross, G.W., Masaki, K.H., Abbott, R.D., Teng, E.L., et al. (1996). Prevalence of dementia in older Japanese-American men in Hawaii: The Honolulu-Asia Aging Study. *Journal of the American Medical Association, 276,* 955-960.

Wilkinson, D.Y., and King, G. (1987). Conceptual and methodological issues in the use of race as a variable: Policy implications. *Milbank Quarterly, 65,* 56-71.

Williams, J.E., Massing, M., Rosamond, W.D., Sorlie, P.D., and Tyroler, H.A. (1999). Racial disparities in CHD mortality from 1968-1992 in the state economic areas surrounding the ARIC study communities. *Annals of Epidemiology, 9,* 472-480.

Yamada, M., Sasaki, H., Mimori, Y., Kasagi, F., Sudoh, S., Ikeda, J., et al. (1999). Prevalence and risks of dementia in the Japanese population: RERF's adult health study Hiroshima subjects. *Journal of the American Geriatrics Society, 47,* 189-195.

Yeo, G., Gallagher-Thompson, D., and Lieberman, M. (1996). Variations in dementia characteristics by ethnic category. In G. Yeo and D. Gallagher-Thompson (Eds.), *Ethnicity and the dementias* (pp. 21-30). Washington, DC: Taylor and Francis.

Zekraoui, L., Lagarde, J.P., Raisonnier, A., Gerard, N., Aouizerate, A., and Lucotte, G. (1997). High frequency of the apolipoprotein ε4 allele in African pygmies and most of the African populations in sub-Saharan Africa. *Human Biology, 69,* 575-581.

Zhang, M., Katzman, R., Salmon, D., Jin, H., Cai, G., Wang, Z., et al. (1990). The prevalence of dementia and Alzheimer's disease in Shanghai, China: Impact of age, gender and education. *Annals of Neurology, 27,* 428-437.

Zuckerman, M. (1990). Some dubious premises in research and theory on racial differences: Scientific, social, and ethical issues. *American Psychologist, 45,* 1297-1303.

Section II

Two Key Conceptual and Methodological Challenges

5

The Life-Course Contribution to Ethnic Disparities in Health

Clyde Hertzman

Do the following observations belong together?

- Observation 1: Protective early life factors

Birth cohort studies have shown that early life factors contribute to the risk of coronary heart disease, non-insulin-dependent diabetes, obesity, elevated blood pressure, age-related memory loss, and schizophrenia later in life (Barker, 1992, 1994, 1997; Barker and Osmond, 1986; Blane et al., 1996; Davey Smith, Hart, Blane, Gillis, and Hawthorne, 1997; Davey Smith, Hart, Blane, and Hole, 1998; Eriksson et al., 1999; Frankel, Elwood, Sweetnam, Yamell, and Davey Smith, 1996; Kuh and Ben-Shlomo, 1997; Marmot and Wadsworth, 1997; Osmond and Barker, 2000; Ravelli, Der Meulen, Osmond, Barker, and Bleker, 1999; Ravelli, Stein, and Susser, 1976; Susser et al., 1996).

- Observation 2: Birthweight differences

In a recent study of birthweights among U.S.-born blacks, African-born blacks, and U.S.-born whites in Illinois (1980-1995), the mean birthweight of 44,046 infants of U.S.-born whites was 3,446 grams; of 3,135 infants of African-born blacks, 3,333 grams; but of 43,322 U.S.-born blacks, only 3,089 grams (Davis and Collins, 1997).

- Observation 3: Health status differences

Another recent study (Fang, Madhavan, and Alderman, 1996) showed that the health status of blacks living in New York City as adults was associated with their place of origin: the northern United States, the southern United States, or the Caribbean. The health status of those from the Caribbean was similar to New York City whites, and better than those from the northern United States; in turn, those from the northern United States had better health status than those from the southern United States.

• Observation 4: Infant mortality, Aboriginal population

Infant mortality among the Aboriginal population in British Columbia (BC), Canada, is substantially higher than the non-Aboriginal population. At the same time, life expectancy is lower than the rest of the BC population. However, what is most striking is that, in both cases, there are very large regional differences among Aboriginal populations residing in different parts of the province—variations much larger than for the non-Aboriginal population. As shown in Figures 5-1 and 5-2, the regions with the "best" Aboriginal health status are close to, or overlap with, the

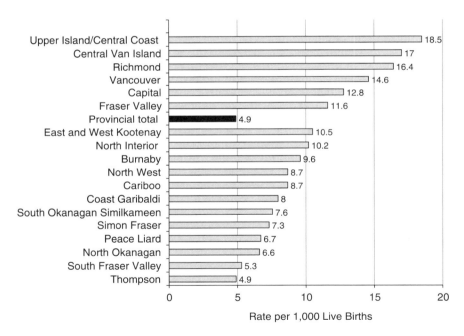

FIGURE 5-1 Infant mortality by health region for status: Indians, British Columbia, 1991-1999.
SOURCE: British Columbia Vital Statistics Agency (2001).

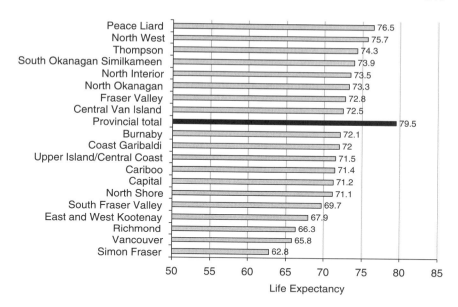

FIGURE 5-2 Life expectancy by health region for status: Indians, British Columbia, 1995-1999.
SOURCE: British Columbia Vital Statistics Agency (2001).

overall population average (British Columbia Vital Statistics Agency, 2001).

• Observation 5: Teenage suicide rates, Aboriginal population

Rates of suicide among Aboriginal teenagers in BC are, on average, much higher than the non-Aboriginal population. However, when the 196 reserve communities across BC are grouped according to the degree of local control they currently exercise over land, health, education, cultural, and other governmental services, the rate of teen suicide falls monotonically as the number of factors under local control goes up (Figure 5-3), such that the teenage suicide rate on reserves that control all these factors is lower than the non-Aboriginal rate for the province (Chandler and Lalonde, 1998).

This chapter contends that these observations, although diverse, form a consistent pattern that is comprehensible from a population health perspective and that can help to explain ethnic disparities in health status.

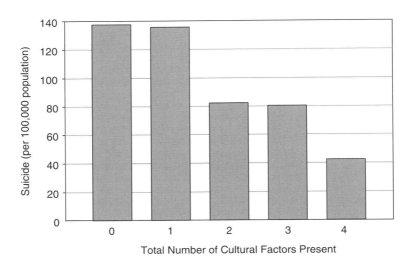

FIGURE 5-3 Aboriginal youth suicide rates by number of factors present in the community.
SOURCE: Chandler and Lalonde (1998).

POPULATION HEALTH PERSPECTIVE

Regarding the life-course dimension of ethnic disparities in health, the population health perspective begins with an incumbent hypothesis: that systematic inequalities in health status among distinct ethnic groups within a society are a product of the interaction between the developmental opportunities and vulnerabilities at each stage of the human life-course, on the one hand, with widely varying attributes of experience at the intimate, civic, and socioeconomic levels of society, on the other. Developmental stages are universal across human populations, notwithstanding ethnicity. In contrast, the nature of day-to-day life experience may differ systematically among ethnic groups. Systematic differences in health status emerge, primarily because some life-course interactions with life experiences are more health enhancing than others. The hierarchy of health status among different ethnic groups in society reflects the rank order of the average quality of life-course/societal interaction experienced by each ethnic group.

According to this hypothesis, ethnic differences in health status emerge from the same sort of nature-nurture interactions that produce socioeconomic differences in health status across the life-course. To produce systematic differences in health status, ethnic differences must be associated with systematically different developmental experiences, and systematically different "qualities" of interaction between the developing individual and his or her intimate, civic, and socioeconomic environment.

From this perspective it is possible to see how the following five introductory observations fit together:

- Observation 1: Protective early life factors
- Observation 2: Birthweight differences
- Observation 3: Health status differences
- Observation 4: Infant mortality, Aboriginal population
- Observation 5: Teenage suicide rates, Aboriginal population

The first three observations listed are examples of the protective effects of early experience: those who grew up in a society where they were not a stigmatized ethnic minority enjoyed health protection, both in adulthood and in the intergenerational transmission of birthweight. Those with the same racial/ethnic background, who grew up as a stigmatized minority in a white-dominated society, were not similarly protected. These examples, of course, are potentially confounded by differential migration according to health status, differential access to health care, and residual genetic/constitutional differences within nominally common "racial" groups (to be discussed).

The latter two observations listed are examples which deal exclusively with nonmigrants (indeed, "original peoples") in a jurisdiction with no financial barriers of access to medical care. Moreover, the Aboriginal peoples of BC fall into several different "nations" that, in turn, have different customs and traditions and, because of the physical barriers of mountains and ocean, had little tendency to interbreed before the era of modern transportation. Despite this, variations in health status across the province do not follow any known intra-Aboriginal national pattern, and huge differences by region are the rule. The nearly fourfold variation in infant mortality shown in Figure 5-1 is also unrelated to proximity to medical care. This range of mortality is a proxy for variations in the "quality" of the reproductive and early child environments encountered by the Aboriginal population. The teenage suicide example is the most direct for our current purposes. The degree of local control of the civic environment in Aboriginal communities is a measure of their liberation from external domination by white society. Figure 5-3 shows that the "degree of liberation" has a dose-response relationship to a key outcome of "healthy child development": teenage suicide.

UNDERSTANDING THE LIFE-COURSE

Life-course factors are now well understood to affect a diverse range of outcomes, from general well-being to physical functioning and chronic diseases (Keating and Hertzman, 1999; Kuh and Ben-Shlomo, 1997; Marmot and Wadsworth, 1997). Exposure to both beneficial and adverse circumstances over the life-course will vary for each individual and will constitute a unique "life exposure trajectory" that will manifest itself in different expressions of health and well-being.

Although this general perspective is noncontroversial, there are large problems of operationalization. Perhaps the most significant is the way in which early life phenomena are studied under the rubric of "development" whereas later life phenomena are studied under the rubric of "aging." Unlike the shorter lived primates, whose complete life-course and those of their offspring can be studied during a "normal" 30-year research career, human longevity poses a problem of how to "stitch together" longitudinal observations from early, middle, and late life into a coherent and credible whole. Because this process of stitching together has not been taken very far, development and aging research often appear to be in conflict. The output of developmental studies of health is often interpreted to claim that, by a certain (undefined) age, future health status has been predetermined, and the rest of the life-course merely reveals what the early years have fated. On the other hand, aging research often seems to treat the individuals who enter middle-aged and elderly cohorts as blank canvases on which later life events will be imprinted.

These separate solitudes need to be brought together. The next several paragraphs present the determinants of health from a developmental perspective, and will appear to some readers as though they reinforce the schism just described. To compensate for this weakness, the succeeding paragraphs will try to connect the developmental perspective to the aging perspective.

Biological Basis

The biological basis for life-course relationships to health arises from the similarity of human development to that of other primate and nonprimate species. From these sources we know that brain structures and functions can develop differently in differing early environments. The developing brain is an environmental organ that sculpts itself according to experience (Cynader and Frost, 1999). Differential experiences are closely associated with systematic differences in the function of at least three important physiological control systems: the HPA axis (the hypothalamic-pituitary-adrenal system, which controls cortisol secretion), the SAM axis (the sympatho-adrenal-medullary system, which controls epinephrine and norepinephrine secretion), and the PNI axis (the psycho-neuro-immune axis; that is, central nervous system influences on immune system function and blood-clotting factors). The SAM, HPA, and PNI axes all have a "life" within individuals in society, which, in turn, has an empirically demonstrable role in producing systematic differences in health over the life-course

(Hertzman, 2000). The hypothesis here is that early life experience profoundly shapes the ways these axes develop; that these body-regulatory and defense systems, in turn, experience the environment and respond to it in radically different ways in different individuals according to the differences in their early experiences; that these responses influence the lifelong health of the individual; and finally, that systematic differences in these responses across population groups in a society (whether defined by socioeconomic status, ethnicity, or geography) contribute to health disparities. The interest here is in the interplay—day to day, hour to hour, moment to moment—between the environments where people live, work, and grow up, on the one hand, and the development and responses of the SAM, HPA, and PNI axes, on the other, which lead to systematically differing health expectancies over a lifetime.

There are, of course, an infinite number of ways in which exposure to expression relationships can unfold over time. In some instances, there will be contemporaneous exposure and expression. If a piano falls on one's head, the exposure and the effects on health and well-being are simultaneous, unequivocal, and easily measured. But in most cases the connections from exposure to expression will be more subtle and will play out over long stretches of the life-course. The possible long-term exposure to expression relationships cluster into three generic patterns: "latency," "cumulative," and "pathway" (Hertzman and Wiens, 1996; Hertzman, Power, Matthews, and Manor, 2001; Power and Hertzman, 1997).

Latency

"Latency" means a relationship between an "exposure" at one point in the life-course and the probability of health "expressions" years or decades later, *irrespective of intervening experience*. The following examples validate the concept of latency.

Barker's "fetal origins hypothesis" posits that several chronic diseases in adult life originate from permanent changes in the structure, physiology, and metabolism of the fetal body as an adaptation to undernutrition (Barker, 1997). Studies of British records from early in the 20th century show associations of birthweight, placenta size, and weight gain in the first year of life with cardiovascular disease in the fifth decade (Barker, 1992, 1994). Fetal growth also has been associated with the development of insulin resistance in mid-life and onset of diabetes in the sixth and seventh decades of life (Osmond and Barker, 2000). Evidence of the relationship between birthweight and cardiovascular risk factors, such as hypertension, has now been found in numerous populations (Huxley, Shiell, and Law, 2000).

Studies of the Dutch Hunger Winter (1944-1945) showed that maternal nutritional deficiency in pregnancy was associated with an increased risk of antisocial personality disorder (ASPD) and schizophrenia among offspring in adult life (Neugebauer, Hoek, and Susser, 1999; Susser et al., 1996). These effects appeared to depend on the timing of prenatal insult: men exposed to severe maternal nutritional deficiency during the first and/or second trimesters of pregnancy had a risk of ASPD that was 2.5 times that of men who had not been exposed prenatally (Neugebauer et al., 1999).

Perhaps the quintessential example of latency arises from longitudinal studies, not of humans, but of rats. In several rat species, the degree of early suckling and licking of the newborn by its mother has a lifelong effect on a range of functions, most notably stress response, learning, and memory (Francis, Diorio, Liu, and Meaney, 1999). Maternal licking and suckling early in life influence the expression of certain genes that regulate the development of the HPA axis, which regulates the amount and pattern of cortisol that the rat's body produces in response to stressful life circumstances. Cortisol has a wide range of effects on physiological functioning. In the short term, it makes the rat more alert and ready to cope with danger. Over the long term, however, high levels of cortisol have the effect of accelerating the aging process in various organs within the body (Sapolsky, 1992). Infrequently suckled baby rats tend to develop, permanently, a highly reactive HPA axis. Frequently suckled rats develop a "down-regulated" HPA axis. The implications of these differences are far reaching. Having a down-regulated HPA axis is associated with better decision-making functions, quicker task learning, and a slower rate of loss of learning and memory functions. Thus, the frequently suckled baby rats acquire a lifelong advantage as a result of a systematic difference in early nurturant experience (Francis et al., 1999).

Cumulative Effects

"Cumulative" refers to multiple exposures over the life-course that have combined effects on health. Vulnerability and/or resiliency can combine over time through cumulating injuries/risk factors or cumulating privileges/protective factors. In some cases, cumulation will occur in a dose-response manner. For example, duration of exposure to adverse socioeconomic circumstances affects childhood growth, with persistent poverty increasing the risk of childhood stunting (low height for age) and wasting (low weight for age), whereas single-year income measures do not (Miller and Korenman, 1994).

Duration of exposure to particular socioeconomic circumstances shows a cumulative effect on several health outcomes in adulthood. In the 1958 British birth cohort, the occupational class of the male parent over the first three decades of life was found to be strongly predictive of health status in early adulthood (Power, Manor, and Matthews, 1999). Figure 5-4 shows a dramatic direct relationship between the risk of poor health and a score that is constructed by combining occupational status at four points in the life-course (with the lowest score indicating continuous high occupational status, and the highest score the reverse). The lifetime score represents cumulative duration and intensity of material/social privilege or deprivation. Those who were always in the lowest occupational class were approximately four times as likely to report poor health as those who were always in the highest. "Lifetime" occupational class is a stronger predictor of poor health than occupational class at any single point in time, indicating that duration of exposure to poor socioeconomic circumstances matters a great deal. Moreover, for both men and women, the risk increases monotonically with increasing lifetime scores (Figure 5-4). In other words, circumstances at each life stage build on one another. Similar patterns have been found by others (Lynch, Kaplan, and Shema, 1997).

Another variant would see different factors over the life-course add to effects of factors from early life. This might be described as a "multiple factor additive" variant. In the 1958 British birth cohort, chronic illness and disability at age 33 were predicted by factors in early life (childhood socioeconomic disadvantage and height), in adolescence (behavioral adjustment), and in adult life (injury and underweight/overweight) (Power, Li, and Manor, 2000).

Pathways

Finally, "pathways" refer to the ways in which individuals get onto well-worn life-course trajectories that carry with them a set of "health

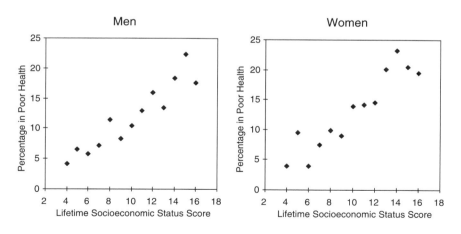

FIGURE 5-4 Poor health includes subjects who rated their health as fair at age 33 and cumulative socioeconomic circumstances (birth to age 33).
SOURCE: Power, Manor, and Matthews (1999).

chances" based on the socioeconomic and psychosocial circumstances that prevail along them. This occurs because a sequence of experiences at one stage of the life-course will influence the probability of other experiences later in the life-course. For those using different terminology, it should be recognized that social mobility is a function of the pathways model. There is a dominant sequence of events that unfolds as follows:

1. At first, early life social origins influence readiness for school (Ross and Roberts, 1999). Studies among preschool-age children in Canada and the United States have demonstrated that the circumstances of the family early in the child's life (income, education, single parenthood, and parenting style), neighborhood (safety, cohesion, and socioeconomic ghettoization), and social institutions (access to "quality" child care arrangements) are powerful determinants of cognitive and behavioral development (Duncan and Brooks-Gunn, 1997, 2000; Duncan, Brooks-Gunn, and Klebanov, 1994; Kohen, Hertzman, and Brooks-Gunn, 1998).

2. Cognitive, emotional, and behavioral readiness for school have consequences for school success and social adjustment. School readiness, as measured by cognitive and social-emotional competencies, is important because children who are not ready for school are more likely to experience school failure, conditions of unemployment, criminality (Tremblay, 1999; Tremblay, Masse, Perron, and LeBlanc, 1992), and psychological morbidity in young adulthood (Power et al., 1991). Intervention studies have demonstrated that improvements in the childhood environment can provide a long-lasting benefit to an individual's life-course trajectory (Hertzman and Wiens, 1996). The Perry Preschool Project demonstrated that an intensive child care and home visiting intervention at ages 3 and 4 could improve high school graduation rates, reduce teenage pregnancy, increase income, reduce dependence on social services, and reduce criminal activity by age 27 among socially disadvantaged children. From the standpoint of the pathway model, the most interesting observation was that the long-term benefits seemed to accrue from the manner in which the intervention improved the children's transition to school (Schweinhart, Barnes, and Weikart, 1993).

3. Next along the pathway, there is abundant evidence that people with a poorer education have more harmful health-related behaviors than those with a better education. Evidence for this pattern is found in relation to smoking, diet, wearing seat belts, and seeking preventive health care, such as immunization and PAP smears (Davey Smith et al., 1998; Winkleby, 1992).

4. Adult socioeconomic circumstances, also closely associated with educational attainment, have an impact on health in adult life (Drever and Whitehead, 1997; Evans, Barer, and Marmor, 1994; Kunst, Geurts, and van

den Berg, 1995; Kunst, Groenhof, Mackenbach, and Health, 1998). International studies of European, American, and Canadian populations demonstrate poorer self-reported health and mortality of the least educated groups (Feldman, Makuc, Kleinman, and Cornoni-Huntley, 1989; Kunst et al., 1995; Pappas, Queen, Hadden, and Fisher, 1993). Thus, social origins can have their effect on health status through their influence on social destinations.

Figure 5-5 (adapted from Hertzman et al., 2001) is meant to illustrate how latent, cumulative, and pathway effects combine with current circumstances to help "explain" health status across the life-course. The arrow in the figure represents the life-course, intersecting with the bulls-eye that represents society. Society is illustrated by three concentric circles representing increasingly broader levels of social aggregation where determinants of health are found: the personal social support network (most intimate), civil society (intermediate), and the socioeconomic environment (broadest). Despite problems of visual representation, the arrow is meant to intersect the bulls-eye at the most intimate level, and does so continuously on a day-to-day basis throughout the life-course. Thus, the figure represents the idea that health status is an emergent property of the ongoing interactions between the individual (at each stage of development across the life-course) and the conditions they encounter in the intimate, civic, and broader socioeconomic environments.

The example illustrated in Figure 5-5 uses this model, in a somewhat reduced form, to display findings from the 1958 British Birth Cohort study. In particular, it shows how experiences during the first 16 years of life

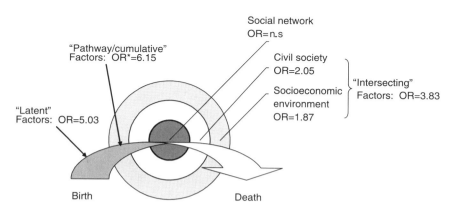

FIGURE 5-5 Contributions to self-rated health at age 33, 1958 birth cohort. OR = odds ratio. For interpretation, please see text. n.s. = not significant (p > 0.05).

affect self-rated health by age 33. In this model, the latent effects were the proportion of adult height the child had obtained by age 7, the regularity with which parents read to the child up to age 7, and the degree of socioemotional adjustment to school by age 7. These variables represent the three principal dimensions of early child development: physical, cognitive, and social-emotional-behavioral. In the model they were statistically independent of one another and of factors that came later in the life-course. The odds ratio of 5.03 suggests that those who have relatively rapid early growth, who were read to consistently, and who adjusted easily into school were one-fifth as likely to be in a state of fair or poor health by age 33 as those who grew slowly, were not read to consistently, and had trouble adjusting to school.

The statistically independent cumulative and pathway effects were: cumulative socioeconomic status at age 0, 7, 11, and 16; socioemotional adjustment to school at ages 11 and 16; and end-of-school qualifications. The model suggests that those who were always in the lowest socioeconomic category throughout childhood, who had ongoing trouble adjusting to school, and who dropped out without formal qualifications were approximately six times more likely to be in a state of fair or poor health by age 33 than those with the opposite status on each of these factors.

In addition, the model shows the extent to which current circumstances, at age 33, contribute to health status above and beyond the contributions of the earlier life-course. The odds ratio for fair/poor self-rated health is 1.87 comparing the lowest and highest current social class; 2.05 for those least affiliated to most affiliated in their local communities; and 3.83 for those with the least sense of control at work and in life, compared with those with the most.

I am unaware of analyses that parallel these by ethnic group in any of the world's large birth cohort studies. In particular, none of the American birth cohort or child longitudinal studies have attempted this sort of analysis. A great deal of work has been done trying to explain educational and developmental differences by nominal ethnic category in the United States, but little of this work has been further linked to health status in adulthood. I would propose that this be a priority to help understand the life-course contribution to ethnic differences in health status in the United States.

BRINGING DEVELOPMENT AND AGING TOGETHER

So far, this analysis covers only the period from birth to early adulthood. How does the developmental perspective link to aging? Here, I propose that four key points of tangency call out for further empirical investigation.

The Shakespearean Connection

In the soliloquy "All the World's a Stage," Shakespeare presented to the Western world a story of the human life-course as a rise (during early life) and a fall (during late life). Although there are more humanistic ways to view the life-course (such as the traditional Japanese notion of life being a voyage that ends at a final destination), the Shakespearean model is more suited to the biological realities. In this model, development is the rise and aging is the fall. Thus, the health and well-being of a given individual on the downward slope of the life-course would, in principle, be determined by two parameters: first, the height at the top of the rise—that is, how success-ful the process of development had been; and second, the rate of decline along the downward slope of aging. From this perspective, then, develop-ment and aging are tied together by the accumulation of "reserve capacity" during development and also by the prospect that early developmental experiences may influence the later life rate of decline.

Similarity of Life-Course Processes

Latent, pathway, and cumulative processes apply late in life, just as they do in early life. The example of the rate of cognitive decline in late life, the incidence of dementia, and their association with level of education earlier in life is a case where all three processes are relevant (Evans et al., 1993). Those with greater levels of education early in life may have slower rates of cognitive decline later in life because of a neurochemical reserve brought about as a result of the education process (a latent effect); or due to the social mobility/enhanced self-esteem associated with greater education (a pathway effect); or due to an association between greater education and greater cognitive stimulation throughout the working life (a cumulative effect).

Similarity of the Determinants of Healthy Aging and Healthy Child Development

Socioeconomic status, social integration, social support (Seeman and Crimmins, 2001), self-esteem (Seeman et al., 1995), and a sense of control or powerlessness at work and in life (Seeman and Lewis, 1995) have all been shown to influence the aging process, either through direct effects or through buffering or exacerbating of existing vulnerabilities. Many of these factors are also important influences in early life, and are reflected in Figure 5-5. Thus, notwithstanding the "rise and fall" dichotomy, the factors that affect the height of the rise and the rate of the fall may well be held in common.

The Life of the Host Defense Systems in Human Society

In our work on the early life-course, we have coined the term "biological embedding" to refer to the process whereby systematic differences in life experience translate into systematic differences in the response of the body's host defense systems to stress that, in turn, will affect organ-system aging and health status in later life (Hertzman, 2000). In the aging field, a highly complementary concept of "allostatic load" has been developed and operationalized to a much greater extent than biological embedding. Allostatic load is composed of a group of metabolic variables that, taken together, represent the metabolic set point of each aging individual's defense/stress response system (Seeman and McEwan, 1996). Allostatic load, stress, and aging can then be likened to a spring. As a spring is repeatedly used, its position at rest may become altered, altering its response to force bearing, and reducing its elasticity over time. In humans the metabolic set point (allostatic load) interacts with environmental stressors (analogous to force bearing). If allostatic load is not optimal, physiologic elasticity (that is, the ability to mount an effective physiological response to stress and return to baseline) may be lost at an accelerated rate, leading to accelerated biological aging. *The key point of tangency, and the key issue for life-course research, is the extent to which the process of biological embedding can "explain" individual or group differences in allostatic load, as they are first measured in adulthood.* The leading hypothesis would be that adverse early experiences would lead, through biological embedding, to a high-risk allostatic load in mid-life and late life.

OPPORTUNITIES FOR ETHNICITY TO AFFECT DEVELOPMENTAL TRAJECTORIES

Latency and Ethnicity

In theory, there are three ways that ethnic differences could translate into latent effects on health across the life-course. First, there is the potential for prenatal transmission of socioeconomic or psychosocial stresses through transplacental transmission of maternal experience via the secretion of cortisol and other stress hormones. The hypothesis here is that pregnant women from relatively deprived ethnic backgrounds will be more likely to find themselves under some form of uncontrollable socioeconomic or psychosocial stress during pregnancy. It has been shown that increased HPA axis activity during pregnancy can be reflected in increasing circulating cortisol in the fetus, both in humans and nonhuman primates (Gunnar and Barr, 1998; Post and Weiss, 1997). Fetal cortisol, in turn, has been shown to be active in neurobiological development. In Coe's (1999) work on rhesus monkeys, a randomized, controlled trial of increasing the level of uncontrollable maternal stress for short bursts during pregnancy (keeping all other aspects of gestational environment constant) led to developmental delays in their offspring. The Dutch Hunger Winter studies and several studies of the risks of low-birthweight and small-for-gestational-age babies have demonstrated that prenatal stress can affect birth outcome. However, I am unaware of any studies that directly connect ethnicity, circumstances during pregnancy, transplacental transmission of maternal experience, and developmental outcome.

Second, there is the potential for ethnic differences in parenting style to make a difference in early cognitive and social development. It is well known, and reasonably well documented, that different ethnic groups tend to have different bonding and attachment styles with their newborns; different values and beliefs regarding when and how to talk with young children and read to them; and parenting styles that can vary from the interactive to the apathetic to the authoritarian. It is now clear that each of these differences can make a difference in the cognitive and social development of the child. For example, it has been shown that the acquisition of vocabulary follows a dose–response relationship according to the degree of oral fluency in the home (Hart and Risley, 1995). I am not aware of any systematic measurements of ethnic differences in oral fluency and reading in the home. Anecdotally, however, these are thought to be large in Canada, with Aboriginal homes believed to be relatively lacking in verbal interchange.

In the Canadian National Longitudinal Survey of Children and Youth, apathetic and authoritarian parenting styles were strongly associated with developmental delay (both social and cognitive), even after other factors were taken into account (Willms, 2000). Once again, we have little useful information on how parenting styles vary by ethnicity. At the forefront of research in early language acquisition is the potential synergy between language and social development, and the degree to which visual contact with a parent or caregiver during language acquisition helps define its social meaning. This latter may be very relevant to ethnicity and early development. For example, Bornstein and Cote (2001) have shown that different cultural groups around the world tend to orient their babies differently when they are being held and carried. In North America, we tend to orient babies outward toward the world, whereas in Japan, they tend to face inward toward the parent.

Finally, there is the prospect that ethnicity is associated with transmission of systematically different messages regarding one's place in the social hierarchy during the neurobiological developmental phases of host defense and higher executive functions. The primitive structures in the mid-brain that sense and initiate physiological responses to threat develop over the first few years of life and, between the third and tenth year of life, form extensive synaptic connections with the executive functions of the prefrontal cortex. Both the early conditioning of the mid-brain and the nature of the connections to the prefrontal cortex appear to be highly conditioned by the environment in which the child develops. At present, we do not know the extent to which parents' perceptions of being a stigmatized group within society can be transmitted to the child during early development or the extent to which a strong family network can buffer such putative effects. We do know that children who grow up in physically abusive environments tend to have a lowered threshold for the recognition of, and physiological reaction to, threat in adult faces (Pollak, Cicchetti, and Klorman, 1998). This is evidence, albeit fragmentary, that early transmission of place in the social hierarchy can occur and can endure.

Children growing up in unsafe, noncohesive, and low socioeconomic ghetto neighborhoods tend to reflect these conditions in cognitive and social development delays by age 4 (Kohen et al., 2002). In Canada, Aboriginal children tend to grow up in such neighborhoods and in the United States black and Latino children tend to do so as well. But once again, the principal research question is unanswered: To what extent is ethnicity associated with differences in early childhood environments that condition key sensing and executive response systems in ways that influence health and well-being across the life-course? One excellent research opportunity here would be a life-course study of the factors that contribute to higher blood pressure among American blacks than whites.

Pathways and Ethnicity

The story of pathways and ethnicity is, first, the story of what happens when a visible ethnic status becomes a social constraint (or social opportunity). The ways in which visible status can affect educational and social mobility through the perceptions and actions of powerful individuals and institutions are too numerous and well known to review here. Insofar as these perceptions have been prejudicial to visible minorities, limiting their trajectories of income, education, and/or occupation, they can be taken to be relevant determinants of ethnic differences in health status, because adult socioeconomic status carries powerful health expectations with it.

The second large factor is readiness for school. When systematic differences in early childhood experiences lead to differences in children's readiness for school, a negative pathway effect is probable. It is well known that children who enter school developmentally unready are themselves at risk of school failure. Classroom composition also appears to affect the educational trajectories of those who come into school fully ready for the experience. Our work in Vancouver shows that the proportion of kindergarten children who are developmentally vulnerable entering school varies sixfold among neighborhoods. Our data suggest that a high proportion of children not "ready for school" seem to hold back the "ready-for-school" children (Mustard and Picherack, 2002). Presumably, this is a classroom pacing effect. In Vancouver, the neighborhoods most heavily populated by Aboriginal children are those with high rates of crime, commercial sex, and drugs; high proportions of children entering school in a developmentally vulnerable state; and low levels of subsequent educational success. Although similar data on readiness for school are yet to be collected in American cities, it is well known that the neighborhoods heavily populated by Latino and black children have similar characteristics to those populated by Vancouver Aboriginals.

Other aspects of the pathway effect include the role of parental expectations on children's developmental trajectories and local levels of environmental enrichment: neighborhood programs supporting parenting and development, school quality beyond classroom composition, and the availability of successful role models during the teenage years and adulthood. Sweden and Japan have been successful in compressing socioeconomic gradients in achievement of basic literacy and numeracy skills by introducing flexibility into the transition from preschool to school. In Sweden this is accomplished through a flexible transition from play-based to formal learning styles. In Japan it is based on flexible teaching and learning styles in the primary grades, especially with respect to quantitative concepts.

It should be reemphasized here that early life conditions affect social mobility through cognitive, social-emotional-behavioral, and physical readiness for school according to the pathway model. To the extent that ethnic differences in school readiness exist, and are related to early life experiences, there will be a social mobility effect (or, for that matter, a social immobility effect) on later health status. To the extent that ethnicity differentially affects early physical development, subsequently affecting school performance and social mobility, there could be a reverse causality effect.

Cumulative Effects and Ethnicity

The most obvious cumulative effect is that associated with the duration and intensity of socioeconomic deprivation among those ethnic groups who tend to be deprived. Here, the literature on socioeconomic deprivation and health per se can simply be read into the record. However, a variety of other "positive" cumulative effects may apply to specific ethnic groups. In Texas first-generation Mexican families have much better health status than would be expected based on their socioeconomic conditions. This has been attributed, in passing, to the protective effects of belonging to a strong, traditional extended family that, after a generation in America, begins to break down. There is also a well-known phenomenon in Canada and the United States of increased late-life survivorship among those ethnic groups whose early life survival rates are relatively low, particularly a tendency for supplementary life expectancy beyond age 70 to be higher among African Americans and Canadian Aboriginals than the white population, despite their lower life expectancy at birth.

A second prospect, which undoubtedly will be receiving increased attention in coming years, is disjunction between genetic susceptibilities and environmental exposures. This can become relevant either when an ethnic group migrates to a new place with a mixture of biological, physical, chemical, cultural, and nutritional characteristics to which it has not been historically adapted or when a host population is overtaken by an in-migrating population that gains hegemony with respect to the biological, cultural, nutritional, or chemical environment. The roles of smallpox and tuberculosis in wiping out host populations in North America during the early years of European colonization are examples of the latter. The spread of syphilis to the European population and the loss of the adaptive value of sickle cell trait to malaria among the American black population are examples of the former. As of this writing, a key issue in Canada is the role of Western diet in the epidemic of diabetes mellitus among the Aboriginal population. Traditional Aboriginal diets were largely absent of unrefined carbohydrates, so the leading hypothesis is that the increasing penetration of Western diet has created an invidious interaction between diet and genetically determined metabolic processes in Aboriginals that are easily overwhelmed by large carbohydrate loads. However, it is likely that, like most chronic diseases, the full explanation will turn out to be more multifactorial in nature.

COMPLEMENTARY EXPLANATIONS FOR ETHNIC DIFFERENCES ACROSS THE LIFE-COURSE

Four groups of explanations could potentially account for ethnic differences in health status across the life-course through population selection processes that are not usually considered to be life-course phenomena. I label them differential migration, differential social mobility, genetic mono-causation, and differential utilization of health services. This section will briefly show how difficult it is, in practice, to make a clear-cut distinction between life-course and non-life-course phenomena. Something that at first glance appears to "confound" life-course may actually be a contributor to it.

Differential Migration

Take, for example, the differential migration hypothesis: Populations that migrate around the world seeking freedom and opportunity are systematically different from both the populations they left behind and those that they encounter when they arrive in their new homes. Also, populations that move voluntarily are systematically different from those that are subject to forced migration. They, in turn, are systematically different from those they leave and those they encounter when they arrive at their involuntary destination. A wealth of evidence supports the existence of each of these phenomena from around the world. Moreover, the first two observations, protective early life factors and birthweight differences, given in this chapter could be accounted for by the fact that Caribbean and African blacks in the United States are voluntary migrants, whereas American-born blacks are either nonmigrants or, if ones' historical memory is long enough, forced migrants.

As a "non-life-course" hypothesis, differential migration has the potential to conceal important information by avoiding the question of how migrants differ from the rest of the population and how these differences evolve over time. For example, there is evidence that over the generations, the children of black Caribbean immigrants to the United States start to develop an American black "racialized" identity that strips them of certain beneficial effects of their parents' identities (Waters, 1999). In other words, what appears at first to be a characteristic of the migrant may be a characteristic of the migrant-environment interaction during vulnerable phases of social development over the life-course. Another example of differential migration revealing a life course dimension concerns cancer in Japanese migrants to California. They arrived in California with the typical Japanese ratio of stomach-to-colon cancer risk that, within two generations, converted to the typical North American pattern (Doll and Peto, 1981). By following migrant families over several generations, it was possible to conclude that an environmental/life-course interaction was decisive in what, initially, looked like a fixed population difference between migrant and host population.

Differential Social Mobility

Differential social mobility is well known to be influenced by early social and economic factors shaping the life-course trajectory. However, critical appraisal requires consideration of the prospect that differential mobility may also be based, to some extent, on biological characteristics differentially distributed by ethnicity that make some groups more (or less) adaptable to the socioeconomic and psychosocial environments of modern society. This hypothesis would suggest that the social destinations of different ethnic groups are (to some extent) predetermined, and thus the health characteristics of these social destinations are predetermined, too. This hypothesis rests on old and highly politically charged premises that, when articulated, rarely lead to useful investigation.

Whatever the role of predestination, two counterfactuals must be stated. First, the more we know about brain development, the clearer it becomes that the developing brain is an environmental organ and is profoundly adaptable according to early environmental experiences. That is, phenomena that might be seen as static characteristics of a given ethnicity may turn out to be products of interactions between environment and life course. Second, with the passage of decades and centuries, privileged and deprived ethnic groups tend to change places with one another, and with these changes come parallel changes in the image of their capabilities as a group. One relevant example is the radical transformation of the image of Asian peoples in North America during the 20th century.

Genetic Mono-Causation

Genetic mono-causation refers to the effects of genetic differences between ethnic groups that are uninfluenced or modified by the physical or social environment, past or present. Where these exist, they could, in theory, lead to systematic differences in health status among ethnic groups that would be unchangeable over place and time. Although there are plenty of well-known examples of health conditions that are found in disproportionate numbers in particular ethnic groups, these conditions are all comparatively rare and cannot explain large differences in health status by ethnicity. For genetic mono-causation to play a significant role, there would need to be something on the order of a senescence gene (or gene complex) that accelerated or slowed the aging of cells across a variety of organ systems, and it would need to be nonrandomly distributed by ethnicity. Although such genes may exist, and may be distributed in a nonrandom fashion among different ethnic groups, it is worth noting that during the 20th century the average life expectancy of the citizens of the world's 25 wealthiest countries rose by 30 years, irrespective of ethnic differences and without recourse to genetic change. There is no evidence that genetic mono-causation has played a significant role in explaining the differences in health status among different ethnic groups that exist today, and it is likely that the role of genetic mono-causation will remain marginal in the future.

Differential Utilization of Health Services

Finally, there is the issue of differential utilization of health care services, by ethnic groups, that are unrelated to differences in health status. These certainly exist. Language barriers of access to care have been documented in many jurisdictions and are strongly associated with ethnicity. For example, in the early 1990s in inner-city Vancouver, 25 percent of surveyed parents who had not taken their primary school-aged children to a dentist in the past year cited "language barriers" as the reason (Hertzman, McLean, Kohen, Dunn, and Evans, 2002). Similarly, cultural factors may inhibit access to care. In Canada, an important subject of investigation and service innovation is ensuring timely access to health care for immigrant women from cultures where women have traditionally played a subordinate social role. Once again, this cannot be construed as a clear-cut non-life-course process because differential utilization of health care early in life can influence health status throughout the balance of the life-course.

AN AGENDA FOR RESEARCH

The framework of understanding presented here strongly implies an agenda for research, and several examples of it have been scattered throughout this chapter. In broad terms, this research agenda hinges on four strategies:

1. There needs to be better exploitation of migrator studies in ways that can estimate the influences of early life factors, social construction of identity, sense of coherence, health selection, and the other categories mentioned. Canada and the United States are two obvious places where such research is feasible because of high rates of immigration, diversity of sources of immigrants, and easy access to second-, third-, and fourth-generation migrant populations. Cooperation must be developed between the research community and the immigration authorities in order to find ethical ways to gain access to sensitive administrative data and direct access to immigrants. In Canada, these relationships are gradually being developed through persistent efforts by population and health researchers to earn the trust of immigration officials for research in the public interest.

2. There needs to be better strategic exploitation of birth cohort studies to understand nature-nurture differences by ethnic status across the life-course. In the United States the primary source for this work is the National Longitudinal Study of Youth (NLSY). It has been used by several investigators cited in this chapter (Duncan and Brooks-Gunn, 1997; Guo and Harris, 2000) to study socioeconomic and neighborhood effects on child development. This data source, in particular, has been used to show how contextual factors have affected differential development among American black and white children. This work needs to be followed forward in time to the ages at which health outcomes become prevalent. To *assist this process, it would be of great value to create a strategic partnership with the Panel Study of Income Dynamics (PSID).* The PSID is an ongoing annual survey of several thousand households that began in 1968 and has been refreshed over time (Lavis, 1997; McDonough, Duncan, Williams, and House, 1997). It has been a rich source of information on labor market

dynamics in relation to adult health outcomes because of its focus on a middle age range. Analysis of early childhood experiences of the PSID cohorts should be carried out in relation to their health outcomes in mid-life. This would form a powerful complement to the NLSY and inform it about the direction that adult follow-ups should take.

Moreover, there is a need for American, British, Canadian, New Zealand, and continental European birth cohort studies (and other child longitudinal studies) to develop common protocols for defining different ethnic groups and comparing their life-course trajectories in different societies. This, of course, is easier said than done. Despite the large size of many of these studies, the number of children of a specific ethnic group in any sample may be too small for analysis. Also, developing common international protocols of coordinated analysis runs up against funding asymmetries, researcher resistance, and other factors. UNICEF may have a role here. It has shown a strong interest in child development in different societies, especially those in transition, and may be a powerful platform for brokering useful international, intercohort comparisons.

3. An area in which "quick wins" may be possible would be to construct case studies of successes versus failures of melting pots—working backward from health status to understand why some melting pots support good health status among specific ethnic groups, while others do not. For example, although Canada's black population is far smaller, as a proportion of the total, than America's, there has never been a discourse of black health disadvantage in Canada. If Canada-U.S. cooperation like that developed for the recent income inequality and mortality studies were established, it would be possible to subject this to rigorous empirical test, working backward to try to understand any systematic differences found. A similar attempt could be made with Canadian and American Aboriginal populations. Here, we know that although America's treatment of its native population was harsher than Canada's in the 17th to 19th centuries, Canada's policies of forced assimilation were more draconian during the 20th century. Do these differences make a difference with respect to current health status? As it currently stands, it is comparatively easy to capture Aboriginal mortality in Canada, but much more difficult in the United States. Overcoming the obstacles to Canada-U.S. comparisons in this respect should be a priority.

4. Finally, we need to mobilize those who work on the neurobiology, endocrinology, and immunology of human development to understand better how ethnic differences and different forms of ethnicity-society interaction can embed themselves in human biology so that systematic differences in health status can occur. For example, some forms of ethnic-society interactions (material and psychosocial) appear to be harmful to health, and

others do not. In another example, it seems to be worse to be black than brown in America despite the visibility of both. Also, it seems that the effects of ethnicity are more pronounced for black men than women in America, at least in terms of economic success and survival through the late teenage years and young adulthood. The field of resiliency (Grotberg, 1995; Werner, 1989) needs to be brought into the discussion here. There is evidence from many manmade and natural disaster zones around the world that a relatively large proportion (approximately 30 percent) of children seem to be strengthened, rather than weakened, by their negative early experiences. They are deemed to be the resilient children. Resiliency seems to accrue to those who have a strong sense of self-efficacy and the sense that they are loved and supported by significant others. Whether or not resiliency can be taught, or engendered through social initiative, may be of great significance in relation to ethnic disparities in health over the life-course and to the biological embedding of adverse early experiences.

REFERENCES

Barker, D.J.P. (1992). *Fetal and infant origins of adult disease.* London: BMJ Books.

Barker, D.J.P. (1994). *Mothers, babies and disease in later life.* London: BMJ Books.

Barker, D.J.P. (1997). Fetal nutrition and cardiovascular disease in later life. *British Medical Bulletin, 53,* 96-108.

Barker, D.J.P., and Osmond, C. (1986). Infant mortality, childhood nutrition, and ischemic heart disease in England and Wales. *The Lancet, 1,* 1077-1081.

Blane, D., Hart, C.L., Davey Smith, G., Gillis, C.R., Hole, D.J., and Hawthorne, V.M. (1996). Association of cardiovascular disease risk factors with socioeconomic position during childhood and during adulthood. *British Medical Journal, 313,* 1434-1438.

Bornstein, M.H., and Cote, L.R. (2001). Mother-infant interaction and acculturation: I. Behavioural comparisons in Japanese American and South American families. *International Journal of Behavioural Development, 25,* 549-563.

British Columbia Vital Statistics Agency. (2001). *Regional analysis of health statistics for status Indians in British Columbia 1991-1999.* Victoria, Canada: Ministry of Health Services.

Chandler, M.J., and Lalonde, C. (1998). Cultural continuity as a hedge against suicide in Canada's first nations. *Transcultural Psychiatry, 35,* 191-219.

Coe, C. (1999). Psychosocial factors and psychoneuroimmunology within a lifespan perspective. In D. Keating and C. Hertzman (Eds.), *Developmental health and the wealth of nations* (pp. 201-219). New York: Guilford Press.

Cynader, M.S., and Frost, B.J. (1999). Mechanisms of brain development: Neuronal sculpting by the physical and social environment. In D. Keating and C. Hertzman (Eds.), *Developmental health and the wealth of nations* (pp. 153-184). New York: Guilford Press.

Davey Smith, G., Hart, C., Blane, D., Gillis, C., and Hawthorne, V. (1997). Lifetime socioeconomic position and mortality: Prospective observational study. *British Medical Journal, 314,* 547-552.

Davey Smith, G., Hart, C., Blane, D., and Hole, D. (1998). Adverse socioeconomic conditions in childhood and cause specific adult mortality: Prospective observational study. *British Medical Journal, 316,* 1631-1635.

Davis, R.J., and Collins, J.W. (1997). Differing birthweight among infants of US-born blacks, African-born blacks, and U.S.-born whites. *New England Journal of Medicine, 337,* 1209-1214.

Doll, R., and Peto, R. (1981). *The causes of cancer.* Oxford, England: Oxford University Press.

Drever, F., and Whitehead, M. (1997). *Health inequalities.* (DS #15, The Stationery Office). London: Office for National Statistics.

Duncan, G.J., and Brooks-Gunn, J. (Eds.). (1997). *Consequences of growing up poor.* New York: Russell Sage Foundation.

Duncan, G.J., and Brooks-Gunn, J. (2000). Family poverty, welfare reform, and child development. *Child Development, 71,* 188-196.

Duncan, G.J., Brooks-Gunn, J., and Klebanov, P.K. (1994). Economic deprivation and early childhood development. *Child Development, 65,* 296-318.

Eriksson, J.G., Forsen, T., Tuomilehto, J., Winter, P.D., Osmond, C., and Barker, D.J.P. (1999). Catch-up growth in childhood and death from coronary heart disease: Longitudinal study. *British Medical Journal, 318,* 427-431.

Evans, D.A., Beckett, L.A., Albert, M.S., Hebert, L.E., Scherr, P.A., Funkenstein, H.H., and Taylor, J.O. (1993). Level of education and change in cognitive function in a community population of older persons. *Annals of Epidemiology, 3,* 71-77.

Evans, R.G., Barer, M.L., and Marmor, T.R. (Eds.). (1994). *Why are some people healthy and others not? The determinants of health of populations.* New York: Aldine de Gruyter.

Fang, J., Madhavan, S., and Alderman, M.H. (1996, November). The association between birthplace and mortality from cardiovascular causes among black and white residents of New York City. *New England Journal of Medicine, 335*(21), 1545-1551.

Feldman, J.J., Makuc, D. M., Kleinman, J.C., and Cornoni-Huntley, J. (1989). National trends in educational differentials in mortality. *American Journal of Epidemiology, 129*(5), 919-933.

Francis, D., Diorio, J., Liu, D., and Meaney, M.J. (1999). Nongenomic transmission across generations of maternal behavior and stress responses in the rat. *Science, 286,* 1155-1158.

Frankel, S., Elwood, P., Sweetnam, P., Yarnell, J., and Davey Smith, G. (1996). Birthweight, body-mass index in middle age, and incident coronary heart disease. *The Lancet, 348,* 1478-1480.

Grotberg, E. (1995). *A guide to promoting resilience in children: Strengthening the human spirit.* The Hague, The Netherlands: Bernard van Leer Foundation.

Gunnar, M.R., and Barr, R. (1998). Stress, early brain development, and behavior. *Infants and Young Children, 11,* 1-14.

Guo, G., and Harris, K.M. (2000). The mechanisms mediating the effects of poverty on children's intellectual development. *Demography, 37,* 431-447.

Hart, B., and Risley, T.R. (1995). *Meaningful differences in the everyday experience of young American children.* Baltimore: Paul H. Brookes.

Hertzman, C. (2000). The biological embedding of early experience and its effects on health in adulthood. *Annals of the New York Academy of Sciences, 896,* 85-95.

Hertzman, C., and Wiens, M. (1996). Child development and long-term outcomes: A population health perspective and summary of successful interventions. *Social Sciences and Medicine, 43,* 1083-1095.

Hertzman, C., Power, C., Matthews, S., and Manor, O. (2001). Using an interactive framework of society and lifecourse to explain self-rated health in early adulthood. *Social Sciences and Medicine, 53,* 1575-1585.

Hertzman, C., McLean, S., Kohen, D., Dunn, J., and Evans, T. (2002). *Early development in Vancouver: Report of the Community Asset Mapping Project (CAMP).* Available: http://www.earlylearning.ubc.ca [Accessed September 10, 2003].

Huxley, R.R., Shiell, A.W., and Law, C.M. (2000). The role of size at birth and postnatal catch-up growth in determining systolic blood pressure: A systematic review of the literature. *Journal of Hypertension, 18*, 815-831.

Keating, D., and Hertzman, C. (1999). *Developmental health and the wealth of nations.* New York: Guilford Press.

Kohen, D.E., Brooks-Gunn, J., Leventhal, T., and Hertzman, C. (2002). Neighbourhood income and physical and social disorder in Canada: Associations with young children's competencies. *Child Development, 73*, 1844-1869.

Kuh, D.L., and Ben-Shlomo, Y. (1997). *A life-course approach to chronic disease epidemiology: Tracing the origins of ill health from early to adult life.* Oxford, England: Oxford University Press.

Kunst, A.E., Geurts, J.J.M., and van den Berg, J. (1995). International variation in socioeconomic inequalities in self-reported health. *Journal of Epidemiology and Community Health, 49*, 117-123.

Kunst, A.E., Groenhof, F., Mackenbach, J.P., and Health, E.W. (1998). Occupational class and cause specific mortality in middle aged men in 11 European countries: Comparison of population based studies. *British Medical Journal, 316*(7145), 1636-1642.

Lavis, J.N. (1997). *An inquiry into the links between labour-market experiences and health.* Doctoral dissertation, Harvard University.

Lynch, J.W., Kaplan, G.A., and Shema, S.J. (1997). Cumulative impact of sustained economic hardship on physical, cognitive, psychological, and social functioning. *New England Journal of Medicine, 337*(26), 1889-1895.

Marmot, M.G., and Wadsworth, M.E.J. (Eds.). (1997). Fetal and early childhood environment: Long-term health implications. *British Medical Bulletin, 53*, 3-9.

McDonough, P., Duncan, G.J., Williams, D., and House, J. (1997). Income dynamics and adult mortality in the United States, 1972 through 1989. *American Journal of Public Health, 87*, 1476-1483.

Miller, J., and Korenman, S. (1994). Poverty and children's nutritional status in the United States. *American Journal of Epidemiology, 140*, 233-243.

Mustard, F., and Picherack, F. (2002). *Early child development in British Columbia: Enabling communities.* Toronto, Canada: Founders' Network.

Neugebauer, R., Hoek, H.W., and Susser, E. (1999). Prenatal exposure to wartime famine and development of antisocial personality disorder in early adulthood. *Journal of the American Medical Association, 282*, 455-462.

Osmond, C., and Barker, D.J.P. (2000). Fetal, infant, and childhood growth are predictors of coronary heart disease, diabetes, and hypertension in adult men and women. *Environmental Health Perspectives, 108*(Suppl. 3), 545-553.

Pappas, G., Queen, S., Hadden, W., and Fisher, G. (1993). The increasing disparity in mortality between socio-economic groups in the United States, 1960 and 1986. *New England Journal of Medicine, 329*, 103-108.

Pollak, S., Cicchetti, D., and Klorman, R. (1998). Stress, memory, and emotion: Developmental considerations from the study of child maltreatment. *Development and Psychopathology, 10*, 811-828.

Post, R.M., and Weiss, S.R. (1997). Emergent properties of neural systems: How focal molecular neurobiological alterations can affect behavior. *Development and Psychopathology, 9*(4), 907-929.

Power, C., and Hertzman, C. (1997). Social and biological pathways linking early life and adult disease. *British Medical Bulletin, 53*(1), 210-221.

Power, C., Manor, O., and Fox, A.J. (1991). *Health and class: The early years.* London: Chapman Hall.

Power, C., Manor, O., and Matthews, S. (1999). The duration and timing of exposure: Effects of socio-economic environment on adult health. *American Journal of Public Health, 89*(7), 1059-1066.

Power, C., Li, L., and Manor, O. (2000). A prospective study of limiting longstanding illness in early adulthood. *International Journal of Epidemiology, 29,* 131-139.

Ravelli, A.C., Der Meulen, J.H., Osmond, C., Barker, D.J., and Bleker, O.P. (1999). Obesity at the age of fifty in men and women exposed to famine prenatally. *American Journal of Clinical Nutrition, 70*(5), 811-816.

Ravelli, G.P., Stein, Z.A., and Susser, M.W. (1976). Obesity in young men after famine exposure in utero and early infancy. *New England Journal of Medicine, 295*(7), 349-353.

Ross, D.P., and Roberts, P. (1999). *Income and child well-being: A new perspective on the poverty debate.* Ottawa, Canada: Canadian Council on Social Development.

Sapolsky, R.M. (1992). *Stress, the aging brain, and the mechanisms of neuron death.* Cambridge, MA: MIT Press.

Schweinhart, L.J., Barnes, H.V., and Weikart, D.P. (1993). Significant benefits: The High/Scope Perry preschool study through age 27. *Monographs of the High/Scope Educational Research Foundation, 10.*

Seeman, M., and Lewis, S. (1995). Powerlessness, health and mortality: A longitudinal study of older men and mature women. *Social Sciences and Medicine, 41,* 517-525.

Seeman, T.E., and Crimmins, E. (2001). Social environment effects on health and aging. *Annals of the New York Academy of Sciences, 954,* 88-117.

Seeman, T.E., and McEwan, B.S. (1996). Impact of social environment characteristics on neuroendocrine regulation. *Psychosomatic Medicine, 58,* 459-471.

Seeman, T.E., Berkman, L.F., Gulanski, B.I., Robbins, R.J., Greenspan, S.L., Charpentier, P.A., and Rowe, J.W. (1995). Self-esteem and neuroendocrine response to challenge: Macarthur studies of successful aging. *Journal of Psychosomatic Research, 39,* 69-84.

Susser, E., Neugebauer, R., Hoek, H.W., et al. (1996). Schizophrenia after prenatal famine: Further evidence. *Archives of General Psychiatry, 53,* 25-31.

Tremblay, R.E. (1999). When children's development fails. In D. Keating and C. Hertzman (Eds.), *Developmental health and the wealth of nations* (pp. 55-71). New York: Guilford Press.

Tremblay, R.E., Masse, B., Perron, D., and LeBlanc, M. (1992). Disruptive behaviour, poor school achievement, delinquent behaviour, and delinquent personality: Longitudinal analyses. *Journal of Consulting and Clinical Psychology, 60,* 64-72.

Waters, M.C. (1999). *Black identities: West Indian immigrant dreams and American realities.* Cambridge, MA: Harvard University Press.

Werner, E.E. (1989). Children of the garden island. *Scientific American, 260*(4), 106-111.

Willms, D. (2000). *Vulnerable children in Canada.* Edmonton, Canada: University of Alberta Press.

Winkleby, M.A. (1992). Socioeconomic status and health: How education, income, and occupation contribute to risk factors for cardiovascular disease. *American Journal of Public Health, 82,* 816-820.

6

Selection Processes in the Study of Racial and Ethnic Differentials in Adult Health and Mortality

Alberto Palloni and Douglas C. Ewbank

This chapter examines the potential influence exerted by selection processes in the estimation of racial and ethnic differentials in health and mortality. Selection is important because it may influence the direction and magnitude of observed racial and ethnic differentials. In addition, selection processes may exaggerate (attenuate) estimates of effects of membership in a racial or ethnic group that occur due to the existence of intervening mechanisms. We do not undertake this task with the presumption that selection processes are the only or even the most important mechanisms that generate observed racial and ethnic disparities in health and mortality. Instead, we argue that the formulation of sensible inferences and a richer understanding of these disparities require that we consider them explicitly, on an equal explanatory footing, with other possible interpretations. Giving short shrift to or dismissing selection processes on the grounds that they are of trivial importance or because they have been invoked at times in ill-advised applications of social Darwinism only obfuscates the problem. Indeed, some selection processes at least involve mechanisms through which social and economic disparities within racial or ethnic groups are reproduced over time and across generations. To the extent that these mechanisms are empirically relevant for health and mortality, selection processes become an integral part of the production of racial and ethnic disparities. Therefore, they should be treated adroitly instead of being portrayed as a nuisance. We will show that, far from negating the role that material, cultural, social, and behavioral factors have in the production of health and mortality inequalities, explanations that invoke selection mechanisms identify alternative paths through which these factors may influence health and mortality. Thus, interpretations based on selection arguments can serve to identify social and economic processes that perpetuate social stratification in societies at large as well as within racial and ethnic groups.

In this chapter we introduce terminological clarifications and examine some examples of selection processes. We provide a precise definition of selection processes that pertain to health and mortality inequalities, and introduce a simple taxonomy to classify them. We examine strategies for conceptualizing selection processes within the literature on health and mortality. We review a broad array of arguments regarding selection, from those that promote it as a universal cause of all social and economic inequalities in mortality and health, to those that consider it as the intellectual debris of genetic determinism. We examine in some detail three classes of selection processes that are relevant in the area of racial and ethnic health disparities. Using a mixture of simulated and empirical data, we estimate the potential magnitude of their effects and show that, in some cases at least, the impact of selection processes can be quite large—large enough to lead to misinterpretation of observable data and to erroneous policy prescriptions. The chapter ends with a brief discussion of alternative approaches that address conceptual and empirical problems associated with the identification of selection processes.

CONCEPTUAL CLARIFICATION: NATURE OF SELECTION PROCESSES

Conceptualization and Examples

The observed association between an individual's social class or position and health status and mortality risks can be due to two different processes. The first is one whereby influences on health and mortality result from the action of characteristics intrinsic to the social position. Individuals are endowed with these characteristics only by virtue of having attained the social position. For example, members of higher social classes may experience lower mortality because they command more wealth or have attained higher educational levels, and either of these traits is conducive to better health and lower mortality risks.

The second process occurs because individuals have traits or attributes that simultaneously increase their likelihood of accessing (leaving) social positions and exert an influence on their health status and mortality risks. For example, attributes that enhance an individual's health status during adulthood may also contribute to more advantageous earning profiles and to higher educational attainment. In this case the observed association between social position or class, on the one hand, and health status and mortality risks, on the other, is at least partially the result of the mechanics of accession processes, not the consequence of endowments of the social position or class conferred to individuals when they reach it. The observed association between social class and health or mortality is a consequence of a "health selection process" whereby those sharing a particular social position are disproportionately "selected" from among members of the population who also share particularly low (high) values of the health-relevant traits or attributes.

The literature on social class and racial and ethnic health and mortality differentials has conventionally focused on mechanisms of the first type and seeks to quantify the direct effects of social stratification on health and mortality differentials. However, because of the presence of the second mechanism alluded to earlier, inferences regarding the direct effects of membership in certain social positions cannot be based solely on observed correlations. First, identification of selection mechanisms and estimation of their contribution to observed correlations is an important endeavor that leads to more precise estimation of the direct effects of social classes or social positions. In statistical jargon, accounting for selection is necessary to obtain consistent estimates of the effects of social class on health status and mortality. Second, except in the case when traits relevant for both health and social stratification are allocated at random, mechanisms involving health selection are part of the overall process whereby social stratification generates health and mortality inequalities and thus should also be a focus of study for researchers interested in the genesis of health and mortality differentials.

We now review examples of selection processes.

The "Healthy Worker" Effect

The "healthy worker" effect refers to cases when individuals are able to occupy a place in an occupational hierarchy by virtue of their superior health status. For example, a study relating work activities and heart disease (Paffenbarger, Laughlin, and Gima, 1970) showed that the optimal job allocation strategy among stevedores required careful matching of physical demands associated with job duties and individuals' characteristics. As a result individuals in superior health were more likely to be assigned to the most demanding and risky jobs. This could lead to the paradoxical situation whereby individuals who occupy more demanding, stressful, and risky positions are in better health. In this case, the observed association between, say, a measure of occupational risk or exposure to stress, on the one hand, and health and mortality, on the other, is less than the true association. The fact that incumbents of occupational positions with higher exposure to illnesses and disability are drawn from among the healthiest members of the population can lead to an **attenuation and even reversal** of the true association between risk exposure and prevalence of illness or disability. Clearly, one cannot infer from observation that more stressful and physically strenuous jobs are more beneficial for individuals' health. Although in this example the allocation of positions according to health status takes place through an explicit decision-making process, this rarely will be the case. Invariably it will occur via the operation of mechanisms that are latent, complex, influenced by time lags, and hardly ever explicitly manifested or justified.

In another study focusing on the association between mortality and exposure to radiation hazards, it was shown that mortality was lower among employees working within a nuclear facility than among the population living in the surrounding area (Voelz et al., 1978). But this observation cannot be construed to suggest that exposure to higher levels of radiation is immaterial for mortality risks. This is because individuals who worked in the nuclear facility may have been highly selected for characteristics or traits that affect their overall exposure to the risk of cancers and other chronic conditions. Thus, like the first example, possession of traits that enable accession to the occupation also influence their health status, but were part of the individuals' endowment before accession to the social position.

But, unlike the first example, there is an additional mechanism that could create the observed association between occupation and cancer incidence. This mechanism operates via the existence of traits or behaviors acquired **after** accession to the position that contribute to reducing mortality risks. Behavioral modifications adopted to minimize exposure to alternative carcinogens (smoking) may be the direct consequence of occupancy, part of a conscious deployment of individual behaviors to offset increased exposure to known risks. Healthier profiles that result from behavioral management designed to compensate for increased exposure at work will create an observed association between (lower) mortality risks and health status that is genuinely produced by occupancy of the social position itself. These relations contribute to the observational correlation between social position and mortality, **but are not selection effects as defined earlier.** Instead, they should be genuinely attributable to the occupancy of the position.

The "Healthy Migrant" Effect

Migration is an action through which some individuals living in one residential area accede to another area. As other acts of accession to social positions, individual migration requires the possession of individual traits, some of which may be personal (e.g., intelligence, risk tolerance, time pref-

erences) and others may involve membership in a group (e.g., social connections, social support etc.). Except for some types of migration such as
forced relocation and refugee flows, migration requires decision making
that is heavily dependent on the previously mentioned individual attributes.
Some, though not all of them, may be connected to health status. Selection
through migration goes beyond the fact that migration rates among the
disabled, mentally ill, or other population categories with obviously impaired health status are lower than among the rest of the population. Individuals who migrate may be more educated, less risk averse, more aggressive and entrepreneurial, more resilient, with low discount rates of the
future, and better prepared to face stressful situations. The net result could
be that the distribution of health status in the migrant population at destination will look quite different from the health status distribution of a
random sample of the population of origin.

A healthy migrant effect leads to the same potential misinterpretation
identified previously in the case of the healthy worker effect. A comparison
between members of the migrant group and the population at origin will
reveal health status disparities. But this cannot be used to infer effects
associated with adoption of traits and behaviors at destination or, alternatively, with the act of migration itself. Similarly, comparisons between the
migrant group and the population at destination do sometimes reveal unex-
pectedly low differences. But these should not automatically lead one to
infer the importance of cultural advantages (disadvantages) of the migrant
over the native group.

The healthy migrant effect has been examined in a number of contexts.
It is a prime target of epidemiological studies seeking to isolate the effects of
environment on health status. One of the earliest and best studied examples
was the case of Japanese migrants in California who experienced lower
incidence of gastric cancers than the Japanese in Japan (Dunn and Buell,
1966). The most obvious interpretation is that reduced rates of gastric
cancers are associated with a newer diet in the place of destination; thus, an
environmental effect might be inferred (see also Kasl and Berkman, 1983).
But this may overlook the fact that Japanese migrants to California were
not a random sample of the Japanese population, either in terms of social
class or in terms of region of residence or their own ethnicity. A second
study found that Japanese living in Japan as well as those living in Hawaii
and Los Angeles displayed serum cholesterol levels that were directly related to the percentage of calories supplied by fats in their diet; this provides
added evidence for the environmental hypothesis (Keys et al., 1957). A
third study, also among Japanese living in the United States and in Japan
(Marmot, Adelstern, and Bulusu, 1994; Marmot and Syme, 1976), shows
that those living in the United States (particularly in California) displayed
higher rates of coronary heart disease than those living in Japan. Although

this finding could be associated with different intensity of exposure to key risks factors such as stress, it also can be attributed to characteristics of the "new position" (e.g., stress of being a migrant in the United States, newer and more deleterious lifestyle). But it could just as easily be explained by the fact that migrants are more likely to be drawn from a population that experiences higher risk of coronary diseases and blood pressure anywhere, regardless of migration status—namely, type A personalities (Graham and Graham-Tomasi, 1985; Rosenman, Friedman, and Strause, 1964). An important finding that tilts the balance toward the environmental interpretation is that coronary heart disease is lower among Japanese migrants who adhere more strongly to Japanese culture, a behavioral strategy that may offset some of the added risks imposed by increased environmental stress (Marmot and Syme, 1976; Marmot et al., 1994).

A number of studies of migrants' health status show the recurrent finding that migrants to an area display lower mortality rates than those in the origin population. This is a distinctive marker of migrant selection, and though it does not prove its existence, it certainly suggests its presence (Kasl and Berkman, 1983; Marmot et al., 1994; Swallen, 1997b). An important exception to this regularity is the classic study of Irish migrants living in Boston and their siblings living in Ireland. This study found no important differences in death rates due to cardiovascular disease across the groups (Trulson et al., 1964).

Finally, the "Hispanic paradox" in the United States refers to the fact that Mexican and some non-Mexican Hispanics experience similar or better health status and lower adult mortality rates, and their infants are born at higher weights than African Americans and non-Hispanic whites (Palloni and Morenoff, 2001). These regularities have been attributed to a number of factors, all the product of traits and endowments that migrants may bring with them or acquire during their stay at a destination. These include more favorable behavioral profiles in terms of diet, smoking, and alcohol consumption (Abraido-Lanza et al., 1999; Markides and Coreil, 1986; Sorlie et al., 1993); more cohesive social networks; and superior social support (Frisbie, Cho, and Hummer, 2001). But it is just as likely to be the result of superior health status of migrants that preceded and facilitated the act of migration.

Social Stratification and Health Status

There are mechanisms other than the "healthy worker" effect that facilitate or impede individuals' accession to positions in the social stratification system. Even if, for example, earnings and income differentials were largely explained by educational attainment (and they are not), the question remains about the degree to which educational attainment, and more generally, cognitive abilities and other market-related skills commanding higher salaries and wages are influenced by health status experienced by individuals early in their lives. The possibility that health status may play a nontrivial role in the allocation of individuals across the social stratification system is strengthened by findings that suggest that earnings are tightly related to unconventional skills, those that are not part of the bundle of labor inputs in a standard production function (Bowles and Gintis, 2000). Some of these factors are related to health status early in life. Relatively recent work on the effects of early childhood on lifecycle trajectories (see Chapter 5, this volume) suggests new insights into the mechanisms that may link health status and earnings potential. Although some of these relations have been suspected for a long time (Goldberg and Morrison, 1963; Harkey, Miles, and Rushing, 1976; Illsley, 1955), efforts to incorporate them as an integral part of the study of social class mortality and health differentials are of more recent origins (Case, Fertig, and Paxson, 2003; Goldman, 2001; Palloni and Milesi, 2002; Power, Fogelman, and Fox, 1986; Power, Manor, and Fox, 1991; Power and Matthews, 1997; Power, Matthews, and Manor, 1996; Stern, 1983; West, 1991).

Because the relevant processes may be spread out over a lifetime, involve long time lags, and are mediated by a number of intervening mechanisms, the resulting effects are referred to in the epidemiological literature with the rather unfortunate label of "indirect selection effects." This is apparently to distinguish from "direct selection effects," which are more akin to reverse causality (to be reviewed).

Dilution of Mortality Excesses and Closing Ethnic Mortality Gaps: Heterogeneity

It has been observed that comparisons of mortality levels between two racial or ethnic groups could lead to different inferences depending on the age interval to which they refer. This occurs when age-specific mortality rates of the groups being compared either converge toward each other or cross over at some point. The explanations for this pattern of differentials are diverse and include the possibility of data artifacts, the presence of mechanisms with age-specific effects, and selection processes. We will review three examples of this phenomenon. Not all of them are pure examples of selection processes, but all were, at one time or another, attributed to selection processes.

The first example involves the comparison of black and white mortality rates in the United States. What intrigued most researchers was the fact that mortality rates for blacks converged toward that of whites at older ages (Manton, Poss, and Wing, 1979; Manton and Stallard, 1984). As we know now, most of the convergence is due to a data artifact produced by poor quality of age declaration (overstatement) among blacks both in death certificates and in Censuses or other population registers used to calculate the rates (Coale and Kisker, 1990; Preston et al., 1998). But for some time, the idea that the convergence was real and not the product of data errors dominated the discussion. One explanation proposed at the time that did not receive much support was that factors that determine mortality in each group are not invariant with age, and a few of them that could have been harmful (beneficial) early on become protective (deleterious) later in life. Factors may include lifestyle and affluence.

The most influential explanation for the apparent convergence is that, as a result of mortality differentials early in life, the composition by health status of surviving members changes more drastically in one racial group than in the other. Thus, because blacks are exposed to a more severe mortality regime early in life, the survivors to older ages may be healthier, or less frail, than their white counterparts, and their average mortality risk closer to that of whites than earlier in the life course. The underlying mortality differentials between the two races remain unchanged, while the one we observe suggests that differentials change across the age span.

A second example of convergence involves mortality risks of Hispanics and non-Hispanic whites in the United States. These tend to converge at older ages even though Hispanic mortality is considerably lower than non-Hispanic white mortality at younger ages (Palloni and Arias, 2003). Here, too, there is the possibility that convergence is an artifact of age misstatement, but, unlike the case of the black-white crossover, the evidence to support this conjecture is not strong. As argued by researchers trying to explain a similar convergence of infant and child health status, the pattern could be an outcome of assimilation and adoption of harmful behavioral profiles among Hispanics or due to the cumulated effects of lower quality health care that are seen as duration of residence in the United States (and, with it, age of incumbents) increases (Morenoff, 2000; Rumbaut and Weeks, 1991; Scribner, 1996). Another possibility we will explore as an example of reverse causality is that at older ages, there is substantial return migration to Mexico by Mexican immigrants with poor health status.

Alternatively, it could just as easily be the result of a selection process similar to that invoked to explain the black-white mortality convergence. The only difference in this case is that it is the relatively more severe early mortality regime to which non-Hispanic whites are exposed that could drive the convergence toward the lower mortality rates of that of Hispanics.[1]

A final example of heterogeneity involves comparisons by risk groups. Recent work on disease and mortality in a regional sample of Hispanics reveals that obesity—a risk factor for diabetes, cardiovascular diseases and circulatory problems, among other chronic conditions—is associated with lower, not higher, odds of mortality at older ages (Markides et al., 2001).

Similar findings have been associated with cancer morbidity (Woodbury and Manton, 1977). The robustness of these findings remains to be decided and obvious competing hypotheses—such as the fact that the contrast group includes individuals with very low body mass due to the presence of severe illnesses—need to be eliminated, but these outcomes could be the result of selection processes analogous to those invoked to explain mortality crossover. Individuals who are obese do indeed experience higher mortality risks at some ages. But those who escape higher mortality and survive to older ages may be selected for factors that are protective: Survivors from the pool of individuals with higher mortality risks associated with obesity, cancer, or other co-morbidities are disproportionately drawn from a subpopulation with a more beneficial health profile that confers them protection against higher risks associated both with obesity (or cancer or other morbidity), diabetes, and other conditions.

In these examples, the observed differentials between groups (race, ethnic, risk group) shift as individuals age. Except for the case of the black-white crossover, the shift is real and observed, not an illusion. However, the shift cannot be interpreted as a consequence of changes in the differentials across groups (which, in all examples given earlier, may have been fixed). The variability in the magnitude and direction of differentials is an outcome of processes of selective survival that are different across the groups being compared. The commonality in all these examples is this: As in the illustrations of selection posed earlier, there are traits (underlying individual health) that affect the likelihood of individuals' promotion to positions (surviving to older ages) and that simultaneously influence the mortality risks experienced in those positions (underlying risks at older ages). The key phenomenon common to all these examples is selection on some health-relevant traits among individuals who survive to an older age. This type of selection effect is referred to in the literature as **heterogeneity**.

Reverse Causality, 'Drift' or Social Mobility Through Ill Health

There are situations in which severe health limitations and impairments constrain individuals affected by them to occupy a much narrower range of occupations or social positions than the general population. The best known examples involve physical limitations such as blindness or psychiatric conditions such as schizophrenia, both of which severely limit possible jobs, occupations, and social positions. But the relatively worse health status of these individuals is a cause rather than a consequence of their social positions.

A subtler and more commonly found class of reverse causation includes situations in which deterioration of health status directly leads to erosion of an individual's social and economic positions. Individuals make decisions about labor supply that partially depend on their current or anticipated health status. Thus, those who retire and leave the labor market due to health reasons will forego income and may endure fast erosion of savings to keep desired standards of living. Disinvestments and asset dilution are phenomena that can occur as a result of health deterioration. Similarly, large out-of-pocket expenses to defray caring costs of chronic illnesses and disability may be more or less common depending on illness, disability, and type of insurance coverage.

A third example of reverse causality appears in the analysis of health and mortality differentials involving migrants when return migration flows are possible and of some demographic relevance. This is because immigrants who return to the place of origin may be disproportionately drawn from among those who are affected by ill health or disability. As in the cases described previously, the change of social status (from immigrant to outmigrant) is a direct consequence of actual or anticipated health status. Admittedly this type of reverse causation is relevant for only some migrant groups, not all.

The common feature in all three examples of reverse causality described previously is that the observed total correlation between social position and health and mortality will be partially influenced by a subset of individuals who occupy positions as a result of their preexisting health status. Thus, it may be that the overall negative association between, say, occupational prestige and mortality is attenuated once we take into account the fact that individuals with physical or psychiatric impairments can only occupy low-prestige occupations by virtue of their impairments. Or, the observed strong and negative association between wealth and mortality will diminish considerably once we account for the fact that chronic illnesses result in wealth dilution. Or, finally, the observed advantageous health status of migrant relative to native population at older ages may disappear altogether once we account for return migration of the most frail among return migrants.

In all these examples, the observed association between health and social position is a result of the direct effect of health status on social mobility. Unlike the healthy migrant or healthy worker effect, the observed association is not a product of traits that **simultaneously influence both** health status and social mobility. Like the healthy migrant and healthy worker effect, the observable association does not reflect the influence of characteristics or traits of social positions on the health status or mortality risks of individuals.

In the epidemiological literature, these relations and their observational features are referred to as "direct selection effects" or "drift" (West, 1991) and have been treated mostly by enhancing the observational plan (Fox, Goldblatt, and Jones, 1985). In the social sciences and economic literature, these relations are referred to as reverse causality or endogenous effects and have been treated with a combination of more powerful and well-grounded theoretical models and better observational plans. Thus, work on savings motives, on the dynamic of wealth accumulation over the life course, and on their relation to health status is becoming better integrated in economists' lifecycle models (Lilliard and Weiss, 1996; Smith, 1999). Recent empirical work confirms that there are important effects of individuals' antecedent health status on subsequent wealth accumulation or dilution. The relation operates through a variety of intervening mechanisms, including, but not limited to, saving decisions (Adams et al., 2003; Smith, 1999).

Selection Effects and Their Relevance for Assessment of Racial and Ethnic Disparities

Taxonomy

In the examples described previously there is a fundamental distinction between effects associated with characteristics of a social position (or age) and those associated with individual traits that influence both individuals' health status and subsequent mortality risks and his or her ability or potential to occupy the position. These are all processes that can be represented with a causal diagram such as the one in Figure 6-1a. Although in the more

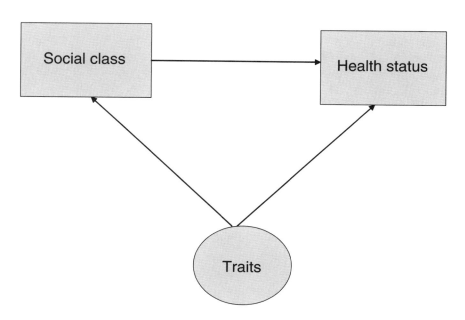

FIGURE 6-1a Relations involved in health selection effects.

statistically inclined literature these are referred to as cases of "causal spu-
riousness" or "endogenous effects," we will follow the literature on health
differentials and refer to these as **health selection effects** (Goldman, 2001;
West, 1991). Because in real-life situations there also will be direct effect of
traits associated with social position on health and mortality, Figure 6-1a
also displays a direct connection between social position and health status.
The observed correlation between social position and health status is a
result of both the direct and the spurious linkage. The analyst has the task
of sorting out their respective contributions.

If social mobility were impossible, antecedent health-related traits could
still induce a spurious correlation between social position and health or
mortality risks by altering the health status composition within each group
at different ages. This is the key feature of processes involving **heterogeneity.** They can also be represented by Figure 6-1a as long as one keeps in
mind that in the case of heterogeneity, the social position refers to an age
category.

The causal diagram appearing in Figure 6-1b depicts a situation where
past health status directly influences the social position. In this case health
status at some point in time directly influences the social position an individual may occupy subsequently. Although in the literature on health differentials this is referred to as "direct selection" or "drift" (West, 1991), we
will refer to it as an example of **reverse causality.**

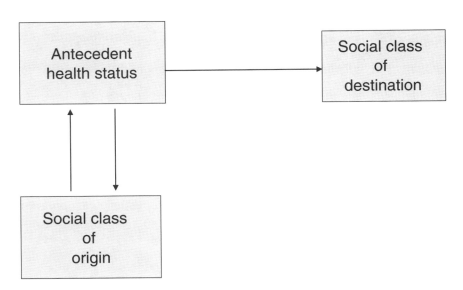

FIGURE 6-1b Relations involved in reverse causation.

In this document all three processes will be treated as examples of **selection processes**, although strictly speaking, only health selection effects and heterogeneity should be classified as such. It is often difficult to draw a precise distinction between empirical examples of these processes, particularly those involving reverse causality and health selection effects proper. However, in the interest of conceptual clarity and because it has direct methodological implications, we will always keep them separate.

Why Do Selection Processes Deserve Attention?

Why should selection processes be considered at all in evaluating the magnitude and direction of ethnic health and mortality disparities at older ages? The connection between some selection processes described earlier and ethnic disparities is transparent in some cases, but is much less so in others.

The Hispanic paradox, a possible outcome of both health selection effects and reverse causality, is a key phenomenon in the assessment of differentials in health and mortality for Hispanics in general, but also for other ethnic groups heavily affected by migration inflows. According to recent estimates, the Hispanic population aged 65 and over represents about 4.1 percent of the total U.S. elderly population. Given current age distributions and projected net migration inflows, this fraction will increase substantially in the near future (National Center for Health Statistics, 2000). Combined with the fact that this population displays what is considered by many to be peculiar profiles of health status and mortality, this implies that we have much to gain from considering explicitly the relevance of selection processes.

Heterogeneity in health and mortality can produce observed trajectories of mortality and health status for any group that are deceiving in the extreme. To the extent that the impact of heterogeneity differs by ethnic groups—and, as we show later, there are very good reasons to suspect that they will—comparisons of health and mortality across race or ethnic groups may yield misleading conclusions and misguided policy prescriptions. Heterogeneity affects all cross-group comparisons of health status and mortality, not just those of one or two ethnic groups, and must be regarded as a key component in any research on the subject.

The case for a serious examination of health selection effects for groups other than those heavily composed by migrants is less obvious. By definition these effects occur only by virtue of the fact that social mobility may be a function of preexisting health conditions. It is then, and only then, that observed contrasts by social groups can produce erroneous inferences about mortality and health status. But if racial or ethnic groups are closed to inflows and outflows from and to other ethnic groups, the problem would seem to be purely academic. This is not so for two reasons. First, one of the important tasks that analysts must perform to assess the magnitude of ethnic and racial differentials is to obtain measures of effects that can be attributed to membership in ethnic groups, as distinct from effects associated with the within-ethnic-group composition by other health-relevant attributes, such as income, wealth, education, and the like. Assume, for example, we wish to test the hypothesis that black-white differentials in health and mortality are associated with social discrimination in the supply of health care. For this purpose, it is important to eliminate the fraction of the total black-white gap in mortality or health associated with income differentials, as income is a known determinant of access to health care. But in doing so, we are introducing the possibility of health selection effects because accession to relevant social positions (in this case reflected in income categories) may be different across ethnic groups. If so, the estimated effects associated with income and, as a result, the "net" effect associated with membership in an ethnic group will be affected by health selection effects. How large these effects can be, or if they exist at all, is a matter to be decided by empirical research and should not be neglected on the basis of a priori judgments.

Second, the composition of some ethnic groups is, to some extent at least, affected by identification of individuals who belong to them (Guend, Swallen, and Kindig, 2002). Increased fluidity in the composition of racial and ethnic groups will be a first and most important consequence of changing criteria for classification of the population by race and ethnicity. These changes will make possible social accession into racial or ethnic groups in much the same way as these are possible for social classes or other social positions in an open society. To the extent that racial or ethnic mobility is health related, the researcher will face problems analogous to those generated by health-related social mobility.

SELECTION PROCESSES IN THE LITERATURE ON HEALTH AND MORTALITY DIFFERENTIALS

The literature on selection processes as "producers" of health and mortality inequalities has a long and variegated pedigree. Arguments about health selection effects are found early on in discussions about U.S. mortality differentials by occupation (Perrott and Collins, 1935). There is indirect reference to it in Britain (Stevenson, 1923) and more detailed discussion appears in the work of Illsley and others (Goldberg and Morrison, 1963; Illsley, 1955). More recently, the issue of health selection effects and some types of reverse causality have resurfaced, but have also become more contentious and controversial, often pitting polarized positions against each other, from those who believe that virtually all social class differentials in health and mortality are attributable to health selection processes and reverse causality (Illsley, 1986; Stern, 1983) to those who believe they are completely irrelevant (Wilkinson, 1986). It may be neither.

A Brief History of Research Traditions on Selection Issues

Discussion of selection processes in past research has progressed through several stages well summarized by West (1991). The origin of systematic discussion of selection processes in the literature on health and mortality differentials is associated with the so-called black report on social class differentials in British mortality (Townsend and Davidson, 1982), in which selection processes (mainly health selection effects and reverse causality) are considered as one of four possible mechanisms producing social class differentials in mortality. The authors of the report did not find the argument about selection very convincing nor did they think that the evidence was consistent with its presence. But their rendition of health selection effects and reverse causality had a distinctively Darwinian tone to it and lost sight of the possibility that selection processes could operate through market demand for individual traits influenced by factors that also contribute to adult health status. Also, as argued by Goldman (2001) in relation to similar empirical evidence invoked against selection elsewhere in the literature, the data analysis that led to dismiss the selection argument does not stand up to evidence constructed via simulated data.

Stern (1983) revisits the claims made in the black report, and in a curiously overlooked paper, he convincingly illustrates the simple claim that health-dependent social mobility inevitably leads to exaggeration of social class differentials in health and mortality. Stern's arguments found empirical support in earlier work by Illsley (1955), who had already produced empirical evidence suggesting that comparison of health effects using parental social class and achieved social class led to very different patterns of health differentials. Illsley's results are consistent with Stern's simplified numerical exercise documenting the influence of intergenerational mobility on cross-sectional health differentials.

More recent discussion of selection processes falls into two distinct categories of research. The first of these focuses almost entirely on reverse causation. These studies seek to identify the effect of a limited number of diseases, such as schizophrenia (Goldberg and Morrison, 1963), epilepsy (Harrison and Taylor, 1976; West, 1991), chronic bronchitis (Meadows, 1961), or mental and physical impairments (West, 1991), on occupational achievement. Some of these studies analyze occupational class differentials under the prism of reverse causality, that is, aiming to identify processes of "drifting" into lower status occupations among individuals who are in poor health (Fox et al., 1985).

The second category of research includes studies that examine more carefully the linkages between early health status and early childhood conditions, on the one hand, and adult health status and adult socioeconomic conditions, on the other (Barker 1991; Ben-Shlomo and Kuh, 2002; Forsdahl, 1978; Koivusilta et al., 1998; Kuh and Ben-Shlomo, 1997; Lundberg, 1986, 1991; Wadsworth, 1991). These are studies that focus more on health selection effects and less on reverse causality, and rely on evidence made possible by the availability of longitudinal follow-ups of several birth cohorts in a number of countries (Lundberg, 1986, 1991; Power et al., 1986, 1990; Wadsworth, 1986; Wadsworth and Kuh, 1997). Similarly, analyses of the Panel Study of Income Dynamics (PSID) and National Longitudinal Surveys in the United States have taken the place of true cohort studies, and important research has already examined links between early conditions and adult health and social class.[2]

As suggested in a review of findings available a decade ago (Blane, Smith, and Bartley, 1993), the record from type of research on selection processes is mixed at best, as differences in procedures, conceptualization, and measurement lead to different conclusions. Some suggest important effects (Wadsworth, 1986), whereas others conclude that health selection effects are weak at best (e.g., Power et al., 1990). A more recent review indicates that the relations could be strong and suggests the possibility of nontrivial health of selection effects (Palloni and Milesi, 2002; see also Case et al., 2003).

The most influential work on heterogeneity emerges in the Unites States, where a flurry of research activity identifies inferential problems that the so-called "unmeasured" heterogeneity poses.[3] Most of this literature (Manton and Woodbury, 1983; Manton, Stallard, and Vaupel, 1981; Vaupel and Yashin, 1985) deals with mortality directly, but the problem is more general and can affect any survival process where attrition of individuals depends on some unmeasured characteristic (Heckman and Singer, 1982; Trussell et al., 1985). The literature contains important warnings about the influence of unmeasured traits on observed differences in mortality (or prevalence) among individuals belonging to two or more groups. Like the problems associated with health selection effects, those associated with heterogeneity have attracted attention, but have not yielded entirely satisfactory solutions.

Bringing Selection Processes Back In

The tenor of the dispute about health selection effects, particularly in the context of British studies, has distracted researchers from the key issues on which all parties in the dispute should agree (Blane et al., 1993; West,

1991). The issues, when they are relevant, are that health selection effects and reverse causality are part and parcel of the object being studied—namely, the processes through which certain social and economic traits that individuals acquire and the health conditions to which they are exposed interact to produce observed differences by groups in health and mortality.

In a thorough review of mechanisms responsible for health and mortality inequality, Goldman (2001) adopts the most reasonable position, namely, to place health selection effects (and reverse causality) on the same analytical level as other factors that are potential determinants of health and mortality. Tests of hypotheses regarding the relevance of each of them must recognize the possibility of effects associated with the others. Similarly, West (1991) cogently argues for a framework that, while directing attention to social class attributes, should also include consideration of selection processes (mostly health selection effects and reverse causality):

> In a fundamental sense, health selection [health selection effects and reverse causality] does not occur in a social vacuum; it is the outcome of an interaction between more or less valued attributes of individuals and the opportunity structures and the institutions and social agencies which control social access to and process within them. In this [. . .] formulation of the issue, all health selection is discrimination of one kind or another, some of which like sex and race discrimination may be judged unfair and wrong (West, 1991, p. 380).

One does not need to go as far as to suggest that health selection effects and reverse causality may be likened to discrimination. But, as labor economists have amply recognized (Bowles and Gintis, 2000), different social systems at different points in time will experience higher demand for some traits than others. Some of these traits may not only command higher incomes and privileges, but also depend on health status. If this is so, health selection effects will be more likely. But this does not make the social stratification system any less real nor does it deny that some characteristics of high-paying jobs, such as health insurance or behavioral profiles, may be genuine conduits to much better health status and to lower mortality risks. As reviewed elsewhere (Case et al., 2003; Palloni and Milesi, 2002), there are grounds to believe that early conditions (health status as well as socioeconomic characteristics) are implicated in early adult socioeconomic status attainment. If, as some literature in labor economics suggests, this relation proves to be more than tenuous—and this can only be determined empirically—then health selection effects must be part and parcel of research on health and mortality differentials by social class or by racial and ethnic groups.

The case for a revisionist position regarding reverse causality effects has been made stronger by recent economic work on lifecycle savings (to be discussed). The processes examined should not be reduced to the case of rare physical or mental impairments, but must include a whole range of actual and anticipatory individual behaviors that are conduits for effects of health status on social and economic standing. We are likely to study these processes more thoroughly as more and better longitudinal data sets become available.

Finally, it is unlikely one requires additional admonitions to warn against the influential effects of (unmeasured) heterogeneity. Like the case of health selection effects and of reverse causality, we have made important strides in understanding ways to identify the presence of unmeasured heterogeneity and to construct adjustment factors to attenuate its effects. As before, this involves a mixture of strategies, including novel study designs and advances in formal modeling.

SELECTION PROCESSES RELEVANT FOR RACIAL AND ETHNIC DISPARITIES

In this section we review evidence from empirical studies and from simulations about the magnitude of effects associated with some selection processes. Our main conclusion is that these effects are not trivial. They should be taken seriously when examining disparities across social classes or across racial and ethnic groups in the United States and in other societies where social and physical mobility is an important feature. We draw from empirical evidence documenting the plausibility of selection effects, and also from simulated exercises that permit the calculation of ranges for estimates of effects under a number of conditions. Although the results of simulation exercises do not constitute evidence per se for or against any hypothesis, they provide a baseline for judgment. If the effects obtained through simulations are large and if the conditions defining the corresponding simulated scenarios are judged to be realistic, we can at least conclude that selection effects must be modeled explicitly before assessing the extent of health and mortality disparities.

The section is organized as follows. First, we examine the so-called Hispanic paradox and assess the claim that it may be the result of health selection effects and reverse causality. Second, we discuss the importance of heterogeneity in the case of black and white mortality disparities in the United States. Finally, we evaluate the potential significance of biases induced by health selection effects and reverse causality.

The Hispanic Paradox[4]

Background

The finding that migrants to the United States tend to show either similar or much better adult mortality experience than native populations is quite pervasive. Rogot and colleagues (1992) find that foreign-born persons who migrated to the United States have lower mortality than do U.S.-born individuals. In a previous study using birthplace statistics, Kestenbaum (1986) detected a similar finding, namely, that those born outside the United States have lower mortality than U.S.-born individuals. In a number of studies on mortality patterns among Puerto Ricans and other Hispanics living in the United States Rosenwaike (1987, 1991) finds systematic differences that favor the migrants over the U.S.-born population. Although they do not perform a complete analysis—because they do not compare Hispanic population in the United States and the corresponding populations of origin—the patterns they observe are fairly regular and consistent. This finding is an element of the so-called Hispanic paradox.

Studies by Markides and colleagues (1997) and by Smith and Kington (1997a, 1997b) review patterns of differentials in health status and, although the evidence is more ambiguous there than in the case of mortality, they too detect a more favorable situation among Hispanic origin populations than among the native U.S. population. The Hispanic health and mortality advantage can be a result of genuinely better health and mortality conditions among migrants, the product of more favorable behavioral profiles and more protective social support networks. But it could also reflect the impacts of health selection and reverse causality.

Health selection through migration can occur as individuals who reach the United States and become more or less established residents are more likely to be drawn from a population that is less frail than the one that does not migrate. Migrants are more likely to be endowed with traits (skills and abilities, risk aversion, time preferences, social connections) that increase their likelihood of success in job markets and that are themselves, or the conditions producing them, strategic determinants of health status. The rigor of the selection process may be related to a number of conditions. But costs of migration and ease of journey are prominent among them. Selection is more likely to occur when the overall costs (and likely payoff) of the move are steeper. Depending on how rigorous selection is, this mechanism can go a long way toward explaining lower mortality and morbidity among U.S. Hispanic immigrants.

A number of complicating factors need to be taken into account. First, age at migration makes a difference. For example, individuals who migrate relatively young out of areas characterized by poorer health conditions will be exposed them for shorter periods than individuals who migrate later in life. This means that, keeping everything else constant, younger migrants are more selected than older ones. Thus information about the age distribution of migrants is a crucial piece of information.

Second, if the effect of early exposure to deleterious conditions does not manifest itself until later in life, selection of healthier members at young ages will be reflected in two regularities: better health and mortality levels soon after migration, and a deteriorating health status and worsening of mortality as individuals age in the country of destination. These effects will mimic those produced by adaptation and assimilation as duration of residence in the host country increases, two processes that seemingly lead to adoption of potentially harmful lifestyles.

Reverse causality ("salmon bias") can also contribute to health and mortality disparities between Hispanics and non-Hispanic whites at older ages. It is suspected, though it has never been shown conclusively, that Hispanic return migrants are drawn disproportionately from a population of individuals whose health status has deteriorated, and who will experience higher mortality risks. The results of such a process will be to generate a disparity in health and mortality that favors Hispanics living in the United States over non-Hispanics. Because this phenomenon is more likely to occur at older ages, the advantage should be more visible and detectable then (Palloni and Arias, 2003).

Magnitude of Biases: Health Selection Effects

We first calculate the magnitude and direction of biases that may affect estimates of adult mortality and health status when there is health selection of migrants. A similar exercise for a number of migrant populations was already performed by Swallen (1997a). Our approach differs from Swallen's only in that we provide a closed expression for the magnitude of the biases. Her conclusions are very similar to ours.

To simplify exposition, we concentrate on mortality and narrow our inquiry to the case where the force of mortality for individual is above some arbitrary age, say x, and can be represented as follows:

$$\mu_i(y) = \delta_i \, \mu_o(y) \quad \text{for } y > x \text{ and } \delta_i > 0 \tag{1}$$

where $\mu_o(y)$ is a baseline hazard and δ_i is an individual frailty factor for individual i, which, for simplicity, we assume to be gamma distributed with mean $\forall/\exists$. It is well known (Vaupel et al., 1979) that under these conditions, the average probability of surviving to age z is given by:

$$S(z) = \exists^\forall \, (Ho(z) + \exists)^{-\forall} \tag{2}$$

where $Ho(z)$ is the integrated baseline hazard up to age z. The average force of mortality at age z is simply

$$\mu(z) = -S(z)'/S(z) \tag{3}$$

where $S(z)'$ is the first derivative of the survival function at age z.

Consider now the case of two subpopulations, one (nonmigrants) where values of 8_i are drawn using the entire distribution, and one (migrants) where the values are drawn from a truncated distribution, *say with* $8_i<8o$. The lower the value of $8o$ the more significant is migrant selectivity in terms of frailty. Under such conditions, one can show that the average probability of surviving to age z among migrants, $S_m(z)$, is given by:

$$S_m(z) = S_n(z) * G_1(z,8o)/G_2(z,8o) \qquad (4)$$

where $S_n(z)$ is the average probability of surviving to age z among nonmigrants, $G_1(z,8o)$ is the distribution function of a gamma random variable with parameters $(\forall, (Ho(z)+\exists))$, and $G_2(z,8o)$ is the distribution function of a gamma random variable with parameters $(\forall, \exists)$.

Under these conditions one can show that $S_m(z)>S_n(z)$ for all z, except those at the tail end of the age span when the probability of surviving drifts to 0. It follows that mortality rates in the migrant population will be lower than in the nonmigrant population. The bias associated with health selection of migrants will tend to vanish over time, as the migrants become older. This is because the compositions by frailty of the migrant and nonmigrant population will converge toward each other and the initial truncation of frailty becomes irrelevant. Thus, convergence of migrant and nonmigrant mortality rates could be expected even in the absence of adaptation or assimilation or of any other change in behavioral profiles or exposure that makes migrants more like the host population.

To illustrate the magnitude of the biases, Figure 6-2a displays the ratios of mortality rates by 5-year age groups in the interval 30-80 that would be observed under different regimes of frailty truncation or health selection. Figure 6-2b displays the ratios of the survival curves. The underlying frailty distribution has a mean and variance equal to 1. The most extreme regime in the graph is one where $8o = 0.25$ and the most benign is one where $8o = 5$. Note that in the first case, the observed mortality rates among migrants are less than half the magnitude than among nonmigrants, and that even in a regime where selection is relatively mild (when $8o$ is 3 or 4) the ratios of hazards are fairly low, particularly at younger ages. This means that even under a mild selection regime, the observed mortality ratios will be consistent with a "Hispanic" advantage that becomes diluted at older ages.

These results suggest a strategy, albeit precarious, to identify health selection effects. If the age pattern of migrant mortality tends to converge (from more advantageous to less advantageous) toward the pattern of nonmigrant mortality, there is *prima facie* evidence of health selection associated with migration. If, on the other hand, the convergence begins at younger ages, it is more likely that other mechanisms are at work. However, as we will show, this identification strategy is precarious because

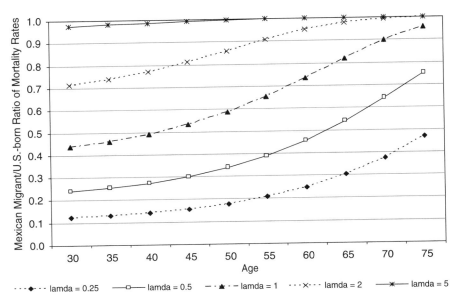

FIGURE 6-2a Effect of selection due to migration on estimated ethnic group differences in mortality: mortality rates.

convergence at older ages also can be consistent with other mechanisms. Furthermore, and depending on the prevailing selection regime, convergence may become measurable only at very old ages, when precise measurement of mortality rates becomes a hazardous enterprise.

This exercise is suggestive and illustrates the potential magnitude of health selection effects. Its results are also consistent with the fact that life expectancy at adult ages (over 45) among Hispanics living in the United States is at least 3 to 4 years higher than the life expectancy at age 45 in countries of origin (Palloni and Arias, 2003). Yet the exercise is stifling and excessively formalistic. It lacks a theoretical motivation to answer a key question, namely, why should one expect more or less health selection, higher or lower values of δ, among migrants?

Perhaps the best way to provide substantive interpretation for this exercise is to rely on economic theory. Grossman's (1972a,b) adaptation of the human capital model to understand demands for health provides a first step. There are two important predictions from this model. The first is that individuals in ill health are less likely to attain a given level of education or, equivalently, be in command of a given endowment of skills. The second is that individuals with higher levels of education or skill endowment will be more efficient health producers. The second step is to introduce a simple

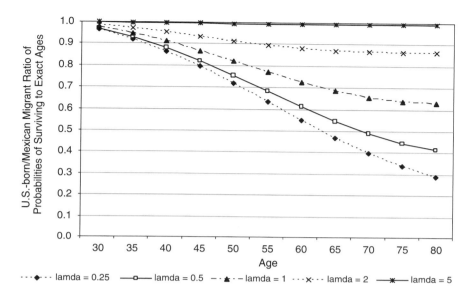

FIGURE 6-2b Effect of selection due to migration on estimated ethnic group differences in mortality: survival functions.

model of migration decision making (see Chapter 7, this volume). The cornerstone of the model is that migration costs bound the level of skills or skill endowment of potential migrants, and that these are more likely to become actual migrants the larger the disparities in skill prices across countries. The most important prediction from this simple representation is that migrants will be selected on health, and that health selection will increase if the costs of migration increase and if skill prices in the area of origin are lower relative to skill prices at destination. The answer to the original query about 8o is now straightforward: the higher the migration costs and the wider the skill price disparities, the lower the value of 8o will be of origin relative to those at destination. This is certainly not the only interpretation, but it is a compelling one for which some empirical evidence has already been gathered (see Chapter 7, this volume).

Magnitude of Biases: Reverse Causality

In our description we emphasized that the contrast in adult mortality levels between Hispanics and non-Hispanics could be associated with reverse causality. This may occur because return migrants are more likely to be in ill health and experience higher mortality risks than migrants who stay. If so, the comparison between those remaining in the United States and the non-Hispanic population will lead to incorrect inferences.

To assess empirically the magnitude of effects due to reverse causality, we perform an empirical exercise using the so-called National Health Interview Survey-National Death Index (NHIS-NDI) data set. This data set consists of records from the NHIS fielded during the years 1989 through 1997 and linked to the NDI (see Palloni and Arias, 2003). We employ a standard parametric hazard model to estimate effects on the 9-year follow-up for males aged 35 and above at the time of the baseline survey.[5] Throughout, we assume that a Gompertz model represents well the profile of mortality increase for ages (approximately) 30 and above. The main model is as follows:

$$:i \ (t \mid X_i; Z_i \ ) = :o \ (X_i+t) \ \exp(\exists Z_i) = \forall \ \exp(((X_i+t)) \ exp(\exists Z_i)) \qquad (5)$$

where $:i \ (t \mid X_i, Z_i)$ is the hazard rate t years into the study for an individual i aged X_i at the outset and characterized by a vector of attributes Z_i, $:_o(X_i+t)$ is the standard Gompertz mortality rate evaluated at age-duration X_i+t, $\exists$ is a vector of effects, $\forall$ is the Gompertz constant, and exp is the Gompertz ancillary parameter or the slope of the hazard rates above age 35. Ethnicity is captured with four dummy variables referring to Puerto Ricans, Cubans, Mexicans, and other Hispanics. The reference group is the non-Hispanic white population. Other variables contained in vector Z include marital status, education, income, and employment status (Palloni and Arias, 2003).

We introduce two modifications to the standard model. First, we scale the baseline hazard so that the Gompertz's constant is an estimate of mortality at age 35 among the reference ethnic group, the non-Hispanic whites. Second, because of the large heterogeneity of initial ages in the sample, we modify the standard formulation of the hazard to account for initial age. This enables us to avoid nonproportional effects. The resulting expression becomes:

$$:i \ (t \mid X_i; Zi) = \forall \ \exp(> (X_i-35)) \ \exp(t) \ exp(\exists Z_i) \qquad (6)$$

and, to be consistent with a Gompertz formulation, we constrain $>$ to be identical to (t). In this model the estimate of $\forall$ is an estimate of the mortality rate at age 35.

Estimates of the simplest model for males are displayed in Table 6-1. These estimates reveal a number of features revealing a satisfying fitting power. Among others the estimated parameters fit well with observed mortality rates and the rate of increase of mortality with age. Note that the Hispanic advantage—negative coefficients of dummies for ethnic groups—

TABLE 6–1 Estimates of Gompertz Hazard Models, White Males Ages 35 and Older, NHIS-NDI: 1989-1997

	Model 1	Model 2	Model 3
Constant (alpha)	−6.08(06)*	−6.17(0.08)	−6.17(0.08)
Slope (gamma)	0.067(0.00)*	0.072(0.00)	0.071(0.00)
Ethnicity			
Puerto Rican	−0.118(0.11)	−0.118(0.10)	−0.117(0.10)
Cuban	−0.050(0.14)	−0.041(0.12)	−0.041(0.12)
Mexican	−0.220(0.05)	−0.163(0.05)*	−0.060(0.10)
Other Hispanic	−0.380(0.10)*	−0.323(0.10)*	−0.640(0.17)*
(X_i-35) (delta)	0.067(00)*	0.072(0.00)*	0.071(0.00)*
Breage		−0.148(0.07)*	−0.148(0.07)*
Int_age		−0.101(0.03)*	
Int_age(mex)			−0.301(0.13)*
Int_age(hisp)			0.410(0.33)
Sample size	17,940	17,940	17,940
Log likelihood	5,602.0	−5,594.0	5,590.0

*refers to $p < 0.001$.

is confined to Mexicans and other Hispanics and does not appear to apply to either Cubans or Puerto Ricans. The estimated magnitude of the advantage is lower for Mexicans than it is for other Hispanics. In fact, while the former group experiences a mortality regime with rates that are $\exp(-0.22)$ ~0.80, or about 80 percent as high as those of non-Hispanic whites (model 1, column 1), the latter group experiences mortality rates not larger than $\exp(-0.38)$~0.68, or slightly more than two-thirds of those of the reference group. These effects are large and statistically significant.

What does this advantage equal to? We can translate the differences among Mexican, other Hispanic, and non-Hispanic white mortality rates into differences in life expectancy. The male advantage estimated before translates into a surplus of residual life expectancy at age 45 of about 2 years for Mexicans and about 4 years for other Hispanics. Because male life expectancy at age 45 in the Unites States is roughly 39.7, the relative advantage for males is in the order of 5 and 10 percent for Mexicans and non-Mexican Hispanics, respectively. Though modest, these differences are somewhat paradoxical.

Although the magnitude of the differences favoring Hispanics, particularly Mexicans and other Hispanics, is admittedly large, it falls well within the bounds of what would be expected via health selection (as discussed previously). One does not need excessively large values of 80 to produce "advantages" amounting to between 2 and 5 years of life expectancy at age 35. Yet, this does not prove the case for health selection effects. It merely raises a red flag. We can, however, provide approximate estimates of the biases induced by reverse causality via return migration.

How can we tell if the estimated Hispanic advantage is produced by a reverse causality process whereby unhealthy Hispanic migrants return to the country of origin? There is an indirect way of answering the question that relies on the following reasoning: If return migrant effects are prevalent, we would expect the Hispanic advantage to be proportionately larger at older ages. Furthermore, because the magnitude of these effects is a function of return migration rates, it is more likely to occur among Mexicans than among other Hispanics whose country of origin is less easily accessible. Return migration costs are part of the individual calculus in migration decision making and here, as it was in the case of the healthy migrant effect, the lower the costs of return migration, the higher the selection will be. For this reason we expect the difference in the advantage by age to be trivial for other Hispanics, but significant for Mexicans.

To test this conjecture, we define a new dummy variable, "breage," to be 0 if age at the onset of the study is younger than age 65; we set it equal to 1 if the age is older than 65. We then estimate two models, one where the effects of an interaction term between ethnicity (Mexican and other Hispanic) and the dummy variable for age group are identical for both Mexicans and other Hispanics, and a second model where the effects of the interaction term are unconstrained. The results are displayed in the second and third columns of Table 6-1. The constrained model (model 2, column 2) yields a negative and significant effect of the interaction term (int_age). This means that, as expected when there is a return migrant effect, the advantage is larger for those who were aged 65 and above at the beginning of the study. The unconstrained model (model 3, column 3) shows that the effect of older age applies to Mexicans, but not to other Hispanics. This pattern is as conjectured: If return migration effects are present, they are more likely to occur among Mexicans than among other Hispanics. In fact, the main effects associated with Mexicans vanish, and what remains is the result of relatively lower mortality rates for those at older ages. By contrast, the advantage for other Hispanics remains intact and cannot be accounted by return migrant effects.

Admittedly, however, these findings are consistent with an alternative explanation that would seek the root of ethnic contrasts in differences in mortality regimes by migrant cohorts. To have some credibility, however, such an explanation should identify the factors that result in mortality shifts across cohorts, and convincingly explain why such patterns are present among Mexicans, but not other Hispanics.

Although there are alternative ways of testing the hypotheses regarding return migration[6] (Palloni and Arias, 2003), we have enough evidence to pose a key question: How "real" can the Hispanic advantage be if we are able to dispose of it by using a device that would be inconsequential if the impact of return migration were unimportant? This proves our main point, namely, that selection effects are of sufficiently large import to cast doubts on conventional inferences and interpretations regarding ethnic disparities.

Heterogeneity

Two regularities deserve attention as they affect inferences about race and ethnic disparities. First, variability of mortality rates at young or early adult ages is more widespread than variability of mortality rates at older ages (Vaupel et al., 1979). Comparisons of mortality rates for two ethnic groups or social classes yield discrepancies that attain maximum values at adult ages and decline steadily thereafter (Manton et al., 1979; Nam and Okay, 1977; Strehler, 1977; Vaupel et al., 1979). In particular, the so-called black-white mortality crossover in the United States attracted considerable attention because it lends itself to such radically different interpretations. Does the observed convergence of mortality patterns for blacks and whites in the United States constitute prima facie evidence of the influence of effects that change during individual's lifetimes? Are elderly blacks better cared for than elderly whites? Do they have healthier individual behaviors than whites? Or is the observed convergence a result of poor data among blacks, with artificially depressed rates at older ages being the product of age exaggeration (Coale and Kisker, 1990; Preston, Elo, and Stewart, 1999; Preston et al., 1998)? It is now fairly well established that, except at very old ages, virtually all convergence between black and white rates is associated with faulty age declaration. Despite this we will continue to use the example to illustrate some of the strategies to identify the existence of unmeasured heterogeneity.

Second, research on health and mortality among migrant groups generally finds that health and mortality disparities between migrants and nonmigrants (at destination) tend to erode as migrants' duration of stay increases. **When age of the population is kept constant**, these duration effects can be interpreted as the result of assimilation or adaptation, processes that have the potential to undermine initial advantages that migrants may enjoy by equalizing risk profiles of migrants and nonmigrants. Any return migration effect is working against convergence of the migrant mortality pattern to the nonmigrant mortality pattern, as it depletes the migrant population of its least healthy individuals. None of these effects can be associated with heterogeneity.

However, duration effects observed in the **absence of controls for age** (current or at the time of entry) may admit a different interpretation. In fact, they may be the result of stronger heterogeneity in the population with the highest mortality, in this case the nonmigrant population. That is, the population that is exposed to higher mortality levels earlier in life (non-migrant) sheds its most frail members. As a consequence its composition by frailty resembles more closely the population with the initial mortality advantage (migrants).

How influential is unmeasured heterogeneity in the evaluation of ethnic and race inequalities? There are a number of ways to calculate approximate estimates for the magnitude of effects associated with heterogeneity. As was the case for the healthy migrant effect, we are stepping on fragile terrain for, by definition, we need to focus on quantities that are unmeasured and, more generally, unmeasurable. The best we can do is to offer ranges that apply under reasonable scenarios. We will do this to study the problem of black-white mortality convergence. With suitable modifications, similar procedures can be employed to examine the convergence of migrants' mortality rates by duration of stay.

A Multivariate Parametric Approach

Let us focus on the black-white disparity in the United States. Other than the PSID, the National Longitudinal Survey of Men (NLSM) is the longest follow-up of individuals of both races where mortality can be studied. The follow-up period started in 1966 and ended in 1991, and included men in the labor force aged 45 and above at the time of first interview. The use of this data set has one advantage and one shortcoming. The advantage is that observed age patterns of mortality will not be affected by age misstatement because special care was placed in confirming age at death and at the onset of the survey. The shortcoming is that the sample includes only the population in the labor force at the time of the initial interviews. It thus excludes the most infirm members of the population, those whose absence from the labor market is associated with ill health. To the extent that the exclusion is more significant for blacks than it is for whites, this peculiarity of the sample will lead to underplaying any convergence of mortality patterns between the two races. If selection out of the labor force due to health status is very strong, it will lead to underestimating the black-white mortality differential at the outset and to underplaying the rate of convergence of the respective mortality patterns.

To estimate black-white disparities (among men only), we use a hazard model identical to equations (1) and (2), with suitable modifications for variables reflecting ethnic group and with a minimum initial age of 45 instead of 35. The model is fitted to observed rates throughout the 25-year follow-up. The ratios of black to white death rates among those aged 45 to

54 and 55+ at the outset are displayed in Figure 6-3. Note that these ratios do not suggest obvious signs of age-dependent convergence. If anything, the fact that the ratios for the older cohort are higher than those for the younger cohort may well imply divergence of rates.

We start from a model that includes age at the onset of the study as well as race. Although this model reveals average race disparities, it tells us nothing about convergence of mortality patterns. The second model allows for the possibility of convergence by forcing the slope parameter of the Gompertz baseline to be a function of race. If there is convergence driven by a more severe mortality regime early in life among blacks, we should see a deceleration in the rate of increase of mortality rates for blacks, but much less so for whites. Thus, the first test is to verify that the slope for the Gompertz function is lower for black males than it is for white males.

The heterogeneity argument suggests that if one were able to "control" for factors that cause variance in frailty or underlying health, we would not observe a convergence in the mortality patterns. We can test for this in our data set by reestimating the hazard model with a Gamma-distributed error term.[7] If the effects of unmeasured traits can be suitably captured by a Gamma-distributed random component, and if such traits and their effects on mortality are fixed, we should be able to observe that the effect of race on mortality is increased. Furthermore, the estimated effect should be roughly equivalent to the effect estimated when the slope of the Gompertz

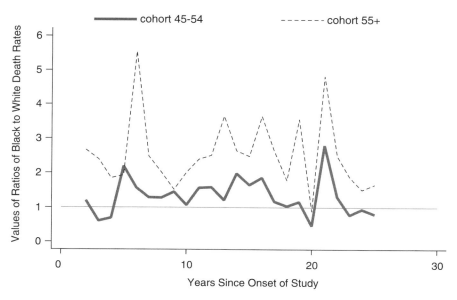

FIGURE 6-3 Ratios of black to white death rates for two cohorts.

is allowed to be a function of race. Thus, the second test is to verify that the effects of race change after we account for unmeasured heterogeneity.

The results are displayed in Table 6-2. The first column shows the effects on mortality of being black: the relative risk is equivalent to exp(0.39)~1.41, that is, mortality among black men is nearly 41 percent higher than among white males. The slope parameter (~0.09) is near to the midpoint of a plausible range for populations such as those in the United States (0.06-0.012). The second column shows the results of estimating the same model with a Gamma heterogeneity component. Here the effect of race is virtually unchanged and the estimated variance of the Gamma-distributed trait is near to 0. This indicates that the race effect estimated in column 1 is uncontaminated by selection via survival. The second test we have suggested does not confirm the existence of heterogeneity.[8]

To perform the first check we have described, we estimate a model with a slope parameter defined as a function of race. Consistency with the previous result requires that the effect of race on the slope be vanishingly small. The third column of the table confirms that this is indeed the case: The estimated effect of race on the slope is virtually 0. The first test we have suggested is also negative and does not confirm the presence of heterogeneity effects.

With an important caveat, the main conclusion from this exercise is that, as suggested initially by Figure 6-3, there are no signs of even weak convergence of black and white mortality patterns. There is no empirical

TABLE 6-2 Hazard Models for Mortality of Males in the NLSM, 1966–1991

Variable		Parameter (std error)		
		Model 1	Model 2	Model 3
Constant		−5.62(0.08)	−5.63(0.08)	−5.66(0.09)
Slope		0.091(0.00)	0.091(0.00)	
	A*			0.092(0.00)
	B*			−0.005(0.006)
Delta		0.091(0.00)	0.091(0.00)	0.092
Black		0.33(0.05)	0.33(0.05)	0.32(0.05)
1/K**			0.0003(0.0006)	
n		4,317	4,317	4,317
LL		−3,414	−3,413	−3,412

*A and B refer to the constant and the effects of being black in a function defining the Gompertz slope parameter as a linear function of the dummy variable for race (slope = A + B * race).

**1/K is the estimated variance of the gamma-distributed unmeasured trait.

evidence that the disparity estimated from the relative risks of blacks is an understatement of the true disparity. The caveat is that the sample on which the conclusion is based is a peculiar one for it excludes individuals who are not in the labor force and are likely to have worse health status than those included.

The Relative Risk Approach

In a series of papers (Ewbank, 2000; Ewbank and Jones, 2001), Ewbank suggests alternative approaches to evaluate the magnitude of effects associated with heterogeneity. Some of these have been proposed to understand the relation between observed risks for cohorts and the underlying or baseline risks (Caselli, Vaupel, and Yashin, 2000; Vaupel et al., 1979; Yashin et al., 1999). Ewbank (2000) applies various procedures to the study of mortality disparities between individuals with different genotypes. One can adapt one of these strategies to assess approximately the effects of heterogeneity on estimates of black-white mortality differentials. A similar approach could be used to assess biases in estimates of disparities between any two racial or ethnic groups.

We start from a slightly modified version of expression (1) above:

$$_{:wi}(y) = \delta_i \,_{:wo}(y) \quad \text{for } y > x \text{ and } \delta_i > 0 \qquad (7)$$

The subscript "w" indicates that the expression is for the force of mortality among whites. Assume that blacks are subject to the same heterogeneity regime, but to a different mortality pattern:

$$_{:bi}(y) = \delta_i \, R \,_{:wo}(y) \quad \text{for } y > x \text{ and } \delta_i > 0 \qquad (8)$$

where R is a constant factor representing excess mortality among blacks relative to whites. For simplicity we assume that R is age invariant. If, as before, we assume that δ_i is Gamma distributed with mean 1 and variance $1/\exists$, it follows that the observed ratios of black mortality to white mortality rates will be given by (approximately)

$$\Delta_x = R \, [S_w(x)]^{(R-1)/\exists} \qquad 9)$$

where $S_w(x)$ is the observed (average) survival function among whites. If $\exists$ is large, Δ_x will be a consistent estimator of R. When the variance of heterogeneity is large ($\exists$ is small), $\Delta_x < R$ and the observed ratios (Δ_x's) of black to white mortality will be a downwardly biased estimate of the true value of R. Or, equivalently, we will understate the black-white disparities and increasingly so for older ages. To give a sense of magnitude, we estimate alternative values of Δ_x associated with different values of $\exists$. We use the U.S. (male) life tables for 1990 and begin calculations at age 40.[9] The survival function $S(x)$ is unity for age 40 and the value of R is estimated to be equal to the ratio of black to white mortality at age 40. Figure 6-4a displays the resulting estimates of Δ_x associated with each value of ∃ and the observed values of Δ_x. Note that observed value of Δ_x is consistent with high variances (low values of ∃) in the first part of the age span and with lower values at older ages.[10]

Figure 6-4b reveals the same uncertainty about race disparities in mortality using a slightly different device: This figure plots the ratios of the underlying mortality patterns (unaffected by heterogeneity) that prevail for each value of ∃. Note that if ∃ were between 0.5 and 1 (corresponding to variances of 2 and 1, respectively), the ratios would be much flatter than observed, indicating that disparities are larger than those observed.

The main point that these figures illustrate is that inferences about mortality disparities that rely on observed ratios of death rates are subject to a great deal of uncertainty unless we know more about the parameters of the distribution of unmeasured traits on which selection is occurring. As in the case of the Hispanic paradox reviewed before, we cannot state with certainty the magnitude of the impact of heterogeneity on estimates of

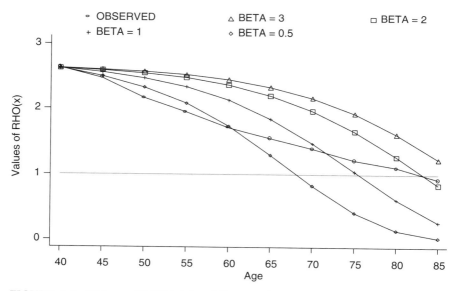

FIGURE 6-4a Values of RHO(x) for different values of BETA.

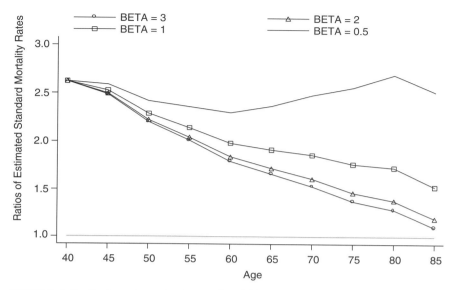

FIGURE 6-4b Ratios of standard rates for different values of BETA.

racial and ethnic mortality (or health status) disparities. But Figures 6-4a and 6-4b suggest that it is unlikely to be trivial.

Health Selection Effects Associated with Social Class

The case of the Hispanic paradox examined earlier illustrates the importance of at least two types of selection, health selection effects ("healthy migrant effect") and reverse causality ("return migration effects" or "salmon bias"). Examination of patterns of black-white mortality differentials produces more ambiguous results regarding unmeasured heterogeneity. In one case we find no support for the idea that convergence of mortality patterns takes place at all. In the second case, the data support the conjecture that selection via survival may exert some influence.

We now turn to selection processes associated with inferences about health and mortality differentials by social classes. We address three issues: (1) Are the potential effects of health selection into social class worth considering if our object is to make inferences about health and mortality disparities by racial or ethnic groups? (2) What are the processes that lead to health selection into social classes and what type of biases do they introduce in the estimation of racial and ethnic differentials? (3) What is the empirical evidence regarding the existence of these processes?

Are Health Selection Effects Relevant for the Examination of Racial and Ethnic Disparities?

Even when interethnic or interrace mobility is unimportant or impossible, health selection effects implicating membership in social classes within each racial or ethnic group are relevant. The reason is that attribution of health or mortality effects to a racial or ethnic group normally requires controls for a number of confounding factors, including social class or indicators of social class such as income education. However, estimates of such net effects will be biased if health selection effects are different within racial or ethnic groups. Let us compare black-white mortality rates. Assume that education level is the best indicator of social class and that health selection into higher levels of education is stronger among blacks than among whites. This means that blacks who attain higher levels of education are drawn from among those who, on average, exhibit better health status than whites who attain the same levels of education. It follows that race disparities in mortality and health status among highly educated individuals will contain a downward bias because, by assumption, the composition by health status at high levels of education favors blacks. At lower levels of education, whites' health status may be better than among blacks of equivalent education because their average health status is higher. Because the observed black-white disparity in mortality is a weighted average of the within-education categories of race disparities, its overall value will depend on differential fertility rates by education and on educational mobility rates as much as it does on true race mortality disparities. The final result is that observed measures of race disparities will be functions of factors not directly related to health status.[11]

To show that the magnitude of biases associated with these selection processes is not trivial, we employ a direct and an indirect assessment of effects.

Indirect estimation. Instead of simulating a situation that replicates the conditions given in the example above, we rely on estimates from two simulations designed to assess the effects of selection under slightly different conditions. The first of these was designed to assess the impact of health selection on education on estimates of disparities in the prevalence of low-birthweight infants among Hispanic migrants and the U.S. non-Hispanic population (Palloni and Morenoff, 2001). This simulation involves two health selection processes, one operating through migration and one influencing educational attainment at a time preceding the decision to migrate. The conclusion of the exercise is that both selection processes are important and they can both exert powerful influences on the estimates of education and migrant status on health status. They suggest that, if only education selection operates, one could **underestimate** true race disparities by as much as 55 percent.

The simulation exercise was designed by Goldman (1994) to evaluate the magnitude of biases associated with estimates of mortality differentials between married and nonmarried individuals produced by health selection on marital status. Her simulations are general, but her results and conclusions are similar to the ones reached with the narrower simulations by Palloni and Morenoff—namely, health selection effects, even of small magnitude, can have a large impact on estimates of the impact of other variables on mortality levels.

In summary, there is indirect evidence that one should exercise caution against optimistic assessments about the potentially trivial magnitude of selection effects.

Direct estimation. We now turn our attention to an assessment of the potential magnitude of health selection effects proper, that is, processes through which individuals are allocated to various social classes by virtue of traits acquired early in life that affect both risk of accession to the social positions and health status and mortality.

In an insightful but overlooked account of the misleading inferences that the presence of health selection may produce, Stern (1983) performed a simple exercise to quantify the magnitude of health selection effects. He assumed two social classes and three possible health statuses. He then proceeded to estimate the observed health status (and associated mortality) differentials under scenarios with different regimes of social mobility, including no mobility as well as mobility associated with health status with which the offspring generation was randomly endowed. Stern's main conclusion was that health status and mortality differentials by social class of incumbents will be exaggerated if social mobility is partially driven by the health status of incumbents to social positions. To avoid this bias, the social class position of the parental generation should be considered.

In this section we perform the exercise suggested by Stern, with three important modifications. The first is that we only examine the distribution of individuals by social class that results after the system has achieved a steady state. This is important because the distribution of individuals by social class and health status will depend not just on the actual regime of social mobility, but on the initial distribution of the population by social class and health status as well. We are more interested in evaluating intrinsic properties of the system, hence those associated with steady state distributions rather than in transient characteristics of the stratification regime.

Second, we allow for inheritance of health status of individuals so that those born to a social class are distributed by health status according to rules reproducing alternative situations. In one of them offspring health status is random relative to parental health status; in another there is perfect correlation between parents and offspring health status. In a third situation, a stronger correlation exists between parent-offspring health status in low social-class families than in high social-class families. This modification to Stern's exercise is not intended to reflect a belief that offspring literally inherit parental health status. Instead, it is meant to capture the possibility that parents pass on conditions to offspring that influence their health and that both parents and offspring may be subject to shared environments determining their health status.

Third, we allow members of a social class to have differential fertility and natural rates of increase to reflect cases where there is unequal growth by social class of origin.

This exercise is a severely stylized representation of real relations and thus has a number of limitations. For example, we must assume that, if it occurs at all, social mobility takes place only once and does so sometimes early in individuals' careers. We also assume that inheritance of health status leads to immutable adult health status and that no improvement or deterioration will take place by virtue of membership in a particular social class. These assumptions are confining, but they enable us to perform calculations that are revealing of the magnitude of effects attributable to health selection effects.

As Stern does, we assume two social classes, high and low, but unlike Stern we only include two categories of health status, good and poor. We impose three types of rules: (1) the first regulates probabilities of moving from one social class to another as a function of health status; (2) the second regulates the relation between health status across two generations; and (3) the third determines fertility differentials by social class. Table 6-3a displays eight matrices containing several versions of the rules. Matrix M1 represents the case where there is only limited health-dependent mobility, M2 represents the case where there is strong health-related mobility, and M3 represents the case of no mobility. H1 is for the case when there is perfect inheritance of health status, H2 when there is none, and H3 when inheritance of health status is stronger in the low social class. Finally, F1 and F2 represent the case of stationary and growing populations, respectively. The latter assumes that net fertility is higher among members of the low social class.

The main results, summarized in the first panel of Table 6-3b, are in the form of average health status by social class and their respective ratios. Poor health status is assigned a value of 1 and good health status a value of 2. The overall health status of a social class is calculated as the weighted average of the health status of its members. The results in Table 6-3 lead to three main inferences:

TABLE 6-3a Matrices to Calculate Population by Social Class and Health Status*

Matrices

A. Mobility matrices

M1: limited health-dependent mobility; M2: expanded health-dependent mobility; M3: expanded non-health-dependent mobility

$$M1 = \begin{bmatrix} 1 & 0.05 & 0 & 0 \\ 0 & 0.95 & 0 & 0 \\ 0 & 0 & 0.95 & 0 \\ 0 & 0.05 & 0 & 1 \end{bmatrix}$$

$$M2 = \begin{bmatrix} 1 & 0 & 0.2 & 0 \\ 0 & 0.7 & 0 & 0.2 \\ 0 & 0 & 0.8 & 0 \\ 0 & 0.3 & 0 & 0.8 \end{bmatrix}$$

$$M3 = \begin{bmatrix} 0.7 & 0 & 0.2 & 0 \\ 0 & 0.7 & 0 & 0.2 \\ 0.3 & 0 & 0.8 & 0 \\ 0 & 0.3 & 0 & 0.8 \end{bmatrix}$$

B. Health status matrices

H1: perfect health inheritance; H2: no health inheritance; H3: health inheritance that differs by social class

$$H1 = \begin{bmatrix} 1 & 0 & 0 & 0 \\ 0 & 1 & 0 & 0 \\ 0 & 0 & 1 & 0 \\ 0 & 0 & 0 & 1 \end{bmatrix}$$

$$H2 = \begin{bmatrix} 0.5 & 0.5 & 0 & 0 \\ 0.5 & 0.5 & 0 & 0 \\ 0 & 0 & 0.5 & 0.5 \\ 0 & 0 & 0.5 & 0.5 \end{bmatrix}$$

$$H3 = \begin{bmatrix} 1 & 0.2 & 0 & 0 \\ 0 & 0.8 & 0 & 0 \\ 0 & 0 & 0.2 & 0 \\ 0 & 0 & 0.8 & 1 \end{bmatrix}$$

C. Net reproductive values by social class and health status

F1: stationary population; F2: growing social class, higher net growth in low social class

$$F1 = \begin{bmatrix} 1 & 0 & 0 & 0 \\ 0 & 1 & 0 & 0 \\ 0 & 0 & 1 & 0 \\ 0 & 0 & 0 & 1 \end{bmatrix}$$

$$F2 = \begin{bmatrix} 1.8 & 0 & 0 & 0 \\ 0 & 1.8 & 0 & 0 \\ 0 & 0 & 1.1 & 0 \\ 0 & 0 & 0 & 1.1 \end{bmatrix}$$

* All matrices are 4-by-4 matrices and rows and columns represent transition probabilities of moving from any of four states into any of the others. The first two rows (and columns) represent low class (poor and good health); the second two rows (and columns) represent high class (poor and good health).

1. When there is no health-related social mobility (or no mobility at all), health status differentials by social class will be accurately reflected by observed differentials.

2. When social mobility is a function of health status, health status differentials by social class will be exaggerated in direct proportion to the strength of the connection between social mobility and health status.

3. When health status is strongly inheritable, observed health disparities will exaggerate intrinsic health disparities **even when social mobility is only weakly related to health status.**

The second panel of Table 6-3b includes consideration of race by adding two race groups subjected to the same regimes of mobility and health status inheritance as before. This addition enables us to see what health selection can do to obfuscate observed race differentials. As predicted before, the stylized regimes we impose here indicate that differentials by race can be exaggerated if one race is more affected by health selection effects than the other, and if members of the lower classes within the race group with heavier selection are endowed with a higher natural rate of increase.

The matrix representation suggested here can be generalized to capture more complex scenarios, and analyses of steady state distributions and properties should yield important insights not revealed by examining simple indicators of health disparities. For the time being, the simplified version of the model used above suffices to reinforce Stern's conclusions. This was **not** that race or social class disparities do not exist or that they are an illusion produced by health selection effects. The conclusion one reaches is this: **Observed social class disparities in health and mortality reflect two kinds of effects—those attributable to characteristics with which incumbents of a position are endowed once they accede to that social class and those attributable to individuals' traits that facilitated access to a social class.** Over time observed health and mortality differentials by social class will reflect the influence of both sets of characteristics, but their relative contribution will change as a function of the regime of social mobility, the degree of relations between parents' and offspring's traits, and even the reproduction regime within social classes.

What Mechanisms or Processes Produce Health Selection into Social Classes?

Having illustrated that race comparisons can be affected by health selection into social classes, the task remains of identifying those processes that result in health selection effects. Two bodies of research address the issue of interest. The first grows out of the literature on health and mortality whereas the second is anchored in economic theory.

TABLE 6-3b Ratio of Health Status in High to Low Class for Different Social Mobility Regimes*

Scenario	Ratio	Scenario	Ratio
Baseline	1.0	Limited health department mobility Class difference in inheritance	
Limited health department mobility No health status inheritance		Stationary regime	0.82
Stationary regime	0.97	Expanded health department mobility Class difference in inheritance	
Expanded health department mobility No health status inheritance		Stationary regime	0.50
Stationary regime	0.84	Expanded nonhealth department mobility Class difference in inheritance	
Expanded nonhealth department mobility No health status inheritance		Stationary regime	1.0
Stationary regime	1.0		
Limited health department mobility Perfect health status inheritance			
Stationary regime	0.77		
Expanded health department mobility Perfect health status inheritance			
Stationary regime	0.52		
Expanded nonhealth department mobility Perfect health status inheritance			
Stationary regime	1.0		

Comparison for two race groups

Case I:
Group 1 regime: Limited health department mobility, no health inheritance, stationary
Group 2 regime: Expanded health department mobility, no health inheritance, stationary

Group I average health status = 1.5   Group 2 average health status = 1.5

Case II:
Group 1 regime: As before
Group 2 regime: Expanded health department mobility, no health inheritance, growing population

Group I average health status = 1.5
Group 2 average health status = 1.1

*These results are all from steady state distributions.

Early childhood effects. In his paper on health selection effects, Stern (1983) drew attention to the possibility that health selection effects could be responsible for artificially inflated effects of social class and, furthermore, that these effects were more pervasive than those more commonly attributable to reverse causality. Stern goes further to suggest a mechanism that could lead to this outcome by adopting Grossman's model for health stocks. His argument is that educational attainment, a trait that exerts a strong influence on earnings and adult social class position, could, in fact, be determined by early health status. Power and colleagues (1986) followed this idea with the formulation of a more complete model where social class position influences health and mortality, and where early health status and, more generally, early childhood conditions, affect the acquisition of traits relevant for social mobility.

Recent economic research echoes early preoccupation with skills and traits that do not enter into standard accounts of earnings and income, and launched an offensive to consider them more seriously (Bowles, Gintis, and Osborne, 2000). Some of these traits, such as entrepreneurship, independence, and work habits, may be related to but are not fully captured by formal education. Others, such as physical attractiveness, autonomy, and leadership, are not necessarily related to education or cognitive skills per se but appear to have independent effects on earnings. In all cases, early childhood environments may account for variability in these traits in populations entering the labor market.

Because childhood environments (and early child health status) are partly determined by parental social class, the connection between early health status and subsequent earning potential provides a means to explain persistent intergenerational earning inequalities. Thus, the relation is not just of a mechanism through which a subset of selection processes may have an impact on observed adult health and mortality disparities, but also a process that reproduces social stratification and social inequalities.

Some empirical evidence links early onset of chronic conditions and disability and labor market performance (Blane et al., 1993; Wadsworth and Kuh, 1997; West, 1991). In these cases, the relation between health status and social class is akin to reverse causality: Early experiences with health status lock individuals into life-course paths with poor prospects of status mobility. But this evidence pertains to rare conditions and cannot possibly explain much of the large observed social class differentials in health and mortality among adults.

There is also empirical evidence supporting the existence of a relation between some chronic ailments with characteristic late onset and early life conditions (Barker, 1991). But even though the empirical evidence for the postulated connection between early life conditions and adult morbidity is suggestive, we lack convincing confirmation that the relevant chronic conditions strongly influence job market prospects and wealth accumulation. Without empirical evidence supporting the latter conjecture, the paths suggested by Barker cannot be invoked to even suspect health selection effects.

Finally, up until recently the record of empirical evidence supporting complex relations spanning multiple life stages in the life of individuals has been somewhat tenuous and controversial (Blane et al., 1993; Power et al., 1986, 1990; Power, Matthews, and Manor, 1998; Wadsworth, 1986; Wilkinson, 1986). Of particular note is the evidence derived from a handful of relatively new cohort studies supporting the existence of some relations between early health and early labor market potential (Case, Lubotsky, and Paxson, 2002; Case et al., 2003; Kuh and Wadsworth, 1989; Nystrom Peck, 1992; Nystrom Peck and Lundberg, 1995; Nystrom Peck and Vagero, 1987; Persico, Postlethwaite, and Silverman, 2001; see Palloni and Milesi, 2002, for a more complete review of studies).

In summary, the evidence gathered for the various intervening mechanisms or processes is fragile, and the case for health selection effects operating through individual traits shaped early in life remains a suggestive but elusive hypothesis. Yet, because the magnitude of effects may not be trivial, the conjecture must be considered side by side with other hypotheses rather than being relegated summarily to the dustbin of implausible alternative explanations.

Early adult health and wealth accumulation. A second strand of literature deals with the effects that individual health stock may have on wealth accumulation over the life-cycle. This research is more preoccupied with relations between health and social class spawned later in the life-cycle of individuals rather than early on as described above.

Life-cycle models attempt to incorporate effects of individuals' health and health expectations on savings, bequests, retirement, and other labor supply decisions (Hurd, 1987; Hurd and Wise, 1989; Lilliard and Weiss, 1996; Smith, 1999). In theory, these models can be deployed to represent a host of complex relations between health and economic standing that span early and late adult stages in the life of individuals. However, most of the empirical work in economics that rests on one or another version of these life-cycle models has been applied to individuals who are in postretirement stages (or very close to retirement) and attempts to capture reverse causality, such as effects of changes in late adult health status on wealth and labor force status. Thus, the avenue of research opened up by the formulation of economic life-cycle models is promising, but has not yet offered evidence for or against the existence of health selection effects emerging during the early phases of the occupational careers of individuals.

Empirical Evidence for the Relevance of Health Selection Effects

Through indirect and direct estimates, we established that health selection effects can be consequential for inferences about health and mortality disparities by racial and ethnic groups. We also identified intervening processes through which the relations producing health selection effects could operate. But all of this remains suggestive until we find evidence to support the existence of such intervening processes. Here is where we lack more than superficial information.

Studies based on two British cohorts uncover mixed evidence, some suggesting strong connections between early child health status and subsequent adult social class (Case et al., 2003; Wadsworth, 1986), others showing weak effects of early adolescent health on adult social class (Power et al., 1990). In an isolated study that explicitly poses reciprocal connection between socioeconomic status (SES) and health, Mulatu and Schooler (2002) reveal evidence suggesting that the causal path from SES to health status is stronger then the reverse causal path. Quite apart from the fact that the investigators do not distinguish between relations established early on in the life-cycle of individuals and those that are more accurately represented by reverse causality, the estimated effects are fragile, the health outcome studied not the optimal one, and the sample too small to make strong generalizations.

Only through systematic work with true cohort studies and through the adoption of more comprehensive and rich models to describe the relations involved (such as life-cycle models) will we increase our ability to assess the actual importance of intervening processes that are potential generators of health selection effects.

Reverse Causality

Reverse causality has been examined with some detail by epidemiological studies of the relation between occupation and mortality. Thus, for example, the studies based on the Office for Population Censuses and Surveys (OPCS) Longitudinal Study of Mortality (Fox et al., 1985) showed that apparent attenuation of the occupational gradient, a result expected if strong reverse causation was present, disappeared over time. Shallower occupational class gradients were replaced over time by strong association for adults during both the preretirement and postretirement periods. This led to the conclusion that if selection effects cum reverse causality (via health-related displacement from the labor force) took place, they were transient and had only a minor impact on ultimate occupational class gradients.

Economic studies enriched by the adoption of life-cycle models and taking advantage of panel designs, Health and Retirement Study (HRS), Asset and Health Dynamics (AHEAD) uncover potent relations produced by reverse causality, some working through out-of-pocket expenses for medical care, others through labor supply, while most of the observed association remains unexplained (Lilliard and Weiss, 1996; Smith, 1999). Other studies using similar data sets but different techniques to infer causality are more sanguine, and suggest that the causal connections indeed could exist, but may depend on the nature of the causative health shock (Adams et al., 2002).

Application of simple techniques to extant longitudinal data can offer unusually rich glimpses into the potential effects of reverse causality. Once again, we employ the National Longitudinal Survey of Men, a panel survey that provides information on the mortality experience of U.S. adult males between 1966 and 1991. We attempt to test the following two implications of reverse causality:

1. If reverse causality processes are important and work late during the life course, then a time-varying wealth effect on mortality should be considerably attenuated relative to a time-invariant wealth effect, where wealth reflects conditions early in the life of the cohorts (such as assets at the onset of the study in 1966, an indicator of wealth that cannot be affected by health in the subsequent 25 years).

2. If reverse causality processes are important and work continuously late during the life course, then the effects on mortality of both a measure of fixed assets (as of 1966) and that of time-dependent assets must be considerably attenuated once we control for health status at the onset of the study. Note that it is likely to be the case that if there are any health selection effects that manifest themselves late in the life of individuals, a control for health status will also reduce their impact. The final outcome is that we could overestimate the impact of reverse causality if we compare estimates of wealth before and after controlling for preexisting health.[12]

We use a conventional parametric (Gompertz) hazard model (see expression (1)) and control for race, education, and occupation of the individual. We measure wealth (fixed or time dependent) using three dummy variables to represent from the lowest to the highest quartile of the wealth (assets) distribution. Finally, we measure health status using individuals' health self-reports. Table 6-4 displays estimated relative mortality risks associated with the first to third quartiles of the asset distribution in four different models. Model I includes a measure of fixed assets (in 1966), but does not control for health status at the outset of the panel study. Model II adds the controls for health status. Model III includes assets as a time-varying covariate, but without controls for health status. Model IV is like Model III, but includes controls for self-reported health status.

TABLE 6-4 Effects of Fixed and Time-Varying Assets With and Without
Controls for Self-Reported Health Status (NLSM: 1966-1991)

Variable	Estimates and Statistical Significance			
Fixed Assets	Model I	Model II	Model III	Model IV
Quartile 1	0.37**	0.31**	—	—
Quartile 2	0.18**	0.13	—	—
Quartile 3	0.08	0.07	—	—
Time-Varying Assets				
Quartile 1	—	—	0.56**	0.30**
Quartile 2	—	—	0.41**	0.30**
Quartile 3	—	—	0.23**	0.19**

NOTE: All models contain controls for race, education, marital status, and occupation
(first, as of first interview, and longest). To avoid cluttering, estimates for these variables and
ancillary parameters have been omitted.
*Significant with $p<.05$.
**Significant with $p<.01$.

First, note from Model I that the effects of wealth on mortality are
strong and in the proper direction. Individuals in the lowest quartile experience mortality risks that are 45 percent higher than those in the richest
quartile (exp[0.37]). Those between the first and second quartile experience
mortality risks that are about 20 percent higher (exp[0.18]). Second, although some of these effects are attenuated once self-reported health status
is controlled for (Model II), the main effect associated with the poorest
quartile remains unaltered. Third, the effects of time-varying assets are
much larger than those associated with assets measured as fixed covariates.
Fourth and finally, the estimated effects of variable assets are considerably
reduced, though they do not disappear, when controlling for self-reported
health status.

The fact that effects of time-varying assets are at least 40 percent higher
than those associated with fixed assets is an important sign of either health
selection effects or of reverse causality of the type discussed by Smith (1999)
with HRS and AHEAD. To the extent that assets are diluted due to health
shocks and that the dilution is reflected in continuous measures of individuals' wealth, there will be a more powerful correlation between time-dependent assets and mortality risks than will be the case with fixed-assets measures. This will occur even if the variable that measures assets refers to
wealth experienced in a period just prior to the time when mortality risks
are evaluated. Second, the fact that a control for prior health status attenu-
ates the effects of assets (of both types) is also an indication that some of the
association, at least, is attributable to the possible effects of prior health

status on wealth. In this case, antecedent health status reflects past health status with effects on current wealth.

This empirical exercise suggests that at least part of the relation between wealth and mortality must be attributed to dilution of wealth caused by changes in health status. Because this evidence pertains to older adults, it can be used legitimately to complement the findings of Smith (1999), Adams et al. (2003), and other researchers. But because it does not address the issue of whether health early in life influences economic status of individuals during the early part of their labor market experience, it is simply not pertinent for health selection effects of the type investigated before.

In summary, although it is too early to make strong statements about the exact nature of these relations, the estimated effects obtained so far are important and, at the very least, suggest that overlooking the direct influence of health on wealth in late life may result in misinterpretations of the nature of the relation between socioeconomic position and health status.

APPROACHES TO MODEL SELECTION PROCESSES

Are there feasible solutions to the problems identified in the previous section? Can they be deployed to produce better estimates of health and mortality differentials by racial and ethnic groups? Can some or all of the problems associated with selection processes be addressed to produce robust estimates of effects of race and ethnicity? Answers to these questions will vary and will depend largely on the nature of the problem. Therefore, we will proceed by first evaluating briefly generic strategies proposed in the literature, then we will examine solutions to more circumscribed problems.

There are two common features shared by all solutions we will discuss. First, they are all dependent on the formulation of an explicit model with testable propositions. Observed relations cannot be interpreted in a cogent way unless we do so on the basis of a well-defined model about how reality works. Second, in most cases the models cannot be properly tested with the data available. In those cases we will be forced to make amendments, and introduce shortcuts and simplifications. In the end, these changes to the original model may lead to ambiguities in the interpretation of results. This is nothing new. But when dealing with the problems at hand, it behooves the investigator to supply enough information to calibrate the degree of uncertainty associated with inferences from the preferred model and the data available.

Following Social Class Gradients Over Time: What Not to Do

It is commonplace to find in the literature that identification of a selection process is obtained on the basis of observations about the persistence or intensification of a given social class gradient (on health or mortality). Thus, for example, it is believed that if health selection into a social class is an important contributor to the relation, the social class gradient would then attenuate as individuals became older. As we indicated before, this type of pattern will occur even in the absence of health selection effects. All it takes is additional selection through survival. This problem is ubiquitous: In most cases, a particular outcome for the gradient will be consistent with multiple interpretations. Unless we have an explicit identification procedure to select from among alternative interpretations, we should not delude ourselves into believing that we produce evidence for or against a particular hypothesis. This is corroborated by simulation models. For example, Goldman (1994) has shown that the range of patterns for mortality gradients generated by different health selection processes is much broader than what researchers have speculated. Although Goldman's simulations were tailored to deal with the problem of marriage selection, her results are equally valid for social class gradients.

This suggests what not to do: Unless we have a clear model about what selection processes are at work and how they are operating, we should refrain from interpreting simple patterns of social class gradients as evidence for or against them.

Addressing Reverse Causality

Far from being insoluble, the two examples of reverse causality discussed in this chapter are quite tractable. In all cases tractability requires satisfying two conditions. The first is that there should be an explicit model reflecting expected theoretical relations. The second is that there should be adequate data to test the model. A good example of these two conditions is available in the work by Adams et al. (2003) as well as in the brief analyses presented by Smith (1999). In both cases the researchers impose structure on the data from theoretical expectations about how reverse causality can work, for example, by identifying the mechanisms that make it happen. Then they use the data to test the presence of such mechanisms. One may disagree with the cogency of these models or quarrel with a few or all of the assumptions made. But because these are in the open, one will not be led astray. The only problem with these models is that they require panel data, and are simply not identifiable through cross-sectional information.

The example of return migration among Hispanics suggests alternative methodologies to identify reverse causation. The test described in this chapter is just one among many other candidates. One of them is to retrieve information on the health status and mortality patterns of Mexicans who recently returned to Mexico from the United States, then compare these patterns with those of migrants who stay in the United States. The test demands a binational data set, one that is more expensive and complex than the more commonly available data on migrants and migration to the United States.

Addressing Health Selection

In some cases microsimulation models can be of great help by enabling us to test for the existence of effects and to verify relations expected from theory. Seldom, however, will they be useful for more than establishing boundary conditions and ranges of values for parameter estimates. This is exactly how these models were used when dealing with the Hispanic paradox (Palloni and Morenoff, 2001), or with the issue of health selection and mortality differentials by marital status (Goldman, 2001). In these two cases, microsimulation models were used to estimate the magnitude of uncertainty associated with a process with a given set of observable relations. This is a first and, in some cases, the only, line of attack when health selection effects are suspected.

A second strategy is to directly model the health selection process of interest, that is, to explicitly represent it as a set of relations between measurable quantities. Although this is possible, the strategy is rarely a feasible one. The reason is that these models are plagued by identification problems that make estimation of relevant parameters from observable relations a difficult endeavor, and that frequently require assumptions that stifle interpretations.

The identification problem could be minimized if the information available is appropriate. The data demands to deal with health selection effects addressed in this chapter are high because the researcher requires information over the life course of individuals. Although a growing number of research projects are being designed to collect and make available data for birth cohorts, the required information continues to be a scarce commodity. But one should not necessarily be confined to waiting for a new cohort study to begin or for those already in the field to reach a more mature stage. As argued by Ewbank (1998), it is possible to estimate parameters of complex models employing different and independent data sets, each of them informing a different aspect or set of relations among the total set of relations the researcher would like to represent. For example, in a recent review document (Palloni and Milesi, 2002), different data sets are used to estimate the amount of variance in earnings that could be explained by early child health status. The procedures are not yet completely worked out and many difficulties remain to be resolved, but they are promising and worth exploring further.

Addressing Unmeasured Heterogeneity

There are two known characteristics of models for heterogeneity or selection via survival. The first is that estimates of parameters are somewhat sensitive to the specification of distributional properties of the unmeasured traits. Recall that selection through survival is attributable to individual traits that increase (decrease) chances of surviving from one point in time to the next and, simultaneously, affect subsequent health and mortality. In the examples examined in this chapter we employed the assumption that unmeasured traits or attributes could be represented by a gamma-distributed random variable. The problem is that the choice of distribution is not as mundane as we made it out to be. Indeed, inferences about the process we are studying may not always be very robust to violation of assumptions about the distributions of the trait causing heterogeneity in the population (Heckman and Singer, 1982; Trussell and Richards, 1985; Vaupel and Yashin, 1985).

Although lack of robustness may be limiting in some problems and in data sets, not all is lost. In some cases it is possible to establish with some degree of confidence the type of distribution that is more appropriate for the data, and even venture a range of values for the associated parameters of such distributions. An interesting example in which this is convincingly demonstrated is discussed by Ewbank and Jones (2001) in their research on the APOE-4 gene.

The second, and perhaps more devastating, property of these models is that even if one were to adopt a conservative stance and impose no parametric form on the unmeasured trait (Heckman and Singer, 1982), thus escaping the first problem, estimates could still be sensitive to the form of the underlying risk (Trussell and Richards, 1985). This would not be an important issue if we knew well the age pattern of progression of events at older ages. But, contrary to what most demographers thought, this is not even true for the case of mortality, let alone for the study of other, much lesser understood, phenomena such as disability or morbidity associated with chronic illness.

An important limitation of both parametric and nonparametric approaches to unmeasured heterogeneity is that they rest the questionable assumption that factors or traits that account for heterogeneity are fixed over time and may not change regardless of what health events an individual may experience throughout his or her life. Needless to say, this is a somewhat unsatisfactory assumption. Recent progress on parametric models suggests that there are ways of relaxing the assumption of invariance, although more experimentation is needed to understand the properties, advantages, and shortcomings of these models (Weitz and Fraser, 2001).

In summary, a model-based approach combined with conventional longitudinal data will not solve the problem of inferences in the presence of selection via survival. However, a combination of data expansion and model formulation offers potential advantages.

Data Expansion

Conventional information on events of interest, such as timing and occurrence of deaths or disability, refer to individuals and, at best, to the household they belong or to the larger community where they reside. The fact that some traits responsible for heterogeneity are frequently shared by related individuals makes it possible to at least neutralize their effects. This requires information on survival (or disability or illness), not just for the individuals who are targets of investigation, but for those related to them who may share some of the unmeasured traits. For example, information on spouses can be used to attenuate the effects of unmeasured conditions shared by spouses. Information on siblings can be used to neutralize the effects of traits shared by siblings who grew up together or apart, including some shared genetically related frailty. Information on twins has been conventionally used to draw inferences about environmental effects net of genetic endowments. The methods for estimating parameters with these kinds of expanded data sets exist and have been tried many times, some with more success than others. An interesting illustration of how estimates of unmeasured heterogeneity derived from twin studies can be applied to solve problems posed by heterogeneity in a completely different setting is discussed by Ewbank (2000) and Caselli and colleagues (2000). Another example is the estimation of unmeasured heterogeneity using spouse data and its application to the assessment of mortality differentials by social class (Mare and Palloni, 1986).

Model-Based Approaches

Ewbank and Jones (2001) suggest a number of model-based and data expansion approaches to measure individual variance or heterogeneity of mortality risks. One of them is tantamount to data reduction and yields estimates of the distribution of individual mortality risks attributable to factors known to affect mortality included as measured characteristics in the data set. Estimates of the variability under model specifications that differ in terms of the covariates included can produce information on how the distribution of unmeasured traits behaves. This information could conceivably be used in other data sets when some of the covariates known to affect mortality are not available.

An Important Recommendation

Investing efforts to identify selection processes in the study of racial, ethnic, and social-class mortality and health disparities is not tantamount to denying the importance of race or social class. As we argued before, if they are relevant at all, these processes may reveal rather than obscure a number of mechanisms that perpetuate racial, ethnic, and social-class inequalities. The first condition for identification is to recognize that some selection processes may be at work and that they could be relevant for the problem being investigated. The second condition is to explicitly include a description of the relations implied by the selection process. The third and final condition is to estimate, reveal, and discuss pertinent measures of uncertainty. We do not refer to conventional assessment of variability of estimates **given the appropriateness of a model**, but to measures that reflect the range of possible estimates when competing models are equally plausible.

ENDNOTES

1. Duration effects that are invariant to controls for age at entry into the United States are not as easy to interpret as a partial product of selection effects and are probably attributable to health differences across migrant cohorts.

2. For a review of pertinent studies, see Palloni and Milesi (2002).

3. Although the term "unmeasured heterogeneity" mostly refers to issues of selection through survival, it often has been used to refer to the so-called mover-stayer problem, or "state-dependent heterogeneity." This is a situation in which a subset of individuals under observation can never experience the event of interest or their risk of experiencing it is low. To simplify terminology and unless otherwise stated, we use the term "unmeasured heterogeneity" to refer to selection processes through survival only. However, research that requires the formulation of multistate hazard models must face up to both "heterogeneity" problems.

4. This section of the chapter is a summary of findings reported by Palloni and Morenoff (2001).

5. Our initial intention was to study the mortality experience at ages above 40. Because individuals who are younger than 40 at baseline will contribute variable amounts of exposure at ages 40 and above during the follow-up period, we opted for a compromise solution and included individuals who at baseline were aged 35 and older.

6. In particular, one can test for differences in the slope of the hazard rates. Slope differences are a natural way in which gradual shifts in the composition of population by health status are manifested in mortality data.

7. The literature on heterogeneity suggests that a Gamma-distributed frailty captures well the effects on unmeasured traits that influence mortality (Ewbank, 2000; Ewbank and Jones, 2001; Vaupel et al., 1979; Yashin et al., 1999) but other specifications are equally plausible.

8. The absence of evidence for unmeasured heterogeneity does not mean there is none. It simply tells us that **within the age range we are examining**, it is immaterial. Its presence may be felt more heavily at older ages.

9. We will evaluate expressions above age 40 and ignore the effects of mortality dynamics prior to this age.

10. It should be noted that, as a rule, the examination of period instead of cohort life tables is likely to underplay the role of selection via heterogeneity in frailty.

11. Arguments analogous to these can be invoked to justify attention to health selection via reverse causality, or processes whereby health status directly impacts the risk of social mobility.

12. This data set is not ideal for our purposes. As mentioned already, it has the important shortcoming of only including men who were in the labor force at the outset of the study. The effect will be to underestimate the impact of reverse causality.

REFERENCES

Abraido-Lanza, A.F., Dohrenwend, B.P., Ng-Mak, D.S., and Turner, J.B. (1999). The Latino mortality paradox: A test of the "salmon bias" and health migrant hypotheses. *American Journal of Public Health, 89*(10), 1543-1548.

Adams, P., et al. (2002, October 10-11). *A re-examination of the Hispanic mortality paradox.* Paper presented at the Center for Demography and Ecology 40th Anniversary Symposium, Madison, WI.

Adams, P., Hurd, M.D., McFadden, D., Merrill, A., and Ribeiro, T. (2003). Healthy, wealthy, and wise? Tests for direct causal paths between health and socioeconomic status. *Journal of Econometrics, 112,* 3-56.

Barker, D.J.P. (1991). The fetal and infant origins of inequalities in health in Britain. *Journal of Public Health Medicine, 13*(2), 64-68.

Ben-Shlomo, Y., and Kuh, D. (2002). A life course approach to chronic disease epidemiology: Conceptual models, empirical challenges and interdisciplinary perspectives. *International Journal of Epidemiology, 31,* 285-293.

Blane, D., Smith, G.D., and Bartley, M. (1993). Social selection: What does it contribute to social class differences in health? *Sociology of Health and Illness, 15*(1), 1-15.

Bowles, S. and Gintis, H. (2000). *The inheritance of economic status: Education, class, and genetics.* Working paper no. 01-01-005, University of Massachusetts, Department of Economics.

Bowles, S., Gintis, H., and Osborne, M. (2000). *The determinants of earnings: Skills, preferences, and schooling.* University of Massachusetts, Department of Economics. Unpublished manuscript.

Case, A., Lubotsky, D., and Paxson, C. (2002). Socioeconomic status and health in childhood: Origins of the gradient. *American Economic Review, 92*(5), 1308-1334.

Case, A., Fertig, A., and Paxson, C. (2003). *From cradle to grave? The lasting impact of childhood education and circumstance.* Center for Health and Wellbeing, Princeton University. Unpublished manuscript.

Caselli, G., Vaupel, J., and Yashin, A. (2000). Longevity, heterogeneity and selection. *Atti della XL Riunione Scientifica della Società Italiana di Statistica,* 49-72.

Coale, A.J., and Kisker, E.E. (1990). Defects in data on old age mortality in the United States: New procedures for calculating mortality schedules and life tables at the highest ages. *Asian and Pacific Population Forum, 4*(1), 1-31.

Dunn, J.E., Jr., and Buell, P.E. (1966, September 19). *Gastro-intestinal cancer among the ethnic groups in California.* Paper presented at the meeting of Third World Congress of Gastroenterology, Tokyo, Japan.

Ewbank, D. (1998). *APOE and the risks of Alzheimer's disease and ischemic heart disease: A demographic meta-analytic model.* Philadelphia: University of Pennsylvania Population Studies Center.

Ewbank, D.C. (2000). *Mortality among the least frail: Lessons from research on the APOE gene.* Philadelphia: University of Pennsylvania Population Studies Center.

Ewbank, D.C., and Jones, N. (2001, March 29). *Preliminary observations on the variations in the risk of death*. Paper presented at the meeting of the Population Association of American, Washington, DC.

Forsdahl, A. (1978). Living conditions in childhood and subsequent development of risk factors for arteriosclerotic heart disease. *Journal of Epidemiology and Community Health, 32*, 34-37.

Fox, A.J., Goldblatt, P.O., and Jones, D.R. (1985). Social class mortality differentials: Artifact, selection or life circumstances? *Journal of Epidemiology and Community Health, 39*, 1-8.

Frisbie, W.P., Cho, Y., and Hummer, R.A. (2001). Immigration and the health of Asian and Pacific Islander adults in the United States. *American Journal of Epidemiology, 153*(4), 372-380.

Goldberg, E.M., and Morrison, S.L. (1963). Schizophrenia and social class. *British Journal of Psychiatry, 109*, 785-791.

Goldman, N. (1994). Social factors and health: The causation-selection issue revisited. *Proceedings of the National Academy of Sciences, 91*(February), 1251-1255.

Goldman, N. (2001). Social inequalities in health: Disentangling the underlying mechanisms. In M. Weinstein, A.I. Hermalin, and M.A. Stoto (Eds.), *Population health and aging: Strengthening the dialogue between epidemiology and demography*. New York: New York Academy of Sciences.

Graham, S., and Graham-Tomasi, R. (1985). Reviews and commentary: Achieved status as a risk factor in epidemiology. *Journal of Epidemiology (Formerly American Journal of Hygiene), 122*(4), 553-558.

Grossman, M. (1972a). On the concept of health capital and the demand for health. *Journal of Political Economy, 80*(2), 223-255.

Grossman, M. (1972b). *The demand for health—a theoretical and empirical investigation*. New York: National Bureau of Economic Research.

Guend, A., Swallen, K.C., and Kindig, D. (2002). *Exploring the racial/ethnic gap in healthy life expectancy: United States, 1989-1991* (Center for Demography and Ecology Working Paper 2002-02). Madison: University of Wisconsin Press.

Harkey, J., Miles, D.L., and Rushing, W.A. (1976). The relation between social class and functional status: A new look at the Drift Hypothesis. *Journal of Health and Social Behavior, 17*, 194-204.

Harrison, R.M., and Taylor, D.C. (1976). Childhood seizures: A 25 year follow-up. *Lancet, 1*, 948-957.

Heckman, J., and Singer, B. (1982). Population heterogeneity in demographic models. In K. Land and A. Rogers (Eds.), *Multidimensional mathematical demography*. New York: Academic Press.

Hurd, M. (1987). Savings of the elderly and desired bequests. *American Economic Review, 77*, 298-312.

Hurd, M., and Wise, D. (1989). Wealth depletion and life-cycle consumption by the elderly. In D. Wise (Ed.), *Topics in the economics of aging*. Chicago: University of Chicago Press.

Illsley, R. (1955). Social class selection and class differences in relation to stillbirths and infant death. *British Medical Journal, 2*, 1520-1526.

Illsley, R. (1986). Occupational class, selection and the production of inequalities in health. *The Quarterly Journal of Social Affairs, 2*(2), 151-165.

Kasl, S.V., and Berkman, L. (1983). Health consequences of the experiences of migration. *Annual Review of Public Health, 4*, 69-90.

Kestenbaum, B. (1986). Mortality by nativity. *Demography, 23*(1), 87-90.

Keys, A. (1957, April 10). *Lessons from serum cholesterol studies in Japan, Hawaii and Los Angeles*. Paper presented at the Symposium on the Pathogenesis of Coronary Heart Disease, Boston.

Kuh, D., and Wadsworth, M. (1989). Parental height: Childhood environment and subsequent adult height in a national birth cohort. *International Journal of Epidemiology, 18,* 663.

Lilliard, L., and Weiss, Y. (1996). Uncertain health and survival: Effect on end-of-life consumption. *Journal of Business and Economic Statistics, 15*(2), 254-268.

Lundberg, O. (1986). Class and health: Comparing Britain and Sweden. *Social Science and Medicine, 23,* 511-517.

Lundberg, O. (1991). Childhood living conditions, health status, and social mobility: A contribution to the health selection debate. *European Sociological Review, 7*(2), 149-162.

Manton, K., and Stallard, E. (1984). *Recent trends in mortality analysis.* New York: Academic Press.

Manton, K.G., and Woodbury, M.A. (1983). A mathematical model of the physiological dynamics of aging and correlated mortality selection. Application to the Duke Longitudinal Study. *Journal of Gerontology, 38*(4), 406-413.

Manton, K.G., Poss, S.S., and Wing, S. (1979). The black/white mortality crossover: Investigation from the perspectives of the components of aging. *Gerontologist, 19,* 291-299.

Manton, K.G., Stallard, E., and Vaupel, J.W. (1981). Methods for comparing the mortality experience of heterogeneous populations. *Demography, 18*(3), 389-410.

Mare, R.D., and Palloni, A. (1986). *Selection bias and program assessment in the job training Longitudinal Survey, Part II: Design for modeling and statistical analysis.* Paper prepared for U.S. Bureau of the Census, Survey Methods Division.

Markides, K.S., and Coreil, J. (1986). The health of Hispanics in the southwestern United States: An epidemiologic paradox. *Public Health Reports, 101*(3), 253-265.

Markides, K.S., et al. (1997). Health status of Hispanic elderly. In L.G. Martin and B.J. Soldo (Eds.), *Racial and ethnic differences in the health of older Americans* (pp. 285-300). Committee on Population, Commission on Behavioral and Social Sciences and Education, National Research Council. Washington, DC: National Academy Press.

Markides, K.S., Black, S.A., Ostir, G.V., Angel, R.J., Guralnik, J.M., and Lichtenstein, M. (2001). Lower body function and mortality in Mexican American elderly people. *The Journals of Gerontology: Series A: Biological Sciences and Medical Sciences, 56*(4), M243-M247.

Marmot, M.G., and Syme, L.S. (1976). Acculturation and coronary heart disease in Japanese-Americans. *American Journal of Epidemiology, 104*(3), 225-247.

Marmot, M.G., Adelstein, A.M., and Bulusu, L. (1994). Lessons from the study of immigrant mortality. *Lancet, 1,* 1455-1458.

Meadows, S.H. (1961). Social class migration and chronic bronchitis. *British Journal of Preventative Social Medicine, 15,* 171-176.

Morenoff, J.D. (2000). *Unraveling paradoxes of public health: Neighborhood environments and racial/ethnic differences in birth outcomes* (Ph.D. dissertation). Chicago: University of Chicago Press.

Mulatu, M.S., and Schooler, C. (2002). Causal connections between socio-economic status and health: Reciprocal effects and mediating mechanisms. *Journal of Health and Social Behavior, 43,* 22-41.

Nam, C.B., and Okay, A. (1977). *Factors contributing to the mortality crossover pattern.* Paper presented at the XVII General Conference of the International Union for the Scientific Study of Population, Mexico City.

National Center for Health Statistics (NCHS). (2000). *Healthy people 2000.* Hyattsville, MD: Author.

Nystrom Peck, A.M. (1992). Childhood environment, intergenerational mobility and adult health: Evidence from Swedish data. *Journal of Epidemiology and Community Health, 46,* 71-74.

Nystrom Peck, A.M., and Vagero, D.H. (1987). Adult body height and childhood socio-economic group in the Swedish population. *Journal of Epidemiology and Community Health, 41.*

Nystrom Peck, M., and Lundberg, O. (1995). Short stature as an effect of economic and social conditions in childhood. *Social Science and Medicine, 41*(5), 733-738.

Paffenbarger, R.S., Jr., Laughlin, M.E., and Gima, A.S. (1970). Work activity of longshore-men as related to death from coronary heart disease and stroke. *New England Journal of Medicine, 282,* 1190-1214.

Palloni, A., and Arias, E. (2003). *The Hispanic paradox of adult mortality revisited.* (Center for Demography Working Paper 2003-01). Madison: University of Wisconsin Press.

Palloni, A., and Milesi, C. (2002, October 24-27). *Social classes, inequalities and health dispari-ties: The intervening role of early health status. Ethnic variations in intergenerational conti-nuities and discontinuities in psychosocial features and disorders.* Paper presented at the Jacobs Conference, Zurich, Switzerland.

Palloni, A., and Morenoff, J.D. (2001). Interpreting the paradoxical in the Hispanic paradox: Demographic and epidemiologic approaches. In M. Weinstein, A.I. Hermalin, and M.A. Stoto (Eds.), *Population health and aging: Strengthening the dialogue between epidemi-ology and demography.* Demography and Epidemiology: Frontiers in Population Health and Aging. New York: New York Academy of Sciences.

Perrott, G. St. J., and Collins, S.D. (1935). Relation of sickness to income and income change in 10 surveyed communities. Health and Depression Studies No. 1. *Public Health Re-ports, 50,* 595-622.

Persico, N., Postlewaite, A., and Silverman, D. (2001). *The effect of adolescent experience on labor market outcomes: The case of height.* (PIER working paper). Philadelphia: Depart-ment of Economics, University of Pennsylvania.

Power, C., and Matthews, S. (1997). Origins of health inequalities in a national population sample. *Lancet, 350,* 1584-1589.

Power, C., Fogelman, K., and Fox, A.J. (1986). Health and social mobility during the early years of life. *Quarterly Journal of Social Affairs, 2*(4), 397-413.

Power, C., Manor, O., and Fox, A.J. (1990). Health in childhood and social inequalities in health in young adults. *Journal of the Royal Statistical Society, Series A, 153*(1), 17-28.

Power, C., Manor, O., and Fox, A.J. (1991). *Health and class: The early years.* London: Chapman and Hall.

Power, C., Matthews, S., and Manor, O. (1996). Inequalities in self rated health in the 1958 birth cohort: Lifetime social circumstances or social mobility. *British Medical Journal, 313,* 449-453.

Power, C., Matthews, S., and Manor, O. (1998). Inequalities in self-rated health: Explana-tions from different stages of life. *Lancet, 351,* 1009-1014.

Preston, S.H., Elo, I.T., Foster, A., and Fu, H. (1998). Reconstructing the size of the African-American population by age and sex: 1930-1990. *Demography, 35,* 1-21.

Preston, S.H., Elo, I.T., and Stewart, Q. (1999). Effects of age misreporting on mortality estimates at older ages. *Population Studies, 53,* 165-177.

Rogot, E. (1992). *A study of 1.3 million persons by demographic, social and economic factors: 1979-1985 follow-up* (National Institutes of Health Pub. No. 92-3297). Bethesda, MD: National Institutes of Health.

Rosenman, R.H., Friedman, M., and Strause, R. (1964). A predictive study of coronary heart disease: The Western Collaborative Group Study. *Journal of the American Medical As-sociation, 189,* 15-22.

Rosenwaike, I. (1987). Mortality differentials among persons born in Cuba, Mexico and Puerto Rico residing in the United States, 1979-1981. *American Journal of Public Health, 77*(5), 603-606.

Rosenwaike, I. (1991). *Mortality of Hispanic populations*. New York: Greenwood Press.

Rumbaut, R.G., and Weeks, J.R. (1991). *Perinatal risks and outcomes among low-income immigrants*. Final Report for the Maternal and Child Health Research Program. Rockville, MD: U.S. Department of Health and Human Services.

Scribner, R.A. (1996). Paradox as paradigm—the health outcomes of Mexican Americans. *American Journal of Public Health, 86*(3), 303-305.

Smith, J. (1999). Healthy bodies and thick wallets: The dual relation between health and economic status. *Journal of Economic Perspectives, 13*(2), 145-166.

Smith, J.P., and Kington, R.S. (1997a). Demographic and economic correlates of health in old age. *Demography, 34*(1), 159-170.

Smith, J.P., and Kington, R.S. (1997b). Race, socioeconomic status, and health in late life. In L.G. Martin and B.J. Soldo (Eds.), *Racial and ethnic differences in the health of older Americans* (pp. 105-162). Committee on Population, Commission on Behavioral and Social Sciences and Education, National Research Council. Washington, DC: National Academy Press.

Sorlie, P.D., Backlund, M.S., Johnson, N.J., and Rogat, F. (1993). Mortality by Hispanic status in the United States. *Journal of the American Medical Association, 270*(20), 2464-2468.

Stern, J. (1983). Social mobility and the interpretation of social class mortality differentials. *Journal of Social Policy, 12*(1), 27-49.

Stevenson, T.H.C. (1923). The social distribution of mortality from different causes in England and Wales. *Biometrika, 15*, 382-400.

Strehler, B.L. (1977). *Time, cells, and aging*. New York: Academic Press.

Swallen, K.C. (1997a, March). *Cross-national comparisons of mortality differentials: Immigrants to the US and stayers in common countries of origin*. Paper presented at the meeting of the Population Association of America. Washington, DC.

Swallen, K.C. (1997b). Do health selection effects last? A comparison of morbidity rates for elderly adult immigrants and US-born elderly persons. *Journal of Cross-Cultural Gerontology, 12*(4), 317-339.

Townsend, P., and Davidson, N. (1982). *Inequalities in health: The black report*. London: Pelican.

Trulson, M.F., Clancy, R.E., Jessop, W.J.E., Childers, R.W., and Stare, F.J. (1964). Comparisons of siblings in Boston and Ireland. *Journal of the American Dietetic Association, 4*, 225-229.

Trussell, J., and Richards, T. (1985). Correcting for unmeasured heterogeneity in hazard models using the Heckman-Singer procedure. *Sociological Methodology, 15*, 248-276.

Trussell, J., et al. (1985). Determinants of birth-interval length in the Philippines, Malaysia, and Indonesia: A hazard-model analysis. *Demography, 22*, 145-168.

Vaupel, J., Manton, K., and Stallard, E. (1979). The impact of heterogeneity in individual frailty on the dynamics of mortality. *Demography, 16*(3), 439-454.

Vaupel, J.W., and Yashin, A.I. (1985). Heterogeneity's ruses: Some surprising effects of selection on population dynamics. *The American Statistician, 39*(3), 176-185.

Voelz, G.L., et al. (1978, March 13-17). International symposium of the late biological effects of ionizing radiation. International Atomic Energy Agency, Vienna. [Paper presented].

Wadsworth, M.E.J. (1986). Serious illness in childhood and its association with later-life achievement. In R.G. Wilkinson (Ed.), *Class and health* (pp. 50-74). London: Tavistock Institute.

Wadsworth, M. E. J. (1991). *The imprint of time: Childhood, history and adult life*. Oxford, England: Clarendon Press.

Wadsworth, M.E.J., and Kuh, D.J.L. (1997). Childhood influences on adult health: A review of recent work from the British 1946 National Birth Cohort Study, the MRC National Survey of Health and Development. *Paediatric and Perinatal Epidemiology, 11,* 2-20.

Weitz, J.S., and Fraser, H.B. (2001). Explaining mortality rate plateaus. *Proceedings of the National Academy of Sciences, 98*(26), 15383-15386.

West, P. (1991). Rethinking the health selection explanation for health inequalities. *Social Science and Medicine, 32*(4), 373-384.

Wilkinson, R.G. (1986). Socioeconomic differentials in mortality: Interpreting the data on size and trends. In R.G. Wilkinson (Ed.), *Class and health: Research and longitudinal data* (pp. 1-20). London: Tavistock.

Woodbury, M.A., and Manton, K.G. (1977). A random walk model of human mortality and aging. *Theoretical Population, Biology, 11,* 37-48.

Yashin, A.I., et al. (1999). Genes, demography, and life span: The contribution of demographic data in genetic studies on aging and longevity. *American Journal of Human Genetics, 65,* 1178-1193.

7

Immigrant Health:
Selectivity and Acculturation

*Guillermina Jasso, Douglas S. Massey, Mark R. Rosenzweig,
and James P. Smith*

Despite overall improvements in health, there is renewed concern that racial and ethnic disparities in health persist and in some cases may have expanded. Ethnic health disparities are inherently linked to immigration because ethnic identities are traced to the country of origin of an immigrant or his or her ancestors. The average healthiness of the original immigrants, the diversity in health status among immigrants, and the subsequent health trajectories following immigration both over the immigrants' lifetime and that of their descendants all combine to produce the ethnic health disparities we observe at any point in time. Identifying the determinants of the original health selection of migrants and the forces that shape health paths following immigration is critical to understanding ethnic health differences.

According to the 2000 U.S. Census, there are 32 million foreign-born people now living in this country, constituting about one in nine of the total population. The foreign-born population has been growing rapidly as the numbers of immigrants has been rising in recent decades, reaching rates that rival the number of arrivals at the beginning of the 20th century. Moreover, immigration will be the driving force in accounting for the future growth of the American population. Recent estimates indicate that the American population will increase by 120 million people over the next 50 years, 80 million of who will be the direct or indirect consequence of immigration (see Smith and Edmonston, 1997). These demographic trends suggest that the health status of immigrants and their descendants will play an increasingly central role in shaping health outcomes of the American people. The importance of immigrant health is not limited to an American setting. The United States is only an average country in terms of the fraction of its residents who are foreign born, and increasing rates of international migration make this issue one that transcends borders.

Immigrants potentially offer some significant analytical advantages for understanding the origins of health disparities in any population. Most importantly, by definition immigrants have changed regimes, moving from an environment with one set of health risks, behaviors, and constraints into another one that may contain a quite different mix. Given the number of sending countries, the diversity of health regimes from which immigrants flow may be enormous. Because isolating meaningful variation in health environments can be problematic within a domestic-born population, scholars from several disciplines have been eager to use immigrant samples to measure the impact of environmental factors such as diet, health care systems, and environmental risks. But these perceived advantages of immigrant samples do not come without a cost, as immigrant samples also raise difficult analytical issues about the extent of health selectivity and the nature of the appropriate counterfactual.

This paper is divided into six sections. The first, section one, provides a simple descriptive comparison of some salient health outcomes of foreign-born and domestic-born Americans. Relying on the existing scientific literature, the section that follows highlights some key findings and the hypotheses these findings generate about the health status of the foreign-born population. Two of the more central questions that have emerged involve the mechanisms shaping health selectivity and the determinants of health trajectories following immigration. With this in mind, the next section outlines some simple theoretical models of health selectivity of immigrants and their subsequent health trajectories following immigration. The following section uses data from the New Immigrant Survey to provide new information on the diversity of health outcomes of new legal immigrants to the United States. New empirical models that estimate the determinants of health selectivity and health trajectories following immigration are presented in the next section. The final section summarizes our views on the principal research and public policy questions about immigrant health that are high priority. It also contains our recommendations about how scientific funding agencies may best assist the research community in answering these questions.

HEALTH OF THE NATIVE BORN AND FOREIGN BORN: AN OVERVIEW

How do the native born and foreign born compare in terms of their overall health? Two widely used measures of health outcomes are self-reports of general health status based on a five-point scale ranging from excellent to poor and prevalence rates of important chronic conditions. Table 7-1 compares the self-reports of native and foreign-born individuals using the 1996 National Health Interview Survey, and Table 7-2 provides a similar comparison for some common chronic conditions.[1] Because immigrants are on average much younger than the native born and health is strongly related to age, the data in these tables are also stratified by age.

Using self-reports of general health status in Table 7-1, the foreign-born population in the United States appears to be in slightly worse health than the native born. These differences are concentrated in the higher end of this health scale. For example, conditioned on age, the fraction of foreign born who report themselves in either excellent or very good health is about four or five percentage points lower than that of the native born. The principal exception occurs among those ages 61 to 80; a considerably higher fraction of the foreign born say they are in either fair or poor health.

There is growing evidence that residents of different countries use different response thresholds when placing themselves within scales that involve ranking along general well-being criteria, including self-reported health (see Banks, Kapteyn, Smith, and Van Soest, 2004; King, Murray, Solomon, and Tandon, 2003). For this reason, it is useful to also examine other measures of health outcomes that may not be as susceptible to the problem of international differences in response thresholds.

The picture is quite different when disease prevalence rates are used instead as the health index. Across all conditions and in every age category listed in Table 7-2, the foreign born have much lower rates of chronic conditions than the native born. For example, for the two most prevalent chronic diseases—arthritis and hypertension—disease prevalence rates are nearly 50 percent higher among the native born. Although these differences

TABLE 7-1 Self-Reported Health Status of Native and Foreign-Born Individuals

| | Age Category | | | | |
	21-30	31-40	41-60	61-80	All Ages
Born in United States					
Excellent or very good	73.9	71.4	60.4	42.7	62.4
Good	21.1	21.4	25.7	32.9	25.1
Fair or poor	5.0	7.2	13.8	24.4	12.5
# of observations	6,750	8,484	12,185	6,642	34,061
Foreign born					
Excellent or very good	68.7	66.5	56.6	38.9	59.7
Good	25.7	25.9	29.0	30.1	27.5
Fair or poor	5.6	7.7	14.4	31.0	12.8
# of observations	1,747	1,918	2,268	900	6,833

SOURCE: Calculations by authors from 1996 National Health Interview Survey.

TABLE 7-2 Prevalence of Chronic Conditions by Nativity Status

	Age Category				
	21-30	31-40	41-60	61-80	All Ages
Arthritis					
U.S. born	2.7	6.7	18.5	42.0	16.9
Foreign born	2.1	2.2	11.4	41.9	11.2
Diabetes					
U.S. born	0.4	1.5	4.1	11.0	4.1
Foreign born	0.0	1.3	3.5	10.7	3.2
Hypertension					
U.S. born	3.7	5.9	17.0	36.2	15.3
Foreign born	1.4	4.6	12.9	34.7	10.8
Heart disease					
U.S. born	3.5	5.1	8.7	19.5	8.9
Foreign born	0.9	2.9	6.2	20.7	6.1
Asthma					
U.S. born	6.9	5.3	4.6	5.5	5.4
Foreign born	3.7	2.5	3.8	4.8	3.5
Diseases of the lung					
U.S. born	9.1	7.3	9.9	13.1	9.7
Foreign born	2.4	5.8	6.3	7.4	5.3

SOURCE: Calculations by authors from the 1996 National Health Interview Survey. Note that because questions on specific chronic conditions were given to one-sixth of the sample, the number of observations in this table are approximately one-sixth of those in Table 7-1.

are smaller in the other conditions contained in this table (diabetes, heart disease, asthma, and diseases of the lung), in every case lower rates are found in the foreign-born population. When considered together, the data in Tables 7-1 and 7-2 suggest that foreign-born populations may self-report themselves in worse health than the native born do given their objective health circumstances. An alternative view is that self-reports of specific health conditions are underreported in foreign-born populations perhaps due to their less frequent contact with Western medical diagnostics. Cultural, language, and institutional differences across nations may also have a significant impact on what people know and what they report about their illnesses. We return to these issues later in this chapter.

Once again, there is some evidence in Table 7-2 of a reversal in ranking among older households. Reported rates of heart disease actually are slightly higher among the oldest foreign-born group listed, and there is a noticeable tendency for differences to converge to near equality among the older populations in all conditions other than diseases of the lung. This apparently more rapid disease progression across age groups among the foreign born in Tables 7-1 and 7-2 is one source of the view that immigrant populations tend to experience more rapid health deterioration over their stay in the United States than is typical of the native-born population.[2]

For several reasons, such a conclusion would be at best premature. As the demographic and labor economics literature has argued and demonstrated repeatedly, patterns obtained from cross-sectional age stratifications may not reveal actual lifecycle realities for anyone (see Smith and Edmonston, 1997). The within-age cell populations in Table 7-2 are members of distinct immigrant cohorts who may differ among other factors in their underlying health. A cross-sectional age pattern inherently cannot separate across-cohort differences from those that represent the pure effects of aging or staying longer in a location. Compounding this problem, there are nontrivial rates of emigration from these immigrant cohorts, and any health selectivity associated with such emigration would add more complexity. Finally, there is no obvious reason why health trajectories of the native-born U.S. population are representative of the health-age profiles that immigrants would have experienced if they had decided not to immigrate. We will return to a fuller discussion of these issues.

The immigrants who arrive in any year may also be influenced by forces unique to that year, such as the current state of relative economic conditions in the sending or receiving countries, new legislative changes in the rules governing immigration, or a specific refugee crisis. Consequently, the year immigrants migrate may matter in terms of their initial health outcomes. To illustrate this point, Table 7-3 lists self-reported health status in calendar years 1991 and 1996 among those who last immigrated to the Untied States less than 5 years ago. Health status appears to be lower among the immigrants of the early 1990s compared to those who immigrated during the late 1980s. In every instance in Table 7-3, the fraction that report in fair or poor health is larger in 1996 than in 1991. This variation in health status among immigrants arriving only 5 years apart

TABLE 7-3 Self-Reported Health Status by Time Since Immigration and Calendar Year

	Age Category				
	21-30	31-40	41-60	61-80	All Ages
0-5 years in United States in 1991					
Excellent or very good	71.9	67.2	52.9	40.6	65.7
Good	23.3	26.9	30.9	34.4	26.2
Fair or poor	4.8	5.9	16.2	25.1	8.2
# of observations	702	364	273	62	1,401
0-5 years in United States in 1996					
Excellent or very good	68.3	61.7	43.1	47.6	60.9
Good	24.3	30.3	37.8	14.7	27.9
Fair or poor	7.4	8.1	19.1	37.7	11.2
# of observations	521	256	182	42	1,001

SOURCE: Calculations by authors from 1996 National Health Interview Survey.

sends a warning signal that research conclusions drawn from studies of immigrant cohorts from different times in American history may be generalized only with considerable risk.

Stratification by age does not provide a direct test of the impact on health of different levels of exposure by immigrants to the U.S. environment. Table 7-4 provides a more direct test by arraying prevalence rates of chronic conditions by length of reported stay in the United States. Because sample sizes are quite thin in any single NHIS year, the data are pooled across all years of the NHIS between 1991 and 1996 inclusive.[3] If (controlling for age) all immigrant cohorts were identical at time of entry into the United States, then the patterns observed across time since immigration would inform us about the impact of different durations of exposure to the American health environment. Unlike the age patterns discussed earlier, these data do not speak unambiguously about any effects of differential duration of stay in the United States. For example, among those over age 50, hypertension is most prevalent among those in the 0 to 5 years since immigration group, lung disease is most prevalent among those in the 6- to 10-year group, and arthritis is most common among those with 11 to 15 years of exposure to the United States. In addition to sampling variability, this array is confusing partly because the ceteris paribus of all immigrant cohorts being alike at time of entry is unlikely to be correct. The relatively high rates of hypertension among recent immigrants over age 50 may simply indicate that there is differential health selection by age.

The availability of multiple cross-sections from the National Health Interview Surveys (NHIS) allows one to mimic an analysis that has become one of the mainstays in the labor economics literature regarding immigrant assimilation. By appropriately arraying the data by year since immigration and by age, one can in principle track cohorts as they age. This stratification is the basis of Table 7-5, which lists self-reported health status by time

TABLE 7-4 Rates of Chronic Conditions of New Immigrants

	0-5			6-10			11-15		
	All	25-44	50+	All	25-44	50+	All	25-44	50+
Hypertension	6.3	2.7	31.8	5.1	3.5	17.0	7.4	3.2	27.6
Diabetes	1.4	0.8	6.1	2.1	1.0	8.2	1.9	0.9	8.0
Cancer	0.2	0.1	1.3	0.1	0.0	1.2	0.2	0.1	0.8
Lung disease	2.1	1.9	3.7	3.2	3.2	5.9	3.2	3.2	3.8
Arthritis	5.3	2.8	23.1	5.3	2.1	24.7	7.0	2.5	26.3
Heart disease	3.7	1.9	18.0	3.7	1.6	11.5	2.6	2.7	14.5
Asthma	1.1	1.3	1.9	2.6	2.7	3.1	2.3	2.2	2.8

NOTE: For each condition, the numbers of observations are about 1,300 to 1,400 in the "All" column for each of the times since immigration, about 800-900 for the 25- to 44-year-old age group and about 200 for the 50+ age group.
SOURCE: 1991-1996 NHIS combined files.

TABLE 7-5 Self-Reported Health Status by Time Since Immigration

Age Category in 1991	% in Excellent or Very Good Health		% in Fair or Poor Health	
	1991	1996	1991	1996
0-5 years since immigration in 1991				
21-30	71.9	67.5	4.8	5.9
31-40	67.2	65.7	5.9	10.1
41-60	52.9	46.3	16.2	28.4
6-10 years since immigration in 1991				
21-30	67.8	61.1	6.4	7.2
31-40	62.0	69.2	8.3	6.9
41-60	55.2	54.8	10.8	15.7
Born in the United States				
21-30	75.4	71.9	4.9	6.5
31-40	72.8	67.0	6.3	9.7
41-60	60.4	54.5	13.5	17.8

NOTE: There are about 55,000 observations in the U.S. born data and roughly 1,300 in the 0-5 and 6-10 years from immigration cells.

since immigration and age where both are indexed by their 1991 values. To illustrate, the first entry in the 1991 column refers to those foreign born aged 21 to 30 in 1991 who had migrated to the United States within the previous 5 years. Of that group, 71.9 percent said they were in excellent or very good health. The number adjacent to it under the 1996 column (67.5) represents the self-reported health status of those who were 26 to 35 years old in 1996 and who had last migrated to the United States 6 to 10 years ago. Because both age and time since immigration have been incremented by 5 years, the 1991 and 1996 numbers would refer to the same group of people if the immigrant group was closed. Data are presented separately for those who in 1991 had migrated 0 to 5 years ago and 6 to 10 years ago. The final panel represents those born in the United States.

Not surprisingly given that respondents are necessarily getting older, the general tendency for all groups included in this table is that their health deteriorated somewhat between 1991 and 1996. More germane to our topic is the relative profiles of immigrants compared to those born in the United States. Although initial health levels are higher for the native born, there does not appear to be any systematic differential rate of deterioration at the higher health levels between the most recent arrivals (0 to 5 years) and the native born. However, there is some evidence of a greater movement of recent immigrants into the fair or poor category. When we compare the native born to those whose reported 1991 time of arrival was 6 to 10 years ago, if anything immigrant health deterioration may be less than the native born.

Table 7-6 performs a similar analysis using prevalence rates of chronic conditions. Two findings stand out from this table. First, by far the most

TABLE 7-6 Rates of Chronic Conditions of New Immigrants

Foreign Born				
Age	25-44	30-49	50+	55+
Years in United States	0-5	6-10	0-5	6-10
Hypertension	2.7	3.9	31.8	18.2
Diabetes	0.8	1.7	6.1	8.8
Cancer	0.1	0.0	1.3	0.7
Lung Disease	1.9	2.6	3.7	8.1
Arthritis	2.8	3.8	23.1	29.5
Heart Disease	1.9	2.2	18.0	14.6
Asthma	1.1	2.9	1.3	4.6
Age	25-44	30-49	50+	55+
Years in United States	6-10	11-15	6-10	11-15
Hypertension	3.5	4.8	17.0	28.1
Diabetes	1.0	1.2	8.2	11.2
Cancer	0.0	0.7	1.2	0.8
Lung Disease	3.2	3.5	5.9	3.1
Arthritis	2.1	4.6	24.7	29.7
Heart Disease	1.6	2.9	11.5	17.5
Asthma	2.7	2.3	3.1	3.3
U.S. Born: Age	25-44	30-49	50+	55+
Hypertension	6.4	9.1	31.4	33.9
Diabetes	1.5	2.0	8.8	9.8
Cancer	0.6	0.9	0.8	6.8
Lung disease	8.3	8.5	11.8	12.1
Arthritis	6.3	8.7	37.0	40.6
Heart disease	5.0	6.2	22.8	25.5
Asthma	4.9	4.8	4.7	4.6

NOTE: See Table 7-4 for explanation on number of observations.
SOURCE: 1991-1996 NHIS combined files.

salient pattern involves health selectivity of immigrants. No matter what duration since immigration is examined, prevalence rates among immigrants are much less than those for the U.S. born. As we will argue, strictly speaking the U.S. native-born population is not the appropriate comparison group to use when evaluating health selection of migrants. Rather, health selection of migrants involves a comparison between the health of migrants and stayers in the sending countries at the time of immigration. This comparison would be extraordinarily difficult given the number of sending countries and the state of health data in most of the sending countries. However, the United States can be used indirectly for this comparison. Because the health of the U.S. native born is so far in excess of those in most migrant sending countries, if migrants to the United States have better health than the U.S. native born, they surely have better health than those who stayed in the sending countries.

Using this argument, the extent of this health selectivity is especially strong among younger migrants and for more serious health conditions. For example, prevalence rates for cancer, heart disease, and diseases of the lung are far less for recent migrants than for the U.S. born. Second, if we examine changes in prevalence rates with increasing age (and time since immigration), there is little evidence that the foreign born are doing worse compared to native-born Americans. An important caveat to the analysis contained in Tables 7-5 and 7-6 is that they are examining health changes over short increments in duration of stay. For many illnesses, one would want to examine health changes over much longer durations of stay than 5 years to better capture the impact of changing geographic location.

Moreover, the limitations of this analysis implicit in Tables 7-5 and 7-6 are serious when it comes to tracking immigrants. First, immigrant cohorts are not closed, because there is substantial emigration from the original immigrant cohort. For example, up to a third of Mexican immigrants who are in one decennial Census appear to have emigrated by the next. These rates of emigration differ significantly by nationality and across time. Second, the question on time since immigration asked in surveys is subject to considerable ambiguity. The specific question in the NHIS—"In what year did you come to the United States to stay?"—is quite ambiguous. Immigrants typically take many trips to the United States with uncertain intentions about how permanent their residence will be. For example, some may have come for temporary reasons, but subsequently decided to live permanently in the United States. Since they initially did not come to stay, it is unclear how they should answer the NHIS question.

MAIN FINDINGS FROM THE LITERATURE

There is a vast scientific literature on immigrant health differentials and their determinants that would be impossible to fully summarize here. Instead, we focus our review on that part of the literature that deals centrally with the main issues of the initial health selectivity of immigrants and the subsequent health trajectory following immigration.

Epidemiology has a long tradition of using migrant studies to isolate environmental effects on health. Put most simply, the basic notion is that if disease rates change when you move from one place to another, it is indicative of a role for environmental factors. A good example is Marmot's observation that deaths by motor accidents are high both in France and among French immigrants to England, suggesting that the French bring their "accidents" with them (Marmot, Adelstein, and Bulusu, 1984).

A typical epidemiological study examines some health outcome in three populations that presumably differ in a significant way in their environments—people in the host country, the sending country, and migrants. Differences among them then are used to test the impact of some type of "environmental" exposure along a dimension where the groups are believed a priori to differ significantly. Although many differences may exist in their respective environments, the hope is that the design of the study has isolated and measured a small subset of salient differences. These epidemiological studies often examine patterns obtained from specific diseases where knowledge about the origins and progression of disease can be used to help isolate the migrant effect. As a practical matter, these comparisons are often limited to small geographical areas, especially in the host country. As we will see, the substantial heterogeneity in health among immigrants cautions that the use of small geographic areas to capture the representative migrant may be quite perilous.

A simple illustrative example of such studies is cited by Kasl and Berkman (1983) and relates to cancer. For example, mortality rates from breast cancer are low among both the Issei (Japanese migrants to the United States) and the Nisei (those born in the United States to Japanese parents), suggesting a genetic interpretation, while colon cancer rates among both the Issei and the Nisei are near the U.S. rates, from which a stronger environmental influence was inferred.

Perhaps the most influential of these studies has involved the health of Japanese immigrants to the United States.[4] As a typical example of such studies, Marmot and Syme (1976) provide data showing that among men of Japanese ancestry, while all-cause mortality is higher among Japanese men (with cancer as the primary cause of death difference), the risks and occurrence of coronary heart disease (CHD) are lowest among those living in Japan, intermediate among those in Hawaii, and highest among those living in California. Moreover, while attenuated, these differences persisted among nonsmokers and among men with similar levels of cholesterol and/or blood pressure. Marmot hypothesized that the remaining differences may be due to cultural differences between the United States and Japan. Traditional Japanese culture is more characterized by group cohesion and social stability, which may be stress reducing and thus protective in reducing heart disease. Marmot examined health outcomes of Japanese living in and around the San Francisco Bay area, stratified by the degree of adherence to Japanese culture. Among these Japanese men, the more they adhered to the original Japanese culture, both during childhood and during adulthood, the lower the risks of CHD. This association prevails even when dietary preferences are controlled.[5]

Given its modern migration history with large numbers of migrants from quite diverse cultures (Europe, Asia, and Africa), it is not surprising that Israel has been home to several important studies. The Israel Ischemic Heart Disease Project is a particularly influential research effort. In this study, 10,000 male Israeli government workers aged 40 and over were examined three times during a 5-year period, from 1963 to 1968. These government workers included first generation Israelis from many sending countries. According to the summary provided by Kasl and Berkman (1983), despite the large differences in culture and background across regions of birth, differences in disease rates were surprisingly small. In this case, either large differences in background did not translate into similarly significant health disparities or selection of a specific occupation (government employees) induced too much equality in health outcomes.

Finally, in another prospective epidemiological study of 1,001 middle-aged men of Irish ancestry, the relation between dietary information collected approximately 20 years ago and subsequent mortality from coronary heart disease was examined. Following the typical epidemiological protocol, the men were initially enrolled in three cohorts: one of men born and living in Ireland, another of those born in Ireland who had emigrated to Boston, and the third of those born in the Boston area of Irish immigrants. There were no differences in mortality from coronary heart disease among the three cohorts and only weak evidence that diet is related to the development of coronary heart disease.

In addition to using migrant samples to test the impact of differential environmental exposure, the second issue that has loomed large in the epidemiological studies concerns the health selection effect. In one of the most comprehensive studies of immigration selection, Marmot, Adelstein, and Bulusu (1984) compared mortality rates of migrants to England from Ireland, Poland, Italy, the Indian subcontinent, and the Caribbean to mortality rates for the sending countries. A summary of their findings is contained in Table 7-7, which lists age-standardized mortality rates compared to those who were born in the United Kingdom (UK). For all countries but Ireland, all-cause mortality rates were much lower among migrants compared to those of residents in the country of origin. While there are no controls for duration of stay, their data are suggestive of quite strong health

TABLE 7-7 Standardized Male Mortality Rates for Selected Immigrants to England and Wales (rates relative to United Kingdom)

	Migrants	Country of Origin
Ireland	114	99
Poland	95	107
Italy	77	91
Caribbean	94	119
Indian subcontinent	98	NA

SOURCE: Adapted from Marmot et al. (1984, Table 1).

selection effects among migrants to the UK. The exception of Ireland is also of interest in part because it indicates that health selection effects may vary systematically across countries. The cost of moving between the UK and Ireland is relatively low, and as we will demonstrate, in such situations health selection should be weaker. In addition, our model predicts that healthy Irish migrants should be found in much more distant places.

Latinos represent an important special case for research on immigrant health. In part the attention given to Latino health reflects their place as the numerically largest immigrant ethnic group, a dominance that will grow more pronounced in the future. But it also stems from scientific interest in the reasons for the so-called "Hispanic paradox"—by many measures Hispanic health is far superior to what one might expect given their socioeconomic status. In particular, although they share similar economic positions, Hispanic health levels are far better than those of African Americans and are often above those of non-Hispanic whites, whose economic resources are far superior. The Hispanic paradox is illustrated in Table 7-8. Age-adjusted death rates for the two leading causes of death—diseases of the heart and malignant neoplasms—are 50 percent lower among Hispanics than among African Americans. With the exception of diabetes, Hispanic age-adjusted death rates are actually lower for all diseases than those of non-Hispanic whites. The only group that outperforms Latinos on these measures is Asians/Pacific Islanders, whose overall lower mortality rate is due principally to low rates of death from heart disease.

The reasons underlying the Hispanic health paradox have been a source of considerable research and debate. Two themes have dominated that debate, but they are the same as those highlighted in this chapter. The first is the healthy migrant effect, where Latino migrants are seen as inherently healthier. This literature is largely silent on whether this better health due to selection mostly reflects the generally superior health habits, behaviors, and conditions in the Latino sending countries relative to the United States or

TABLE 7-8 Age-Adjusted Death Rates by Cause of Death: 1998

	Hispanic	Non-Hispanic White	African American	Asian/ Pacific Islander
All	596.4	862.7	1,135.7	516.8
Diseases of heart	175.6	271.7	340.6	154.4
Malignant neoplasms	123.7	203.0	255.1	124.2
Lower respiratory disease	18.6	44.8	30.8	17.2
Cardiovascular diseases	39.1	58.0	80.1	50.6
Diabetes	32.1	21.1	22.1	16.9
Injuries	30.2	34.6	39.5	17.6
Suicide	6.3	12.8	5.8	6.6
Homicide	8.8	3.1	22.6	3.5

SOURCE: Centers for Disease Control and Prevention (2001).

whether it is principally due to health selectivity among migrants compared to those who stayed. The problem with a heavy reliance on the generally superior health behaviors and conditions in the sending countries is that on standard health outcome measures such as mortality and morbidity, the major Latino sending countries rank below the United States.

The second theme concerns the protective effects of culture and norms within Latino families and communities. The argument is that there is cultural buffering, which is characterized by norms proscribing risky behaviors and promoting good ones, such as a healthier diet and stronger family support networks (Vega and Amaro, 1994). There is evidence that Latinos do have lower prevalence rates of some of the more common risk factors for good health. For example, rates of cigarette smoking are lower among foreign-born Latinos. The notable exception to better Latino health behaviors involves excessive weight and obesity. During the 1988-1994 time period, 24.4 percent of Mexican men and 36.1 percent of Mexican women were obese, much higher rates than observed among non-Hispanic whites. Similarly, 70 percent of Mexican women were reported as overweight compared to only 47 percent of non-Hispanic white women (see Centers for Disease Control and Prevention, 2001). Such weight-related problems no doubt have much to do with the high prevalence of diabetes among Hispanics.

With increased acculturation, however, the argument continues that the protective cultural buffering begins to dissipate, and with it Latino health deteriorates toward the U.S. norm. This deterioration becomes even more severe as we pass through the generations. As just one illustration among many, second generation Hispanic women fare worse than the first generation in terms of adolescent pregnancy and having low birthweight children (Vega and Amaro, 1994).

The final generic issue raised in the literature is that the very act of migration may also directly affect immigrant health. This effect is associated with the process of migration itself, which is often viewed as quite stressful with negative psychosocial impacts (Kasl and Berkman, 1983). This form of health impact of migration suggests that health problems of migrants should eventually be manifested in specific diseases. Cardiovascular diseases are known to be sensitive to prolonged exposure to high levels of stress, so that relatively high rates of heart disease among the foreign born associated with length of stay may be indicative of such a mechanism. More recently, heart disease has played an increased role in these studies. Migrants' rates of heart disease are intermediate between sending and host country and converge with time since immigration (Kasl and Berkman, 1983). Repeated exposures of immigrants to prejudice and discriminatory acts in the host country are also cited as a reason for stress and its eventual toll on health (Vega and Amaro, 1994).

The emphasis in the epidemiological literature on specific diseases is important and should become a more standard part of analyses by social scientists. The early concerns about immigrant health had to do with the externalities associated with the spread of communicable diseases. Although this concern is much diminished today, tuberculosis tests and medical exams are required before admittance to permanent residence in the United States.

THEORETICAL ISSUES

There are two perennial themes to the literature on migration and health outcomes—the nature of the health selectivity of international migrants and the impact of migration on the subsequent health trajectory of migrants. Although these themes have appeared in the scientific literature for many decades and across several academic disciplines, there has been remarkably little theoretical guidance about the likely nature of the selectivity or on the mechanisms through which health trajectories may be altered by migration. In this section, we present a simple theoretical framework within which these questions can be investigated. A latter section summarizes our empirical estimates of these models.

Migration Model of Initial Health Selectivity

Will migrants be positively selected on their health, and if so what are the personal and environmental factors influencing the extent of this selection? Although one of the most often mentioned empirical findings regarding international migration concerns the possible health selectivity of migrants, there has been little formal theoretical investigation of this relationship. In this section, we develop a simple framework adapted from Jasso, Rosenzweig, and Smith (2001) that illustrates the main issues.

The decision to migrate can be viewed as a balance between the gains and costs of migration. For simplicity, these gains can be thought of as the difference in income received in the receiving and sending country. Income is the product of the skill of the individual (k), the rate of utilization of skill (or labor supply) (l), and a country-specific price of skill (w). All prices, skills, and utilization rates may be country specific.

Thus, an individual will migrate if:

$$w_a \, k_{ia} \, l_{ia} - w_j \, k_{ij} \, l_{ij} > c_{aj} \tag{1}$$

where c_{aj} is the cost of moving from country j to country a. These costs may include not only any monetary costs associated with mobility, but also any nonpecuniary costs (utility), such as any cultural differences between the sending and receiving country, the quality and availability of good health care, being away from family and friends, and the like. Individual skills may not be perfectly transferable across countries, a relationship that may be summarized by $k_{ia} = \alpha_j k_{ij}$ where α_j is index of transferability from country j to country a. Similarly, the relation of skill prices across countries can be written as $w_j = \beta_o + \beta_j w_a$ and the relation of labor supply across countries is $l_{ia} = c_j l_{ij}$. Substituting these intercounty associations into equation (1), an individual migrates if

$$w_a k_{ij} l_{ij} \left(\alpha_j c_j - \frac{\beta_o}{w_a} - \beta_j \right) > c_{aj} \qquad (2)$$

Before bringing health into this model, we mention some predictions for both number of migrants and skill selectivity of migrants who do come. First, an increase in the cost of migration (c_{aj}), whether due to monetary or nonmonetary factors, will reduce the number of migrants. Given skill prices, increases in migration costs also imply greater selectivity on either skill or labor supply. That is, when migration costs are greater, migrants must be either more skilled or harder workers or both. Second, countries with higher skill prices (β_j) will also send fewer migrants to the United States, but once again these migrants should be more selective on labor effort or skill. Finally, migration rates will increase when rates of skill transferability (α_j) are higher, but migrants who do come will be of lower skill or work effort.

Health can enter this model in several ways. The most direct pathway is that health enhances earnings capacity. It is widely acknowledged that health is an important component of an individual's human capital (Grossman, 1972), so that skill levels are generally greater among healthier people. Healthier individuals are generally more energetic and robust, so that skill utilization (or labor supply) and health are also positively correlated. Because health increases both k_{ij} and l_{ij}, healthier individuals will gain more from migration and migrants will be positively selected on their health.

Health will interact with the other determinants of migration we have mentioned. Where the costs of migration between two countries are greater, migrants will self-select on better health to a greater extent. Thus, countries that are more distant from each other, either geographically or culturally, will (other things equal) be more positively selected on migrant health. Similarly, migrants from countries with lower skill prices relative to those in the United States will be less positively selected on migrant health. Finally, when skill transferability is lower, migrants will more positively select on health.

Holding everything else equal, equation (2) indicates that there is a minimum health level that would make migration worthwhile. Because health varies so much among sending countries, this implies that the dispersion in health outcomes among migrants should be less than that which exists across sending countries and that the magnitude of health selection is negatively related to health levels in the sending countries.

To this point, we have highlighted health effects that operate principally through labor market earnings. Migrants may also be attracted to countries with higher quality health care or healthier environments. These factors may be incorporated into the model as part of the nonpecuniary costs of migration. For example, if the United States offers a healthier environment or lower cost health care of a given quality than that which exists in the sending country, more migrants will come, but the marginal migrant will be less healthy.

Labor market considerations are less important for older migrants who may have either short or no remaining tenure in the labor market. The factors relating to skill levels, utilization, and prices may be of no importance for new migrants over age 60 who do not plan to work. In contrast, the better health care available in the United States may be of far greater concern among older migrants. This indicates that health selection effects may be quite different among older migrants, a point consistent with the age stratifications in the data presented earlier.[6] It also suggests the importance of time because migration is a key control in examining the health of older migrants. Older migrants consist of two groups—those who have migrated at a much younger age and who were presumably positively selected on their health and those who migrated at much older ages, when the migration selection may have been reversed.

Comprehensive evidence on the extent of health selection of migrants is difficult to obtain. In principle we would like to know how migrants compare at the time of their initial migration with residents in their sending country. The data contained in Table 7-7 do suggest that the migrant health selection effect may be strong, but there is no control for duration of stay in the United Kingdom.

As a first step toward gauging the importance of health selectivity, Table 7-9 ranks countries by numbers of legal male migrants to the United States in 1995, and then provides for each country the levels of male life expectancy and the probability of a male dying between ages 15 and 59. The later index is provided because it is presumably less affected by infant mortality and more closely approximates the ages when migration takes place. The story told by these two death indexes is quite similar, so we will concentrate our discussion on the more conventional life-expectancy measure. The variance in male life expectancy across these major sending countries is enormous, with a range of more than 25 years. Three countries have higher life expectancy than the United States, while overall life expectancy in 14 of the countries is lower than in the United States. A weighted (by

TABLE 7-9 Life Expectancies of Major Sending Countries

Country	Number of Migrants (000's)	Male Life Expectancy	Male Probability of Dying Between Ages 15 and 59
Mexico	89.9	71.0	0.194
Philippines	51.0	64.6	0.232
Vietnam	41.8	66.7	0.225
Dominican Republic	38.5	65.5	0.177
China	35.5	68.9	0.170
India	34.7	59.8	0.275
Cuba	17.9	73.7	0.143
Ukraine	17.4	62.6	0.326
Jamaica	16.4	75.8	0.135
Korea	16.0	70.5	NA
Russia	14.6	59.4	0.352
Haiti	14.0	49.7	0.481
Poland	13.8	69.2	0.242
Canada	12.9	76.0	0.104
United Kingdom	12.4	74.8	0.111
Guatemala	11.7	63.5	0.326
Columbia	10.8	67.2	0.221
United States	—	73.9	0.148
Immigrant weighted average		67.1	

NOTE: Countries with more than 10,000 migrants to the United States in 1995.

SOURCES: Life expectancies were obtained from Harvard Burden of Disease Unit Research Paper No. 8. Probabilities of men dying between ages 15 and 59 obtained from *The World Health Report 2000*, World Health Organization.

number of migrants) average of life expectancies from these major sending countries is 67.1 years, nearly 7 years less than that in the United States.

Thus, the typical legal migrant comes from a country where average health is far below that in the United States, but the typical migrant to the United States is much healthier than the typical native-born resident. In our view, this is convincing evidence not only that there is a health selection effect for migrants to the United States, but also that the average magnitude of the health selection effect is very large. For some countries, the presumption must be that health selection is even larger. For example, the average male life expectancy in India is less than 60 years. The typical Indian migrants to the United States would clearly not expect such a life expectancy either in India or in the United States. Table 7-9 also suggests that the extent of health selection varies considerably across sending countries. The real question is whether that variability is systematically related to the factors highlighted in the model outlined in this section.

Progress on this issue has been limited because we typically do not know the health of immigrants at time of first arrival, which is the only time when selectivity can be unambiguously evaluated. Health selectivity involves a comparison at the time of immigration between the health of movers and the health of stayers in the sending country; it has nothing directly to do with health of the native born of those in the receiving country.

Table 7-10 attempts to partially remedy this situation by placing the 17 countries listed in Table 7-9 into three groups based on the average male life expectancy in the sending country. Group 1 includes migrants from the five countries with the longest male lifespan, while Group 3 includes migrants from the six countries with the shortest male lifespan. Group 2 includes those from countries that fall between the other groups. This grouping discriminates well among the sending countries in this dimension. Men in Group 2 countries live an average of nearly 5 fewer years than men in Group 1 countries, while those in Group 3 countries live almost 9 fewer years than those in Group 2.

The remaining columns in Table 7-10 measure health outcomes of new legal immigrants to the United States approximately at the time of their arrival. Using the general health status scale, new immigrants from Group 1 countries self-report themselves in much better health than the two other country groups. However, the difference between Group 2 and 3 immigrants is not large (and may even slightly favor Group 3) in spite of the 8-year difference in male life expectancy between them. Moreover, there appear to be very small differences between these three groups in the overall prevalence rates of conditions.[7] These data suggest that especially among Group 2 and 3 countries, there is considerably less heterogeneity among new immigrants than there is among health outcomes in the sending countries. This confirms the theoretical prediction that the variance in health among migrants is much smaller than the variance in health in sending countries.

Table 7-11 provides additional evidence on the issue of health selection. Swallen (2002) has computed male life expectancy by ethnic group for the native born and foreign born in the United States. Her data demonstrate

TABLE 7-10 Comparisons of New Legal Immigrants with Life Expectancy in Country of Origin

Country of Origin Grouping	Male Life Expectancy	% in Excellent or Very Good Health	% in Fair or Poor Condition	% with any Chronic Condition	% with any Serious Condition
1	72.3	57.1	14.1	20.6	7.0
2	67.5	43.4	29.4	23.9	6.4
3	58.7	52.9	22.1	23.4	6.9

NOTE: The three country groupings are based on the list of 17 countries in Table 7-9, ordered by levels of male life expectancy. Group 1 includes the five sending countries that rank highest in male LE while Group 3 includes the six countries that rank lowest in male LE. The health outcome measures in the 3rd through 6th columns are from the New Immigrant Survey-Pilot.

TABLE 7-11 Life Expectancies by Nativity

Age	White male		Asian male			Hispanic male		
	U.S born	Foreign born	U.S. born	Foreign born	Home country	U.S. born	Foreign born	Home country
5	68.2	66.9	73.5	74.2	65.2	68.1	70.3	67.5
45	30.8	31.6	35.2	35.7	29.8	31.8	34.1	32.5
65	15.1	15.9	15.8	18.7	14.3	16.1	18.0	17.0

SOURCES: Data for U.S. born and foreign born are obtained from Swallen (2002). These data are for 1990 life tables. Data for Home Country are immigrant weighted averages of the data contained in Table 7-9. These data are for 2000 life tables.

that within broad ethnic categories, the foreign born have longer life expectancies than the U.S. born and implicitly the foreign born have longer expectancies than residents in the sending countries (by comparison with Table 7-9). This comparison is made more explicit by including immigrant-weighted average life expectancies in the sending countries for Asians and Hispanics. The latter numbers are for calendar year 2000, while the nativity numbers for the United States are for 1990, so the home country numbers are inflated by a few years of mortality improvement compared to the nativity life expectancy (LE) numbers. These comparisons show that for Asian immigrants life expectancies in the United States (at age 5) may be as much as 10 years greater than the average in the Asian sending countries. This must mean that health selection among Asians is very large or that the United States is a much healthier place to live than the typical Asian sending country. Although Asian life expectancies are lower in the second generation, they remain much higher than in the Asian sending countries.

The data in Table 7-11 show that positive health selection also exists among Latino immigrants, but that it is much smaller in magnitude. Adjusting for the secular improvements in mortality, the LE differential between Latino migrants and their home countries is about 5 years. Once again, LE falls in the second generation, but would still remain above the sending countries after adjusting for the secular improvements in mortality.

Migration Model of Subsequent Health Trajectory

The second most prominent subject concerns what happens to immigrants' health subsequent to their arrival in the United States. The dominant empirical conclusion appears to be that trajectories of immigrant health are less positive than they would have been if they had not migrated. Once again, these findings coexist with little assistance from formal theory, but the usual reasons cited include a less healthy environment in the United

States or the adoption by migrants of the alleged poorer health habits that exist in America.

A useful place to introduce some theory is the health production function—the relationship between various inputs and the stock or commodity "health" (H_t):

$$H_t = f(H_{t-1}, G_o, B_t, MC_t, ED, E_t) \tag{3}$$

Health in time period t, H_t, is the result of the stock of health in the time period $t-1$, H_{t-1}, depreciation, and investments to improve health in the previous time period. Health is produced by several different inputs, including the use and quality of medical care (MC_t), the adoption of good personal health behaviors (good diet, exercise), and the avoidance of bad ones (smoking, excessive drinking) (B_t), and a vector of country-specific environmental factors (E_t), such as the air pollution level or prevalence rates of contagious diseases.

Education may enter this production function because it affects the way individuals can transform inputs into good health. For example, more educated households may choose more qualified doctors, be more aware of the harmful health effects of behaviors such as smoking or environmental risks, or be better able to provide preventive self-care to prevent illness or to mitigate its more harmful effects. Finally, family background or genetic endowments (G_o), which are typically unobserved by the researcher, have played an important role in contemporary research on this topic. For example, Rosenzweig and others have argued that the existence of these unobserved background factors that can often be traced to early childhood may seriously bias estimates of this production function.[8]

In this framework, health changes over the life course and the trajectory of these changes are the result of the stock of health in the time period $t-1$, H_{t-1}, depreciation over the previous time period, and investments to improve health in the previous time period.[9] The current inputs and behaviors chosen are investments that produce increments to the stock of health. These inputs, such as the demand for medical care, are "derived" demands: valued not directly but only because of their impact on health. Because the purchase of these inputs or the adoption of health-related behaviors are choices individuals or families can make, they are, in the parlance of economics, "endogenous" variables.

$$H_t = H^*(H_{t-1}, P_{mc}, P_o, ED, E_t, Y_t, G_o) \tag{4}$$

Equation (4) expresses current health as a function of the price of medical care (P_{mc}), the price of other inputs (P_o), education of each family member (ED), and household income (Y_t).

If we let period $t-1$ be the time of immigration, we can solve equation (4) sequentially to obtain the health trajectory subsequent to immigration. Conditional on health at the point of immigration, this health trajectory is a function of all relevant prices and incomes subsequent to immigration. Solving sequentially

$$H^m_t = H^*(H_{t-1}, P_{mc}, P_o, ED, E_t, Y_t, G_o) \qquad (5)$$

(where ~ indicates a time series vector of values).

Because equation (5) describes the health trajectory if a person immigrates, the relevant prices, incomes, and environmental factors are those that exist in the United States. There is a corresponding equation that would be obtained if the person chose not to immigrate:

$$H^{nm}_t = H^*(H_{t-1}, P_{mc}, P_o, ED, E_t, Y_t, G_o) \qquad (5')$$

(where prices, incomes, and environmental influences are now those that exist in the sending country).

Combined, equations (5) and (5') suggest that there are several pathways through which health may be altered by immigration. First, higher incomes may promote better health. Jasso et al. (2001) show that the typical economic gain from legal immigration to the United States is large but quite variable across immigrant attributes. For example, the mean economic gain at the time of green card receipt was about $15,000 per year. Economic gains of this magnitude could eventually translate into improved health trajectories. The variability of economic gains suggests similar variability in improved health outcomes.

An advantage of immigrant samples for this issue concerns its ability to separate out the effects of changes in relative and absolute incomes, two quite distinct hypotheses of why income may affect health. Relative income position is thought to affect health by the stress associated with lower hierarchical position, while absolute income may alter health through access to care. Many immigrants may experience a large absolute increase in income while finding themselves at a lower point in the income distribution in the United States than they were in their country of origin. These distinct effects of relative and absolute income position are quite difficult to separate in domestic population samples.

Turning to country-level environmental attributes, equations (5) and (5') represent a comparison of country-specific attributes that promote or hinder health. Because there are more than 100 different sending countries, it indicates that individual studies such as those of Japanese immigrants are not capable of being informative about the experiences of other immigrants from other countries or of those who arrived at a different time. A good deal of the emphasis in the Japanese studies rests on the comparative benefits of a Japanese diet or culture over an American one, a comparison that would not carry over to other side-by-side contrasts.

Equations (5) and (5') also indicate that simple summary statements—such as that living in the United States is bad for immigrant health—are misplaced. Across all the environmental factors that influence health, America is unlikely to rank as either the best or worst health environment. What is more relevant is measuring the specific environmental factors—diet, specific health behaviors, health environment, health care system—that distinguish subsequent health outcomes.

Equations (5) and (5') raise the fundamental question of what the appropriate counterfactual is. We are interested in a comparison of what happens to an immigrant as he/she stays in the United States compared to what would have happened in the sending country if no migration had taken place. Although often used in the literature, an appropriate counterfactual is not what is happening to the health of a native-born U.S. resident. Rather, the effect on the health of an immigrant changing countries involves a comparison of the health trajectory of an immigrant in the receiving country with the health trajectories of "similar" people in the sending countries.

Equations (5) and (5') do not represent a complete characterization of the problem, which has a form similar to that developed by Willis and Rosen (1979), where individuals now self-select as migrants or nonmigrants. The migrant selection rule was described in equations (1) and (2), earlier illustrating that although often discussed separately, health selection and subsequent health trajectories are not orthogonal processes. Current and perhaps expected future health profiles influence the decision to migrate so that migrants are not a random sample of the population at risk either in terms of their current health or its expected trajectory.

Finally, health selection is not independent of the subsequent health trajectory. To this point we have modeled selection in a cross-section. But consider a sending country with the exact same distribution of health as that which exists in the United States. In our theoretical model (supported by the empirical facts to follow), immigrants of working age still should be quite positively selected on their health—so we see very low rates of serious illness (heart disease, cancer, diabetes, and the like) among new immigrants to the United States. But because you can only self-select based on something you know about or at least suspect, differences in health outcomes of immigrants and the native born in onset of disease 10 or 20 years after immigration should show much smaller differences, or maybe none at all. Therefore, by a simple process of regression toward the mean, disease rates of the foreign born will necessarily converge to the U.S. norm. For a similar reason, the health of the second generation will tend to fall relative to the first generation. A good deal of the current literature interprets a decline in immigrant health, with length of stay or across generations as indicative of problems in American health environments.[10] But all it may be is the necessary consequence of strong health selection effects and regression toward the mean.

THE HEALTH OF NEW LEGAL IMMIGRANTS

In this section, we present results obtained from the New Immigrant Pilot Survey (NIS-P), a panel survey of a nationally representative sample of new legal immigrants. These legal immigrants were admitted to legal permanent residence to the United States during the months of July and August of 1996 (for details, see Jasso, Massey, Rosenzweig, and Smith, 2000). This sample was based on probability samples of administrative records of the U.S. Immigration and Naturalization Service (INS) representing all those who received their green cards during those months. The NIS-P links survey information about immigrants' pre- and postimmigration labor market, schooling, health, and migratory experiences with data available from INS administrative records, including the visa type under which the immigrant was admitted. The NIS-P consists of a baseline survey, a 3-month follow-up of half of the original sample (to evaluate whether periodicity affected attrition), a 6-month follow-up of all original sample members, and a 1-year follow-up, also of all original sample members.[11]

Given the brief 15-minute telephone interviews, the health information collected in the NIS-P was limited—largely self-reported general health status, the prevalence of selected chronic conditions, some health behaviors, the utilization of medical services, and how that care was paid. Yet, even this limited health information proves to be quite valuable. The reason is that the problems that plagued monitoring the economic success of new legal immigrants also have affected current research findings on immigrant health. These problems include the lack of any true national representative samples and the inability to follow this appropriate sample over time.

Table 7-12 lists the distribution of self-reported health status of these new legal immigrants alongside distributions for the native born obtained in the same year from the NHIS. Using this index, once again the health of new legal immigrants to the United States is generally quite good. Fewer than one in seven report themselves as being in fair or poor health. If we compare all adult immigrants to native-born Americans, the data indicate that the only noticeable difference that emerges takes place among older immigrants. This age pattern among legal immigrants is additional evidence that the nature of health selection is very different among older immigrants.

Table 7-13 lists rates of chronic conditions for respondents in the NIS-P. To examine the possibility that any disparities with the native born are

TABLE 7-12 Health Status of New Legal Immigrants and the U.S. Native Born

	NIS			1996 NHIS: Born in U.S.		
	All	25-44	50+	All	25-44	50+
Excellent or very good	59.6	66.2	29.9	62.4	71.2	46.8
Good	26.8	26.9	27.7	25.1	21.5	30.9
Fair or poor	13.6	7.0	42.5	12.5	7.3	22.3
# of observations	972	588	127	34,061	16,024	13,105

SOURCES: New Immigrant Pilot Survey and born in the United States from 1996 NHIS.

due to age, rates are also listed for those 25 to 44 years old and for those over age 50. To provide a benchmark, the middle three columns provide rates for native-born Americans from the 1996 NHIS and the last three columns for those who said they had arrived within the past 5 years. The latter group is most similar to respondents in the NIS-P in terms of duration of stay in the United States, but will include, in addition to legal immigrants, nonimmigrants (e.g., students, those on temporary visa) and illegal immigrants. Reported rates of chronic conditions of new legal immigrants are quite low, especially compared to the native born. Among the younger sample (those between ages 25 and 44), these differences are particularly large in the more severe conditions. For some diseases such as hypertension and diabetes, health selection may actually reverse among older, new legal immigrants.

It is sometimes argued that these low rates of chronic conditions among the foreign-born population simply reflect the lower degree of contact with doctors and hospitals. Without such contact, a condition would not be diagnosed. To check this possibility, we look in Table 7-14 at rates conditional on having seen a physician or having been hospitalized during the past year. In fact, rates of contact with Western medicine among new legal

TABLE 7-13 Rates of Chronic Conditions of New Legal Immigrants

	NIS			Native Born			0-5		
	All	25-44	50+	All	25-44	50+	All	25-44	50+
Hypertension	10.8	4.6	40.6	16.9	6.0	33.3	6.3	1.4	31.6
Diabetes	2.5	0.6	13.3	4.1	1.5	8.9	1.4	0.0	3.4
Cancer	0.7	0.6	1.8	2.3	0.6	5.9	0.2	0.1	1.3
Lung disease	1.9	1.4	4.6	9.7	4.1	12.4	2.1	2.0	0.0
Arthritis	7.4	3.1	27.3	16.9	6.3	36.3	5.3	3.1	21.4
Heart disease	3.0	1.0	15.1	8.9	5.9	19.9	3.7	0.0	19.9
Asthma	3.4	2.8	3.6	5.4	6.0	5.0	1.1	1.3	0.0

SOURCES: Native born and 0-5 from NHIS and from New Immigrant Pilot Survey. For number of observations, see Table 7-12.

TABLE 7-14 Prevalence Rates of Chronic Conditions for Those Who Saw a Doctor or Were Hospitalized During the Past Year

| | 25-44 | | 50+ | |
	0-5 Years	U.S. Born	0-5 Years	U.S. Born
Hypertension	3.9	7.7	38.1	35.7
Diabetes	1.4	1.9	7.1	10.2
Cancer	0.2	0.8	1.1	6.7
Lung disease	2.7	10.4	4.7	13.2
Arthritis	3.2	7.3	31.2	40.1
Heart disease	2.7	6.1	23.9	26.1
Asthma	2.3	5.9	1.4	5.3

immigrants are quite high; 62 percent of the new legal immigrants said they had seen a doctor during the past year. Even among those who had such contact, reported rates of chronic conditions are much lower among new immigrants than among the native born. This indicates that this source of reporting bias may not be able to explain the better health of immigrants.[12]

This comparison with native-born Americans hides the far more interesting story about the considerable variation in health that exists among immigrants. One dimension of that diversity concerns the countries from which they came. These data are listed for general health status in panel A of Table 7-15 and for the more important chronic conditions in panel B of

TABLE 7-15 Diversity of Immigrant Health Outcomes by Place of Last Residence

A. Self-Reported Health Status

Place of origin	Excellent or Very Good	Good	Fair or Poor
Europe	52	30	19
South America	69	18	13
Asia	57	29	14
Africa	70	29	1
Mexico	49	34	16
Other North America	74	16	10

B. Prevalence Rates of Selected Chronic Conditions

Place of origin	Hypertension	Arthritis	Diabetes
Europe	17.4	12.0	3.7
South America	8.5	4.6	3.0
Asia	5.5	6.6	1.4
Africa	9.5	2.4	2.4
Mexico	11.0	7.1	4.8
Other North America	13.5	6.2	1.0

SOURCE: New Immigrant Pilot Survey.

the same table. While nearly three quarters of immigrants from North America (except Mexico) are in excellent or very good health, this fraction drops to about half among Europeans and Mexicans. A similar degree of heterogeneity holds when we examine type of visa. For example, hypertension is particularly common among Europeans (about 1 in 6) and much more rare among new Asian migrants (about 1 in 20).

Another dimension of this heterogeneity exists by visa category. This dimension is important because visa status—the legal reason why an immigrant was allowed into the United States—is one of the principal policy levers that can be used to change the types of immigrants who arrive. The A panel of Table 7-16 lists the distribution of self-reported health status by the major categories of admission to legal status in the United States. The health of immigrants in the two largest visa categories—employment and spouses of U.S. citizens—is generally excellent and much better than that of the typical native-born American (see Table 7-1). The situation is not as sanguine in the other groups listed in this table. To illustrate, the other immigrant visa category where individuals qualify through marriage—spouses of permanent resident aliens—report themselves in much poorer health than those people who married U.S. citizens. However, one group of immigrants stands out in terms of their relatively bad health status—refugees and asylees. Shortly after the time of their green card receipt, one-third of refugees self-report as being in fair or poor health.

Panel B of Table 7-16 illustrates this diversity by visa status by listing prevalence rates for the more common chronic conditions. As before,

TABLE 7-16 Diversity of Immigrant Health Outcomes by Visa Status

A. Self-Reported Health Status

Visa status	Excellent or Very Good	Good	Fair or Poor
Principal employment	76	18	6
Spouse of U.S. citizen	74	20	6
Spouse of permanent resident	51	37	14
Diversity	46	38	17
Refugee or asylee	38	30	32

B. Prevalence Rates of Selected Chronic Conditions

Visa status	Hypertension	Arthritis	Diabetes
Principal employment	5.3	4.2	0.5
Spouse of U.S. citizen	4.8	4.0	0.0
Spouse of permanent resident	9.7	4.8	3.2
Diversity	14.6	4.1	4.2
Refugee or asylee	25.3	17.7	5.1

SOURCE: New Immigrant Pilot Survey.

chronic conditions vary across types of immigrants. In every single visa category, prevalence rates are smaller—and often considerably smaller— among new immigrants. For example, a quarter of all refugees and asylees have hypertension, while nearly one in five were diagnosed with arthritis. The ability of such data to isolate health problems of some immigrants by a known characteristic may turn into an important public health tool in targeting health interventions.

To this point, our data on the health status of new legal immigrants has concentrated on when they arrived. The question of what happens subsequently has absorbed much recent research on immigrant health. Most scholarship in this field argues that on average, immigrant health actually deteriorates with length of stay in the United States. The reasons for this relative deterioration are debated, but there is general acceptance that living in the United States may not be all that good for your health.

The difficulty with the "years" is that we do not have good national data that track immigrants over time. Although the NIS-P only monitors health changes over a short period of about a year, these early years may be a critical time in health evolution. The "all" row in Table 7-17 examines changes in self-reported health status for the full NIS sample. Contrary to the widespread view, on average immigrant health actually improved during the first year of the survey. For example, at the time of the 6-month interview, 18 percent of respondents reported themselves in fair or poor health. Roughly 9 months later, only 14 percent reported the same status.

There are two main hypotheses about our two salient findings: First, immigrant health is better than that of native-born Americans, and second, it actually improves over time. The explanations generically fall into two

TABLE 7-17 Short-Run Changes in Health Status

	Initial			Final		
	Excellent or Very Good	Good	Fair or Poor	Excellent or Very Good	Good	Fair or Poor
All	56	26	18	59	27	14
Saw doctor						
Yes	56	25	19	60	26	14
No	66	28	16	70	28	12
Place of origin						
Asia	53	24	23	54	29	14
Europe	54	28	19	52	30	18
South America	63	23	13	71	17	10
Other North America	63	25	13	74	16	10
Mexico	42	38	19	49	34	16

camps. The first explanation is that it is a real phenomenon and immigrants are much healthier. Just as immigrants were highly selective on other traits, this explanation claims that immigrants are selective on their health. In part, this health selectivity may result from medical screening exams given prior to entry, although there is some legitimate question about how rigorous those exams are. More importantly, immigrants may self-select themselves on their health.

One explanation for this improvement is that it results from reporting biases, of which three are often mentioned. The first reporting issue relates to language—the effect of limited English-language ability and changes in that ability over time. Some immigrants may not fully understand the question and as their language ability improves, they report health improvements even though no change has occurred. To examine this possibility, the next row in Table 7-17 examines only immigrants whose English ability was very good when they arrived and did not change. Even in this sample where language is good and unchanging, health status got better over time. The second reporting bias concerns contact with Western medical diagnosis. The next two rows in Table 7-17 list changes in health status by whether or not the respondent had seen a health care provider in the past year. Once again, short-run improvements in health appear to exist independently of physician contact.

The third type of reporting bias involves the reference comparison implicitly being made. If a person says his or her health is very good, the natural question is compared to whom? This is a particularly salient issue for immigrants, whose reference group may be changing with the very act of migration. For example, if an immigrant comes from a place where the average health is much worse than in the United States, he or she may downgrade this evaluation when he or she begins to discover that average health is much better in the United States. A symmetric argument holds for places where average health is above that in the United States. One way of testing this hypothesis is to examine changes across place of origin. The final rows in this table do exactly that. Health status improves across all countries of origin. Moreover, there does not appear to be any relation of health change to whether one arrives from a place where the average health was either low or high. The arguments were not meant to imply that reporting biases in health do not exist. However, these biases appear not able to explain the principal health patterns observed for immigrants. In general, immigrant health is quite good and it appears to improve over time, at least in the short run.

EMPIRICAL MODELS OF HEALTH SELECTIVITY AND HEALTH TRAJECTORIES

In this section, we present new empirical models estimating the determinants of health selectivity of migrants to the United States. and short-run health changes subsequent to immigration. Both models rely on data obtained from the New Immigrant Pilot Survey, which was described in detail in the previous section. We first present our analysis of health selectivity of migrants and conclude this section with a simple model of short-run health changes following immigration. The basic idea behind these analyses is that skill and health are complements—those factors that induce more skilled immigrants to emigrate to the United States also induce healthier immigrants. Skill and health go together for two reasons. First, those immigrants with more skill have higher incomes and thus can "purchase" better health, a proposition we will test directly based on the change in income of the immigrants. Second, those who tend to invest in human capital do so with respect to both investments in health and in labor market skills.

Health Selectivity of Immigrants

The theoretical model in an earlier section highlighted some central factors that should influence both the skill and health selectivity of immigrants. The parallel nature of the predictions for skill and health argues for the estimation of models of both outcomes at the same time with the same set of covariates. Therefore, to carry out an analysis motivated by the theoretical framework discussed earlier, we focus on the home country earnings and health outcomes of adult immigrants aged 21 through 64 who obtained visas as employment immigrants or as spouses of U.S. citizens or U.S. permanent resident aliens. We chose these categories principally because such immigrants are able to immigrate without having a blood relative in the United States—a very different kind of selection effect than the one that concerns us here. This nonnepotistic immigration is thus an option for all individuals born and residing outside the United States. In contrast, the left-out group is very heterogeneous, including refugees, parents, and adult unmarried children. In addition, we select people within this working-age group (ages 21 to 64) because the data presented earlier indicate that the health selection process is quite different for older immigrants.

We examine two outcomes that address the selectivity of immigrants—their last earnings in the sending countries and their self-reported health status indexed by an ordinal five-point scale ranked from excellent to poor. We use the immigrant's earnings in his or her home country rather than the U.S. wage because the former is not affected by possibly imperfect skill transferability. A unique feature of the NIS-P is that it provides information on the earnings of the immigrants in their last job before coming to the United States. More than 77 percent of the immigrants had worked in a foreign country in the 10 years prior to the survey. We converted the earnings in the last job abroad, provided by the immigrants in native currency units, to dollar amounts based on estimates of the country-specific purchasing power of the currencies from the Penn International Comparisons Project, described by Summers and Heston (1991). These conversion factors are explicitly designed to take into account differences in the "cost of living" across countries and to avoid the distortions associated with exchange rate regimes in order to facilitate cross-country comparisons. Table 7-18 contains our estimated models for these two outcomes—Generalized Least Squares (GLS) estimation for the ln of purchasing power parity (PPP)-full time earnings in the sending country and ordered logit estimation for the self-reported health index (scaled from 1 = excellent to 5 = poor). This scale is used to parallel work where mortality is the health outcome.

Our basic migration model with worker skill heterogeneity and country skill-price differentials implies that high skill-price countries will send fewer but more skilled and healthier immigrants. How can we measure variation across countries in skill prices? In terms of the observable correlates of skill prices, among workers residing in countries with the same output per worker, those workers residing in countries where workers have higher average skill levels receive lower skill prices, while among workers in countries with the same average worker skill levels, those in countries with higher output per worker will receive higher skill prices. Given immigrant skill heterogeneity and selectivity due to home country skill-price variation, these results imply that immigrants from countries with high output per worker and with low average levels of schooling will have the highest skill levels and best health among immigrants with identical own schooling levels.

To measure skill prices in accordance with the model, we used the real (PPP-converted) Gross Domestic Product (GDP) *per worker* estimates from the Penn World Table, Mark 5.6 supplemented with updated 1995 estimates from the ICP, and estimates of the average schooling levels of the population aged 25 and over in origin countries from Barro and Lee (1993). Average schooling estimates are available for a large but not complete subset of countries for which there are PPP GDP estimates. For those countries for which there are no schooling stock estimates, we constructed a variable indicating that schooling was missing and set the schooling variable to zero. Similarly, home country average health is indexed by female life expectancy, with an indicator variable for the few countries for which we were unable to obtain a value.

TABLE 7-18 Determinants of Log of Immigrants' Home Country Earnings and Health Status

Sample	Home Country Earners	Health Status from Excellent (1) to Poor (5)
Variable/Estimation Procedure	GLS	Ordered Logit
Home country characteristic		
Ln (real GDP/worker)	1.27	−.4329
	(7.71)*	(1.92)
Ln (average schooling in years)	−0.91	0.6527
	(2.55)	(1.85)
Distance to closest U.S. port of entry (miles × 10⁻⁴)	0.157	0.429
	(0.42)	(0.68)
Border country	−0.258	1.014
	(1.22)	(2.93)
U.S. military base	−0.0751	0.4748
	(0.31)	(1.51)
English an official language	0.719	−1.138
	(3.89)	(3.44)
Schooling missing	−1.00	1.607
	(1.76)	(2.17)
Ln life expectancy	0.372	−3.197
	(0.42)	(2.11)
Life expectancy missing	2.088	−12.73
	(0.42)	(1.91)
Characteristic of worker		
Schooling (years)	0.0441	−0.0788
	(2.79)	(2.94)
Years in the United States	0.1237	−0.0221
	(1.43)	(0.17)
Years in the United States squared	−0.0182	0.0051
	(1.86)	(0.41)
Age	0.0763	−0.0367
	(2.17)	(0.64)
Age squared	−0.00061	0.0009
	(1.52)	(1.29)
Year last worked in home country	0.0464	—
	(2.42)	
Female	−0.114	0.0620
	(0.90)	(0.30)
Visa		
Spouse of U.S. citizen	−0.575	0.2551
	(3.13)	(0.85)
Spouse of U.S. permanent resident alien	−0.331	1.728
	(1.11)	(4.17)
Spouse of employment immigrant	−0.393	0.1599
	(2.24)	(0.55)
Constant	−9.53	
	(1.87)	
Number of immigrants	342	327
Number of countries	58	
Adjusted R^2	0.445	0.1065

*Absolute value of t-ratio adjusted for country cluster effects in parentheses in column.

We have several measures related to the costs of immigration. The first is whether the immigrant is from a border country to the United States (Mexico or Canada), while the second variable is the distance of the origin country's capital to the closest major entry city in the United States. The third is an indicator variable taking on the value of one if the country was a host to a U.S. military base in the 5 years preceding the NIS-P survey. Military bases are enclaves of U.S. citizens abroad, many of whom are young and single so that the cost of obtaining entry by marrying a U.S. citizen is lower. The selection framework suggests that countries with military bases, border countries (Mexico and Canada), and countries generally not located at great distances from the United States have lower U.S. immigration barriers or costs and should, given skill prices, be disproportionately sending countries for low-skill and less healthy immigrants.

Worker attributes included in these models include own schooling measured in years, number of years in the United States because some of these immigrants obtained their green cards while living in this country, a quadratic in age, sex (an indicator variable set to one for women), and the year last worked in the home country (for the home country earnings equation model only). In addition, three indicator variables for type of visa are included: whether the immigrant obtained a visa as a spouse of a U.S. citizen, a spouse of a permanent resident alien, or a spouse of a principal employment visa immigrant.

In column 2 of Table 7-18, we report GLS estimates of ln (national log) home country earnings in a model that includes the country-specific skill price determinants—the log of real GDP per worker and the log of the average schooling of workers—and the individual worker's individual observable skill attributes. A parallel ordered logit model for self-reported health status is listed in the third column. These specifications also include visa category variables, geographic proximity variables, and years of U.S. residence as determinants of home country earnings to assess how earnings and health selectivity can obscure interpretations of the determinants of the U.S. earnings and health of immigrants. Because the geographic location of a country relative to the United States, the U.S. visa status of an immigrant, and his or her U.S. experience are unlikely to have direct effects on home country earnings or health, the coefficients on these variables mainly reflect selectivity.

In conformity to the model, the coefficient on the log of per-worker country output is positive for home country earnings and negative for our health index (with poor health at the top of this index). Similarly, the sign of the coefficient on the measure of average worker skill in the country is negative for ln earnings and positive for health status. Combined, these results indicate that immigrants from countries with high skill prices are, as predicted, positively selected both on their skill and their overall health.

Not surprisingly, immigrants from countries where the average health status is better (as measured by average life expectancy) are healthier. These effects are not quantitatively trivial. For example, a doubling of GDP/worker (holding everything the same), which is equivalent to a doubling in the skill price, would increase the proportion of immigrants in "excellent" health by 20 percent and reduce the proportion in "fair" health by 25 percent. Similarly, a much smaller 10 percent increase in the price of skill increases the proportion of immigrants in "excellent" health by 3 percent and reduces the proportion in fair health by 4 percent.

In contrast, there appears to be no relation between country-specific average life expectancy and home country earnings. This may reflect two offsetting forces. First, average life expectancy is correlated with own health, which should increase earnings. But in the formulation in Table 7-18, average life expectancy also is a (negative) proxy for unobserved skill prices, which should reduce earnings.

There are several measures of the cost of immigration included in these models. A simple measure of geographic distance does not matter in either equation, perhaps because the distance to the nearest point of entry may not be the most relevant measure given the existence of ethnic enclaves in the United States. In contrast, other things equal, immigrants from the two border countries (Canada and Mexico), where the cost of migration is presumably less, send less skilled and less healthy migrants to the United States. We also estimate poorer health status among migrants from countries with military bases, although this effect is not statistically significant at conventional levels.

With respect to effects of personal attributes, our estimates support the conventional finding that own schooling is positively associated with both last home country earnings and with self-assessed health status. Both estimates are statistically significant. The interpretation of the coefficient on U.S. experience is not whether increased time in the United States increases or decreases home country earnings, because home country earnings are measured *prior* to coming to the United States. Rather, this variable should be interpreted as measuring whether immigrants, of given age, who came to the United States earlier have higher or lower levels of skills. Our results indicate no statistically significant effect of time in the United States on home country earnings.

This interpretation is not possible for health status, which is measured instead after arrival in the United States. However, because our results will indicate that health status improves after arrival in the United States, our estimate of a zero net effect of U.S. experience on health in Table 7-18 may indicate that those who come to this country earlier also had worse health on average.

Visa status also captures some aspects of immigrant selection. All effects are estimates compared to the left-out group—those who obtained principal employment visas. Although spouses of U.S. citizens and spouses of those who obtained principal employment visas appear to be negatively selected on their labor market skills, there does not seem to be any selectivity on their health status. In contrast, spouses of permanent resident aliens are in significantly poorer health than immigrants on employment visas.

In sum, the results in Table 7-18 indicate that there exists systematic variation in the skill and health selectivity of immigrants to the United States that in large part conforms remarkably well with the theoretical predictions outlined earlier. In particular, the country-specific factors that positively select on the skills of new immigrants also appear to positively select on their health status. The results imply that increases in the price of skills in countries outside the United States, a common result of economic development, will lead to a more skilled and healthier immigrant population in the United States.

Short-Run Health Trajectories

Although it receives almost no mention in the existing literature on health trajectories, one of the biggest changes attributable to immigration is a very large income gain (Jasso et al., 2001). To the extent that income is an important determinant of health status, there is reason to believe that the economic gains of immigrants can result in health improvements. In this section we use new data on immigrants to examine how economic gains from immigration affect health change. Because long-term panel data that follow immigrants from the start of their immigration process are simply not available, estimating models of health change subsequent to immigration is difficult. Once again a data source that offers some potential for examining health change is the New Immigrant Pilot Survey. The random sample of new legal immigrants of the NIS-P was followed up at three subsequent waves. Self-assessed health status, rated from excellent to poor, was reported by all respondents at the 6-month and 12-month interviews, which were actually about 9 months to 1 year apart. In this analysis, we examine changes in self-reported health status ranked as improved, stayed the same, and deteriorated, again using an ordered logit model. We can think of this model as a fixed effects equation. For example, suppose that health is a lagged function of income and other fixed traits (such as schooling, visa, country of origin attributes). Because we have health and income at two points in time, differencing gives the change in health as a function of the lagged change in income. Age is added to the model to capture nonlinearities in age.

Our results are reported in Table 7-19. The main explanatory variable is the economic gain from immigration—the difference between the earnings received in the United States and amount earned in the last job in the

TABLE 7-19 Ordered Logit of Whether Self-Reported Health Status Improved, Stayed Same, or Deteriorated

	Coefficient	Z
Economic gain	0.0716	3.23
Age	–0.0189	1.23
Cut 1	–2.3600	
Cut 2	0.3231	

sending country. To make earnings in different countries as comparable as possible, as explained earlier, all sending country earnings are adjusted for purchasing power parity. The size and variability of the economic gain from immigration is not trivial. According to the estimates contained in Jasso et al. (2001), the mean economic gain from immigration was about $21,000, around which there was enormous variability. Moreover, the results in Table 7-19 indicate that the income gain associated with immigration positively affects health, so that big gainers are more likely to have subsequently improved health.

Recognizing the real possibility of dual causality, one should be cautious about any interpretation dealing with the relation between health and income (Smith, 1999). But given the magnitude of the gains in income due to immigration, it would be difficult to argue that health changes associated with immigration "caused' these income changes. Most important, the results in Table 7-19 add more reasons for some skepticism about the widely held view that health will decline due to immigration. The impact on one's health of living in a particular place is probably slow and cumulative, and the results in Table 7-19 only measure short-run changes. However, these economic gains at the time of immigration are unlikely to dissipate over time; in fact, the evidence shows that they will most likely expand over time (Jasso et al., 2001). Thus, even though the model estimated in Table 7-19 only predicts short-run health changes, the persistence of these large economic gains over the long term makes one suspect that on this mechanism at least health improvements might also persist. There is a vast literature spanning several disciplines that argues that income strongly promotes improved health. Why the force of this literature is ignored when the topic shifts to immigration is an interesting question.

RECOMMENDATIONS ON RESEARCH PRIORITIES AND FUNDING

There are several recommendations for research priorities and funding that are suggested by the findings in this chapter. First, the data have highlighted the enormous heterogeneity that exists within the foreign-born population. This heterogeneity appears in many dimensions, and immigrant health is certainly no exception. The most direct implication of this heterogeneity is that researchers need data with larger sample sizes of immigrants so that they can conduct country-specific analyses. The current, prominent national social science surveys contain immigrant samples as an addendum, roughly in proportion to their role in the overall population. Consequently, sample sizes for even the larger individual immigrant groups are often severely inadequate for meaningful analysis on the topic of immigrant health. If processes of health selection and acculturation vary across immigrant groups, our current data would not be able to detect either for many ethnic groups.

Second, it is essential that surveys be designed that capture immigrants at the start of the immigrant process. There are several key advantages to such a design. It allows one to more accurately access the extent of health selectivity at the time of immigration, before the environment in the receiving country has had any significant impact on the immigrant's health. It also permits an assessment of subsequent health trajectories from the beginning of the immigration process. Currently available immigrant samples are, at best, representative samples of the currently resident foreign-born population—those members of past immigrant cohorts who remained in the United States. Because we know little about the nature of the health selection of those who emigrated, it is impossible to deduce what health trajectories were for the typical immigrant. The New Immigrant Survey is an important step in the direction of obtaining a sample of immigrants at the beginning of a well-defined point—the receipt of a green card—and following all members of that cohort, whether or not they subsequently emigrated.

Third, in order to investigate the principal unanswered questions about immigrant health, it is necessary to integrate health, economic, social, and demographic measures within a single survey. Although they are quite useful for documenting health disparities, traditional health surveys such as NHIS or the National Health and Nutrition Environmental Survey are not ideal vehicles for understanding root causes because their measures of the economic, social, and demographic environment are quite limited. Similarly, current economic and demographic surveys are too narrow in the scope and depth of the health information they contain. These new surveys must also incorporate measures of the principal pathways that affect health trajectories. Such measures would include diet, income, and cultural support networks. Finally, it would be quite desirable to supplement observational health measures with physical measurements of health conditions.

Fourth, studies of the health outcomes of immigrant children and the children of immigrants also merit high priority on the research agenda. Such research adds an intergenerational component that speaks to possible alternative pathways of health acculturation across generations. Because the outcomes of children are closely tied to the behaviors and constraints faced by their immigrant parents, it is important to include children in the same surveys as their parents. These children are the eventual future legacy of immigration so understanding the determinants of their health addresses the issue of the long-term impact of immigration on the health of the American population.

Fifth, an important insight from the epidemiology literature is that investigations of specific diseases can help elucidate the pathways through which immigration affects health. For example, models that emphasize the impact of psychosocial stress associated with the process of immigration often see the main manifestations of this stress showing up later in diseases of the heart. Similarly, exposures to certain environmental or behavioral risks such as smoking may lead to increased risks of cancers or other diseases of the lung. Consequently, it is important to be able to track specific disease progressions of immigrants that can then be contrasted to those that characterize their native-born counterparts.

Sixth, the subject of immigrant health argues for the value of comparable international comparison studies. One of the arguments in favor of studies of immigrant health is that the diversity of health environments represented by the many sending countries offers an important analytical tool for studying effects of geographical environment on health. A similar agreement can be made about the receiving countries. The United States is not a unique country in terms of its position as an immigrant-receiving nation, and the considerable diversity among receiving countries will also provide much useful information.

Conclusions

In this chapter, we have explored some salient issues concerning immigrant health. Ethnic health disparities are inherently linked to immigration because ethnic identities often are traced to the country of origin of one's immigrant ancestors. Two of the central questions that have dominated the medical and social science literature on immigrant health are the central focus of this chapter. These issues involve the magnitude and mechanisms shaping health selectivity and the determinants of health trajectories following immigration. Health selection—the propensity of immigrants to be much healthier than a representative person in the sending country—is a quantitatively important phenomenon that is fundamental to understanding the most basic patterns that emerge about immigrant health. Immigrants are quite healthy and are very positively selected on this trait. However, great diversity exists among immigrants in the extent of health selection. In addition, the nature of health selection of immigrants appears to be fundamentally different among older immigrants, who have largely passed their prime working years. As part of this chapter, we also developed a theoretical model that attempts to explain the diversity in health selection among immigrants.

One of the consequences of this strong health selection effect is that it makes current evidence of health trajectories following immigration very problematic. For example, the general theme in the literature appears to be that immigration to the United States may have deleterious health consequences. However, this pattern is also easily explained simply by positive health selection on currently observed health traits and outcomes and then the subsequent necessary regression toward the mean. Research on health trajectories following immigration also frequently suffers from some confusion on what the appropriate comparison group should be. The issue is what an immigrant health profile is following immigration compared to what it would have been if he or she did not migrate. Comparisons that have dominated the existing literature that rely principally on how immigrants fare relative to native-born populations do not directly speak to the issue of the effects of immigration on lifetime health profiles.

ACKNOWLEDGMENT

Paper prepared for National Academy of Sciences Conference on Racial and Ethnic Disparities in Health. This research was supported by grants from the National Institutes of Health.

ENDNOTES

1. The National Health Interview Survey (NHIS) is conducted annually by the National Center for Health Statistics, Centers for Disease Control and Prevention. The NHIS annually administers interviews to a nationally representative sample of about 43,000 households, including about 106,000 persons. From each family in the NHIS, one sample adult and one sample child, if any, are randomly selected, and more detailed information on each is collected. To economize on interview length while asking detailed and comprehensive questions about specific conditions, until recent survey waves individuals were randomly assigned into six groups to ask questions about specific chronic conditions.

2. These data are consistent with the classic study by Kitagawa and Hauser (1973), which showed that mortality rates of the foreign born during middle age (35 to 64) were lower than those of the native born, but the reverse was true at older ages.

3. There are only 143 people in the NHIS asked a specific question about diabetes who had migrated within the previous 5 years.

4. This study is referred to as the Japanese-American Coronary Heart Disease Study. It included 11,900 men ages 45 to 69 in Hiroshima, Nagasaki, Honolulu, and the San Francisco Bay area.

5. This does not mean that diet was not important. According to Marmot and Syme (1976), the mean percentage of fat in the diet ranged from 15 percent in Japan to 37.6 percent in California Japanese.

6. One useful addition would be to model return migration where one particular dimension would concern migration back to the source country following retirement. The labor market conditions emphasized in the text would no longer receive great weight. While quality of medical care might encourage staying in the United States, the lower cost of living would make return migration more likely. Another extension would concern the initial and subsequent health of minor children who accompany their parents in the migration process. The extent of health selection is probably muted for minor children because the correlation in health of migrant parents and migrant children is far from perfect. In addition, there is some concern that the social environment in the United States for some immigrants may be quite risky, especially for adolescents. These concerns often center on drugs, alcohol, and gang behavior. Although the health of the children of migrants is an important topic, it is not our main concern here.

7. These conclusions would not change if we control for age.

8. For example, a person who has been generally sickly throughout their lives may require more medical care. If we do not control for this persistent unhealthiness, a regression of current health on medical services will understate the efficacy of medical care.

9. This production function, which summarizes the transformation of these inputs into health outputs, is typically governed by biological considerations.

10. For good examples, see National Research Council (2002).

11. Response rate at baseline was 62 percent and attrition by the 12-month interview was 5 percent. See Jasso et al. (2000) for details.

12. This qualified statement is necessary as having some physician contact may be a quite inadequate control. Immigrants and the native born may differ as well in the many other dimensions of contact, such as the quality of the consultation and the type and depth of the information exchanged. In addition, seeing a physician about one issue (e.g., an eye problem) may not make one aware of others (e.g., hypertension). In addition, doctors may act in a passive role, only treating the specific complaints that individuals report. These types of physician behavior may also vary across countries.

REFERENCES

Banks, J., Kapteyn, A., Smith, J.P., and Van Soest, A. (2004, February). *International comparisons of work and disability*. Paper presented at NBER conference on disability, Charleston, South Carolina.

Barro, R., and Lee, J.W. (1994). International comparisons of educational attainment. *Journal of Monetary Economics, 32*(December), 363-394.

Centers for Disease Control and Prevention. (2001). *Health: United States: 2001 with urban and rural health chartbook*. Hyattsville, MD: National Center for Health Statistics.

Grossman, M. (1972). *The demand for health: A theoretical and empirical investigation*. New York: National Bureau of Economic Research.

Jasso, G., Massey, D., Rosenzweig, M., and Smith, J.P. (2000). The new immigrant pilot survey (NIS): Overview and findings about U.S. immigrants at admission. *Demography, 37*(1), 127-138.

Jasso, G., Rosenzweig, M., and Smith, J.P. (2001). *The earnings of U.S. immigrants: World skill prices, skill transferability and selectivity*. Unpublished manuscript.

Kasl, S.V., and Berkman, L. (1983). Health consequences of the experiences of migration. *Annual Review of Public Health, 4*, 69-90.

King, G., Murray, C. Solomon, J., and Tandon, A. (2003). Enhancing the validity and cross-cultural comparability of measurement in survey research. *American Political Science Review, 98*(1), 567-583.

Kitagawa, E., and Hauser, P. (1973). *Differential mortality in the United States: A study in socioeconomic epidemiology.* Cambridge, MA: Harvard University Press.

Marmot, M.G., and Syme, S.L. (1976). Acculturation and coronary heart disease in Japanese-Americans. *American Journal of Epidemiology, 104*(3), 225-247.

Marmot, M.G., Adelstein, A.M., and Bulusu, L. (1984). Lessons from the study of immigrant mortality. *Lancet, 2,* 1455-1457.

National Research Council. (2002). *Emerging issues in Hispanic health: Summary of a workshop.* Center for Social and Economic Studies, Committee on Population, Commission on Behavioral and Social Sciences and Education. Washington, DC: National Academy Press.

Smith, J.P. (1999). Healthy bodies and thick wallets: The dual relation between health and economic status. *Journal of Economic Perspectives, 13*(2), 145-167.

Smith, J.P., and Edmonston, B. (1997). *The new Americans: Economic, demographic, and fiscal effects of immigration.* Washington, DC: National Academy Press.

Summers, R., and Heston, A. (1991). The Penn World Table (Mark 5): An expanded set of international comparisons, 1950-1988. *Quarterly Journal of Economics, 106,* 327-368.

Swallen, K.C. (2002). *Mortality in the U.S.: Comparing race/ethnicity and nativity.* Unpublished manuscript, University of Wisconsin.

Vega, W., and Amaro, H. (1994). Latino outlook: Good health, uncertain prognosis. *Annual Review of Public Health, 15,* 39-67.

Willis, R.J., and Rosen, S. (1979). Education and self-selection. *Journal of Political Economy, 87*(5), S7-S37.

SECTION III

THE SEARCH FOR CAUSAL PATHWAYS

8

Genetic Factors in Ethnic Disparities in Health

Richard S. Cooper

I very early got the idea that what I was going to do was prove to the world the Negroes were just like other people.—W.E.B. *DuBois*

Biology is being transformed by the advent of technology that allows us to define the molecular basis of genetic variation. Having pushed physics off the pedestal reserved for "big science," biologists have sequenced the genomes of half a dozen organisms, altered the sequence in even more, and cataloged millions of the DNA variants found in humans. The technological capacity to read and manipulate genes has in turn generated speculation that our ability to solve health problems will be transformed in a similarly dramatic fashion. Acknowledging that we are in the early stages of this new era, the practical accomplishments of genetic medicine to date are much more modest, however. Although great success has been achieved with the rare monogenic disorders, for the common chronic illnesses that account for most of the death and disability in our society, genomics has yet to elucidate the pathophysiology in important ways or improve treatment (Cooper and Psaty, 2003; Khoury, 2000; Lander, 1996; Report of the Advisory Committee on Health Research, 2002).

Describing the genetic underpinnings of common chronic diseases is a challenge of infinitely greater complexity than obtaining a sequence of nucleotides or finding single gene mutations. A quantum leap in biology will be required before the genes and the associated physiologic abnormalities that confer susceptibility to chronic disease can be understood. Given the intertwined effects of genes and environment on these conditions, the question remains as to whether or not important genetic causes can even be identified. Nonetheless, the exploration of the genome has accumulated unstoppable momentum and will profoundly alter our understanding of the biological world, even if it does not transform the practice of medicine or public health.

Genomics is connected to public health science through population genetics and epidemiology, and to the everyday practice of public health through race. An important goal of this discussion will be to try to disentangle genomics from race, based on the argument that they are categorically different ways of framing the epidemiologic questions. This is more than an intellectual challenge, however, because deeply held beliefs about the relative influence of nature and nurture on variation in disease patterns between populations bind the two together. After centuries of reliance on race as a surrogate for genes, the impulse has been to merely incorporate molecular data as new details, leaving the accepted framework in place. However, this solution can only be temporary. Among its many consequences, molecular genetics has made the current model of race obsolete and, in the long run, untenable. As a result, through no initiative of its own, public health suddenly has been presented with the opportunity to rethink one of its most intractable problems. Perhaps, one might argue, that will be the most important contribution of genetics to public health: Given our complete inability to devise effective solutions to racial inequalities in health, discarding what now passes for theory could be a salutary development.

The two main dimensions of the race controversy can be discussed separately. First, the "ideological" concept of race informs popular discourse and shapes policy, with a parallel impact in public health. This version of race is defined by social and historical forces and is used to create and justify many of the divisions that exist among people of varying religious, ethnic, or geographic backgrounds. This concept assumes the existence of categories that have no scientific foundation—at least none based on molecular data. This concept has been challenged since Darwin (1981), yet it persists for ideological purposes (Cooper, 1984; Montagu, 1964; Root, 2001). Although everyone in public health needs to be reminded of the importance and illegitimacy of this notion, and those who have not yet heard the news need to be informed, there is little of substantive importance that is really new to add to this debate: We should begin by simply acknowledging that race in the world of politics, and all the nutritional, educational, and social influences it entrains, continues to be the determining influence on ethnic variation in health.

A second use of race has assumed new relevance. As a label for regional populations, race has a long history in population genetics, and in this arena, important opportunities exist to revisit old questions on interethnic variation in health. At stake is whether or not we can move beyond the indirect methods applied in epidemiology or the generalizations built on estimation of genetic distance that have preoccupied population geneticists and anthropologists (Cavalli-Sforza, Menozzi, and Piazza, 1996; Relethford,

1998). Specifically, it is now possible to ask a set of testable questions: Can the global variation in the human genome be aggregated into subunits, and do those units correspond to the categories we call race? Can we assess the relative magnitude of shared and nonshared genetic material among population groups? Is there variation in causal genetic polymorphisms that is associated with important differences in chronic disease risk? Is it possible to conceptualize the collective human genome as a whole, and express that concept in quantitative terms?

Of course, complete answers to these questions are still well beyond our grasp. Some of the questions, like the aggregation of variants within population groups, are likely to be answered in the near future, while others, like the relative frequencies of causal variants for chronic diseases, may never be fully answered. Yet molecular genetics is changing the way we think about human variation, and it is crucial that this change has a positive impact on medicine and public health. Even though the noxious effects of racism—the social and economic consequences of the ideology—will only be eliminated through a political process, it remains the obligation of biological scientists to contribute to this eventual outcome by providing a clear description of the natural phenomena as we understand them. With an eye to history, it will be necessary, first and foremost, to ensure that the mistakes surrounding racial comparisons in the past are not repeated using molecular data.

In its current usage among epidemiologists, who have provided most of what we know about interethnic variation in health, the "common sense" or popular meaning of race is accepted as a given, unsupported by biological evidence, and serves both as a construct that frames research questions and a premise on which explanations are based. This standard application of race has obvious limitations and has resulted in widespread misunderstanding about the potential of genes to influence health (Cooper, Kaufman, and Ward, 2003; Kaufman and Cooper, 1996; Krieger, Rowley, Herman, Avery, and Phillips, 1993). As in society at large, incorporation of these notions into the intellectual grammar of science can lead to racist practice (Cooper and Kaufman, 1998). Thus, one of the aims of this paper will be an attempt to explore the role of scientific racism within the discipline of public health, and examine how that shapes the discourse and the research agenda.

ETHNIC DISPARITIES IN HEALTH STATUS

The focus of this discussion will be on the broad medical syndromes that account for most of the disability and premature mortality in the U.S. population. The first problem that arises when examining the racial/ethnic health patterns is how best to organize the data. As is well known, the definitions used by government agencies are explicitly not based on biological categories (Cooper, 1994; Hahn, 1992; Lott, 1993); instead this system was developed to meet the political obligations of the Census. The designation of "black," "white," "American Indian," and "Asian" are considered races, while "Hispanic" is a language or cultural grouping, and the conglomerate category of "Asian/Pacific Islanders/American Indian" is often used to collapse data from many smaller race groups. There is no way to map these categories directly onto genetic subpopulations, although there is some broad correspondence between the racial/ethnic labels and the continent of origin of the ancestral populations.

With the availability of vital statistics on both Hispanics and Asian/Pacific Islanders, we now have a reasonably clear description of the patterns of common disease in the U.S. racial/ethnic groups (Table 8-1). Health status will be discussed in more detail in other sections of this volume, the more limited purpose here is to frame the specific question that needs to be addressed by a genetic analysis. The first and most striking feature is the heterogeneity that exists among the groups. The most prevalent notion of minority health status in the United States is built on the "deficiency model," that is, an expectation of poorer outcomes for groups other than whites. Dismissed in the past as artifactual, the relative advantage enjoyed by Hispanics, despite similar education and income to blacks, is now undeniable. Characterized as the "Hispanic paradox," an active research agenda exists

TABLE 8-1 Health Status Measures in Racial/Ethnic Groups in the United States, 1998

Cause of Death	Age-Adjusted Death Rates*			
	White	Black	Hispanic	Asian
All causes	450.4	690.9	432.8	264.6
Heart disease	121.9	183.3	84.2	67.4
Coronary heart disease	79.2	92.5	54.7	42.9
Stroke	23.3	41.4	19.0	22.7
Cancer	121.0	161.2	76.1	74.8
COPD	21.9	17.7	8.5	7.4
Pneumonia/influenza	12.7	17.4	9.8	10.3
Liver disease/cirrhosis	7.1	8.0	11.7	2.4
Diabetes mellitus	12.0	28.8	18.4	8.7
HIV infection	2.6	20.6	6.2	0.8
External causes	46.7	68.8	44.7	24.4
Infant Mortality per 1,000	6.0	13.6	5.8	5.5
Life expectancy (years from birth)	77.3	71.3	>80?	>80?

*Per 100,000.
SOURCE: National Center for Health Statistics (2000).

in epidemiology to explain this counterintuitive finding (Markides and Coreil, 1986). Unreported "shoebox" burials were said to contribute to low infant mortality, while a healthy migrant effect and the return of sick elderly to their country of origin accounted for low adult mortality (James, 1993; Markides and Coreil, 1986). A number of cohort studies now document low age-specific death rates in Hispanics, primarily Mexican Americans, which cannot be ascribed to these biases (Wei et al., 1996). This relative advantage is not universal, however; in many Hispanic communities, obesity and diabetes occur at much greater frequencies than among whites (Diehl and Stern, 1989; Harris et al., 1998).

On the other hand, black Americans experience higher rates of all the major causes of death except chronic obstructive pulmonary disease and liver disease (Table 8-1). The excess rates of cardiovascular disease (CVD) have long been recognized as being secondary to the high prevalence of hypertension (Cooper, 1993). Despite high rates of hypertension, coronary heart disease mortality was lower among blacks than whites over the past half century, and it was once widely held that blacks were constitutionally resistant to atherosclerosis (Johnson and Payne, 1984). Rates of coronary heart disease in blacks now exceed whites (Cooper et al., 2001). Asian Americans experience remarkably lower death rates, particularly from CVD (Liao, McGee, and Cooper, 1999). Type II diabetes had been less common in blacks in the first half of the 20th century; it now occurs twice as often among blacks as among whites (Harris et al., 1998; Stamler et al., 1979).

Death rates from common malignant neoplasms are highest among black Americans (Table 8-2). The black excess is found in all the common forms of cancer except myeloma, and the differences are particularly marked in the younger age groups. Potential genetic influences are given considerable attention in studies of prostate cancer, where blacks have an incidence twice that of whites (National Center for Health Statistics [NCHS], 2000;

TABLE 8-2 Death Rates from Malignant Neoplasms in Racial/Ethnic Groups in the United States, 1998

Racial/Ethnic Group	Total*		Lung		Breast
	Men	Women	Men	Women	Women
White	146	106	49.4	27.4	19.0
Black	208	129	70.8	27.2	26.2
American Indian/ Alaskan Native	96	74	33.9	16.5	10.8
Asian/Pacific Islander	91	63	24.6	11.2	9.3
Hispanic	93	64	21.4	8.3	12.5

*Per 100,000.
SOURCE: National Center for Health Statistics (2000).

Robbins, Whittemore, and Thom, 2000). Lung cancer has attracted less speculation, despite a black to white mortality rate ratio of 1.0:1.4; overall, blacks smoke less than whites, so the etiologic forces at work are obscure (NCHS, 2000). Breast cancer mortality is higher in blacks than whites, and at a younger age the excess is twofold; the long-awaited downturn in mortality that began in 1992 has been observed only in whites. Known mutations at the BRCA loci account for a substantial proportion of breast cancer cases only among women of Jewish ancestry.

Deaths from diabetes and liver disease are higher among Hispanics than whites, although total mortality is lower and life expectancy among Hispanics is thought to exceed 80 (Table 8-1). All-cause mortality for Asians is remarkably low—only 38 percent of the rate among blacks. The risk of dying from HIV is 2.4 times higher in Hispanics than whites, but 8 times higher in blacks. Infant mortality is lower in Hispanics and Asians than whites, but more than twice as high in blacks; the persistently higher rates among blacks are driven in large measure by prematurity and low birthweight (Kleinman and Kessel, 1987). The prevalence of diabetes is currently 14 percent among Mexican Americans, 12 percent among blacks, and 7 percent among whites (Harris et al., 1998).

In general, other measures of health status are consistent with this overall picture. Self-reported health is rated lowest by blacks and Native Americans, followed in order by Hispanics, whites, and Asian/Pacific Islanders (McGee, Liao, Cao, and Cooper, 1999). These differences tend to be accentuated with increasing age (McGee, Liao, Cao, and Cooper, 1999). Similar patterns exist for disability (Liao, McGee, Cao, and Cooper, 1998). Higher incidence of Alzheimer's disease has been reported among African Americans, independent of the prevalence of APOE-4 by some investigators (Tang et al., 1998), but not others (Bohnstedt, Fox, and Kohatsu, 1994).

Growing sophistication in descriptive epidemiology, particularly related to CVD and diabetes, has made it possible to model the relationship between risk factor exposures and subsequent disability and disease rates. Measurement of smoking habits, blood pressure, and cholesterol in young adulthood has been shown to predict directly the quality of life and health care experience of persons over 65 (Daviglus et al., 1998). In broad strokes, therefore, health among the elderly can be linked to surveillance data on known exposures. Against this increasingly well-defined epidemiologic background, we are observing growing inequality by social class and geographic region, as well as race/ethnicity (Cooper et al., 2001; Pappas, Queen, Hadden, and Fisher, 1993). Thus, while coronary heart disease rates have been declining at a rate of about 3 percent a year among whites nationwide, CVD mortality has turned upward among blacks in Mississippi (Jones et al., 2000). Blacks in communities located in the center of large cities have also experienced declining health; life expectancy for black men in Atlanta,

Baltimore, St. Louis, Los Angeles, and several other cities was less than 60 years in 1992 (Good, 1998).

The contrasts in disease patterns among U.S. racial and ethnic groups are obviously much more complex than can be described in this brief overview. The relevant question for this discussion is how the influence of genetics on variation in health outcomes among U.S. racial/ethnic groups might be recognized. The syndromes that have attracted the most attention are hypertension, asthma, dementia, low birthweight, renal disease, obesity/diabetes, and prostate cancer among blacks and, to a lesser extent, diabetes in Hispanics and Native Americans; in each instance the markedly elevated incidence ratios, with whites as the reference group, have fueled speculation about potential genetic predisposition. The magnitude and consistency of the ethnic differentials, such as in relation to hypertension and prostate cancer, lends credence to these arguments, although the potential environmental contribution is universally acknowledged.

A focus on specific syndromes can be misleading, however. It is essential to remember that the health disadvantage extends across a range of key public health measures. Although the hypothesis of genetic predisposition may seem plausible taken one disease at a time, when faced with the pattern as a whole, the probability that the black disadvantage is primarily genetic becomes remote. Rather than postulating a genetic cause for each condition, a more parsimonious explanation would suggest a common-source exposure to a disease-promoting environment. Likewise, a universal characteristic of the syndromes that vary across ethnic groups, with the exception of prostate cancer, is a strong social class gradient. Most of these syndromes have also shown marked secular trends in recent decades, and the prevalence changes across generations among migrants (Collins, Wu, and David, 2002). Stated in its complementary form, the entire basis for the genetic predisposition hypothesis lies in the contrasts in disease rates between historically defined racial/ethnic populations living in the same country. Clearly a strong set of assumptions regarding equal levels of exposure to environmental factors is required to sustain this hypothesis.

Although it is subject to many of the same caveats, a different test of the racial predisposition hypothesis is provided by comparisons of genetically related populations in contrasting social settings. All forms of CVD, including hypertension, are low in West Africa, and the levels are equal to U.S. whites in the Caribbean (Cooper et al., 1997a). The evolution of hypertension risk occurs in parallel with changes in known risk factors (Figure 8-1) (Cooper et al., 1997a). The blood pressure gap between blacks and whites is narrow in Cuba (Ordunez-Garcia, Espinosa-Brito, Cooper, Kaufman, and Nieto, 1998) and between blacks and persons of Indian descent in Trinidad (Miller, Maude, and Beckles, 1996). Blacks in Brazil have more hypertension than whites, but the differential is also smaller than in the

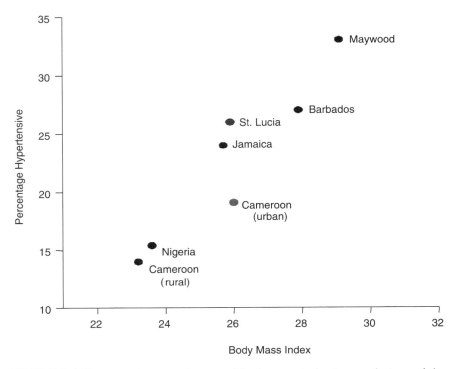

FIGURE 8-1 Hypertension prevalence and body mass index in populations of the African diaspora.

United States (Cooper and Rotimi, 1994; Sichieri, Oliveira, and Pereira, 2001). Obesity and diabetes are infrequent in Africa and among Native American groups not living in U.S. reservations (Cooper et al., 1997b; Esparza et al., 2000; King and Rewers, 1991). Diabetes is less common among blacks than whites in Brazil (Franco, 1992). Asthma and dementia are less common in Africa than among U.S. blacks (Hendrie et al., 1995; Litonjua, Carey, Weiss, and Gold, 1999). The rate of prostate cancer in blacks outside the United States is not yet reliably known, although high rates have been reported from Jamaica (Glover et al., 1986). Foreign-born women of African descent have children whose birthweight on average is close to whites (David and Collins, 1997; Friedman et al., 1993), and the disparity only emerges after a period of residence in the United States (Collins et al., 2002). Life expectancy in Jamaica and Barbados is longer than among U.S. blacks, where the estimated income is 1/30th to 1/5th as high. Although this pattern is still logically consistent with a predisposition inherent in blacks that is unmasked by environmental stimuli in the United States, it demonstrates that genes are not the determining factor in any of these examples. To avoid misunderstanding on this point, however, it must be acknowledged that among members of populations that share a common environment, genetic susceptibility can play a crucial role in determining who develops a particular illness; the issue addressed here has been the variation in aggregate health status among groups across time and place.

In summary, the broad pattern of racial/ethnic variation in disease occurrence seen in the United States has formed the basis for strong arguments in favor of genetic predisposing factors among blacks and, to a lesser extent, Hispanics and Native Americans. However, the competing hypothesis that the root cause is embedded in the historical and social circumstances peculiar to each of these groups is more consistent with the data (Chaturverdi, 2001). Furthermore, the probability that genes account for the general pattern of health disadvantage is untenable and it must follow that the claims made, for example, by investigators studying diabetes, renal failure, hypertension, and prostate cancer regarding genetic predisposition cannot all be true based on this joint probability. Likewise, the presence of a strong environmental hypothesis, based on the overall pattern, creates a prior assumption against genetic predisposition for any given disease. But these arguments are simply logical inferences; the possibility that genes make an important contribution to interethnic variation of a major disease cannot be dismissed. The contemporary standard will require molecular evidence in order to resolve the question of the relative balance of genes versus environment. Nonetheless, as in all other branches of science, the rules require that the null hypothesis is the only legitimate starting point; the burden of proof should fall on those who claim the genetic, not social, content of race is causal.

THE CONTRIBUTION OF GENETIC EPIDEMIOLOGY TO UNDERSTANDING ETHNIC DISPARITIES

The search for nongenetic explanations of racial/ethnic variation has occupied epidemiologists for many years, and this experience has important implications for the study of genetic factors. Traditionally, epidemiology has placed emphasis on studies that use the individual as the unit of measurement. When group variation is of interest, it is modeled as the average of the individuals, rather than through any emergent or higher order properties. Alternatively, a second approach uses ecological analyses and attempts to analyze social and economic forces that impinge on groups, taking as the unit of analysis a community or population subgroup. Although risk factor epidemiology at the individual level has enjoyed enormous success, its limitations as a tool to understand variations in population health have also been recognized (Koopman, 1996). However, the conceptual framework for ecologic studies is less well established, and the proposition that economic inequality and institutionalized racism, for example, should be considered causes of health status variation generally has not been embraced. However, just as the scope of biological problems can be defined at different levels—the molecule, the organism, or the population—the nature of the explanations at these levels must take different forms (Rose, 1998). Variation in health status across racial/ethnic groups uniquely requires consideration of social processes that are not individual traits, but group-level phenomena.

Genetic epidemiology must also confront this dilemma, albeit under different constraints, and fashion methods that are appropriate to understanding variation among both groups and individuals. Unfortunately, while traditional epidemiology makes unwarranted assumptions about the role of the individual in shaping his or her health status independent of social context, the conventional approach to studying genetic influences is guided by the sense that individuals are endowed with intrinsic qualities by virtue of membership in a particular race (Cooper and Kaufman, 1998; Kaufman and Cooper, 2001; Kaufman, Cooper, and McGee, 1997). In both instances, whether standard risk factors or genetic influences are being studied, the emphasis on inherent attributes creates a bias against considering social context (Lewontin, 1995; Rose, 1998). Examples of this effect are particularly apparent in the "pregenomic era" when inferences about genotype were based exclusively on data obtained from examination of the phenotype (Brancati, Kao, Folsom, Watson, and Szklo, 2000; Grim and Robinson, 1996; Robbins et al., 2000).

Indirect Methods of Assessing Genetic Factors as a Cause of Ethnic Disparities

A variety of indirect methods have been used to assess the contribution of genetics to interethnic differences in disease susceptibility (Table 8-3). In one approach the simple demonstration that a trait is heritable, and varies systematically between groups, leads directly to the inference that observed differences might be genetic in origin. Characterized as the "heritability hang-up" by geneticists (Feldman and Lewontin, 1975), these inferences have no logical basis. A trait can be highly heritable in each of two popula-

TABLE 8-3 Methods to Detect Genetic Effects on Interethnic Variation in Health

Approach	Statistical Method
Indirect	Heritability
	The "subtraction method"
Molecular	Genome scan
	Candidate genes

tions, and the mean difference between them could have nothing to do with genetic effects. For example, the proportion of the variance that is familial for height is approximately 80 percent, yet short stature among the Japanese compared to Europeans cannot be ascribed to differential frequencies of genetic variants. When the Japanese move to the United States, or adopt a Westernized diet, attained height increases rapidly with each generation.

The second common indirect method involves the attempt to partial out "environmental" factors by adjusting the trait for covariates and then arguing that "what is left over," or the residual effect after subtracting external exposures, is likely to be genetic (Kaufman and Cooper, 1996). Because this "subtraction method" has become the standard approach in epidemiology and continues to be widely applied, it deserves consideration in some detail. A classic example of this procedure was demonstrated by the analysis of the difference in blood pressures among blacks and whites in the screening phase of the Hypertension Detection and Follow-up Program Cooperative Group (1977). Because a strong social class effect exists for blood pressure, and blacks and whites differ in socioeconomic status (SES), the data were stratified by educational level to examine whether the racial effect persisted (Figure 8-2). In fact, while an SES gradient is observed in both races, a significant gap exists at equivalent educational categories.

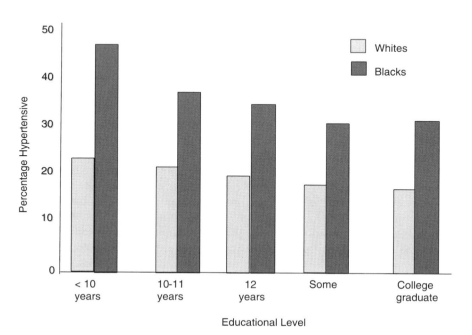

FIGURE 8-2 Hypertension prevalence by education, whites and blacks; Hypertension Detection and Follow-up Program.

The logical basis for the "subtraction method" is deceptively straight-forward. An investigator begins with the recognition that an exposure, which, for example, might be correlated with risk of early mortality, occurs at a higher level in blacks than in whites. Because the relationship between this exposure and the outcome of interest is confounded, adjustment is necessary to make an unbiased comparison. The expectation is that if SES or other exposure variables fully explain the between-group difference, then equal rates of the outcome will be observed. A residual difference can then be attributed to intrinsic attributes of the two races, that is, genetics. For example, when a differential persisted after "controlling for SES," it was concluded that "race-related biologic differences contribute to higher prostate cancer mortality in blacks" (Robbins et al., 2000, p. 493). Noting that "obesity is not a sufficient explanation" of racial differences in diabe-tes, it was inferred that "other factors must be involved, and most likely these are genetic" (Anonymous, 1989, p. 199). Based on similar reasoning, other investigators concurred that "the most straightforward interpretation of the observation that African American race has a strong independent association with diabetes mellitus is that African Americans are more sus-ceptible . . . than their white counterparts" (Brancati, Whelton, Kuller, and Klag, 1996). Noting that blood pressures are higher in "Africans, American Caribbeans and other black populations . . . at the same level of salt intake," the conclusion was reached that this "difference is likely to be genetically determined" (Law, Frost, and Wald, 1991). Similar analyses have been used to suggest that a genetic cause exists for differences in obesity, heart failure survival, birthweight, asthma, osteoporosis, and es-sentially all other traits that vary among racial/ethnic groups (Brancati et al., 1996; Carson, Ziesche, Johnson, and Cohn, 1999; Van den Oord and Rowe, 2000).

The "subtraction method" has been criticized (Kaufman and Cooper, 1996, 1999). Using the empirical measures of SES that are available, such as education, fails to eliminate the difference in exposure to the myriad factors that constitute the social influences on health for U.S. blacks and whites. These weak proxies cannot summarize the influence of lifestyle exposures. If one postulates that only modest residual confounding exists in these models, the results will be highly biased in favor of a "genetic" effect when none exists (Kaufman et al., 1997). Conceptually this approach vio-lates the assumptions necessary in the counterfactual framework used in epidemiologic research (Greenland and Robins, 1986; Kaufman and Coo-per, 1999).

From a technical perspective, the statistical models used in epidemiol-ogy are not designed to address the question being asked by the "subtrac-tion method." The primary goal of observational epidemiology is to gener-ate point estimates of exposure-outcome relationships that can be distinguished from the null, that is, to find effects that meet standard criteria for statistical significance. Although the actual size of this effect may be of some interest, in many cases it is difficult to estimate accurately, given imprecision in measurement of both the exposure and the outcome. Furthermore, simply knowing that an exposure has a noxious effect (e.g., tobacco smoke, environmental lead) can often be sufficient to motivate the policy to remove or curb this exposure. The "subtraction method," on the other hand, presupposes that the variables used in the model capture all or the great majority of the variance attributable to factors in the environment. Clearly this assumption cannot be met, and it will never be possible to measure all of the lifetime contributions of known or unrecognized exposures. Furthermore, the measurement of many exposures is not comparable across groups; for example, earning power at similar levels of education is very different for blacks and whites, and purchasing power is different for similar incomes (Auerbach and Kringold, 2001). Contrariwise, race/ethnicity, as socially defined, is measured with precision and will absorb the information latent in the confounders, an outcome that would be apparent if sensitivity analyses were conducted (Kaufman et al., 1997). The point being made here is not that epidemiologists occasionally rely on fuzzy logic or fall back on loosely formulated generalizations. Instead, it is being argued that an inferential process that can offer no evidence for or against the hypothesis is central to the analysis strategy epidemiologists have used to study race.

In fact, the "subtraction method" has so many limitations and biases that the relevant question becomes, why has it been accepted as the standard approach? Whatever more general speculation might be invited by this question, it seems clear that a strong a priori assumption about the essentialist nature of race is required before the "subtraction method" makes sense as an analytic tool. The contribution of genetics to interethnic variation for most health traits remains completely unknown, making this a legitimate area of controversy. However, the current indirect methods are incapable of generating empirical evidence on this question, any more than alchemy can advance the field of chemistry. Faith in the potential of these methods, and the uncritical willingness to use them, demonstrates instead a belief that race, as currently operationalized in public health, codes for substantial information about genetic factors that influence disease susceptibility.

In addition to the methods that attempt to estimate genetic effects in a semiquantitative way, a substantial literature on racial/ethnic variation in health simply posits a genetic cause and argues that any observed differences could be the explanation. A group of investigators recently justified this approach by pointing out—correctly—that it represents accepted practice: "Because of observed group differences in the risk of hypertension . . .

research continues to treat these groups as distinct biological entities and investigates the genetic factors that might account for the differences . . . " (Brewster, Clark, and van Montfrans, 2000, p. 1541). Within this framework they proceeded to "hypothesize that the genetic factor increasing the ability of black people . . . to develop higher blood pressures . . . is greater total intracellular activity of the central regulatory enzyme of energy metabolism, creatine kinase . . ." (Brewster et al., 2000, p. 1541). Unfortunately for this argument, while racial differences in creatine kinase activity have been reported, no evidence links creatine kinase with hypertension and no genetic mechanisms are identified; why someone would propose this physiologic measure as a cause of black-white differences in hypertension is therefore obscure.

Postulating that any observed group differences could be a cause invites a serious risk of Type I error. For example, similar theories, based on intracellular calcium, telomere length, insulin resistance, renin secretion, kallikrein, beta-hydroxylase, growth factors, melanin, cation transport, and a host of other physiologic traits, all of which lack an established causal relationship to hypertension, have been proposed as "genetic causes" of the excess hypertension in blacks (Cooper and Kaufman, 1998; Cooper and Rotimi, 1994; Fekete et al., 1996; Fray and Douglas, 1993; Gillum, 1979; Saad et al., 1991). In the same manner, a difference in resting metabolic rate between blacks and whites has been advanced as a cause of the excess obesity among blacks, even though no causal link between resting metabolic rate and obesity has been established (Kimm et al., 2002; Morrison, Alfaro, Khoury, Thornton, and Daniels, 1996; Yanovski, Reynolds, Boyle, and Yanovski, 1997). It is hard to conceive of stronger evidence of a commitment to an essentialist notion of race than exemplified by this literature.

Molecular Approaches to the Study of Genes That Could Influence Interethnic Variation in Health

The current challenge in the study of interethnic variation in health is how to move from inferences based on the phenotype, which is a product of the interaction between genes and environment, to those based on genotype. Because this territory is almost entirely uncharted in studies of humans, assumptions must be made about the likely magnitude and distribution of the effects that should be sought (Clayton and McKeigue, 2001). For any given genotype-phenotype relationship, an inverse relationship exists between the size of the effect of a given variant and the number of variants involved. For diseases like hypertension, where many genetic variants are likely to be involved, it therefore follows that the effect of any one variant will be small. Contrariwise, in monogenic disorders a single mutation can have a devastating effect. Because single gene disorders generally confer a selective disadvantage, these mutations are infrequent in number and are maintained at a low rate in the population. Unique among monogenic disorders, sickle cell disease and related red cell defects have attained high frequency in endemic malaria regions. Despite the attention they have received, in industrial societies like the United States these monogenic diseases make a negligible contribution to interethnic variation. Based on the calculation of excess deaths, for example, hematologic disorders account for only 0.3 percent of the black-white differential (Cooper, 1984).

One gene with a large effect is easier to find than many with small effects, and the great successes of molecular genetics to date have been in monogenic disorders. The contradiction between studying the rare genetic disorders and the public support required for "big science" has not been lost on geneticists, however. As noted in a recent editorial, with the Human Genome Project coming to an end, the challenge to biologists is to "make the genome relevant to public health. This relevance will not be found by identifying genes associated with rare hereditary diseases, but by . . . (tackling) . . . the common, complex diseases" (Anonymous, 2002, p. 199). Accordingly, over the past decade, genetic epidemiology has shifted its focus dramatically from monogenic to common chronic diseases, driven in large part by the new opportunities for molecular analysis (Collins, Lonjou, and Morton, 1999; Lander, 1996; Lander and Schork, 1994). Conditions that have public health impact, like hypertension, diabetes, atherosclerosis, obesity, and the common cancers, are now being subjected to intense scrutiny.

Although several variants are assumed to combine to create susceptibility to these traits, whether they are oligogenic (determined by moderate numbers of variants, each with moderate effects) or fully polygenic (many variants, each with small effects) is still unknown. No matter which model is adopted, the search for these variants has been challenging (Chagnon, Perusse, Weisnagel, Rankinen, and Bouchard, 2000; Doris, 2001; Levy et al., 2000; Risch, 2000) and the weak impact of individual variants may be the least of the problem. While most chronic conditions have substantial genetic components, as demonstrated by the familial aggregation, environmental exposures are likely to play the dominant role. Interactions of these environmental factors, many of which may still be unidentified, with the genetic substrate create complex patterns that are still difficult to conceptualize and even harder to measure.

Defining genetic factors that account for interethnic variation in health is dependent on the success of this "gene hunting" operation in a stepwise process. First, influential variants must be identified, and then their effect and frequency compared across groups. Two general approaches are currently being used in this first stage to search for the genetic variants. Anonymous markers that do not code protein sequences are genotyped in family members, and the co-segregation of chromosomal segments with the phenotype is used to localize potential variants. This method, known as the "genome scan," relies on linkage between the marker and the trait, and has been applied with great success to monogenic disorders. At the next stage, "positional cloning" is used to identify the variant itself. A second, complementary approach postulates candidate genes at the outset, from physiology or animal experimental research primarily, and tests specific variants in these genes. The candidate gene approach can use linkage analysis, based on related individuals, or the case-control design, known in genetic epidemiology as an "association study."

Finding Genes: The Genome Scan Approach

A broad experience with genome scans now exists, involving traits that range from blood pressure and height to psychiatric disorders (Doris, 2001; Hirschhorn et al., 2001; Laitinen et al., 2001; Levy et al., 2000; Province et al., 2003; Wu et al., 2002). As already suggested, this method has met with only modest success when applied to complex traits (Altmuller, Palmer, Fischer, Scherb, and Wjst, 2001; Hugot et al., 2001; Risch, 2000; Tavtigian et al., 2001). The statistical power of this method—that is, the ability to find an influential locus if one exists—is limited, while the risk of a Type 1 error—false-positive results—is high. If, for example, the total genetic variance associated with a trait is 30 percent, and 10 genes are involved, then the method needs to have sufficient power to detect average effects of 3 percent. In general, power for most genome scan studies is only adequate for effects in the 10 to 20 percent range. On the other hand, these assumptions may not be entirely realistic because it is unlikely that the impacts of various susceptibility genes are evenly distributed, and there is reason for optimism that some loci influence a good deal more than 3 percent of the variance in some families.

Given the focus here on the potential contribution of genes to interethnic variation in health, a detailed summary of the accomplishments based on the genome scan as an aid to cloning susceptibility genes is not necessary. The application of the genome scan approach is still at the first stage for most conditions—attempting to find reproducible evidence of linkage to particular chromosomal regions (Chagnon, Perusse, Weisnagel, Rankinen, and Bouchard, 2000; Doris, 2001). However, some consistency has begun to emerge. Obesity, a continuously distributed trait with a polygenic inheritance pattern, can serve as an illustrative example. Evidence of linkage using the genome scan approach has emerged in several studies for regions on chromosomes 3 and 7 (Chagnon et al., 2000). In a meta-analysis of 6,800 individuals from four ethnic groups, a region on chromosome 3 was linked to obesity in more than one of the racial/ethnic populations and in the combined sample at a high level of statistical significance (log odds = 3.6) (Wu et al., 2002). With independent replication in multiple population samples, some confidence is warranted in the linkage finding on chromosome 3; the second stage, pulling a causal variant out of a region spanning 10 to 20 million nucleotides, is nonetheless daunting. Hypertension appears to be more resistant to this approach, where even more inconsistency across racial groups has been observed (Doris, 2001; Province et al., 2003), and studies of psychiatric disorders also have been hard to replicate (Pato, Schindler, and Pato, 2000). On the other hand, the number of influential genes may vary across traits, making some easier to unravel than others, and enhanced analytic tools are being developed for both the laboratory and statistical methods that may reduce the technical obstacles.

A more general problem related to genes and ethnic disparities emerges from this literature. The interpretation of genome scans from various ethnic population samples immediately confronts a dilemma: Should we regard these populations as separate entities? In other words, having undertaken a genome scan involving whites and blacks, should we pool the results, or treat them as separate samples? If we find differences between the two samples, should we regard these as an indication that different genetic effects exist in the two groups, or should we conclude simply that they are the result of sampling variation, as might occur with repeated studies in the same ethnic group? Given our ignorance about the existence of subunits within the human species, or their correspondence to groups we label as races, there is no a priori basis for conducting analyses separately. Technical problems arise in linkage analysis when divergent populations are pooled because the allele frequencies of the "microsatellite" markers may vary across groups, but this limitation can be overcome. From this perspective, it is illuminating to observe that all analyses performed to date have carefully adhered to the principle of distinguishing among population groups as if they were genetic categories. Furthermore, some analysts have concluded that different results obtained in samples of blacks and whites provide evidence of different underlying genetic effects (Collaborative Study on the Genetics of Asthma, 1997), a conclusion that, even in the short interval that has passed since the work was conducted, can be recognized as wholly unjustified. As with indirect methods, the internal evidence from within the discipline on the conduct of this research demonstrates a commitment to a concept of race that has its provenance outside science.

Finding Genes: The Candidate Gene Approach

An even more extensive literature exists for candidate genes, given the less demanding technical requirements for this design compared to the genome scan. The approach to this enormous field, as above, must be to focus on an illustrative example. Hypertension is the most common disease trait in our population, with a lifetime risk approaching 90 percent, and a population-attributable risk for mortality of about 10 percent (Vasan et al., 2002). It has been recognized since the 1930s that black Americans have a prevalence rate that is twice as high as found among whites, and hypertension is the largest single contributor to the black-white disparity (Cooper and Rotimi, 1997). Uncontrolled hypertension is a direct cause of stroke, coronary heart disease, renal failure, heart failure, and vascular dementia. The detailed understanding of the physiology of hypertension has made it possible to identify a large number of candidate genes. The renin-angiotensin system (RAS), which plays a key role in regulating salt and water metabolism and maintaining vascular tone, has been particularly well studied. The RAS has four principal components. Angiotensinogen (AGT), the protein substrate produced by the liver, circulates in excess in the plasma and is cleaved by renin to make angiotensin-I (Ang-I). Ang-I is rapidly cleaved by the angiotensin converting enzyme (ACE) to Ang-II, which then interacts with tissue receptors. Heralding a false spring early in the course of candidate gene research, investigators from Utah and France demonstrated that a highly significant association of variants in the AGT gene influenced both circulating AGT levels and risk of hypertension (Jeunemaitre et al., 1992). Identification of an easily typed marker in ACE—the so-called "insertion/ deletion" or "I/D" marker—provoked an outpouring of publications on this gene as well. Subsequent meta-analyses suggested modest effects for variants in these two genes (Soubrier, 1998; Staessen et al., 1999), although much of this literature was negative.

Because it has been well characterized, the RAS provides a useful summary of the current state of knowledge regarding candidate genes and their potential impact on interethnic variation in health. The ACE gene is composed of a sequence of 24,000 nucleotides, of which 75 are known to vary. The first problem confronting the genetic epidemiologist is how to summarize and manage this variation. The vast majority of research to date has used only one variant in a gene to capture all the genetic information, and it is generally not known whether this marker is causal, simply linked physically to (i.e., confounded by the presence of) other causal variants at a neighboring site, or uninformative about hidden causal variants.

Attempting to address these questions immediately provokes the more fundamental question posed earlier: What is the scope of human genetic variation and how do we measure it? Variation can be reasonably summarized in two ways. The most basic unit of genetic information is the base pair, known as the "single nucleotide polymorphism" (SNP) when it is found in more than one form. Given the nature of evolution, and the relative youth of our species, large segments of chromosomes are found in identical "blocks," as one might expect in large families (Reich et al.,

2001). These blocks, sometimes referred to as "haplotypes," span large distances in the genome, and the SNPs within these blocks are inherited in a fixed pattern (i.e., all SNPs in the blocks are in the same form). In many instances only two or three different blocks will be present in the population. In addition to the specific SNPs, the size and distribution of the haplotypes also characterize the diversity within a population, reflecting the combined effects of age and size.

Initial work on ACE linked the I/D variant to circulating levels of the enzyme (Rigat et al., 1990). However, this variant was found in an intron, or a noncoding segment of the gene, and was simply linked to the causal variants. The challenge then became one of dissecting the ACE gene into sufficiently small segments to isolate the causal SNPs. Analysis of the ACE gene in a large number of individuals confirmed previous findings of greater genetic diversity in persons of African origin (Zhu et al., 2000). A total of 28 haplotypes were identified among blacks, while only 3 occurred in moderate frequency among Europeans (Zhu et al., 2000). The high information content available in the African-origin samples in turn made it possible to conduct fine mapping studies, that is, to localize effects within the gene. Two areas were identified that appeared to influence ACE levels. Subsequently these techniques were applied to a sample of Nigerians and a moderately strong association with blood pressure was confirmed in the same manner (Zhu et al., 2001). The limited haplotype diversity present in the European samples at this particular locus would not have permitted similar analyses (Reich et al., 2001; Zhu et al., 2003a), although there is no reason to think that the effect varies between ethnic groups.

Ultimately molecular epidemiology requires identification of the variation in DNA sequence that causes variation in the phenotype. Hundreds of mutations have been found in many monogenic disorders, such as cystic fibrosis and retinitis pigmentosa (Cystic Fibrosis Genetic Analysis Consortium, 1994; RetNet[1]), although a few common variants account for most cases. The impact of these variants on the phenotype can in some instances be little influenced by the environment. In polygenic disorders, however, the effects of different variants within the same gene and variants in different genes are obviously more subtle and complex. Certain effects will be present only in certain environments, and interactions between sets of genetic variants are also likely to occur.

In effect, there is no abstract "genetic effect" because the actions of genes are only detectable by their influence on a phenotype, and therefore the product of a particular environment. Given that the mixture of environment and genetic background may vary across racial/ethnic populations, in many instances it may be difficult to isolate the causal genetic effect separately from the environmental effect. Certainly it will be difficult to summarize all the possible genetic effects into an overall estimate of the relative degree of susceptibility of two populations.

Pharmacogenetics

In addition to the potential role that genetic variation might play in disease susceptibility, there is currently great interest in whether the response to therapeutic drugs can be predicted by genotype. The most important aim of pharmacogenetics is to sort patients into "responders" and "nonresponders," thereby improving the efficiency of the medical encounter. The complementary aim is to identify persons who might be at high risk of severe side effects from a particular drug. A parallel interest exists in whether these responses vary by race. Given the widespread use of drugs for chronic conditions, particularly among the elderly, the public health implications of relative efficacy could be substantial.

The frequencies of polymorphisms affecting drug metabolism do vary among population groups (McLeod, 2001). The critical question, as in other applications of the race concept, is whether this classification scheme improves or harms our understanding of the variation we observe. Using molecular techniques, a direct test can be made of the question of whether or not geographic patterns of genetic variation structure interindividual variation in drug response (Wilson et al., 2001). To test this hypothesis, microsatellite markers, similar to those used in genome scan analyses, were typed on individuals from eight regional populations and the population structure—the degree of genetic relatedness of the groups—was inferred (Wilson et al., 2001). Genotyping was then conducted on polymorphisms in drug-metabolizing enzymes of the cytochrome p450 system. Finally, a comparison was made of the relative accuracy with which variants in the enzymes were predicted using standard ethnic labels versus the genetic clustering algorithm (Wilson et al., 2001). Two important results emerged. First, adding molecular data to the classification process improved prediction over ethnic labels for three of the four enzymes examined. However, both schemes were relatively ineffective at predicting individual responses, reminding us again that variation among individuals is orders of magnitude greater than variation among population groups. Pharmacogenetics confronts the same dilemma faced over the years by epidemiology; despite the perceived meaning of race, and its enormous currency in social life, the genetic content of these categories never meets our expectations.

Focused candidate gene studies have started to yield positive results, however. Hypertension presents an attractive opportunity for pharmacogenomics. Heterogeneity in drug response exists among individuals and across classes of agents and, because lifelong therapy is required, tailored prescribing could be more effective than "trial-and-error" methods. In a sample of 387 patients, the blood pressure response to a therapeutic challenge with a diuretic was examined after stratifying on a marker associated with the "G protein" (Turner, Schwartz, Chapman, and Boerwinkle, 2001). Among persons homozygous for the T allele, the fall in systolic blood pressure was 16 mmHg, compared to 10 mmHg among persons with the opposite genotype (Turner et al., 2001). Although no differences were noted in the degree of response by genotype among blacks and whites, the prevalence of the T allele was much higher among blacks than whites (Turner et al., 2001). A recent report of a nutritional intervention also showed a markedly different response in blood pressure on the basis of a genotype in the AGT gene (Svetky et al., 2001). Again, the "at risk" allele was more frequent in blacks than whites (Svetky et al., 2001). Taken together, these studies suggest that provocative interventions may be more effective at unmasking genetic effects, at least for blood pressure, and open new opportunities to define the role of candidate genes. Likewise, they present the first reasonable evidence that factors conferring genetic susceptibility to hypertension may be differentially distributed among these population groups. However, only limited marker sets were examined in both of these studies and replication certainly will be required (Yancy, 2001).

A related controversy has arisen over the interpretation of differences among ethnic groups in drug response seen in treatment trials. In a post hoc analysis of a randomized trial of ACE inhibitors for heart failure, the drug was found to reduce the rate of hospitalization significantly more in whites than in blacks (Exner, 2001). Reanalysis of two other small heart failure trials also demonstrated nonsignificant racial differences in response to treatment with ACE inhibitors (Carson et al., 1999). Based on this evidence, a request was approved by the Food and Drug Administration to test a non-ACE inhibitor drug for heart failure as the first "race-specific" therapy. Attempts to drop inclusion of ACE inhibitor therapy for blacks as part of quality assurance requirements were also reported (Masoudi and Havranek, 2001). However, the evidence in support of this race-specific effect has been challenged. The original analysis was based on the rate of hospitalization, only one of the nonfatal end points from the large Studies of Left Ventricular Dysfunction (SOLVD) (Exner, 2001). When development of heart failure symptoms was examined in SOLVD, the relative efficacy of the ACE inhibitor was the same in blacks and whites (relative risk 0.58 versus 0.55, respectively) (Dries, Cooper, Strong, and Drazner, 2002). Most likely the original result obtained by Exner (2001) was due to a Type 1 error. Drug choice is increasingly dictated by the evidence from clinical trials; there is currently no basis for thinking that race should override trial evidence. A treatment that has been unequivocally established, like ACE inhibition, must be assumed to work in all subgroups of humans.

WHAT IS THIS THING CALLED RACE?

As evident from the preceding sections, it is being argued here that race is the organizing principle of the debate over genes and ethnic disparities. There is essentially no distinction, it is further argued, between the popular notions of race that are absorbed into consciousness as categories inherent in nature, like gender or species, and the concept of race as applied in biological research. But an external event is now impinging on the social process that creates and maintains this idea—molecular genetics has given us probes that make it possible to explore the biologic reality behind the accepted beliefs. The moment is not too far off when the race concept will acquire an empirical foundation, displacing, or at least challenging, its ideological claims. Can we predict what this concept might look like?

As with all branches of science, accretion of data around a new construct requires a symbolic or metaphorical image to represent the abstract notion that is the organizing principle. Revisiting earlier questions after the excursion through genetic epidemiology, we can now ask, what image should we use to describe the shape of the collective human genome? The sequencing phase of the Human Genome Project has spawned a variety of metaphors, usually related to the basic theme of the "letters in the alphabet of biology" or the "Book of Life." Ignoring the inevitable letdown that followed the "genome hype," the publication of the human sequence has not immediately opened new vistas on the biological world (Anonymous, 2002; Lewontin, 2000). This occurred in part, of course, because we do not know how to read this alphabet. Years of painstaking molecular biology will be required to decipher the individual signals encoded in the genome, most of which are shared across the biological world. On the other hand, current technology is reasonably well suited to the challenge of describing the overall pattern of variation within the species (Reich et al., 2001; Romualdi et al., 2002). This exploration, as argued previously, should inform our understanding of the concept of race.

The technical study of human genetic variation traditionally has fallen within population genetics. A major experimental tool has been the estimation of genetic distance as a means of reconstructing ancestral relationships and the history of geographic dispersion (Cavalli-Sforza et al., 1996). Typically this research program has relied on the metaphor of the tree, placing various modern populations on branches with ever-increasing degrees of separation. As a means of representation, the phylogenetic tree is more of a diagram than a symbolic image, and geneticists are appropriately skeptical of the broad implications of this classification scheme for phenotypic traits. Genetic distance by itself is not meant to imply that populations could not share genetic variants. Given their encounters with data, as well as the past association with eugenics, many geneticists question the value of racial distinctions (McLeod, 2001; Wilson et al., 2001). Nonetheless, the image of the tree places emphasis on degrees of separation and subverts the question of similarity, or the relationship of the parts to the whole.

A different image is more widely used than the phylogenetic tree. In the popular mind, race is accepted as an important, albeit imprecise, proxy for heritable influences on traits ranging from IQ to obesity (Herrnstein and Murray, 1994; Kimm et al., 2002). The image employed is the normal distribution, with the mean of one population group shifted relative to the other. The genome is conceived of as a fixed, independent cause, projected directly onto the phenotype, without the filtering or conditioning effect of environment. By measuring the distribution of a trait, such as height or blood pressure, we can therefore infer the distribution of the underlying genetic determinants. Developed in its most complete form in relation to IQ, but borrowed wholesale by public health, this construct provides the foundation for the hypothesis of discrete "genes for intelligence" or "genes for hypertension" (Muntaner, Nieto, and O'Campo, 1996).

Just as the discovery of microorganisms transformed our understanding of infection, the ability to measure genotype challenges previous concepts of human variation. First and foremost is the question, do racial categories delimit human variation in a meaningful way? Or, as 19th century biologists would say, are we "carving nature at the joints?" Since the first scientific speculation on the genetic composition of our species, the discrete versus continuous nature of variation has been a central controversy. To support his general argument that evolution shaped the biological world and united it as a single whole, Darwin (1981, p. 194) resisted the notion of racial categories:

> [T]he most weighty of all the arguments against treating the races of man as distinct species, is that they graduate into each other, independently in many cases, of their having intercrossed. Man has been studied more carefully than any other organic being, and yet there is the greatest possible diversity amongst capable judges whether he should be classed as a single species or race . . . . This diversity of judgment does not prove that the races ought not to be ranked as a species but it shows that it is hardly possible to discover clear distinctive characters between them. Every naturalist who has had the misfortune to undertake the description of a group of highly varying organisms, has encountered cases precisely like that of man; and if of a cautious disposition, he will end by uniting all the forms which graduate into each other as a single species; for he will say to himself that he has no right to give names to objects which he cannot define.

This question can now be reformulated in the technical language of molecular genetics. A contemporary version is summarized by Templeton (1999, p. 647):

Race is generally used as a synonym for subspecies, which traditionally is a geographically circumscribed, genetically differentiated population. Sometimes traits show independent patterns of geographic
variation such that some combination will distinguish most populations from all others. To avoid making "race" the equivalent of a
local population, minimal thresholds of differentiation are imposed.
Human "races" are below the thresholds used in other species, so
valid traditional subspecies do not exist in humans. A "subspecies"
can also be defined as a distinct evolutionary lineage within a species.
Genetic surveys and the analyses of DNA haplotype trees show that
human "races" are not distinct lineages, and that this is not due to
recent admixture; human "races" are not and never were "pure."
Instead, human evolution has been and is characterized by many lo-
cally differentiated populations coexisting at any given time, but with
sufficient genetic contact to make all of humanity a single lineage
sharing a common evolutionary fate.

The evidence for this common evolutionary lineage, with its origins in
Africa, continues to emerge with increasing clarity as genomic science advances. Recent developments now demonstrate this phenomenon at the
level of the organization of the genome. As described previously, DNA
variants that are physically close to each other tend to be correlated, that is,
two individuals who inherit a particular variant at a locus will tend to share
the variants found at loci in close physical proximity on the same chromosome. This result occurs because "blocks" or pieces of chromosome are
passed down over time through the population (Reich et al., 2001; Stephens
et al., 2001). This pattern of sharing is dissipated as the distance between
variants increases. If, however, race or ethnicity defines a natural unit
within the species, then variants at physically unlinked loci (e.g., on different chromosomes) also should be shared more commonly among members
of that race. A more general way to formulate this question is to ask, to
what degree is there structure in the human genome? Massive genotyping
experiments based on randomly selected segments of the human genome
have made it possible to test this question directly (Gabriel et al., 2002;
Reich et al., 2001; Stephens et al., 2001), revisiting with genetic data
Lewontin's analysis based on variation in proteins (Lewontin, 1972, 1974).
These efforts are ongoing, but, initial results suggest that although the
distribution of variants from representative continental populations cannot
be considered entirely random, the degree of correlation among unlinked
markers is negligible in quantitative terms (Romualdi et al., 2002). Thus,
although variation among populations exists for some genetic variants, this
variation is not aggregated or "packaged" in demographic units, but for the
most part occurs piecemeal or random; it is continuous over space rather
than occurring in discrete categories (Romualdi et al., 2002). One cannot

reliably predict the probability of unknown variants from the frequencies of known variants.

The Practical Implications of Race for Public Health Today

The question that race brings to public health is not whether random polymorphisms aggregate, but whether disease variants aggregate. While it is possible, although unproven, that some individual variants could be particularly influential, it is usually assumed that susceptibility to complex diseases involves the sum of many variants, and these variants occur at a relatively high frequency in the population—the so-called "common disease-common variant" hypothesis (Chakravarti, 1999; Lander, 1996). Distributed across the genome, each locus will have a weak effect, and a complementary set of these variants is necessary to create susceptibility. Alternatively, there could be many rare variants that in combination confer susceptibility (Pritchard, 2001). As noted earlier, the effects of these mutations are likely to be uniformly small, although the possibility does exist that some genes could have moderate to large effects.

These assumptions have considerable relevance for interethnic variation. Common genetic mutations are by necessity old, given the time required for them to become widely distributed, and they are usually found in all ethnic groups (Halushka et al., 1999). The "common disease-common variant" hypothesis would therefore lead to the conclusion that the important disease-susceptibility mutations are distributed in a global pattern. On the other hand, rare variants would have most likely arisen after dispersion from Africa. For example, the mutations underlying Tay-Sachs and cystic fibrosis, which occur frequently in European subpopulations, are rare in Africa. Just as the mutations for these monogenic disorders are unequally distributed in ethnic groups, rare variants with large effects on chronic diseases could be spread unevenly in modern populations. However, if the "common disease-common variant" hypothesis is correct, as seems most likely, multiple polymorphisms would have to be present in one population, but absent in others.

What mechanisms could therefore be involved in generating the clusters of susceptibility variants necessary to create excess risk in an ethnic population? Two plausible mechanisms can be invoked—the play of chance or evolutionary selection. Influential variants could be differentially distributed by chance in particular ethnic groups, and this must occur to some extent. Viewed across all conditions, however, one would expect a balanced pattern of advantage and disadvantage when comparing large populations. As argued earlier, the possibility that chance could have created the pattern of health differentials seen in the United States, particularly the pervasive black disadvantage, is so remote as to be implausible. As the basis for variation in any single disease, chance cannot be ruled out, but it should be an explanation of last resort, particularly if one assumes a combination of several variants is required. In terms of a general principle, we are left with selection as the main organizing theory.

Could selection have created racial variation in susceptibility to the diseases of late adulthood that have emerged in industrialized society? Most of the diseases of public health concern were not subject to selective pressure in the past. Nonetheless, some of the underlying traits—such as blood pressure and body composition—probably were because survival value would be attached to adequate functioning of these systems. Variation in susceptibility to common disease among regional populations therefore could have resulted from differential selective pressure in varying environments. This model, of course, has been used successfully to explain the variation in sickle cell and thalassemia. Likewise, it must apply to skin pigmentation, although the mechanism has been difficult to establish (Robins, 1991). Several attempts have been made to transfer this model to chronic conditions, such as blood pressure and obesity that result from dysregulation of physiologic systems under the stress of the modern lifestyle. The "slavery hypothesis" was developed to explain excess hypertension in blacks based on the proposition that a bottleneck, or a severe restriction of the population diversity, occurred during the "middle passage." This hypothesis states that selective mortality caused by salt-wasting disorders created genetic susceptibility to hypertension among the surviving African Americans who avidly retained salt (Grim and Robinson, 1996; Wilson, 1986). The "thrifty gene" hypothesis argues that the selection advantage against starvation conferred by an ability to store excess calories as fat is the cause of diabetes in Native Americans and Pacific Islanders (Hegele, 2001; Neel, 1999; Ravussin and Bogardus, 1990; Weiss, Ferrell, and Hanis, 1984).

In effect these hypotheses are an attempt to apply the race concept and are subject to the general criticisms outlined previously. In addition, more specific tests can be proposed. For example, the historical evidence does not support high mortality during the "middle passage" of slavery and there is no genetic evidence of a "bottleneck" that narrowed diversity among blacks in the Americas (Curtin, 1992; Gabriel et al., 2002; Zhu et al., 2003b). To the contrary, evidence exists for a demographic bottleneck during the formation of the European population (Reich et al., 2001). The epidemic of obesity and subsequent diabetes has now overwhelmed so many racial and ethnic groups that this particular "thrifty gene" must be a human gene; diabetes occurs at an equally high prevalence among such disparate groups as black Americans, Mexican Americans, Australian Aborigines, Polynesians, Chinese in Mauritius, and Saudi Arabians (Franco, 1992; Harris et al., 1998; King and Rewers, 1991; O'Dea, Spargo, and Nestel, 1982). Despite these shortcomings, the "slavery hypothesis" and the "thrifty gene" struck a responsive chord and have achieved wide acceptance. Again the interesting question becomes, why are these "just so" stories embraced as fact? As with the other examples discussed here, the concept of race creates a belief structure that is receptive to explanations built on genetic determinism.

Race as a Diagnostic Test for Genetic Disorders

Race could serve as a surrogate marker for risk of specific single-gene mutations. In formal terms the precision of "race as a diagnostic test" can be evaluated using the standard clinical measures of sensitivity, specificity, and predictive power. The broadest public health experience with this application lies with postnatal screening for sickle cell (Centers for Disease Control and Prevention, 2003). After the demonstration that penicillin was effective in life-threatening infections in newborns with sickle cell, neonatal screening programs were initiated. In the initial phases only black infants were screened. However, it was soon recognized that sensitivity, or the case detection rate, was not optimal. Black race is not a reliable marker for the prevalence of sickle cell disease in the United States (Table 8-4). In many states universal screening has now been implemented, increasing the number of cases identified by as much as 30 percent (i.e., sensitivity before universal screening was only 70 percent, which is inadequate for a screening procedure).

In a contrary example, the high prevalence of Tay-Sachs among Ashkenazi Jews permits more focused screening for this condition (Khoury, 2000). It may also be possible that other genetic mutations could vary so markedly by race/ethnicity that targeted screening or interventions will be justified, but the nonassortative mating common in multiethnic societies will dilute this effect, and the example of sickle cell is probably more typical.

TABLE 8-4 Racial/Ethnic Variation in the Prevalence of Sickle Cell Disease Among Live Births, 1990

Racial/Ethnic Group	Prevalence*
White	2
Black	289
Hispanic, total	5
Hispanic, eastern states	90
Hispanic, western states	3
Asian	7
Native American	36

*Per 100,000.
SOURCE: CDC, Office of Genetics and Disease Prevention.

It is still difficult, however, to define in practical terms the independent public health role of race as a marker for genetic susceptibility. If it is important to know whether a patient has a variant that confers susceptibility or an unusual drug response, it will have to be measured directly, although targeted screening may be justified in some instances. Community surveillance data on disease incidence, not inference from race, is likely to remain the only reliable measure on which to base public health interventions.

GENETICS AND THE HEALTH STATUS OF BLACK AMERICANS

No discussion of genetic factors and racial/ethnic disparities would be complete without consideration of the contrasts drawn between Africans and non-Africans. The first imperative derives from the undeniable centrality of distinctions between black and white as the basis of the meaning of race. Although the history of assimilation into U.S. society has many chapters, and they all include stories of hard times, discrimination, slavery, and institutionalized racism directed at persons of African descent have inflicted the deepest wounds. Secondly, the public health goal of "eliminating disparities" takes its meaning from the health disadvantage among blacks summarized in Table 8-1. Urgent health problems exist for many U.S. subpopulations, but a uniform pattern of disadvantage, stretching from perinatal health to dementia and reduction of life expectancy, is found only among black Americans. Finally, the impact of race on other aspects of social life, such as housing, education, and employment, is more significant among blacks.

Africa entered the modern world through a distinctive route. Having nurtured the physical development of our species and generated the foundational ideas of "Western culture" in Egypt (Bernal, 1987), Africa fell behind in the development of technologically based societies. Reunited with the mainstream of Western history through the slave trade and colonialism, Africans remain subject to domination by a persistently hostile culture wherever they live (Gilroy, 1993; Gossett, 1973; Oliver and Atmore, 1992). Consequently Africans on the continent have not shared the material benefits of the capitalist economy and the modern nation state, while their descendants abroad have been excluded from full citizenship in the countries that they did so much to build. This historical framework determines not only the current health status of black populations, but the way in which this health status is studied and explicated.

In response to the challenge posed by empirical notions of inheritance, Europeans excluded Africans from the "human race" (Gossett, 1973; Gould, 1981; Montagu, 1964). As the science of genetics matured in technical and theoretical capacity, this position has been subject to growing challenge (Darwin, 1981; Gould, 1981; Lewontin, Rose, and Kamin, 1984; Montagu, 1964). Nonetheless, contemporary Western consciousness, in both the popular and scientific realm, continues to rely heavily on assumptions about the "otherness" and "inferiority" of Africans and their descendants (Gilroy, 2000; Gosset, 1973; Gould, 1981; Montagu, 1964). Without taking account of these two complementary forces—the history of the European encounter with Africa and the intellectual and ideological framework that is used to describe its consequences—an analysis of the health status of African Americans will continue to substitute justification for explanation.

While acknowledging the potential of molecular genetics, the tone in this presentation generally has been one of skepticism or outright rejection of many aspects of research on the genetics of race and health. However, there is one crucial area where a convincing answer to an important question has emerged. As suggested previously in the analysis of candidate gene data, the scope of human genetic diversity can now be modeled with a high degree of sophistication. In analyses based on large numbers of SNPs as well as haplotype distributions, the distinction between African and all non-African populations stands out with unmistakable clarity. Primate evolution occurred over millions of years in Africa (Klein, 1989), yet modern humans migrated to other continents only 50,000 to 100,000 years ago, beginning from an original population of about 10,000 (Harpending et al., 1998; Stephens et al., 2001). These migrations either involved small numbers of individuals, or were subject to severe demographic bottlenecks, as in the case of Europe (Reich et al., 2001). As a result the repository of human diversity within modern African populations is greater than among those outside Africa (Harpending et al., 1998).

Within a pattern that completely overlaps, the haplotypes and genetic variants in populations outside of Africa are a subset of those found in Africa; that is, they are a sample of the African whole (Figure 8-3). Given the small size of the founder populations outside Africa, by chance the frequency of particular haplotypes has been exaggerated in some instances, and other haplotypes have been lost. The development of regional populations can therefore be thought of as small pseudopods or "outpouchings" that became detached, and then increased in size, magnifying the distinctive characteristics of the original sample.

In Figure 8-4 the RAS haplotypes illustrate the relatively even distribution among U.S. blacks, in comparison to the "lumpy" pattern among whites. Africans are therefore the trunk of the phylogenetic tree, the origin of our species, the center, not the outlier or the peculiar "other." Of all of the stories told about race, so far this is the only one with an empirical basis. It is deeply ironic, therefore, that the regional population that is the source of all other populations and today contains the most complete reser-

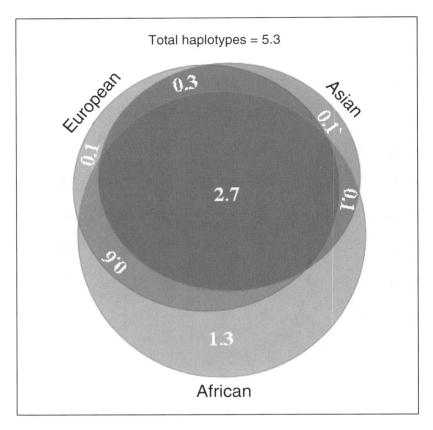

FIGURE 8-3 Distribution and overlap of haplotype blocks in three major continental groups.

voir of human diversity has been repeatedly characterized as uniquely shaped by evolution and "genetically susceptible" to the broad disease syndromes that now occur worldwide.

Perhaps the story of genetic susceptibility should be rewritten. The humans who left Africa took with them a sample of the common genetic variants that had been collected through random mutation over our evolutionary history; a more complete repository of these mutations remained in Africa. The assortment of these variants in a given individual provides the sum of genetic risk for a specific chronic disease manifested in the modern industrialized environment. The distribution of SNPs and haplotypes among racial/ethnic groups does not demonstrate a generalized pattern of "lumping" or shared variance among contemporary regional populations. Although some important susceptibility alleles may be shared unequally, this

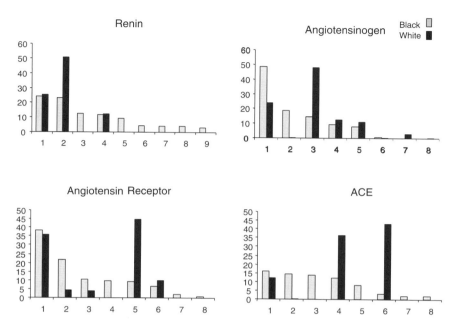

FIGURE 8-4 Frequency distribution of haplotypes in the RAS genes in whites and blacks.

has not been demonstrated yet. Africans share virtually all the common variants found in humanity and should represent the genetic "central tendency" of our species. The image of the genome that suggests itself based on this story is a time-lapse photograph of the sun—a globular whole, fringed with a corona that spurts outward and collapses to the center again.

Studies of population variation in health status will continue to be constrained if deterministic theories like the "thrifty gene" are applied whenever a disease emerges at a higher prevalence in a new ethnic group. The properties of the genome that make it a single unit shared across all regional populations would be a more appropriate premise for comparative analyses.

CONCLUSIONS

The study of genes and variation in the health of populations continues to struggle under two constraints imposed by social reality—one that influences how we frame the questions and the other that determines how people are arranged in the hierarchy. Our notion of race suggests certain answers, thereby prejudicing the questions, and the arrangement of people by race and class structures the environmental exposures, and, by extension, many aspects of health status. Although both constructs—race and inequality—confront us as products of the natural world, they are in fact reflecting an image of what we have made. That image has become nearly impossible to decipher where race and inequality merge.

Stripping away its claims to a natural origin, what is race? A name we call ourselves, *sein finn,* as they say in Irish—we ourselves—or a name for the Other? Until very recently the study of race had never been a possibility for science, despite the depths of its penetration into biology. We now have reason to believe that era is about to end as empirical questions begin to dominate the research agenda. Does race have any meaning beyond geography and history? Does the genome of our species aggregate into subunits? Does it even branch into trees? If we see it as a whole, will it look like the sun? These questions, which can be answered only with molecular data, are now at least "askable."

But scientific questions are not asked in a vacuum. Although it can legitimately be argued that in some instances the results of experimentation describe the shape of nature, questions are patently a human construct, made from materials already available to us in the social environment. Given the potency of race as a cultural idea and its influence on scientific thinking, there is reason for concern about where the attempts to discover the genetic determinants of health and disease will take us. An analogy to history may help frame this dilemma. In questioning the "memory-storage" model of history, attention has been drawn to the variable chance with which events are recorded and archived and how narratives about these events reflect the understanding of the present (Trouillot, 1995). Differential claims on the archive, and differential chances of being the hero of the narrative, are determined by differentials in power. A record of uneven quality, subjected to the filter of ideology, does not yield a description of the past, but rather a context within which we interpret the events of today. Although not a myth, because history makes a different set of claims on reality, the narratives of the past are never true or objective. In that sense, there is no "pastness," only an understanding of what shaped the present.

Genetics, like history, queries the past, attempting to use the record left in the genome to understand how evolution and population dynamics created the current pattern of variation. Although the course of human history—wars, famine, migration, conquest, and slavery—biases and complicates the record, the ability to know all the sequence variation means that the geneticist's archive is far more egalitarian and complete than is the historian's. One need only consider the story of Thomas Jefferson's family to appreciate the gap between what is recorded in history books and what is recorded in our genome (Ellis, 1998; Foster et al., 1998). If in fact the genetic history of our species is essentially complete and unbiased, the opportunities for objective description are limitless, constrained only by the questions we are asking. We can, in a sense, no longer blame our sources, but only ourselves.

But of course, after a moment's reflection, we know this is a false hope; the questions we ask are determined by the history of our consciousness, itself created from the narrative written by those in power today from an inconsistent record of the past. We are returned to the original problem—biological and social history can never be divorced. Biological scientists like to think that they work in an intellectual space uncontaminated by superstition and prejudice and therefore resist the rhetoric of context. But race is a true chimera—part geography, part history, part genes—and neither the idea nor the practice can be understood as anything other than the fantastic creation of the human mind. There is no use of race that isolates the biological from the social.

The study of genes and ethnic variation in health occupies contested territory, where genotype is hidden within phenotype and the biologic is molded by the social. Race attempts to distill and simplify this dialectical process into a linear pattern of cause and effect, obfuscating everything. We are looking to population genetics to give structure to this debate, using empirical observation as the scaffold. Can it relieve us entirely of the concept of race? Races exist only in distinction to each other; "whiteness" is defined by "blackness," and each is endowed with a distinct essence. If in fact there is no "other," then there is no essential difference, and the notion becomes empty of meaning. As on so many other occasions, however, these optimistic pronouncements will have no authority, or, at the very least, they will come too late in Western history. We live in a world where every construct is racialized—citizenship, personal identity, neighborhood, health—and it is unlikely that the evidence of genetics will be sufficient to counterbalance the enormous weight of social ideology. But within the narrow discipline of genetic epidemiology, is it too much to ask that essentialist notions, which molecular data are now demonstrating to be mere superstition, should no longer hold sway?

ENDNOTE

1. Refers to Retinal Information Network. Information can be found at www.sph.uth.tmc.edu/Retnet/home.htm.

REFERENCES

Altmuller, J., Palmer, L.J., Fischer, G., Scherb, H., and Wjst, M. (2001). Genomewide scans of complex human disease: True linkage is hard to find. *American Journal of Human Genetics, 69*, 936-950.

Anonymous. (1989). From the Health Resources and Services Administration. *Journal of the American Medical Association, 261*(2), 199.

Anonymous. (2002). The HGP: End of phase 1. *Nature Genetics, 30*(2), 125.

Auerbach, J.A., and Kringold, B.K. (Eds.). (2000). *Income, socioeconomic status and health: Exploring the relationships.* Washington, DC: National Policy Association.

Bernal, M. (1987). *Black Athena: The Afroasiatic roots of classical civilization.* New Brunswick, NJ: Rutgers University Press.

Bohnstedt, M., Fox, P.J., and Kohatsu, N.D. (1994). Correlates of mini-mental status examination scores among elderly demented patients: The influence of race-ethnicity. *Journal of Clinical Epidemiology, 47,* 1381-1387.

Brancati, F.L., Whelton, P.K., Kuller, L.H., and Klag, M.J. (1996). Diabetes mellitus, race and socioeconomic status: A population based study. *Annals of Epidemiology, 6,* 67-73.

Brancati, F.L., Kao, W.H., Folsom, A.R., Watson, R.L., and Szklo, M. (2000). Incident type 2 diabetes mellitus in African American and white adults: The Atherosclerosis Risk in Communities Study. *Journal of the American Medical Association, 283,* 2253-2259.

Brewster, L.M., Clark, J.F., and van Montfrans, G.A. (2000). Is greater tissue activity of creatine kinase the genetic factor increasing hypertension risk in black people of sub-Saharan African descent? *Journal of Hypertension, 18,* 1537-1544.

Carson, P., Ziesche, S., Johnson, G., and Cohn, J.N. (1999). Racial differences in response to therapy for heart failure: Analysis of the vasodilator-heart failure trials. Vasodilator-Heart Failure Trial Study Group. *Journal of Cardiac Failure, 5,* 178-187.

Cavalli-Sforza, L., Menozzi, P., and Piazza, A. (1996). *The history and geography of human genes.* Princeton, NJ: Princeton University Press.

Centers for Disease Control and Prevention. Available at: http://www.cdc.gov/genomics/activities/newborn/sickle [accessed September 26, 2003].

Chagnon, Y.C., Perusse, L., Weisnagel, S.J., Rankinen, T., and Bouchard, C. (2000). The human obesity gene map: The 1999 update. *Obesity Research, 8,* 89-117.

Chakravarti, A. (1999). Population genetics—making sense out of sequence. *Nature Genetics, 22,* 239-247.

Chaturverdi, N. (2001). Ethnicity as an epidemiology determinant—crudely racist or crucially important? *International Journal of Epidemiology, 30,* 925-927.

Clayton, D., and McKeigue, P.M. (2001). Epidemiological methods for studying genes and environmental factors in complex diseases. *Lancet, 358*(9290), 1356-1360.

Collaborative Study on the Genetics of Asthma. (1997, April). A genome-wide search for asthma susceptibility loci in ethnically diverse populations. *National Genetics, 15*(4), 389-392.

Collins, A., Lonjou, C., and Morton, N.E. (1999). Genetic epidemiology of single-nucleotide polymorphisms. *Proceedings of the National Academy of Sciences of the United States of America, 96,* 15173-15177.

Collins, J.W., Jr., Wu, S.Y., and David, R.J. (2002). Differing intergenerational birthweights among descendants of U.S.-born and foreign-born whites and African Americans in Illinois. *American Journal of Epidemiology, 155,* 210-216.

Cooper, R. (1994). A case study in the use of race and ethnicity in public health surveillance. *Public Health Reports, 109,* 46-52.

Cooper, R., and Rotimi, C. (1997). Hypertension in blacks. *American Journal of Hypertension, 10*(7), 804-812.

Cooper, R., Rotimi, C., Ataman, S., McGee, D., Osotimehin, B., Kadiri, S., Muna, W., Kingue, S., Fraser, H., Forrester, T., Bennett, F., and Wilks, R. (1997a). Hypertension prevalence in seven populations of African origin. *American Journal of Public Health, 87*(2), 160-168.

Cooper, R., Rotimi, C., Kaufman, J.S., Owoaje, E.E., Fraser, H., Forrester, T., Wilks, R., Riste, L.K., and Cruickshank, J.K. (1997b). Prevalence of NIDDM among populations of the African diaspora. *Diabetes Care, 20*(3), 343-348.

Cooper, R., Cutler, J., Desvigne-Nickens, P., Fortmann, S.P., Friedman, L., Havlik, R., Hogeliln, G., Marler, J., McGovern, P., Morosco, G., Mosca, L., Pearson, T., Stamler, J., Stryer, D., and Thom, T. (2001). Trends and disparities in coronary heart disease, stroke, and other cardiovascular diseases in the United States: Findings of the National Conference on CVD Prevention. *Circulation, 102,* 3137-3147.

Cooper, R.S. (1984). A note on the biological concept of race and its application in epidemiological research. *American Heart Journal, 108,* 715-723.

Cooper, R.S. (1993). Health and the social status of blacks in the United States. *Annals of Epidemiology, 3,* 137-144.

Cooper, R.S., and Kaufman, J.S. (1998). Race and hypertension: Science or nescience? *Hypertension, 32,* 813-816.

Cooper, R.S., and Psati, B.M. (2003). Genomics and medicine. *Annals of Internal Medicine, 137,* 576-580.

Cooper, R.S., and Rotimi, C. (1994). Hypertension in populations of West African origin: Is there a genetic predisposition? *Journal of Hypertension, 12,* 215-227.

Cooper, R.S., Kaufman, J., and Ward, R. (2003). Race and genomics. *New England Journal of Medicine, 348,* 1166-1170.

Curtin, P.D. (1992). The slavery hypothesis for hypertension among African Americans: The historical evidence. *American Journal of Public Health, 82,* 1681-1686.

Cystic Fibrosis Genetic Analysis Consortium. (1994). Population variation of common cystic fibrosis mutations. *Human Mutation, 4,* 167-177.

Darwin, C. (1981). *The descent of man.* Princeton, NJ: Princeton University Press.

David, R.J., and Collins, J.W., Jr. (1997). Differing birthweight among infants of U.S.-born blacks, African-born blacks and U.S.-born whites. *New England Journal of Medicine, 337,* 1209-1214.

Daviglus, M.L., Liu, K., Greenland, P., Dyer, A.R., Garside, D.B., Manheim, L., Lowe, L.P., Rodin, M., Lubitz, J., and Stamler, J. (1998). Benefit of a favorable cardiovascular risk-factor profile in middle age with respect to Medicare costs. *New England Journal of Medicine, 339,* 1122-1129.

Diehl, A.K., and Stern, M.P. (1989). Special health problems of Mexican-Americans: Obesity, gallbladder disease, diabetes mellitus, and cardiovascular disease. *Advances in Internal Medicine, 34,* 79-96.

Doris, P.A. (2001). Hypertension genetics, single nucleotide polymorphisms, and the common disease: Common variant hypothesis. *Hypertension, 39,* 323-331.

Dries, D.L., Cooper, R.S., Strong, M., and Drazner, M.H. (2002). Efficacy of ACE-inhibition in reducing progression of asymptomatic left ventricular dysfunction to symptomatic heart failure in black and white patients. *Journal of the American College of Cardiology, 40,* 311-317.

Ellis, J.J. (1998). *American sphinx: The character of Thomas Jefferson.* New York: Vintage Books.

Esparza, J., Fox, C., Harper, I.T., Bennett, P.H., Schulz, L.O., Valencia, M.E., and Ravussin, E. (2000). Daily energy expenditure in Mexican and USA Pima Indians: Low physical activity as a possible cause of obesity. *International Journal of Obesity and Related Metabolic Disorders, 24,* 55-59.

Exner, D.V. (2001). Lesser response to angiotensin-converting-enzyme inhibitor therapy in black as compared with white patients with left ventricular dysfunction. *New England Journal of Medicine, 344,* 1351-1357.

Fekete, Z., Kimura, M., Horiguchi, M., Gardner, J.P., Nash, F., and Aviv, A. (1996). Differences between store-dependent Ca2+ fluxes in lymphocytes from African Americans and whites. *Journal of Hypertension, 14,* 1293-1299.

Feldman, M.W., and Lewontin, R.C. (1975). The heritability hangup. *Science, 190,* 1163-1168.

Foster, E.A., Jobling, M.A., Taylor, P.G., Donnelly, P., de Knijff, P., Mieremet, R., Zerial, T., and Tyler-Smith, C. (1998). Jefferson fathered slave's last child. *Nature, 396,* 27-28.

Franco, L.J. (1992). Diabetes in Brazil: A review of recent survey data. *Ethnicity and Disease, 2,* 158-165.

Fray, J.C.S., and Douglas, J.G. (1993). *Pathophysiology of hypertension in blacks.* New York: Oxford University Press.

Friedman, D.J., Cohen, B.B., Mahan, C.M., Lederman, R.I., Vezina, R.J., and Dunn, V.H. (1993). Maternal ethnicity and birthweight among blacks. *Ethnicity and Disease, 3,* 255-269.

Gabriel, S.B., Schaffner, S.F., Nguyen, H., Moore, J.M., Roy, J., Blumensteil, B., Higgins, J., DeFelice, M., Lochner, A., Faggart, M., Liu-Cordero, S.N., Adeyemo, A., Cooper, R.S., Rotimi, C., Ward, R., Lander, E.S., Daly, M.J., and Altshuler, D. (2002). The structure of haplotype blocks in the human genome. *Science, 296,* 2225-2229.

Gillum, R.F. (1979). Pathophysiology of hypertension in blacks and whites: A review of the basis of racial blood pressure differences. *Hypertension, 1,* 468-475.

Gilroy, P. (1993). *The Black Atlantic: Modernity and double consciousness.* Cambridge, MA: Harvard University Press.

Gilroy, P. (2000). *Against race: Imagining political culture beyond the color line.* Cambridge, MA: Harvard University Press.

Glover, F.E., Coffey, D.S., Douglas, L., Cadogan, M., Russell, H., Tulloch, T., Baker, T.D., Wan, R.L., and Walsh, P.C. (1986). The epidemiology of prostate cancer in Jamaica. *Journal of Urology, 159,* 1984-1986.

Good, G. (1998). *Life expectancy in big cities of the United States, 1992.* Chicago: City of Chicago Department of Public Health.

Gossett, T.F. (1973). *Race: The history of an idea in America.* New York: Schocken Books.

Gould, S.J. (1981). *The mismeasure of man.* New York: W.W. Norton.

Greenland, S., and Robins, J.M. (1986). Identifiability, exchangeability, and epidemiological confounding. *International Journal of Epidemiology, 15*(3), 413-419.

Grim, C.E., and Robinson, M. (1996). Blood pressure variation in blacks: Genetic factors. *Seminars in Nephrology, 16,* 83-93.

Hahn, R.A. (1992). The state of federal health statistics on racial and ethnic groups. *Journal of the American Medical Association, 267,* 268-271.

Halushka, M., Fan, J.B., Bentley, K., Hsie, L., Weder, A., Cooper, R.S., Lipshutz, R., and Chakravarti, A. (1999). Patterns of single-nucleotide polymorphisms in candidate genes for blood pressure homeostasis. *Nature Genetics, 22,* 239-247.

Harpending, H.C., Batzer, M.A., Gurven, M., Jorde, L.B., Rogers, A.R., and Sherry, S.T. (1998). Genetic traces of ancient demography. *Proceedings of the National Academy of Sciences of the United States of America, 95,* 1961-1967.

Harris, M.I., Flegal, K.M., Cowie, C.C., Eberhardt, M.S., Goldstein, D.E., Little, R.R., Wiedmeyer, H.M., and Byrd-Holt, D.D. (1998). Prevalence of diabetes, impaired fasting glucose, and impaired glucose tolerance in U.S. adults: The Third National Health and Nutrition Examination Survey, 1988-1994. *Diabetes Care, 21,* 518-524.

Hegele, R.A. (2001). Genes and environment in type 2 diabetes and atherosclerosis in Aboriginal Canadians. *Current Atherosclerosis Reports, 3,* 216-221.

Hendrie, H.C., Osuntoken, B.O., Hall, K.S., Ogunniyi, A.O., Hui, S.L., Unverzagt, F.W., Gureje, O., Rodenberg, C.A., Baiyewu, O., and Musick, B.S. (1995). Prevalence of Alzheimer's disease and dementia in two communities: Nigerian Africans and African Americans. *American Journal of Psychiatry, 152,* 1485-1492.

Herrnstein, R., and Murray, C. (1994). *The Bell Curve: Intelligence and class structure in American life.* New York: Free Press.

Hirschhorn, J.H., Lindgren, C.M., Daly, M.J., Kirby, A., Schaffner, S.F., Burtt, N.P., Altshuler, D., Parker, A., Rioux, J.D., Platko, J., Gaudet, D., Hudson, T.J., Groon, L.C., and Lander, E.S. (2001). Genomewide linkage analysis of stature in multiple populations reveals several regions with evidence of linkage to adult height. *American Journal of Human Genetics, 69,* 106-116.

Hugot, J.P., Chamailard, M., Zouali, H., Lesage, S., Cezard, J.P., Belaiche, J., Almer, S., Tysk, C., O'Morain, C.A., Gassull, M., Binder, V., Finkel, Y.U., Cortot, A., Modigliani, R., Laurent-Puig, P., Gower-Rousseau, C., Macry, J., Colombel, J.F., Sahbatuou, M., and Thomas, G. (2001). Association of the NOD2 leucine-rich repeat variants with susceptibility to Crohn's disease. *Nature, 31,* 599-603.

Hypertension Detection and Follow-up Program Cooperative Group. (1977). Race, education and prevalence of hypertension. *American Journal of Epidemiology, 89,* 2277-2281.

James, S.A. (1993). Racial and ethnic differences in infant mortality and low birthweight: A psychosocial critique. *Annals of Epidemiology, 3,* 130-136.

Jeunemaitre, X., Soubrier, F., Kotelevtsev, Y.V., Lifton, R.P., Williams, C.S., Charru, A., Hunt, S.C., Hopkins, P.N., Williams, R.P., Lalouel, J., and Corvol, P. (1992). Molecular basis of human hypertension: Role of angiotensinogen. *Cell, 71,* 169-180.

Johnson, K.W., and Payne, G.H. (1984). Report of a working conference on coronary heart disease in black populations. *American Heart Journal, 108,* 633-862.

Jones, D.W., Sempos, C.T., Thom, T.J., Harrington, A.M., Taylor, H.A., Jr., Fletcher, B.W., Mehrotra, B.D., Wyatt, S.B., and Davis, C.E. (2000). Rising levels of cardiovascular mortality in Mississippi, 1979-1995. *American Journal of the Medical Sciences, 319,* 131-137.

Kaufman, J.S., and Cooper, R.S. (1996). Descriptive studies of racial differences in disease: In search of the hypothesis. *Public Health Reports, 110,* 662-666.

Kaufman, J.S., and Cooper, R.S. (1999). Seeking causal explanations in social epidemiology. *American Journal of Epidemiology, 150,* 113-120.

Kaufman, J.S., and Cooper, R.S. (2001). Considerations for use of racial/ethnic classification in etiologic research. *American Journal of Epidemiology, 154,* 291-298.

Kaufman, J.S., Cooper, R.S., and McGee, D. (1997). Socioeconomic status and health in blacks and whites: The problem of residual confounding and the resiliency of race. *Epidemiology, 6,* 621-628.

Khoury, M.J. (2000). *Genetics and public health in the 21st century.* Oxford, England: Oxford University Press.

Kimm, S.Y.S., Glynn, N.W., Aston, C.E., Damcott, C.M., Poehlman, E.T., Daniles, S.R., and Ferrell, R.E. (2002). Racial differences in the relation between uncoupling protein genes and resting energy expenditure. *American Journal of Clinical Nutrition, 75,* 714-719.

King, H., and Rewers, M. (1991). Diabetes in adults is now a Third World problem. *Bulletin of the World Health Organization, 69,* 643-648.

Klein, R.G. (1989). *The human career: Human biological and cultural origins.* Chicago: University of Chicago Press.

Kleinman, J.C., and Kessel, S.S. (1987). Racial differences in low birthweight: Trends and risk factors. *New England Journal of Medicine, 317,* 749-753.

Koopman, J.S. (1996). Emerging objectives and methods in epidemiology. *American Journal of Public Health, 86,* 630-632.

Krieger, N., Rowley, D.L., Herman, A.A., Avery, B., and Phillips, M.T. (1993). Racism, sexism, and social class: Implications for studies of health, disease, and well-being. *American Journal of Preventive Medicine, 9*(Suppl. 6), 82-122.

Laitinen, T., Daly, M.J., Rioux, J.D., Kauppi, P., Laprise, C., Petays, T., Green, T., Cargill, M., Hahtela, T., Lander, E.S., Laitinen, L.A., Hudson, T.J., and Kere, J. (2001). A susceptibility locus for asthma-related traits on chromosome 7 revealed by genome-wide scan in a founder population. *Nature Genetics, 28,* 87-91.

Lander, E.S. (1996). The new genomics: Global views of biology. *Science, 274,* 536-539.

Lander, E.S., and Schork, N.J. (1994). Genetic dissection of complex traits. *Science, 265,* 2037-2048.

Law, M.R., Frost, C.D., and Wald, N.J. (1991). By how much does dietary salt reduction lower blood pressure? *British Medical Journal, 302,* 811-815.

Levy, D., DeStefano, A.L., Larson, M.G., O'Donnell, C.J., Lifton, R.P., Gavras, H., Cupples, L.A., and Myers, R.H. (2000). Evidence for a gene influencing blood pressure on chromosome 17: Genome scan linkage results for longitudinal blood pressure phenotypes in subjects from the Framingham Heart Study. *Hypertension, 36,* 477-483.

Lewontin, R.C. (1972). Apportionment of human diversity. *Journal of Evolutionary Biology, 6,* 381.

Lewontin, R.C. (1974). *The genetic basis of evolutionary change.* New York: Columbia University Press.

Lewontin, R.C. (1995). *Human diversity.* New York: Scientific American Library.

Lewontin, R.C. (2000). *It ain't necessarily so: The dream of the human genome and other illusions.* New York: New York Review Books.

Lewontin, R.C., Rose, S., and Kamin, L. (1984). *Not in our genes: Biology, ideology and human nature.* New York: Pantheon Books.

Liao, Y., McGee, D.L., Cao, G., and Cooper, R.S. (1998). Black-white differences in disability and morbidity in the last years of life. *American Journal of Epidemiology, 149,* 1097-1103.

Liao, Y., McGee, D.L., and Cooper, R.S. (1999). Mortality among US adult Asians and Pacific Islanders: Findings from the National Health Interview Surveys and the National Longitudinal Mortality Study. *Ethnicity and Disease, 9,* 423-433.

Litonjua, A.A., Carey, V.J., Weiss, S.T., and Gold, D.R. (1999). Race, socioeconomic factors, and area of residence are associated with asthma prevalence. *Pediatric Pulmonology, 28,* 394-401.

Lott, J.T. (1993). Policy purposes of race and ethnicity: An assessment of federal racial and ethnic categories. *Ethnicity and Disease, 3,* 221-228.

Markides, K.S., and Coreil, J. (1986). The health of Hispanics in the Southwestern United States: An epidemiologic paradox. *Public Health Reports, 101,* 253-265.

Masoudi, F.A., and Havranek, E.P. (2001). Race and responsiveness to drugs for heart failure. *New England Journal of Medicine, 345,* 767.

McGee, D.L., Liao, Y., Cao, G., and Cooper, R.S. (1999). Self-reported health status and mortality in a multi-ethnic cohort. *American Journal of Epidemiology, 149,* 41-46.

McLeod, H.L. (2001). Pharmacogenetics: More than skin deep. *Nature Genetics, 29,* 247-248.

Miller, G.J., Maude, G.H., and Beckles, G.L. (1996). Incidence of hypertension and non-insulin dependent diabetes mellitus and associated risk factors in a rapidly developing Caribbean community: The St. James survey, Trinidad. *Journal of Epidemiology and Community Health, 50,* 497-505.

Montagu, A. (Ed.). (1964). *The concept of race.* London: Collier-Macmillan.

Morrison, J.A., Alfaro, M.P., Khoury, P., Thornton, B.B., and Daniels, S.F. (1996). Determinants of resting energy expenditure in young black girls and young white girls. *Journal of Pediatrics, 129,* 637-642.

Muntaner, C., Nieto, F.J., and O'Campo, P. (1996). The bell curve: On race, social class, and epidemiologic research. *American Journal of Epidemiology, 144,* 531-536.

National Center for Health Statistics. (2000). *Health, United States, 2000, with adolescent health chartbook.* Hyattsville, MD: Author.

Neel, J.V. (1999). The "thrifty genotype" in 1998. *Nutrition Review, 57,* S2-9.

O'Dea, K., Spargo, R.M., and Nestel, P.J. (1982). Impact of westernization on carbohydrate and lipid metabolism in Australian Aborigines. *Diabetologia, 22,* 148-153.

Oliver, R., and Atmore, A. (1992). *Africa since 1800.* New York: Cambridge University Press.

Ordunez-Garcia, P., Espinosa-Brito, A.D., Cooper, R.S., Kaufman, J., and Nieto, F.J. (1998). Hypertension in Cuba: Evidence of a narrow black-white difference. *Journal of Human Hypertension, 12,* 111-116.

Pappas, G., Queen, S., Hadden, W., and Fisher, G. (1993). The increasing disparity in mortality between socioeconomic groups in the United States, 1960 and 1986. *New England Journal of Medicine, 329,* 103-109.

Pato, C.N., Schindler, K.M., and Pato, M.T. (2000). Genetic analyses of schizophrenia. *Current Psychiatry Reports, 2,* 137-142.

Pritchard, J.K. (2001). Are rare variants responsible for susceptibility to complex diseases? *American Journal of Human Genetics, 69,* 124-137.

Province, M.A., Kardia, S.L.R., Ranade, K., Rao, D.C., Theil, B.A., Cooper, R.S., Risch, N., Turner, S.T., Cox, D.R., Hunt, S.C., Weder, A.B., and Boerwinkle, E. (2003). Meta-analysis combining genome wide linkage scans from four multicenter networks searching for human hypertension genes: The Family Blood Pressure Program (FBPP). *American Journal of Hypertension, 16,* 144-147.

Ravussin, E., and Bogardus, C. (1990). Energy expenditure in the obese: Is there a thrifty gene? *Infusionstherapie, 17,* 108-112.

Reich, D.E., Cargill, M., Bolk, S., Ireland, J., Sabeti, P.C., Richter, D.J., Lavery, T., Kouyoumjian, R., Farhadian, S.F., Ward, R., and Lander, E.S. (2001). Linkage disequilibrium in the human genome. *Nature, 444,* 199-204.

Relethford, J.H. (1998). Genetics of modern human origins and diversity. *Annual Review of Anthropology, 27,* 1-23.

Report of the Advisory Committee on Health Research. (2002). *Genomics and world health.* Geneva, Switzerland: World Health Organization.

Rigat, B., Huyber, C., Alhenc-Gelas, F., Cabmien, F., Corvol, P., and Soubrier, F. (1990). An insertion/deletion polymorphism in the angiotensin I-converting enzyme gene accounting for half the variance of serum enzyme levels. *Journal of Clinical Investigation, 86,* 1343-1346.

Risch, N. (2000). Searching for the genetic determinants in a new millennium. *Nature, 405,* 847-856.

Robbins, A.S., Whittemore, A.S., and Thom, D.H. (2000). Differences in socioeconomic status and survival among white and black men with prostate cancer [Letter]. *American Journal of Epidemiology, 152,* 493.

Robins, A.H. (1991). *Biological perspectives on human pigmentation.* Cambridge, England: Cambridge University Press.

Romualdi, C., Balding, D., Nasidze, I.S., Risch, G., Robichaux, M., Sherry, S.T., Stoneking, M., Batzer, M.A., and Barbujani, G. (2002). Patterns of human diversity, within and among continents, inferred from biallelic DNA polymorphisms. *Genome Research, 12,* 602-612.

Root, M. (2001). The problem of race in medicine. *Philosophy of the Social Sciences, 31,* 20-39.

Rose, S. (1998). *Lifelines: Biology beyond determinism.* Oxford, England: Oxford University Press.

Saad, M.F., Lillioja, S., Nyomba, B.L., Castillo, C., Ferraro, R., De Gregorio, M., Ravussin, E., Knowler, W.C., Bennett, P.H., and Howard, B.V. (1991). Racial differences in the relation between blood pressure and insulin resistance. *New England Journal of Medicine, 324,* 733-739.

Sichieri, R., Oliveira, M.C., and Pereira, R.A. (2001). High prevalence of hypertension among black and mulatto women in a Brazilian survey. *Ethnicity and Disease, 11,* 412-418.

Soubrier, F. (1998). Blood pressure gene at the angiotensin I-converting enzyme locus. Chronicle of a gene foretold. *Circulation, 97,* 1763-1765.

Staessen, J.A., Kuznetsova, T., Wang, J.G., Emelianov, D., Vlietinck, R., and Fagard, R. (1999). M235T angiotensinogen gene polymorphism and cardiovascular renal risk. *Journal of Hypertension, 17,* 9-17.

Stamler, R., Stamler, J., Dyer, A., Garside, R., Cooper, R., Berkson, D., Lindberg, H.A., Stevens, F., Schoenberger, J.A., Shekelle, S., Paul, O., Leeper, M., Garside, D., Tokich, T., and Hoeksema, R. (1979). Asymptomatic hyperglycemia and cardiovascular diseases in three Chicago epidemiologic studies. *Diabetes Care, 2,* 131-141.

Stephens, J.C., Schneider, J.A., Tanguay, D.A., Choi, J., Acharya, T., Stanley, S.E., Jiang, R., Messer, C.J., Chew, A., Han, J.-H., Duan, J., Carr, J.L., Lee, M.S., Koshy, B., Kumar, A.M., Zhang, G., Newell, W.R., Windemuth, A., Zu, C., Kalbfleisch, T.S., Shaner, S.L., Arnold, K., Schulz, V., Drysdale, C.M., Nandablan, K., Judson, R.S., Runao, G., and Vovis, G.F. (2001). Haplotype variation and linkage disequilibrium in 313 human genes. *Science, 293,* 489-493.

Svetky, L.P., Moore, T.J., Simons-Morton, D.G., Appel, L.J., Bray, G.A., Sacks, F.M., Ard, J.D., Mortensen, R.M., Mitchell, S.R., Conlin, P.R., and Desari, M., for the DASH collaborative research group. (2001). Angiotensinogen genotype and blood pressure response in the Dietary Approaches to Stop Hypertension (DASH) study. *Journal of Hypertension, 19,* 1949-1956.

Tang, M.-X., Stern, Y., Marder, K., Bell, K., Gurland, B., Lantigua, R., Andrews, H., Fen, L., Tycko, B., and Mayeux, R. (1998). The APOE-E4 allele and the risk of Alzheimer disease among African Americans, whites, and Hispanics. *Journal of the American Medical Association, 279,* 751-755.

Tavtigian, S.V., Simard, J., Teng, D.H., Abtin, V., Baumgard, M., Beck, A., Camp, N.J., Carillo, A.P., Chen, Y., Dayananth, P., Desrochers, M., Dumont, M., Farnham, J.M., Frank, D., Frye, C., Ghaffari, S., Gupte, J.S., Hu, R., Illiey, D., Janeck, T., Kort, E.N., Laity, K.E., Leavitt, A., Leblanc, G., McArthur-Morrison, J., Pederson, A., Penn, B., Peterson, K.T., Reid, J.E., Richards, S., Schroeder, M., Smith, R., Snyder, S.C., Swedlund, B., Swensen, J., Thomas, A., Tranchant, M., Woodland, A.M., Labrie, F., Skolnick, M.H., Neuhausen, S., Rommens, J., and Cannon-Albright, L.A. (2001). A candidate prostate cancer susceptibility gene at chromosome 17p. *Nature Genetics, 27,* 172-180.

Templeton, A.R. (1999). Human races: A genetic and evolutionary perspective. *American Anthropologist, 100,* 632-650.

Trouillot, M.R. (1995). *Silencing the past: Power and the production of history.* Boston, MA: Beacon Press.

Turner, S.T., Schwartz, G.L., Chapman, A.B., and Boerwinkle, E. (2001). C825T polymorphism of the G protein beta(3)-subunit and antihypertensive response to a thiazide diuretic. *Hypertension, 37,* 739-743.

Van den Oord, E.J.C.G., and Rowe, D.C. (2000). Racial differences in birth health risk: A quantitative genetic approach. *Demography, 37,* 285-298.

Vasan, R.S., Beiser, A., Seshadri, S., Larson, M.G., Kannel, W.B., D'Agostino, R.B., and Levy, D. (2002). Residual lifetime risk for developing hypertension in middle-aged women and men. The Framingham Heart Study. *Journal of the American Medical Association, 287,* 1003-1010.

Wei, M., Valdez, R.A., Mitchell, B.D., Haffner, S.M., Stern, M.P., and Hazuda, H.P. (1996). Migration status, socioeconomic status, and mortality rates in Mexican Americans and non-Hispanic whites. The San Antonio Heart Study. *Annals of Epidemiology, 6,* 307-313.

Weiss, K.M., Ferrell, R.E., and Hanis, C.L. (1984). A New World syndrome of metabolic diseases with a genetic and evolutionary basis. *Yearbook of Physical Anthropology, 27,* 153-178.

Wilson, J.F., Weale, M.E., Smith, A.C., Gratrix, F., Fletcher, B., Thomas, M.G., Bradman, N., and Goldstein, D.B. (2001). Population genetic structure of variable drug response. *Nature Genetics, 29,* 265-269.

Wilson, T.W. (1986). History of salt supplies in West Africa and blood pressures today. *Lancet, 1,* 784-786.

Wu, X., Cooper, R.S., Borecki, I., Hanis, C., Bray, M., Lewis, C.E., Zhu, X., Kan, D., Luke, A., and Curb, D. (2002). A combined analysis of genome-wide linkage scans for BMI from the NHLBI Family Blood Pressure Program. *American Journal of Human Genetics, 70,* 1247-1256.

Yancy, C.W. (2001). Race and response to adrenergic blockade with carvedilol in patients with chronic heart failure. *New England Journal of Medicine, 344,* 1358-1365.

Yanovski, S.Z., Reynolds, J.C., Boyle, A.J., and Yanovski, J.A. (1997). Resting metabolic rate in African-American and Caucasian girls. *Obesity Research, 5,* 321-325.

Zhu, X., McKenzie, C., Forrester, T., Nickerson, D.A., Cooper, R.S., and Rieder, M.J. (2000). Localization of a small genomic region associated with elevated ACE. *American Journal of Human Genetics, 67,* 1144-1153.

Zhu, X., Bouzekri, N., Southam, L., Cooper, R.S., Adeyemo, A., McKenzie, C.A., Luke, A., Chen, G., Elston, R.C., and Ward, R. (2001). Linkage and association analysis of angiotensin I-converting enzyme (ACE) gene polymorphisms with ACE concentration and blood pressure. *American Journal of Human Genetics, 68,* 1139-1148.

Zhu, X., Yan, D., Cooper, R.S., Luke, A., Weder, A., and Chakravarti, A. (2003a). Linkage disequilibrium and haplotype diversity in the genes of the renin-angiotensin system: Findings from the Family Blood Pressure Program. *Genomic Research, 13,* 173-181.

Zhu, X., Yen-Pei, C., Chang, D., Yan, D., Weder, A., Cooper, R., Luke, A., Kan, D., and Chakravarti, A. (2003b). Associations between hypertension and genes in the renin-angiotensin system. *Hypertension, 41*(5), 1027-1034.

9

Race/Ethnicity, Socioeconomic Status, and Health

Eileen M. Crimmins, Mark D. Hayward,
and Teresa E. Seeman

Mounting evidence indicates that racial/ethnic differences in morbidity and mortality are tied to socioeconomic resources (Hayward, Crimmins, Miles, and Yu, 2000; Williams and Collins, 1995). Largely because of data availability, most of this evidence is based on the health experiences of blacks and whites, with much less evidence on the role of socioeconomic factors in understanding racial/ethnic disparities when Americans of Asian or Pacific Island descent, Hispanics, and Native Americans are part of the picture. The potential power of the socioeconomic status (SES) paradigm in understanding health disparities—including racial/ethnic disparities—is evident in the fact that socioeconomic differences in health outcomes have been widely documented for most health conditions in most countries. People who are poorer and who have less education are more likely to suffer from diseases, to experience loss of functioning, to be cognitively and physically impaired, and to experience higher mortality rates (Adler, Boyce, Chesney, Folkman, and Syme, 1993; Adler et al., 1994; Marmot, Kogevinas, and Elston, 1987; Marmot, Ryff, Bumpass, Shipley, and Marks, 1997; Preston and Taubman, 1994; Williams, 1990). In the United States, few health problems are more likely to occur among those who are better off, and some health conditions are particularly sensitive to SES. In recent years socioeconomic differences in health also appear to be increasing in the United States and in other developed countries (Crimmins and Saito, 2001; Feldman, Makuc, Kleinman, and Coroni-Huntley, 1989; Manton, 1997; Marmot, 1994; Pappas, Queen, Hadden, and Fisher, 1993; Preston and Elo, 1995).

The socioeconomic stratification that patterns American life, and differences in life for the major racial/ethnic groups, is assumed to be the root cause of these differences (Adler et al., 1994; Link and Phelan, 1995). People of different social statuses lead lives that differ in almost all aspects—childhood circumstances, educational experiences, work careers, marriage and family experiences, leisure, neighborhood conditions, and health care (Williams and Collins, 1995). Many of the effects of SES on health outcomes are indirect through a variety of life experiences, opportunities, or choices related to SES, beginning in early life and either cumulating or being tempered by later life situations. Health differences are observed throughout the lifecycle, and the general assumption is that differences diminish at older ages. This assumption was questioned recently by Lynch (2003).

Socioeconomic status is obviously related to race and ethnicity in the United States, but the role of socioeconomic factors as a cause of racial/ethnic health differences is complex. Many studies have documented the importance of blacks' low SES as a partial explanation for poor health outcomes relative to whites. Studies have also clarified that socioeconomic differences often do not "explain" all health differences between African Americans and non-Hispanic whites, with black-white differences in health remaining after controlling for socioeconomic conditions (Hayward et al., 2000). Asian Americans' comparatively high SES has been suggested as a cause of this group's better health, but again, other factors also appear to come into play (Lauderdale and Kestenbaum, 2002). The "Hispanic paradox," or the better than expected health experienced by the socioeconomically disadvantaged Hispanic population, is another example of the complexity of the relationships among race/ethnicity, SES, and health outcomes (Abraido-Lanza, Dohrenwend, Ng-Mak, and Turner, 1999).

Ambiguity also surrounds the mechanisms through which SES promotes racial/ethnic differences in health. The issue of whether members of all ethnic groups are able to equally translate increases in SES into health improvements has been raised (Ribisi, Winkleby, Fortmann, and Fiora, 1998; Williams, Lavizzo-Mourey, and Warren, 1994). In addition, researchers have questioned whether the race gap in health is concentrated at the low end of the socioeconomic ladder, with some studies reporting that the race gap in health is strongest among persons with the fewest socioeconomic resources (Lillie-Blanton, Parsons, Gayle, and Dievler, 1996). Other researchers have suggested that the association is more linear, with increasingly better health as SES increases, although there may be some leveling off at the top (Adler et al., 1993; House, Kessler, and Herzog, 1990; Pappas et al., 1993).

Both health and socioeconomic status have many dimensions and can be conceptualized and measured in multiple ways, with measurement often falling far short of the conceptual ideas. This adds to the complexity of synthesizing studies' results relating socioeconomic status, health, and race/ethnicity. In this chapter, our discussion sheds some light on this complexity by briefly exploring how different approaches to conceptualizing both SES and health may affect conclusions about the role of SES in accounting for racial/ethnic health outcomes. As we make clear in our discussion of the major population health surveys, however, no omnibus health survey fully meets the needs of the conceptual issues believed to underlie the racial/ethnic differences in health. Furthermore, we raise the question of whether these major surveys have comparable samples in an attempt to understand one potential source of variation in the empirical associations among race/ethnicity, SES, and health.

Based on these surveys, we then investigate the socioeconomic and health differences among racial/ethnic groups. Our purpose for the empirical analysis is to assess the consistency of key empirical associations among race/ethnicity, the various measures of SES, and multiple dimensions of health (major chronic diseases, physical and cognitive impairment, and mortality). We address two major substantive questions—the extent to which SES factors account for racial/ethnic differences in health and the extent to which the SES gradient in health is shared across the major racial/ethnic groups. When possible, we examine associations for both the prevalence and incidence of a health problem. Prevalence—or the percentage with a health problem at a point in time—is the more commonly used indicator of disease experience, yet it has limitations. Prevalence differences across racial/ethnic groups embody health experiences at earlier ages that have left their stamp on the population (Hayward, Friedman, and Chen, 1996; Schoen, 1988). These experiences, particularly through mortality selection, may also alter the distribution of socioeconomic resources as a cohort ages (Lauderdale, 2001). Incidence—that is, the onset of new cases of health problems—captures health experiences prospectively and points to possible trajectories of health after baseline observation. Incidence allows us to investigate how socioeconomic conditions when individuals do not have a health problem are associated with subsequent health experiences. Our empirical assessment of the associations among race/ethnicity, SES, and health is necessarily cursory, but one that aids in assessing the specificity of associations among race/ethnicity, SES, and a range of health outcomes.

CONCEPTIONS OF SOCIOECONOMIC STATUS

Socioeconomic status can be broadly conceptualized as one's position in the social structure. Sociologists emphasize a Weberian approach that encompasses the notions of class, status, and power. SES is thus more than financial well-being or educational achievement, which are often used as indicators in empirical work; more broadly, it encompasses a lifetime of access to knowledge, resources, and opportunities. In recent work, Oakes and Rossi (2003) suggest that measures of SES should reflect material capital, human capital, and social capital. Although indicators of adult status such as education, current income, wealth, and occupation are often the indicators of SES available for analysis, these may be fairly gross measures of the lifetime accumulation or experience of some types of capital. For example, education represents human and social capital at the beginning of adulthood. Annual income represents only recent accumulation of material capital. Appropriately measuring adult lifetime income may be a better indicator of lifetime material status (Juster and Suzman, 1995). Wealth accumulation may represent total material capital available at the moment, but this may be highly affected by life circumstances, including health.

Sociologists and epidemiologists emphasize the effects of lifetime socioeconomic conditions on health rather than the effects of health on SES. Economists are more sensitive to this latter association, and recent work has documented the link between health problems and reductions in income and wealth at older ages (Smith and Kington, 1997). Importantly, however, the causal direction of the association potentially varies by age, the metric of SES, and likely by specific health conditions. For example, educational attainment is not affected by health for most people because of the lifecycle stage when education is acquired. Of course, for some people with diseases and conditions with childhood onset, educational attainment is influenced by health.

On the other hand, health problems that arise during the working years (e.g., heart condition, diabetes, functional problems, and depression) may significantly affect labor supply, earnings, and wealth accumulation. The cross-sectional relationship of income and current health status among those at the older working ages most likely reflects the combination of the effect of the ability to work on income as well as the effect of earlier income on health (Shea, Miles, and Hayward, 1996). Thus examining this relationship in the cross-section says little about causal effects. In old age, wealth is often consumed by those with health problems in order to provide medical or custodial care, resulting in a negative relationship between health and wealth (Smith, 1999; Smith and Kington, 1997). Most investigations, however, have found that the influence of health on socioeconomic indicators is less important than causation in the other direction, but this cannot be assumed to be true with respect to all relationships between SES and health outcomes across the life course. It is important to consider the potential for interpreting the direction of causation when selecting indicators of SES as well as health outcomes particularly at the older ages.

For an older population, some measures of SES and some health conditions are especially likely to be both causes and consequences of each other.

If older disabled persons move in with their working, middle-aged children in order to cope with disability, they will reside in a family with higher current income. If people stop working at a young age because of disability, they are more likely to have reduced pension funds for the rest of their lives. Because education is not affected by health events after young adulthood, many researchers prefer the use of education as an index of lifetime SES for the adult population. However, because of historical increases in educational attainment among more recent birth cohorts, educational attainment is negatively associated with age in the older population in the cross-section. This makes the SES of people at older ages appear to be less than at younger ages, although the relative meaning of education in terms of lifetime achievement may be affected by the era in which people were educated and careers were developed. For this reason, in some analyses of relationships across ages or time, educational achievement relative to one's peers may be the appropriate metric rather than absolute levels of educational achievement (Pamuk, 1985).

MECHANISMS THROUGH WHICH SES WORKS TO AFFECT HEALTH

Numerous papers have outlined social, psychological, and economic mechanisms through which SES is assumed to affect health outcomes (Anderson, 1995; Hummer, Rogers, and Eberstein, 1998; Kington and Nickens, 2001; Seeman and Crimmins, 2001). We only briefly review some of the implications of this work relevant to the issues addressed in this chapter. In general, among persons of higher SES, exposure to health-threatening conditions should be lower, and resources to buffer health threats should be higher. The influence of SES on health is assumed to begin early in life, perhaps even in the prenatal environment, and continue to accumulate throughout life. Increasing evidence also shows that the effects of some childhood conditions (e.g., infectious diseases) on later life health are only partially mediated by adult achievement processes or lifestyle (Blackwell, Hayward, and Crimmins., 2001; Hayward et al., 2000; Kuh and Davey-Smith, 1997; Preston, Hill, and Drevenstedt, 1998).

Recent work by Warner and Hayward (2002) suggests that childhood circumstances explain a substantial part of the mortality gap between blacks and whites. This led them to propose that the distribution of resources in childhood sets individuals on a path toward stable or deteriorating health. Part of the mechanism is the link between parental and child SES as SES is transmitted from one generation to another. In addition, social capital appears to come into play with a strong health protective effect of early intact families.

Adults of higher SES are more likely to have grown up in childhood homes with better nutrition, fewer health risk behaviors, safer neighborhoods, and more economic resources. As adults, higher SES persons mature in more secure and rewarding career and residential situations. Persons of higher status have a greater ability to access health services and may receive better treatment when served. Higher education provides explicit facts, and leads to attitudes and behaviors that are conducive to better health as well as a willingness to delay gratification in order to achieve desired goals. Persons of higher status smoke less, eat better, and exercise more than persons with fewer resources (Winkleby, Jatulis, Frank, and Fortmann, 1992; Winkleby, Kraemer, Ahn, and Varady, 1998). Higher status brings freedom from some types of worry and stress and enables coping with other types of stress. Lower status is linked to more disruptive life events such as family breakup and unemployment as well as fewer financial resources to cope with such events. Persons of higher status are also more likely to develop psychological resources such as a sense of mastery and control or to experience reduced levels of hostility (Pincus and Callahan, 1995), which are all conducive to better health. Explaining the role of SES in racial and ethnic differences in health thus requires examining the relationship between race/ethnicity and lifetime SES as well as the link between SES and the potential mechanisms through which it works. Most empirical analyses are unable to accomplish this because of a lack of appropriate data.

CONCEPTIONS OF HEALTH AND THEIR RELATIONSHIP TO SOCIOECONOMIC STATUS AND RACE/ETHNICITY

Health has a number of dimensions, including diseases and conditions, functioning loss, disability, and death (Verbrugge and Jette, 1994). The process of health change for populations can be thought of as beginning with the onset of diseases and conditions, which can lead to functioning loss and impairment and eventually disability and death. The development of chronic diseases and conditions—while generally not clinically recognized until at least middle age—is affected by lifelong circumstances that are related to both socioeconomic status and race/ethnicity. Many of these mechanisms have been mentioned already, but additional factors affect the likelihood that people of different ethnic groups and social status groups will not only get diseases, but also whether diseases will result in functioning loss, disability, or death. For example, the stage at which a disease or condition is clinically recognized and reported can vary with the use of health care, which is related to the availability of health insurance and to health care habits. Whether heart disease results in death may depend on how early it is diagnosed and treated, which may, in turn, depend on the provision of health insurance and ascriptive factors such as sex and race. Whether a condition is disabling may depend on the environmental circumstances in which the person lives or works. If job requirements include physical labor, for example, disability may be reported at a level of functioning loss that would not cause disability in a white-collar worker (Hardy and Pavalko, 1986).

Racial/ethnic and socioeconomic differences are greater in some dimensions of health and from some causes than others. For example, black men have higher death rates from heart disease than white men, but they do not differ in the prevalence of reported heart disease (Hayward et al., 2000). Even within the group of diseases classified as cancer, death rates from some cancers appear to be less strongly related to socioeconomic status than deaths from other causes (Pincus, Callahan, and Burkhauser, 1987). Some causes of death and disease are more likely to be affected by the mechanisms through which SES is assumed to work. Stress is believed to be an important factor in heart disease and hypertension. Obesity, a condition more common among those of lower SES, is assumed to pose a risk for diabetes. Differential relationships between diseases and socioeconomic status may be one reason that the relationship between SES and health varies by age. In the young adult years, mortality is dominated by violent death and AIDS, which are both highly related to socioeconomic status. In the middle adult years, deaths due to cancer and heart disease become more prevalent. Early deaths from these causes may be among those with either high vulnerability or lifelong insult. The causes of death and many causes of disability that dominate old age have a long period of development. Racial/ethnic differences in disability are not necessarily the same as those in mortality or in presence of disease (see Chapter 2).

Understanding the time dimension of health outcomes is important for interpreting both socioeconomic and racial/ethnic differences. Many studies focus on the current prevalence of health problems, a measure indicating whether a problem exists at the time of measurement. Current prevalence of health problems is affected by a cohort's entire history of rates of disease onset, durations of conditions, and rates of survival. A difference in the current level of disease between two groups could result from one group having a higher rate of disease than the other, but both groups experiencing the same survival with disease. Or both groups could have the same incidence or onset rate, but different survival rates. Thus, it is not possible to intuit the process by which group differences arise from examining only differences in disease prevalence. Differences in onset and survival are more informative of health processes. For this reason, many investigators prefer to examine the incidence of health problems in a specified period and relate health events in the period to explanatory characteristics that precede the events. It is also difficult to intuit differences in cause-specific mortality for similar reasons. Blacks' higher death rates from heart disease compared to whites, for example, could be a function of higher rates of disease incidence, but similar survival among persons with heart disease. Or the gap in heart disease death rates could be due to a higher death rate for blacks among persons with heart disease, or, the gap could reflect a combination of these morbidity and mortality experiences.

Two additional issues need to be considered in evaluating what we know about socioeconomic and racial/ethnic differences from available data on health outcomes. One issue is the source of the information. Many surveys ask respondents to report if "a doctor has told you" that you have a specified condition. This is affected by contact with doctors; doctors telling patients that they have a condition; and patients correctly interpreting and remembering what they have been told. All of this is likely to be affected by both SES and race/ethnicity. Other health outcomes, such as reports of functional difficulty or self-reports of health status, also depend on the reference group of the respondent. Another issue with much of the current survey data on health is that the severity of the problem is not reported—we know a person has a health problem, but not how severe the problem is. These types of problems with self-report data on health outcomes other than mortality often have resulted in a focus on only mortality or life expectancy in the area of health differentials. As we have clarified, mortality is the end of a process that needs to be better understood in order to meaningfully address racial/ethnic differentials in these various morbid and mortal outcomes.

SOCIOECONOMIC STATUS, AGE, AND HEALTH

As we noted earlier, the importance of socioeconomic status in explaining health differences and even the direction of causation may differ by age if one includes indicators of material well-being. While socioeconomic resources affect health throughout the lifecycle, many scholars report that SES differentials in health are reduced at older ages (House et al., 1994; Marmot and Shipley, 1996). Support for this idea is provided by the fact that racial/ethnic differences in mortality are relatively small at the oldest ages, with some finding that white mortality exceeds that of African Americans and Hispanics at the oldest ages (Liao et al., 1998). Social circumstances may be overwhelmed by biological changes related to aging at the oldest ages, or those who survive may differ from cohort members who did not live until old age. It is not surprising that SES and health are reduced at the older ages when even well-recognized risk factors such as smoking and obesity do not always relate to health outcomes as expected among the older population (Crimmins, 2001).

Health differences among adults by SES and between blacks and whites are thought to be maximal in late middle age (Hayward et al., 2000). However, even examination of the effect of observed socioeconomic differentials in either short-term incidence or prevalence at this age may not fully indicate the overall age pattern of health differences affecting health disparities because the effect is compounded over time. Transformation of standard results from individual-level analyses to clarify group or population differences can sometimes aid in this interpretation. For example, analysis of the relationship of disease onset by educational groups from the Health and Retirement Survey using age-specific schedules of onset provides evidence for the more rapid aging or "weathering" of disadvantaged populations implied by the higher annual rates of disease onset and prevalence experienced by low-status persons. Table 9-1 presents the ages at which three education groups (8 years, 12 years, and 16 years) experience equivalent rates of prevalence and onset of major diseases. Equivalent ages are the ages at which the two higher education groups have the same level of prevalence or annual rate of incidence as that experienced by persons at age 51 in the lowest education group (8 years). Estimated ages are based on logistic models of disease presence and hazard models of disease onset that include education, age, and gender as the independent variables. Those in the middle education group experience the same rates of onset and incidence from 3 to 9 years later, generally in their late 50s. Those in the highest socioeconomic group are able to delay these health experiences into their 60s, from 6 to 19 years later than the lowest education group.

Some of the effect of earlier aging of lower status persons is not captured in this examination of diseases among people in their 50s because a

TABLE 9-1 Age at Which Persons of Different Educational Levels Experience Equivalent Prevalence and Incidence of Specified Diseases: Based on Logistic Models of Prevalence and Hazard Models of Incidence from the Health and Retirement Survey*

Years of Education	8	12	16
Prevalence			
Heart problems	51	54	57
Heart attack	51	58	~64
Hypertension	51	55	58
Stroke	51	56	61
Diabetes	51	57	~64
Chronic lung disease	51	60	~70
Incidence			
Heart problems	52	56	60
Heart attack	52	59	~65
Stroke	52	58	~64
Death	52	57	61

*All models have age and gender controlled. Sample aged 51-61 at wave I. Incidence is between wave I and wave II.

significant number of those with lower SES have been eliminated from the population due to early mortality. Because of mortality before they reached the age of the Health and Retirement Survey, only about three-fourths of men born from 1931 to 1941 lived up to age 60; this figure is probably closer to 40 percent for African Americans (Hayward et al., 2000). Examination of the cause-specific mortality rates of persons in their 40s shows that this differential mortality is strongly reflective of the very early ages at which fatal chronic diseases are prevalent among African Americans. Thus even the study of cohorts beginning in the later working years misses many of the health experiences of the group.

Many studies of health outcomes emphasize the analysis of the onset of health problems among people who do not have the problem at the beginning of the study rather than the prevalence of problems. As noted earlier, this helps in determining cause and effect, but it eliminates additional members of the cohort from analysis—those who get diseases at younger ages. Even in a study of 50-year-olds, the majority of black men and women already will have hypertension and will not be candidates for an incidence analysis. For investigations of health at advanced ages, persons remaining in the population for study are those who survive and often also those who have survived without disease. If survival without diseases differs by SES and race, studies restricted to incidence in the older population miss much of the underlying process leading to the health disparities observed at older ages. Understanding health disparities at the older ages thus requires an understanding of the role of the disease process in selective survival, the prevalence of the disease in a baseline population, and the subsequent morbidity and mortality experiences into advanced ages.

Healthy life expectancy approaches capture the effect of both mortality and morbidity differentials among population groups in a summary indicator. Because the measures can be calculated for any age, they can summarize the effects over the remaining lifecycle fairly simply. Estimates of healthy life by education for blacks and whites in the United States in 1990 have been developed by Crimmins and Saito (2001). Healthy life at age 30 and disabled life at age 30 are shown in Figure 9-1 for persons with less than 9 years of education and for persons with 13 or more years of education. Whites live more healthy years than blacks except for highly educated females. At each level of education, white women live fewer years disabled than black women; for men the difference goes the other way, with white men living more unhealthy years. The third component shown in the figure is the potential years of life that each group loses from the highest observed life expectancy—in this case, highly educated black women. Lost years is the component that is substantially longer for black men and for those with low education. This demonstrates the importance of early mortality in

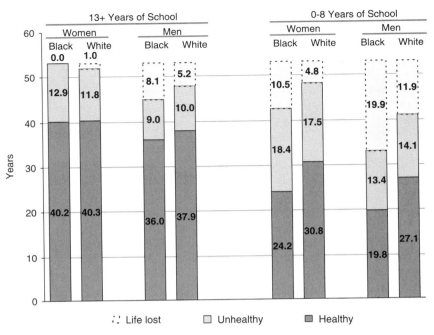

FIGURE 9-1 Years of potential life lost and years of unhealthy and healthy life lived at age 30: sex-race groups with 13+ and 0-8 years of schooling. SOURCE: Crimmins and Saito (2001).

affecting who actually reaches older age to participate in studies of health differentials.

HOW DOES SOCIOECONOMIC STATUS VARY BY RACE/ETHNIC GROUPS IN MAJOR HEALTH SURVEYS?

In this section we address an empirical question: How does socioeconomic status as indicated by educational attainment, family income, and wealth vary across race and ethnicity? Although this is a topic that has been thoroughly addressed elsewhere, we add evidence from a number of the major health surveys of the U.S. population assumed to be nationally representative. We examine these differences in major health surveys of the older or near-retirement-age population in order to clarify the socioeconomic status of the racial/ethnic groups on which generalizations about health differences are often based. We examine whether all of the surveys appear to represent the same populations. Years of education and family income are reported in all surveys and wealth in some. Although these indicators fall far short of capturing the dimensions of SES embodied in most theoretical approaches, they represent what is available in the data. In the next section, we examine relationships between race/ethnicity and health and socioeconomic status using data from these surveys. We separate foreign-born Hispanics from native-born Hispanics in all of our analyses because of the importance of nativity in evaluating observed health differences (see Chapter 6).

The surveys include the Assets and Health Dynamics of the Oldest Old (AHEAD), the National Health and Nutrition Examination Survey III (NHANES III), the National Health Interview Survey of 1994 (NHIS) with some information from its subsample Longitudinal Study on Aging (LSOA II), and the Health and Retirement Study (HRS). The first three of these surveys are representative of the older population and the HRS is representative of people approaching retirement age. AHEAD is initially representative of community dwellers aged 70 and over and was begun in 1993 with an oversample of African Americans and Hispanics to provide the potential for analysis of these groups. The survey also includes an oversample of Florida, which may affect the characteristics of Hispanics studied. The total sample consists of about 7,350 people, of whom slightly over 1,000 are black, 170 are U.S.-born Hispanic, and approximately 240 are foreign-born Hispanic.

NHANES was collected from 1988 to 1994 to address issues of racial/ethnic health differences in the population of all ages. Large samples of African Americans and Hispanics, consisting primarily of persons of Mexican origin, were included in this survey. This sample includes approximately 3,400 people aged 65 and over. This number includes 933 African Americans, approximately 450 U.S.-born Hispanics, and 300 foreign-born Hispanics. The NHIS is a nationally representative survey of the population of all ages, which allows examination of not only the major racial/ethnic groups already listed, but also provides limited information for residents of Asian and Pacific Island origin and Native Americans. It also provides the sample for the LSOA II, which offers additional data on health outcomes. The NHIS contained nearly 12,000 interviews for white non-Hispanic persons 65+ and older, nearly 1,600 African Americans, and 250 each of foreign and native-born Hispanics. There were 156 foreign-born Asians over 64 and 59 U.S.-born Asians in the survey. Nearly 70 older Native Americans were included. The HRS is the parent survey of the AHEAD survey and collected similar information for a slightly younger group: those 51 to 61 in 1992. The HRS has a sample of nearly 7,000 whites, 1,600 African Americans, 400 U.S.-born Hispanics, and 480 foreign-born Hispanics. Inclusion of this survey, which is fairly similar to AHEAD in design and structure, allows comparison of two age groups.

As indicated earlier, each survey provides information on education and current family income, and three provide information on assets. Measurement in the surveys is not identical; because details of the measurement have been discussed in a number of places, they will not be addressed here (Ettner and Crimmins, 2002). Our question is how these racial/ethnic groups compare in SES across these surveys using available indicators of SES. We present medians and interquartile ranges in Figures 9-2 through 9-4 in order to compare the distribution as well as the midpoint of the range.

Examining *education* in the first three surveys for the older population, we see that the median and distribution of education for whites and blacks is fairly similar across surveys (Figure 9-2). There is quite a bit of overlap in the distribution between African Americans and whites even though the median of whites exceeds that of African Americans by 3 or 4 years.

On the other hand, the educational level of Hispanics differs across surveys as does the level and direction of the difference between foreign-born and native-born Hispanics. Although these surveys are generally believed to be "nationally representative," they do not appear to include the same groups of Hispanics. U.S.-born Hispanics have a median education of 6, 7, or 8 years depending on the survey; median education for foreign-born Hispanics ranges from 4 to 10 years. The foreign-born Hispanics in the largely Mexican NHANES have a lower level of education than the foreign-born Hispanics in the NHIS. For comparison we also show education of the foreign born of Mexican origin in the NHIS; this group has an educational level similar to foreign-born Hispanics in AHEAD and NHANES. This comparison makes it clear that the Hispanic population captured in these surveys varies across surveys; it also indicates the importance of considering both nativity and country of origin when analyzing the Hispanic population.

In the NHIS persons of Asian origin have a relatively high level of education, with few persons at low levels of education. The median of the foreign-born Asians aged 65 and over is below that of whites, but above other groups except Native Americans. In contrast to native-born persons of Asian origin, there is a relatively large dispersion in educational level among foreign-born Asians.

The HRS sample is 10 to 20 years younger than the other samples and its higher levels of education indicate change for cohorts over time. The educational level rises in all ethnic groups from that observed for older persons, and the younger groups appear more similar in median education. Median education is within 1 year for whites, blacks, and U.S.-born Hispanics. The middle 50 percent of the educational distribution is smaller for each of these groups in this younger cohort than in the older cohorts, indicating the reduction in dispersion of the middle of the educational distribution in this cohort.

These figures can be compared to figures on education gathered in the U.S. Census (Table 9-2). These do not provide a perfect comparison be-

323

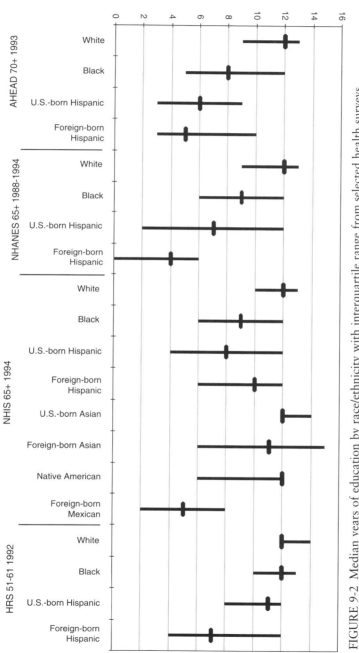

FIGURE 9-2 Median years of education by race/ethnicity with interquartile range from selected health surveys.

TABLE 9-2 Median Education for 65+ Population by Ethnicity:
U.S. Census, 2000

Racial/Ethnic Group	Median Education Level
Non-Hispanic whites	12.0
Blacks	10.3
Hispanics	9.3
Native born	10.2
Foreign born	7.3
Asians	12.0
Native born	12.0
Foreign born	12.0

SOURCE: Calculated from U.S. Bureau of the Census (2000).

cause the Census was taken in 2000, 6 to 7 years later than most of these surveys, but they do provide an indicator of relative educational level for these groups, which can serve as a benchmark.

All the surveys have the same median education for non-Hispanic whites as the Census. Black educational levels appear low in all of the surveys of the older population. The median education reported by the Hispanic samples appears much lower than the level of education reported by the Hispanic population in the Census. An exception to this is the level of education reported by foreign-born Hispanics in the NHIS. In this survey the direction of the differential between foreign born and native born is reversed relative to that in the Census. U.S.-born Americans of Asian origin in the NHIS have the same median education as that reported in the Census, while the median for the foreign born is lower than the comparison group in the Census. While the same data are not available for Native Americans, data for the entire adult population indicates that Native American levels of education are lower than those of whites, not the same for the two groups as reported in the NHIS.

Now we examine reports of income across surveys and compare the relative position of the groups to that reported in the Census and Current Population Survey (CPS). Median family *income* for those 65 and over is always higher for whites than for blacks and both groups of Hispanics (Figure 9-3). Blacks and Hispanics have roughly similar income levels, although Hispanics in the NHANES and the NHIS reports slightly higher levels of income than blacks (Figure 9-3). Asians, both foreign born and native born, are relatively high-income groups with medians exceeding those of whites. As in education, there is great variability in income in the foreign-born Asian group.

Estimates of median income for 1993 can be made using CPS and Census data along with changes in the Consumer Price Index. These indicate that all groups report lower levels of income than would be expected,

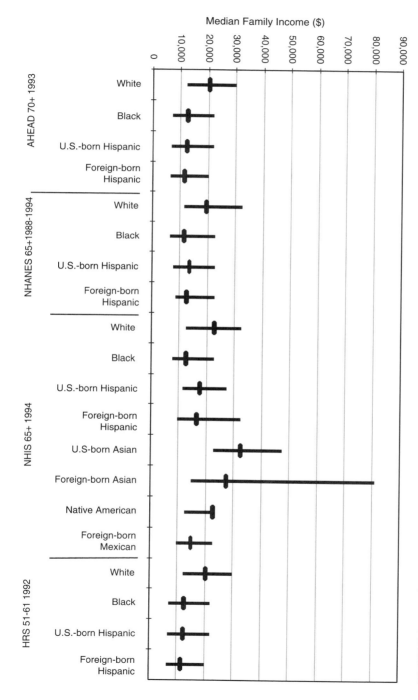

FIGURE 9-3 Median family income by race/ethnicity with interquartile range from selected health survey.

with the exception of Asian Americans and Native Americans. We would expect white median income at ages 65 and older to be about a third higher than that for blacks and Hispanics; the differences between blacks and Hispanics and whites appear to be larger than this in AHEAD. The higher income level for Hispanics relative to blacks reported in NHANES and the NHIS is not expected.

Assets are available from AHEAD, NHIS, and HRS (Figure 9-4). There is more variability in assets among ethnic groups than in income. Americans of Asian and Pacific Island origin have very high levels of assets, and blacks very low. The relative placement of Hispanics varies across surveys. In both AHEAD and HRS, foreign-born Hispanics report very little wealth. In the NHIS, they report wealth similar to U.S.-born Hispanics and higher than that for blacks.

In sum, while there are some indicators of SES that distribute as expected across older racial and ethnic groups in these surveys, there are also instances where the samples appear unrepresentative of the entire population of certain ethnic groups. Sometimes the relative status of blacks and Hispanics differs from what might be expected. The characteristics of Hispanic groups differ markedly across these surveys even though they are usually treated as nationally representative in most analyses of health differences. Asians included in these health surveys, while relatively small in number, indicate high levels of all measures of SES, with wealth being the indicator in which they are relatively highest. Native Americans included in the NHIS are a very small group, but in this survey they report levels of socioeconomic indicators that are close to those for whites, and this raises the issue of representativeness of Native Americans in the NHIS. We believe that further investigation of the issue of drawing survey samples of racial/ethnic groups would be appropriate. When oversamples are drawn using geographic sampling units, members of groups who live in areas of high group concentration are likely to be overrepresented, while those in areas of low concentration will not be. In the case of racial/ethnic differences, this may be an important influence on sample characteristics.

We would like to use the distributions of SES shown in Figures 9-2 to 9-4 to make one additional point. There is a substantial degree of overlap in the distribution of most of the indicators of SES for most subgroups of the population in these large national data sets—with the exception of the education of foreign born Hispanics. Kaufman and Cooper (1999) and Kaufman, Cooper, and McGee (1997) have challenged health researchers by saying that it is impossible to statistically separate the effects of race and SES because the two are so intertwined. While education, income, and wealth may not be adequate representations of all aspects of SES, the evidence indicates that although average values of these indicators vary considerably by race and ethnicity, the distributions generally overlap con-

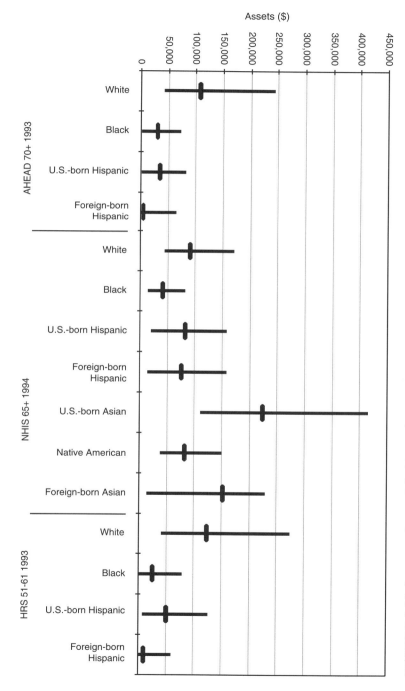

FIGURE 9-4 Median assets by race/ethnicity with interquartile range from selected health surveys.

siderably. This should allow statistical control approaches to separate some of the effects of race/ethnicity and SES. The argument that separation of ethnicity and SES is impossible because of nonoverlapping distributions may have some validity when considering differences between foreign-born Hispanics and other groups or for surveys that are based on community or selected populations.

All of the measures described indicate current SES, although education stays relatively constant over adulthood, and wealth represents the accumulation and maintenance of assets over a lifespan. Two of the surveys—AHEAD and HRS—include indicators of childhood SES: mother's and father's education. These allow some assessment of how closely related current and past educational statuses are for racial/ethnic groups. Table 9-3 shows that racial and ethnic differences in parental education are similar to the differences for the respondent generation. Whites in the AHEAD sample are more than twice as likely as Hispanics to be from a household in which the parents had at least an eighth grade education. The parents of blacks in the AHEAD sample were somewhat more likely to have at least an eighth grade education. The average educational level of parents in the HRS sample is just above 5 years for Hispanics' mothers and fathers and about 10 years for parents of non-Hispanic whites; again the parents of blacks were in the middle. Educational levels are related within and across the generations in each racial/ethnic group. The correlation between years of education of father and mother in the HRS is 0.6 or 0.7 for each of the three groups; the correlation between respondents' own education and that of their fathers

TABLE 9-3 Levels of Parental Education by Race/Ethnicity for HRS and AHEAD Sample Members

HRS (Wave 1): Mean Years of Parental Education

Mother's Education			Father's Education		
White	Black	Hispanic	White	Black	Hispanic
10.0	8.3	5.1	9.7	7.8	5.6

AHEAD (Wave 1): Percentage of Parents with 8+ Years of School

Mother's Education			Father's Education		
White	Black	Hispanic	White	Black	Hispanic
56.9	36.4	22.2	53.5	29.7	24.5

Education of Both Sample Member and Father: Percentage with Low Father's Education (<8) and Low Self-Education (<13)

	White	Black	Native-born Hispanic	Foreign-born Hispanic
AHEAD	37.6	63.6	84.2	67.6
HRS	23.8	48.0	61.9	71.5

and mothers ranges from about 0.35 for blacks to 0.53 for Hispanics (and 0.4 for whites).

One limitation on ability to use the information on childhood SES reported by older persons is that not all respondents know their parents' educations. Parents may have died early in respondents' lives or some respondents may not have had much contact with their parents early in their lives. In the AHEAD sample, 22 percent of blacks did not provide information on their parents; this is true for about half as many Hispanics and non-Hispanic whites.

We also indicate the generational and lifespan nature of SES by looking at the distribution of respondents according to both their own and their father's educational status. The percent of respondents whose father was of low educational status (less than 8 years) and who are themselves of low educational status (less than 13 years) is shown for racial/ethnic groups. This provides some indication of ethnic differences in the likelihood of a lifetime of low status. As expected, minority group members are more likely to both come from backgrounds of low educational attainment and have low educational status themselves. Among the respondents in the AHEAD sample, two-thirds of blacks and foreign-born Hispanics have spent a lifetime in low educational status. This is true for nearly all (84 percent) native-born Hispanics. The differences are somewhat similar in the younger HRS sample, but foreign-born Hispanics were the worst off in this age group.

SOCIOECONOMIC AND RACIAL/ETHNIC DIFFERENCES IN HEALTH

Prevalence of Diseases

Data from these same surveys can be used to examine socioeconomic and racial/ethnic differences in health. Following our earlier discussion of the dimensions of health, we begin with an examination of differences in the prevalence and onset of selected important diseases. These analyses allow us to see whether the relationships among race/ethnicity, socioeconomic status, and disease are the same in the various data sets: how they differ by age and how they differ when incidence rather than prevalence is examined. We include diseases that are among the major causes of death in this age group, as well as arthritis, one of the major causes of disability in the older population. We follow our analysis of disease with an analysis of physical and cognitive impairment. For the longitudinal surveys, death can be examined.

Table 9-4 indicates the risk of having heart disease, heart attack, stroke, diabetes, cancer, hypertension, arthritis, and chronic lung disease by the time of the interview—a prevalence measure—for blacks and native- and

TABLE 9-4 Relative Risk of Disease Prevalence by Race/Ethnicity, Education, and Income

	Relative to Non-Hispanic Whites			Relative to 12 Years of Education			Relative to $20,000-$29,999		
	Blacks	U.S.-born Hispanic	Foreign-born Hispanic	≤8 Yrs	9-11	13+	<$10,000	$10,000-$19,999	≥$30,000
Heart disease									
LSOA 70+									
N=8,333 (1)	0.81*	0.88	0.91						
N=8,206 (2)	0.74*	0.82	0.82	1.24	1.18	0.85			
N=8,206 (3)	0.71*	0.81	0.86	1.19*	1.15	0.86	1.24*	1.00	0.93
AHEAD 70+									
N=7,342 (1)	0.76*	0.75	0.58*						
N=7,342 (2)	0.67*	0.63*	0.49*	1.43*	1.29*	0.98			
N=7,342 (3)	0.66*	0.62*	0.48*	1.39*	1.27*	1.00	1.26*	1.17	1.04
HRS 51-61									
N=9,456 (1)	1.16	0.67	0.71						
N=9,456 (2)	1.06	0.59*	0.60*	1.32	1.35*	0.85*			
N=9,456 (3)	0.95	0.55*	0.56*	1.13	1.24*	0.89	1.72*	1.23	0.83*
Heart attack									
NHANES 65+									
N=4,025 (1)	0.78	0.57	0.43						
N=3,996 (2)	0.77	0.56	0.42	1.09	1.16	1.02			
N=3,516 (3)	0.74	0.54	0.43	1.13	1.08	1.21	1.19	1.20	0.82
AHEAD 70+									
N=7,317 (1)	0.94	0.81	0.91						
N=7,317 (2)	0.79	0.65	0.75	1.42*	1.30	0.74*			
N=7,317 (3)	0.77	0.63	0.72	1.37*	1.28	0.75*	1.28	1.09	1.06
HRS 51-61									
N=8,191 (1)	1.29	0.78	0.88						
N=8,191 (2)	1.10	0.64	0.64	1.64*	1.68*	0.78*			
N=8,125 (3)	0.97	0.61	0.59	1.37*	1.53*	0.83	1.83*	1.03	0.75*
Stroke									
LSOA 70+									

N=8,352 (1)	1.52*	1.12	0.74	1.07	0.89	1.04	1.23	1.25	1.11
N=8,225 (2)	1.41*	1.07	0.72	1.06	0.90	1.03			
N=8,225 (3)	1.38*	1.05	0.72						
NHANES 65+									
N=4,063 (1)	1.83*	1.52	0.52	1.13	0.51*	1.07	2.40*	1.85*	1.29
N=4,032 (2)	1.61*	1.29	0.43	1.04	0.56*	0.98			
N=3,550 (3)	1.33	1.26	0.44						
AHEAD 70+									
N=7,331 (1)	1.36*	1.07	0.62	1.34*	0.84	1.21	1.22	1.23	1.12
N=7,331 (2)	1.19	0.90	0.53	1.31*	0.85	1.20			
N=7,331 (3)	1.18	0.89	0.52						
HRS 51-61									
N=8,191 (1)	2.03*	1.31	1.85*	1.65*	0.78	1.42	2.07*	1.38	0.64*
N=8,191 (2)	1.77*	1.08	1.34	1.25	0.87	1.22			
N=8,125 (3)	1.45*	0.98	1.21						
Diabetes									
LSOA 70+									
N=8,352 (1)	2.10*	1.60*	1.91*	1.42*	0.73*	1.21	1.30*	1.04	0.88
N=8,225 (2)	1.84*	1.41	1.65*	1.34*	0.76*	1.17			
N=8,225 (3)	1.77*	1.39	1.64*						
NHANES 65+									
N=4,063 (1)	1.98*	2.83*	2.74*	1.19	0.68*	1.00	1.18	0.82	0.67*
N=4,033 (2)	1.79*	2.43*	2.22	1.14	0.73*	0.88			
N=3,551 (3)	1.72*	2.23*	2.00						
AHEAD 70+									
N=7,327 (1)	2.38*	2.05*	2.18*	1.20	0.70*	1.21	1.21	1.16	1.14
N=7,327 (2)	2.11*	1.74*	1.92*	1.18	0.70*	1.20			
N=7,327 (3)	2.08*	1.72*	1.89*						
HRS 51-61									
N=8,191 (1)	2.25*	2.23*	1.51*	1.39*	0.91	1.29*	1.51*	1.15	0.87
N=8,191 (2)	2.08*	1.99*	1.25	1.25	0.97	1.23			
N=8,125 (3)	1.92*	1.95*	1.14						
Cancer									
LSOA 70+									
N=8,370 (1)	0.40*	0.85	0.36*	0.88	1.37*	0.89	0.93	1.03	1.05
N=8,242 (2)	0.44*	0.91	0.40*	0.88	1.36*	0.90			
N=8,242 (3)	0.45*	0.92	0.41*						

(continued)

TABLE 9-4 (Continued)

	Relative to Non-Hispanic Whites			Relative to 12 Years of Education			Relative to $20,000-$29,999		
	Blacks	U.S.-born Hispanic	Foreign-born Hispanic	≤8 Yrs	9-11	13+	<$10,000	$10,000-$19,999	≥$30,000
NHANES 65+									
N=4,065 (1)	0.46*	0.29	0.50						
N=4,034 (2)	0.49*	0.31	0.56	0.79	0.80	0.90			
N=3,552 (3)	0.54*	0.24	0.54	0.86	0.70*	0.80	0.69*	0.54*	0.83
AHEAD 70+									
N=7,329 (1)	0.66*	0.86	0.43*						
N=7,329 (2)	0.74*	1.01	0.49*	0.78*	0.79*	1.17			
N=7,329 (3)	0.75*	1.02	0.49*	0.79*	0.80*	1.16	0.99	1.03	1.08
HRS 51-61									
N=8,191 (1)	0.73	1.11	0.32*						
N=8,191 (2)	0.72	1.14	0.36*	0.86	1.32	1.14			
N=8,125 (3)	0.72	1.14	0.36*	0.85	1.31	1.16	1.02	1.10	0.95
Hypertension									
LSOA 70+									
N=8,324 (1)	1.82*	1.07	0.83						
N=8,199 (2)	1.71*	1.01	0.77	1.19*	1.15	0.92			
N=8,199 (3)	1.70*	1.01	0.79	1.13	1.12	0.93	1.34*	1.09	1.09
NHANES 65+									
N=4,047 (1)	1.78*	0.99	0.78						
N=4,017 (2)	1.77*	1.00	0.78	1.02	1.28*	0.96			
N=3,539 (3)	1.70*	0.96	0.77	1.03	1.23*	1.03	1.06	1.04	0.88
AHEAD 70+									
N=7,324 (1)	1.94*	0.98	1.30						
N=7,324 (2)	1.78*	0.84	1.16	1.27*	1.11	0.97			
N=7,324 (3)	1.76*	0.82	1.13	1.24*	1.09	0.97	1.19*	1.07	1.04
HRS 51-61									
N=8,191 (1)	2.39*	1.08	1.15						
N=8,191 (2)	2.31*	1.02	1.04	1.17	1.07	0.93			

N=8,125 (3)	2.18*	0.99	1.00	1.05	1.00	0.96	1.37*	1.03	0.82*
Arthritis									
LSOA 70+									
N=8,286 (1)	1.50*	0.85	0.87						
N=8,158 (2)	1.36*	0.79	0.77	1.28*	1.14*	0.88			
N=8,158 (3)	1.36*	0.77	0.78	1.25*	1.12	0.91	1.18	1.15	0.95
NHANES 65+									
N=4,065 (1)	1.46*	0.95	1.09						
N=4,034 (2)	1.34*	0.85	0.92	1.54*	1.57*	1.18			
N=3,553 (3)	1.24	0.77	0.86	1.57*	1.61*	1.34*	1.17	1.05	0.90
AHEAD 70+									
N=7,326 (1)	2.11*	2.15*	2.93*						
N=7,326 (2)	1.91*	1.85*	2.58*	1.26*	1.13	0.86*			
N=7,326 (3)	1.87*	1.82*	2.51*	1.21*	1.10	0.88	1.25*	1.19*	1.00
HRS 51-61									
N=8,191 (1)	1.14	0.99	0.96						
N=8,191 (2)	1.00	0.812	0.70*	1.63*	1.41*	0.75*			
N=8125 (3)	0.92	0.79	0.66*	1.49*	1.34*	0.79*	1.54*	1.09	0.86*
Chronic lung disease									
AHEAD 70+									
N=7,327 (1)	0.51*	0.61	0.90						
N=7,327 (2)	0.43*	0.49*	0.74	1.43*	1.35*	0.77*			
N=7,327 (3)	0.41*	0.48*	0.72	1.34*	1.30*	0.83	1.19	1.16	0.81
HRS 51-61									
N=8,191 (1)	0.71*	0.97	0.61						
N=8,191 (2)	0.57*	0.71	0.36*	2.25*	1.72*	0.69*			
N=8,125 (3)	0.48*	0.65	0.33*	1.78*	1.51*	0.75*	2.03*	1.40*	0.72*

NOTE: (1) Age and gender controlled; (2) Age, gender, and other specified variables in equation; (3) Age, gender, and other specified variables in equation; missing income in equation for LSOA.
*Significant at .05 level or below.

foreign-born Hispanics relative to non-Hispanic whites. The relative risk is shown without controls for SES (equation 1), then including education, which is represented as a categorical variable with four classes (equation 2), then adding income to the equation as a four-class categorical variable (equation 3). The set of equations allows us to see how much change occurs in the relative racial/ethnic risk with controls for these two aspects of SES. If education and income "explain" racial differences, the effects of the racial/ethnic coefficients should become insignificant with these controls. We use education and income as class variables in order to allow nonlinear effects to become apparent. For example, significance of the coefficient representing the worst off segment of the sample would demonstrate a threshold effect with only this group experiencing worse health. We include education alone in the first equation relating SES and health because it is a better indicator of lifetime SES for people in this age group. Education should be completed before onset of almost all of these diseases and functioning losses as they are very uncommon before late middle age. A relationship between income and these conditions, on the other hand, could either be cause or effect in the case of prevalence. All logistic equations include controls for age and gender.

Blacks are significantly more likely to report having three of these diseases than non-Hispanic whites (Table 9-4). All studies indicate elevated levels among blacks of stroke, diabetes, and hypertension. Also, blacks over 70 have more arthritis.

On the other hand, blacks are less likely than whites to report a number of other conditions (heart disease, cancer, and chronic lung disease). In the younger HRS, there is no significant difference between blacks and whites in reported prevalence of cancer and heart disease.

Both groups of Hispanics, U.S. and foreign born, generally differ in similar ways from non-Hispanic whites. Both groups have significantly higher levels of diabetes. Foreign-born Hispanics report significantly less cancer than non-Hispanic whites, but U.S.-born Hispanics do not differ significantly in cancer levels from non-Hispanic whites.

When education and income are introduced into the equations, some categories of education are significantly related to each health outcome. Lower education is almost always related to more disease; however, for cancer it is persons with higher education who are more likely to have had cancer and to be alive to report it. Income has significant effects—more income is related to better health—in about two-thirds of the equations; the effects are fairly consistent in the younger HRS sample and less so in the older samples.

When socioeconomic status is controlled, few of the already described racial/ethnic health differentials disappear. Although there is generally some reduction in the odds ratios reflecting the link between race/ethnicity and health, the change is generally small. In the case of heart disease and chronic lung disease, the relative likelihood of blacks and Hispanics having these conditions is further reduced.

Findings across surveys are fairly similar, though there are some differences between the HRS and AHEAD. Heart disease and cancer are significantly lower among blacks over 70 (AHEAD), but not older working-age blacks (HRS). The black-white differences in stroke, diabetes, and hypertension are somewhat larger at the younger ages (HRS) than in the older group (AHEAD).

Overall, these findings indicate that the likelihood of having any of these major diseases is related to socioeconomic status, all but cancer negatively. Generally, both education and income show some relationship to these health outcomes, and adding income does not change the relationship between education and the health outcomes. Race/ethnicity is also related to all of the conditions with the exception of reporting a heart attack. Controls for SES do little to change the relationship between race and disease. Foreign-born Hispanics report very low levels of cancer experience. This would potentially be a group who could return home after diagnosis, improving the health of those remaining.

Functioning Loss and Disability

We also examine indicators of the prevalence of physical disability and impaired cognitive functioning from these surveys (Table 9-5). Physical functioning or disability was assessed in terms of reported inability to perform at least one Activity of Daily Living (ADL). Cognitive impairment was defined as scoring below a cutoff value on a battery of performance tests that are only available from the AHEAD survey (Herzog and Wallace, 1997). Blacks are more likely to have both an inability to perform ADLs and to score below the cutoff for cognitive impairment. The odds ratios indicating the risk of physical functioning problems for blacks relative to whites are quite substantial—from 1.6 to 2.4 for the older population and 2.5 for those near retirement age, and blacks are 6 times as likely as non-Hispanic whites to have cognitive impairment, but this is reduced to 3.7 with controls for education and income. U.S.-born Hispanics report more functioning problems and disability than non-Hispanic whites in two of the surveys; foreign-born Hispanics report significantly more functioning problems in three surveys. U.S.- and foreign-born Hispanics have relatively high levels of cognitive impairment. The elevated risk ratios are very similar for blacks and U.S.-born Hispanics, and about half as high for foreign-born Hispanics. Low education is always related to more functioning problems. Not surprisingly, the effect of education is especially strong for cognitive functioning. Cognitive ability early in life could be a determinant of educa-

TABLE 9-5 Relative Risk of Physical Functioning Difficulty and Cognitive Impairment by Race/Ethnicity, Education, and Income

	Relative to Non-Hispanic Whites			Relative to 12 Years of Education			Relative to $20,000-$29,999		
	Blacks	U.S.-born Hispanic	Foreign-born Hispanic	≤8 Yrs	9-11	13+	<$10,000	$10,000-$19,999	≥$30,000
ADL functioning problem									
LSOA 70+									
N=8471 (1)	1.58*	0.87	1.51*	1.40*	1.27*	0.83*			
N=8339 (2)	1.34*	0.78	1.34	1.31*	1.22*	0.85*	1.52*	1.11	1.00
N=8339 (3)	1.27*	0.77	1.33						
NHANES 65+									
N=4066 (1)	2.35*	1.52	2.10	2.47*	1.23	0.76			
N=4035 (2)	1.77*	0.97	1.18	2.43*	1.03	0.82	1.68*	1.14	0.86
N=3553 (3)	1.43	0.92	1.06						
AHEAD 70+									
N=7332 (1)	1.69*	1.79*	1.61*	1.54*	1.27*	0.78*			
N=7332 (2)	1.41*	1.38	1.27	1.23	1.45*	1.23*	0.78*	1.33*	1.17*
N=7161 (3)	1.09	1.37*	1.35						
Disability									
HRS 51-61									
N=8191 (1)	2.48*	2.77*	3.24*	2.69*	1.84*	0.60*			
N=8191 (2)	1.93*	1.90*	1.71*	1.82*	1.45*	0.72*	3.21*	2.08*	0.60
N=8191 (3)	1.46*	1.64*	1.53						
Cognitive impairment									
AHEAD 70+									
N=6565 (1)	6.06*	6.17*	3.77*	5.08*	1.85*	0.87			
N=6565 (2)	3.80*	3.19*	1.88*	4.66*	1.78*	0.88	1.24	0.85	0.86
N=6405 (3)	3.68*	3.18*	1.80*						

NOTE: (1) Age and gender controlled; (2) age, gender, and other specified variables in equation; (3) age, gender, and other specified variables in equation; missing income in equation for LSOA.

*Significant at 0.05 level or below.

tional attainment, so causation could run in both directions for this health indicator. The relative risk of cognitive impairment for both Hispanics and blacks is reduced by half with controls for education and income. The reduction in relative risk of ADL impairment is not as great.

All three minority groups have relatively high risk ratios for disability in the HRS age group. They are higher than the older ages and generally remain significant even with controls for socioeconomic status. In this working age, very low income is linked to higher reports of disability; in this case, the relationship may be partly because persons with disability stop working and earning income. The relationship between both of the SES variables and disability appears stronger in this age group than among the older group.

In summary, the prevalence of diseases, functioning loss, and disability are all related to socioeconomic status; persons of lower status have more problems. Race and ethnicity also are related to all of these dimensions of health, but in complex ways. Education and income appear to partially mediate these relationships, and their roles are greater for functioning loss and disability than for disease.

Disease and Disability Onset

As we noted earlier, investigations of onset of diseases and/or disability that link education and income before the health event are theoretically preferable for understanding the direction of causation. Because the HRS and AHEAD are longitudinal surveys, onset of the same diseases and disabilities can be investigated for those who have not had the disease prior to the initial interview. Smaller samples and fewer onset events result in fewer significant relationships than observed in analysis of prevalence. In Table 9-6 we link race/ethnicity and education and income at the first interview to whether a person has experienced onset of diseases or death during the interval between waves 1 and 2, approximately 2 years.

First we discuss the results for the younger sample. In the HRS sample, onset of all conditions is significantly related to education, with the exception of death. There is less likely to be any relationship with income in this analysis when the income precedes the onset of the disease: Higher income is linked to less heart disease and chronic lung disease. Higher onset rates for blacks are found for the same conditions observed to be higher in prevalence: stroke, diabetes, and hypertension. Blacks are also more likely to die. U.S.- and foreign-born Hispanics have higher levels of diabetes and hypertension onset, but the differences for the foreign born are not significant once controls for education are introduced. There are no onset conditions that are significantly more likely among whites. The observed difference between the prevalence and the onset results for whites would suggest

TABLE 9-6 Relative Risk of Disease Onset by Race/Ethnicity, Education, and Income

	Relative to Non-Hispanic Whites			Relative to 12 Years of Education			Relative to $20,000-$29,999		
	Blacks	U.S.-born Hispanic	Foreign-born Hispanic	≤8 Yrs	9-11	13+	<$10,000	$10,000-$19,999	≥$30,000
Heart disease									
AHEAD 70+									
N=5,008 1	0.94	1.19	0.52						
N=5,008 2	0.84	1.02	0.44	1.36	1.14	0.98			
N=5,008 3	0.85	1.03	0.45	1.34	1.12	1.02	0.90	1.01	0.79
HRS 51-61									
N=7,524 1	1.32	1.33	1.22						
N=7,524 2	1.17	1.13	0.95	1.60*	1.52*	0.97			
N=7,524 3	1.11	1.11	0.91	1.49	1.47*	1.00	1.22	0.48*	0.71*
Heart attack									
AHEAD 70+									
N=6,801 1	1.87	0.63	1.99						
N=6,801 2	0.98	1.94	0.66	1.04	1.44	1.10			
N=6,801 3	0.93	1.84	0.62	0.95	1.38	1.29	1.21	0.86	0.65
HRS 51-61									
N=8,147 1	1.50	1.15	1.61						
N=8,147 2	1.24	1.00	1.07	1.97*	2.41*	0.83			
N=8,147 3	1.04	0.83	0.99	0.78*	1.85*	0.84	1.59	1.05	0.70
Stroke									
AHEAD 70+									
N=6,684 1	1.00	1.32	0.72						
N=6,684 2	1.52	0.57	0.93	1.52*	1.01	0.97			
N=6,684 3	1.08	0.55	0.86	1.35	0.95	1.08	1.70	1.49	0.88
HRS 51-61									
N=8,402 1	2.52*	2.46	2.74						

N=8,402 2	2.18*	1.96	1.92	1.48	1.02	0.52*	1.18	1.36	0.70
N=8,402 3	1.98*	1.84	1.85	1.28	0.93	0.56			
Diabetes									
AHEAD 70+									
N=6,352 1	1.48	1.20	2.12	1.17	0.99	0.77	0.92	1.00	0.93
N=6,352 2	1.34	1.03	1.86	1.17	0.99	0.78			
N=6,352 3	1.35	1.04	1.88						
HRS 51-61									
N=7,712 1	2.99*	3.40*	2.61*	1.72*	1.92*	0.66*	1.75	1.14	0.98
N=7,712 2	2.42*	2.66*	1.84	1.55	1.81*	0.69*			
N=7,712 3	2.22*	2.58*	1.76						
Cancer									
AHEAD 70+									
N=6,314 1	0.65	0.32	1.23	0.95	0.66	0.94	0.92	0.87	1.16
N=6,314 2	0.66	0.31	1.19	1.25	0.99	0.68			
N=6,314 3	0.56	0.69	0.33						
HRS 51-61									
N=8,169 1	0.83	0.84	0.73	1.02	0.98	1.02	0.91	0.71	0.67
N=8,169 2	0.83	0.84	0.72	0.95	0.95	1.07			
N=8,169 3	0.79	0.84	0.70						
Hypertension									
AHEAD 70+									
N=3,662 1	1.45*	0.89	1.07	1.12	1.36	1.00	1.18	0.99	0.75
N=3,662 2	1.38*	0.87	1.05	1.04	1.31	1.07			
N=3,662 3	1.34	0.86	1.00						
HRS 51-61									
N=5,231 1	1.78*	2.01*	1.66*	1.47*	1.32	0.90	1.37	0.67	1.04
N=5,231 2	1.65*	1.74*	1.35	1.48*	1.35*	0.90			
N=5,231 3	1.64*	1.75*	1.32						

(continued)

340

TABLE 9-6 *(Continued)*

	Relative to Non-Hispanic Whites			Relative to 12 Years of Education			Relative to $20,000-$29,999		
	Blacks	U.S.-born Hispanic	Foreign-born Hispanic	≤8 Yrs	9-11	13+	<$10,000	$10,000-$19,999	≥$30,000
Chronic lung disease									
AHEAD 70+									
N=6,498 1	0.56	0.62	0.22						
N=6,498 2	0.51	0.57	0.21	1.13	1.48	0.79			
N=6,498 3	0.47*	0.52	0.19	1.02	1.41	0.83	1.90*	1.18	1.04
HRS 51-61									
N=7,951 1	1.01	0.98	1.45						
N=7,951 2	1.10	0.68	0.60	2.38*	2.13*	0.71			
N=7,951 3	0.92	0.62	0.54	1.88	1.83*	0.79	1.66	1.43	0.61*
Death									
AHEAD 70+									
N=7,332 1	2.06*	1.24	0.58						
N=7,332 2	1.22	1.01	1.02	1.17	1.33*	0.88			
N=7,332 3	1.41	0.88	0.38	1.10	1.09*	0.65	1.55	1.52	0.45
HRS 51-61									
N=8,655 1	1.31*	1.09	1.08						
N=8,655 2	1.73*	0.99	0.41	1.51	1.32	0.55*			
N=8,655 3	1.19*	0.99	1.01	1.14	1.32*	0.89	1.05	0.91	0.88

NOTE: (1) Age and gender controlled; (2) age, gender, and other specified variables in equation; (3) age, gender, and other specified variables in equation; missing income in equation for LSOA.

*Significant at 0.05 level or below.

that survival rates for some diseases differ across races. The onset rates could be the same for heart disease, cancer, and chronic lung disease, but whites may live longer after getting diseases, raising the prevalence of these conditions in the white population.

Now we examine differentials in the older population. There are few significant relationships between disease onset and either indicator of SES or race/ethnicity in the AHEAD or older population. Older blacks are more likely to die before controls for SES are introduced into the equation. They are also more likely to acquire hypertension and less likely to experience onset of chronic lung disease. Stroke and death are more likely among those with low education; chronic lung disease onset is more frequent with low income.

Among those aged 70 and over, onset of functioning problems—both physical and cognitive—is more likely among those with lower education, but neither is related to income (Table 9-7). Onset of ADL problems is greater for all racial/ethnic minority groups, although significantly so only for blacks. Onset of cognitive impairment is more frequent for all three racial/ethnic/nativity groups, although not significantly so for foreign-born Hispanics. With controls for education, the difference between U.S.-born Hispanics and non-Hispanic whites disappears.

Finally, because we have argued that early life experiences are important to late life health, we examined the effect of father's education on the onset of disease and death in the HRS sample (data not shown). When father's education is included as a four-category variable similar to respondent's education, the results indicate that father's education is much less likely to be related to any of the health outcomes. When both own and father's education are included, there is little change in the effect of own education. This indicates that although it may be theoretically desirable, the inclusion of SES of family of origin adds little beyond own education and does not change the effect of own education.

EFFECT OF SOCIOECONOMIC STATUS WITHIN ETHNIC GROUPS

Next we examine the variability in disease and disability prevalence by SES within racial/ethnic group to determine whether the relationships between income and education are the same for all ethnic groups (Tables 9-8 and 9-9). The strongest socioeconomic effects are within the white group. Nearly every disease is significantly more prevalent among whites with low levels of education and income—again cancer is the major exception to this finding (Table 9-8). In general, education does not significantly relate to the prevalence of disease among blacks and Hispanics. There are some exceptions; blacks with lower education have more heart disease in AHEAD and

TABLE 9-7 Relative Risk of Onset of Physical and Cognitive Functioning Problems

	Relative to Non-Hispanic Whites			Relative to 12 Years of Education			Relative to $20,000-$29,999		
	Blacks	U.S.-born Hispanic	Foreign-born Hispanic	≤8 Yrs	9-11	13+	<$10,000	$10,000-$19,999	≥$30,000
AHEAD 70+									
N=3,186 (1)	1.62*	1.08	1.66	1.39*	1.32*	1.11			
N=3,186 (2)	1.49*	1.49	.95	1.29	1.28	1.22			
N=3,121 (3)	1.46	1.57	.97				1.15	1.28	.82
Cognitive functioning problem									
AHEAD 70+									
N=5,027 (1)	4.56*	1.38*	3.68	1.89*	1.67	.45			
N=5,027 (2)	3.42*	.98	2.53*	1.89*	1.65	.50			
N=4,910 (3)	3.06*	.49	2.39				.85	.85	.43

NOTE: (1) Age and gender controlled; (2) age, gender, and other specified variables in equation; (3) age, gender, and other specified variables in equation; missing income in equation for LSOA.

*Significant at 0.05 level or below.

TABLE 9-8 Relative Risk of Prevalence of Disease by Education and Income Within Racial/Ethnic Group

	Relative to 12 Years of Education			Relative to $20,000-$29,999			
	≤8 Yrs	9-11	13+	<$10,000	$10,000-$19,999	≥$30,000	Foreign
Heart disease							
LSOA 70+							
White N=7,003	1.17*	1.20*	0.83	1.26*	0.98	0.92	
Black N=888	1.40	0.81	1.91	1.01	1.28	1.34	
Hispanic N=315	1.15	0.81	0.90	1.48	0.91	1.17	1.03
AHEAD 70+							
White N=5,896	1.33*	1.23*	1.00	1.31*	1.19*	1.03	
Black N=1,023	2.26*	1.90*	0.85	0.78	0.94	1.09	
Hispanic N=406	1.09	1.36	1.08	2.69	1.63	2.22	1.35
HRS 51-61							
White N=5,936	1.21	1.39*	0.89	1.49*	1.12	0.81*	
Black N=1,483	0.82	0.78	0.75	2.21*	1.04	0.80	
Hispanic N=772	1.39	1.31	1.03	2.41	1.77	1.18	1.16
Heart attack							
NHANES 65+							
White N=2,242	1.23	1.10	1.25	1.12	1.12	0.81	
Black N=657	0.83	0.76	1.14	1.56	1.84	0.70	
Hispanic N=520	0.55	0.50	0.99	1.00	1.24	0.88	0.99
AHEAD 70+							
White N=5,890	1.29	1.22	0.73	1.40*	1.10	1.08	
Black N=1,021	2.94	2.45	1.30	0.55	0.81	0.55	
Hispanic N=406	3.21	3.99	1.82	5.99	3.54	5.58	0.89
HRS 51-61							
White N=5,936	1.70*	1.84*	0.88	1.53*	1.07	0.76	
Black N=1,483	0.72	0.62	0.56	2.53	0.86	0.65	
Hispanic N=772	0.61	0.75	0.60	1.63	1.13	0.82	0.89
Stroke							
LSOA 70+							
White N=7,020	1.02	1.04	0.94	1.48*	1.36*	1.24	
Black N=892	1.19	0.93	0.60	0.70	1.07	0.87	
Hispanic N=313	0.94	0.58	—	0.15*	0.29*	0.07*	0.79
NHANES 65+							
White N=2,249	1.03	0.88	0.55*	2.52*	1.83*	1.33	
Black N=661	0.89	1.60	0.81	2.23	1.78	1.78	
Hispanic N=543	0.62	1.20	0.12	2.01	2.50	1.58	0.46
AHEAD 70+							
White N=5,901	1.32*	1.20	0.87	1.26	1.32*	1.11	
Black N=1,024	1.40	1.10	0.70	0.79	0.75	1.07	
Hispanic N=406	0.68	1.61	1.24	4.31	1.49	4.12	1.77
HRS 51-61							
White N=5,936	1.26	1.49	0.91	1.97*	1.45	0.69	
Black N=1,483	0.65	0.68	0.66	2.02	1.48	0.49	
Hispanic N=772	3.44	0.74	1.92	1.39	0.73	0.50	1.04

(continued)

TABLE 9-8 *(Continued)*

	Relative to 12 Years of Education			Relative to $20,000-$29,999			
	≤8 Yrs	9-11	13+	$10,000-<$10,000	$19,999	≥$30,000	Foreign
Diabetes							
LSOA 70+							
White N=7,019	1.44*	1.12	0.80*	1.37*	1.13	0.90	
Black N=892	1.08	1.40	0.67	1.19	0.74	0.95	
Hispanic N=314	0.76	0.82	0.18*	0.47	0.40	0.41	1.31
NHANES							
White N=2,249	1.23	0.89	0.80	1.26	0.73	0.64*	
Black N=660	0.74	0.66	0.56	0.88	1.35	0.38	
Hispanic N=545	2.08	2.18	2.32	2.00	3.08	1.42	0.85
AHEAD 70+							
White N=5,899	1.25*	1.12	0.67*	1.18	1.11	1.09	
Black N=1,023	1.01	1.56	0.98	1.36	1.38	1.31	
Hispanic N=405	1.13	0.32	0.90	1.52	1.48	1.65	0.90
HRS 51-61							
White N=5,936	1.24	1.27	0.99	1.36	1.17	0.82	
Black N=1,483	1.02	1.02	0.73	1.66	1.36	1.17	
Hispanic N=772	1.46	0.99	0.77	1.82	0.77	0.96	1.84*
Cancer							
LSOA 70+							
White N=7,035	0.86	0.92	1.33*	0.92	1.04	1.05	
Black N=892	1.91	0.78	3.45*	1.07	0.84	0.57	
Hispanic N=314	0.62	0.65	1.61	0.43	0.89	1.23	0.46*
NHANES 65+							
White N=2,250	0.89	0.73	0.80	0.76	0.57*	0.88	
Black N=660	0.72	0.25	0.73	0.34	0.62	0.51	
Hispanic N=545	0.38	0.25	0.20	6.19	5.70	26.62	2.73
AHEAD 70+							
White N=5,896	0.84	0.79*	1.17	1.10	1.12	1.09	
Black N=1,022	1.04	1.23	1.64	0.40*	0.35*	0.93	
Hispanic N=406	0.18*	0.22	0.52	1.29	1.69	2.61	2.12
HRS 51-61							
White N=5,936	0.72	1.32	1.18	0.88	1.01	0.87	
Black N=1,483	1.60	1.36	0.88	2.79	2.43	3.30	
Hispanic N=772	0.72	1.15	1.50	0.94	1.51	0.71	3.00*
Hypertension							
LSOA 70+							
White N=6,997	1.09	1.10	0.91	1.37*	1.11	1.09	
Black N=888	1.68*	1.32	1.35	1.02	0.67	0.85	
Hispanic N=314	1.16	1.66	1.05	1.06	1.18	1.73	0.84
NHANES 65+							
White N=2,244	1.08	1.26*	1.07	1.07	1.05	0.86	
Black N=658	1.31	1.53	1.08	0.74	0.70	0.96	
Hispanic N=542	1.57	1.27	0.50	0.68	1.08	1.81	0.96

TABLE 9-8 (Continued)

	Relative to 12 Years of Education			Relative to $20,000-$29,999			
	≤8 Yrs	9-11	13+	$10,000-<$10,000	$19,999	≥$30,000	Foreign
AHEAD 70+							
White N=5,896	1.21*	1.07	0.95	1.14	1.04	1.01	
Black N=1,022	1.47	1.29	1.33	1.44	1.29	1.23	
Hispanic N=406	1.73	2.50	1.25	1.80	1.58	1.78	0.70
HRS 51-61							
White N=5,936	1.07	1.00	1.00	1.21	1.02	0.80*	
Black N=1,483	0.89	1.07	0.76	1.62*	1.16	0.95	
Hispanic N=772	0.98	0.77	0.61	1.44	0.94	0.92	1.03
Arthritis							
LSOA 70+							
White N=6,958	1.24*	1.08	0.91	1.23*	1.20*	0.96	
Black N=887	1.19	0.92	0.72	1.37	0.96	1.00	
Hispanic N=313	1.47	3.83*	1.02	0.30*	0.45	0.38	1.25
NHANES 65+							
White N=2,250	1.69*	1.60*	1.40*	1.56	1.09	0.89	
Black N=660	1.22	1.26	1.12	1.18	0.92	0.96	
Hispanic N=546	0.64	0.77	0.28	0.74	0.58	0.31	1.28
AHEAD 70+							
White N=5,896	1.17	1.14	0.88	1.17	1.09	0.99	
Black N=1,024	1.25	0.98	0.87	1.93*	2.11*	0.81	
Hispanic N=406	1.23	0.98	0.65	1.26	1.49	1.47	0.73
HRS 51-61							
White N=5,936	1.61*	1.40*	0.78*	1.42*	1.08	0.84*	
Black N=1,483	1.37	1.17	0.80	1.76*	0.90	0.93	
Hispanic N=772	0.91	0.86	0.69	1.57	1.64	1.07	1.04
Lung disease							
AHEAD 70+							
White N=5,898	1.41*	1.33*	0.85	1.18	1.16	0.78	
Black N=1,024	1.33	0.99	0.57	1.05	1.11	1.07	
Hispanic N=405	0.32	0.96	0.58	3.99	1.86	4.23	0.70
HRS 51-61							
White N=5,936	1.95*	1.67*	0.74*	2.01*	1.49*	0.76*	
Black N=1,483	1.09	0.78	0.78	1.06	1.13	0.69	
Hispanic N=772	1.04	0.58	0.90	1.75	0.96	0.30*	1.93

*Significant at .05 level or below.

more hypertension in the LSOA. Blacks with higher education report having had more cancer in the LSOA. Among Hispanics, low education is linked to less cancer in AHEAD and more arthritis in LSOA, and more education is linked to less diabetes in LSOA.

Frequently lower income is also linked to higher levels of disease among whites. This is usually true in the HRS sample, perhaps indicating reduced wages among those with diseases. Lower income is also linked to a signifi-cantly higher disease prevalence among blacks in the HRS sample for a number of diseases: hypertension, heart disease, and arthritis.

In the models of functioning and disability, low SES is a strong predic-tor of all problems for whites. Generally, low education is linked to worse physical functioning among older blacks, and low income is related to a higher probability of functioning loss among older Hispanics in AHEAD (Table 9-9). The effect of being in the lowest education group increases the relative risk of cognitive impairment similarly in each of the racial/ethnic groups. Income is strongly related to disability in all groups in the HRS or older working-age sample.

Our results have generally provided support that SES is inversely linked to most aspects of health. The links appear to be stronger before old age; stronger for indicators of functioning than for some diseases; and stronger for education than income.

TABLE 9-9 Effect of Socioeconomic Status on Functioning Problems Within Racial/Ethnic Group

	Relative to 12 Years of Education			Relative to $20,000-$29,999			
	≤8 Yrs	9-11	13+	<$10,000	$10,000-$19,999	≥$30,000	Foreign
ADL functioning difficulty							
LSOA 70+							
White N=7,121	1.32*	1.22*	0.87	1.65	1.16	1.01	
Black N=900	1.67*	1.48	1.04	0.834	0.77	0.72	
Hispanic N=318	0.70	0.73	0.32*	0.96	0.62	1.03	1.69*
NHANES 65+							
White N=2,250	2.65*	0.88	0.82	1.72*	1.01	0.85	
Black N=660	1.74	1.93	0.88	1.76	2.11	0.48	
Hispanic N=546	0.93	2.79	-	0.72	0.67	0.41	1.55
AHEAD 70+							
White N=5,754	1.42*	1.22*	0.77*	1.36*	1.17	1.08	
Black N=1,005	2.16*	1.62	1.09	0.96	1.01	0.99	
Hispanic N=413	0.73	0.71	0.30	2.68*	2.10	1.62	0.95
HRS 51-61							
White N=5,936	2.06*	1.52*	0.75	3.31*	1.77*	0.52*	
Black N=1,483	1.33	1.29	0.64	4.05*	2.92*	0.81	
Hispanic N=772	1.56	1.16	0.61	2.47	3.14*	1.09	0.99
Cognitive impairment							
AHEAD 70+							
White N=5,211	4.23*	1.76*	0.83	1.28	1.06	1.02	
Black N=867	5.44*	1.87	0.51	1.00	0.53	0.47	
Hispanic N=335	4.71*	—	—	1.32	0.49	0.84	0.58

*Significant at 0.05 level or below.

CONCLUSIONS

Socioeconomic status is related to almost all health outcomes. In the United States, people with less education have worse health outcomes. Relationships between education and health among older persons can be interpreted as evidence linking lifetime SES to subsequent health; the direction of causation for income and wealth differentials is less clear. At the older ages particularly, cross-sectional relationships between income and health are a combination of effects from SES to health and health to SES. The role of SES in producing poor health outcomes appears to be less at the older ages than at earlier ages. It is true that groups with different lifetime mortality will have been differentially selected for health as well as SES by old age.

Socioeconomic status better predicts most aspects of health within the white population than within other racial/ethnic groups. If we examine differentials among African Americans and Hispanics, we find that the ability of socioeconomic status to explain differences within these groups is limited. The links in all ethnic groups appear to be greater for functioning loss and disability than for disease or mortality.

Controls for socioeconomic status do little to eliminate some of the racial/ethnic health differences observed. Controlling for SES does more to reduce racial/ethnic differentials in functioning, both physical and cognitive, than in the major diseases that cause death and disability.

Blacks and to some extent Hispanics report high levels of disease that can be characterized as vascular and metabolic. This survey evidence indicates that these are the diseases of focus for reducing adverse health differentials. Functioning loss or disability also is more common among older blacks and Hispanics. Cognitive impairment is significantly higher among both groups and appears highly affected by educational differences.

Some of the observed differences in prevalence, such as higher levels of functioning loss and disability as well as lower levels of heart disease and cancer reported by blacks, may be related to differential likelihood of survival. Conditions that are not highly related to mortality are higher among minority groups and conditions that may benefit the most from treatment are lower in the same groups. This reinforces the need to have further information on racial differences in all aspects of health change and in severity of conditions.

RECOMMENDATIONS

1. We Need Better Information on the Process by Which Health Differentials Arise

This means more details on age and date of onset, severity of condition, treatment, and resolution. Data on ethnic differences that allow understanding of the process of health change in old age are sparse. Much of what we know comes from information on prevalence or mortality. Neither of these indicators inform about the process of health change and the disease stage at which differences occur. In an aging population that is living longer with more diseases, the group with the highest prevalence can be the group with the "best" health. We need to evaluate incidence rates and survival rates in order to interpret the meaning of both prevalence and mortality. Even for the large ethnic groups, very limited information is available on the process of disease onset, life with disease, and resolution of disease.

2. We Need to Better Operationalize Our Theoretical Approach to Understanding Mechanisms Through Which SES Works

Our theoretical understanding of the meaning of SES far exceeds our ability to measure it in a research setting. Much thought needs to be given to how to better incorporate our theoretical ideas of the source of SES health differences into ongoing research. We need to be able to incorporate reasonable measurement of variables that represent the broad range of social, psychological, and financial mechanisms believed to mediate SES effects on health. The sparse evidence we have indicates that social stresses and supports and psychological mechanisms that are related to SES seem to mediate SES differences in health outcomes. Health behaviors also influence health outcomes. Recent work by Singer and Ryff (1999) and Warner and Hayward (2002) represent two successful attempts to incorporate lifecycle circumstances into analyses of adult health outcomes.

3. Greater Specificity of Health Problems Will Add to Our Understanding of Racial/Ethnic and Socioeconomic Differentials in Health

All-cause mortality and general indicators of disability and self-rated health have limited ability to add to understanding the reasons behind differential health. Cause-specific analysis of the different dimensions of health begins to complete a picture of differentials. To reduce poor health outcomes for subgroups of the population, we need to better target the health problems of importance.

4. Existing National Data Should Be Enhanced with Larger Samples of Some Ethnic Groups, More Information on Health Status That Is Not Influenced by Medical Contact or Cultural Differences, and More Information on Potential Mechanisms by Which Socioeconomic and Racial/Ethnic Differences Arise

Understanding the Asian-American health advantage is as important as understanding the disadvantage of other groups. There are challenges to including the racial/ethnic differences in reporting and assessment of health problems, availability and use of medical care, and social and psychological behavior that have only had cursory attention.

5. We Need to Evaluate the Potential for Current Data Collection Efforts to Provide Appropriate Samples That Reflect the Socioeconomic Distribution of Minority Groups

Our largely geographic clustering approach to drawing samples may not provide representative samples of racial/ethnic groups of the population.

6. Health Differentials Need to Be Addressed in a Lifecycle Context

Differentials in the likelihood of reaching old age may be important in understanding differentials in old age.

REFERENCES

Abraido-Lanza, A.F., Dohrenwend, B.P., Ng-Mak, D.S., and Turner, J.B. (1999). The Latino mortality paradox: A test of the "Salmon Bias" and healthy migrant hypotheses. *American Journal of Public Health, 89*(10), 1543-1548.

Adler, N., Boyce, T., Chesney, M., Folkman, S., and Syme, S. (1993). Socioeconomic inequalities in health: No easy solution. *Journal of the American Medical Association, 269*(24), 3140-3145.

Adler, N., Boyce, T., Chesney, M., Cohen, S., Folkman, S., Kahn, R., and Syme, L. (1994). Socioeconomic status and health: The challenge of the gradient. *American Psychologist, 49*, 15-24.

Anderson, N.B. (1995). Behavioral and sociocultural perspectives on ethnicity and health: Introduction to the special issue. *Health Psychology, 14*, 589-591.

Blackwell, D., Hayward, M.D., and Crimmins, E. (2001). Does childhood health affect chronic morbidity in later life? *Social Science and Medicine, 52*, 1269-1284.

Crimmins, E. (2001). Mortality and health in human life spans. *Experimental Gerontology, 36*, 885-897.

Crimmins, E., and Saito, Y. (2001). Trends in healthy life expectancy in the United States, 1970-1990: Gender, racial, and educational differences. *Social Science and Medicine, 52*, 1629-1641.

Ettner, S.L., and Crimmins, E.M. (2002). *Economic measures in health surveys* (Background paper). Bethesda, MD: National Institutes of Health.

Feldman, J.J., Makuc, D., Kleinman, J.C., and Coroni-Huntley, J. (1989). National trends in educational differences in mortality. *American Journal of Epidemiology, 129*, 919-933.

Hardy, M.A., and Pavalko, E.K. (1986). The internal structure of self-reported health measures among older male workers and retirees. *Journal of Health and Social Behavior, 27*, 346-357.

Hayward, M.D., Friedman, S., and Chen, H. (1996). Race inequities in men's retirement. *Journals of Gerontology—Series B: Psychological Sciences and Social Sciences, 51B*(1), S1-S10.

Hayward, M.D., Crimmins, E.M., Miles, T.P., and Yu, Y. (2000). The significance of socioeconomic status in explaining the racial gap in chronic health conditions. *American Sociological Review, 65*, 910-930.

Herzog, A.R., and Wallace, R.B. (1997). Measures of cognitive functioning in the AHEAD study [special issue]. *Journals of Gerontology—Series B: Psychological Sciences and Social Sciences, 52B*, 37-48.

House, J.S., Kessler, R.C., and Herzog, A.R. (1990). Age, socioeconomic status, and health. *The Milbank Quarterly, 68*(3), 383-411.

House, J.S., Lepkowski, J.M., Kinney, A.M., Mero, R.P., Kessler, R.C., and Herzog, A.R. (1994). The social stratification of aging and health. *Journal of Health and Social Behavior, 35*, 213-234.

Hummer, R.A., Rogers, R.G., and Eberstein, I.W. (1998). Sociodemographic differentials in adult mortality: A review of analytic approaches. *Population Development Review, 24*, 553-578.

Juster, T., and Suzman, R. (1995). Overview of the health and retirement study. *Journal of Human Resources, 30*, S7-S56.

Kaufman, J.S., and Cooper, R.S. (1999). Seeking causal explanations in social epidemiology. *American Journal of Epidemiology, 150*, 113-120.

Kaufman, J.S., Cooper, R.S., and McGee, D.L. (1997). Socioeconomic status and health in blacks and whites: The problem of residual confounding and the resiliency of race. *Epidemiology, 8*, 621-628.

Kington, R.S., and Nickens, H.W. (2001). Racial and ethnic differences in health: Recent trends, current patterns, future directions. In N. Smelser, W.J. Wilson, and F. Mitchell (Eds.), *America becoming: Racial trends and their consequences* (pp. 253-310). Washington, DC: National Academy Press.

Kuh, D., and Davey-Smith, G. (1997). The life course and adult chronic disease: An historical perspective with particular reference to coronary heart disease. In D. Kuh and B. Ben-Shlomo (Eds.), *A life course approach to chronic disease epidemiology.* New York: Oxford University Press.

Lauderdale, D.S. (2001). Education and survival: Cohort, period, and age effects. *Demography, 38*, 551-561.

Lauderdale, D.S., and Kestenbaum, B. (2002). Mortality rates of elderly Asian American populations based on Medicare and Social Security data. *Demography, 39*, 529-540.

Liao, Y., Cooper, R.S., Cao, G., Durazo-Arvizu, R., Kaufman, J.S., Luke, A., and McGee, D.L. (1998). Mortality patterns among older Hispanics: Findings from the National Health Interview Survey (1986 to 1994). *Journal of the American College of Cardiology, 30*, 1200-1205.

Lillie-Blanton, M., Parsons, P., Gayle, H., and Dievler, A. (1996). Racial differences in health: Not just black and white, but shades of gray. *Annual Review of Public Health, 17,* 411-448.

Link, B.G., and Phelan, J. (1995). Social conditions as fundamental causes of disease. *Journal of Health and Social Behavior, 36,* 80-94.

Lynch, S.M. (2003). Cohort and life course patterns in the education-health relationship: A hierarchical approach. *Demography, 40*(2), 309-331.

Manton, K.G. (1997). Changes in the age dependence of mortality and disability: Cohort and other determinants. *Demography, 34,* 135-157.

Marmot, M. (1994). Social differentials in health within and between populations. *Daedalus, 123*(4), 197-216.

Marmot, M., Kogevinas, M., and Elston, M. (1987). Social/economic status and disease. *Annual Review of Public Health, 8,* 111-135.

Marmot, M., Ryff, C., Bumpass, L., Shipley, M., and Marks, N. (1997). Social inequalities in health: Next question and converging evidence. *Social Science and Medicine, 44,* 901-910.

Marmot, M.G., and Shipley, M.J. (1996). Do socioeconomic differences in mortality persist after retirement? 25 year follow-up of civil servants from the first Whitehall study. *British Medical Journal, 313,* 1177-1180.

Oakes, J.M., and Rossi, P.H. (2003). The measurement of SES in health research: Current practice and steps toward a new approach. *Social Science and Medicine, 56,* 769-784.

Pamuk, E. (1985). Social class inequality in mortality from 1921 to 1972 in England and Wales. *Population Studies, 39,* 17-31.

Pappas, G., Queen, S., Hadden, W., and Fisher, G. (1993). The increasing disparity in mortality between socioeconomic groups in the United States, 1960 and 1986. *The New England Journal of Medicine, 329,* 103-109.

Pincus, T., and Callahan, L.F. (1995). What explains the association between socioeconomic status and health: Primarily access to medical care or mind-body variables? *Advances: Journal of Mind-Body Health, 11,* 4-36.

Pincus, T., Callahan, L.F., and Burkhauser, R. (1987). More chronic diseases are reported more frequently by individuals with fewer than 12 years of formal education in the age 18-64 U.S. population. *Journal of Chronic Diseases, 40,* 865-874.

Preston, S., and Elo, I. (1995). Are educational differentials in adult mortality increasing in the United States? *Journal of Aging and Health, 7,* 476-496.

Preston, S., and Taubman, P. (1994). Socioeconomic differences in adult mortality and health status. In L. Martin and S. Preston (Eds.), *Demography of aging* (pp. 279-318). Washington, DC: National Academy Press.

Preston, S., Hill, M.E., and Drevenstedt, G. (1998). Childhood conditions that predict survival to advanced ages among African-Americans. *Social Science and Medicine, 47,* 1231-1246.

Ribisi, K.M., Winkleby, M.A., Fortmann, S.P., and Flora, J.A. (1998). The interplay of socioeconomic status and ethnicity on Hispanic and white men's cardiovascular disease risk and health communication patterns. *Health Education Research, 13,* 407-417.

Schoen, R. (1988). *Modeling multigroup populations.* New York: Plenum Press.

Seeman, T.E., and Crimmins, E.M. (2001). Social environment effects on health and aging: Integrating epidemiological and demographic approaches and perspectives. *Annals of the New York Academy of Sciences, 954,* 88-117.

Shea, D., Miles, T.P., and Hayward, M.D. (1996). The health and wealth connection: Racial differences. *The Gerontologist, 36*(3), 342-349.

Singer, B., and Ryff, C. (1999). Hierarchies of life histories. *Annals of the New York Academy of Sciences, 896,* 96-115.

Smith, J.P. (1999). Healthy bodies and thick wallets: The dual relation between health and economic status. *Journal of Economic Perspectives, 13,* 145-166.

Smith, J.P., and Kington, R. (1997). Demographic and economic correlates of health in old age. *Demography, 34,* 159-170.

U.S. Bureau of the Census. (2000, March). *Educational attainment of people 25 years and over by nativity and period of entry, age, sex, race, and Hispanic origin.* Washington, DC: Author.

Verbrugge, L.M., and Jette, A.M. (1994). The disablement process. *Social Science and Medicine, 38,* 1-14.

Warner, D.F., and Hayward, M.D. (2002, May). *Race disparities in men's mortality: The role of childhood social conditions in a process of cumulative disadvantage.* Paper presented at the 2002 Annual Meeting of the Population Association of America, Atlanta.

Williams, D.R. (1990). Socioeconomic differentials in health: A review and redirection. *Social Psychology Quarterly, 53*(2), 81-99.

Williams, D.R., and Collins, C. (1995). U.S. socioeconomic and racial differences in health: Patterns and explanations. *Annual Review of Sociology, 21,* 349-386.

Williams, D.R., Lavizzo-Mourey, R., and Warren, R.C. (1994). The concept of race and health status in America. *Public Health Reports, 109,* 26-41.

Winkleby, M.A., Jatulis, D.E., Frank, E., and Fortmann, S.P. (1992). Socioeconomic status and health: How education, income, and occupation contribute to risk factors for cardiovascular disease. *American Journal of Public Health, 82,* 816-20.

Winkleby, M.A., Kraemer, H.C., Ahn, D.K., and Varady, A.N. (1998). Ethnic and socioeconomic differences in cardiovascular disease risk factors: Findings for women from the Third National Health and Nutrition Examination Survey, 1988-1994. *Journal of the American Medical Association, 280,* 356-362.

10

The Role of Social and Personal Resources in Ethnic Disparities in Late-Life Health

Carlos F. Mendes de Leon and Thomas A. Glass

The past three decades have witnessed a proliferation of research on overall health and well-being of the oldest segments of the population, generally defined as adults aged 65 years and over. An important theme of this research has been to document the existence of disparities in health and well-being across groups defined by race/ethnicity or socioeconomic status (SES) (National Research Council, 1997). As described in detail elsewhere in this volume (see Chapter 3 by Hummer), minority seniors have, on average, higher mortality rates and poorer self-ratings of health (Ferraro and Farmer, 1996; Hummer, 1996), as well as a higher prevalence of physical disability and cognitive function, when compared with the majority population of non-Hispanic whites (Fillenbaum et al., 1998; Froehlich, Bogardus, and Inouye, 2001; Mendes de Leon et al., 1995, 1997; Tang et al., 1998).

Increasingly, the field has moved toward a deeper understanding of the mechanisms and processes that lead to these disparities. In this chapter, we consider the role of personal and social resources in explaining the origins and consequences of racial/ethnic disparities in late-life health. From a lifespan developmental perspective, individuals actively regulate personal and social resources as they "age" for the purpose of personal growth and adaptation (Baltes and Lang, 1997; Lang, 2001; Lang, Featherman, and Nesselroade, 1997; Ryff, 1991). This process is modulated in important ways by the sociocultural environment, which, through prevailing norms, values, and expectations, shapes and reinforces an individual's resources that optimize adaptation (Verbrugge and Jette, 1994). These contextual influences are likely to differ substantially across racial and ethnic groups because race and ethnicity are critical determinants of the residential segregation and social stratification that characterize American society. The relatively unique social experiences and conditions of racial and ethnic sub-populations may lead to important variations in the personal and social resources that are accumulated throughout life. Thus, to the extent that they affect age-related health and well-being, variations in these resources may be an important aspect of understanding and alleviating ethnic disparities in late-life health.

TOWARD A CONCEPTUAL FRAMEWORK

For the purpose of this chapter, we will conceptualize social and personal resources as a series of assets that accrue to individuals as a result of their linkages or interactions with other individuals. The focus will be on those resources that have received the attention of social gerontologists and that are hypothesized to be associated with tangible health benefits. Investigation of these resources may help us to achieve a deeper understanding of the origins of health disparities across race/ethnic lines in late life. Figure 10-1 presents

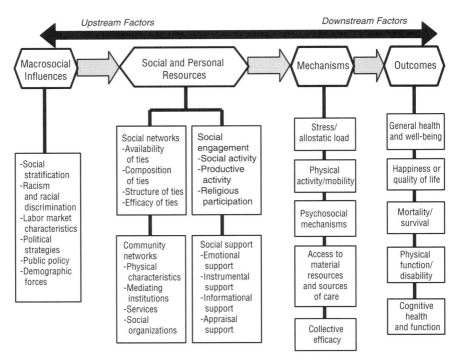

FIGURE 10-1 Conceptual model of the impact of personal resources on health outcomes.
SOURCES: House (1987), Pearlin (1985), and Link and Phelan (1995).

an organizing framework for understanding the role of social and personal resources in the cascade of social and individual-level processes that affect health. This framework will be used as a tool to organize existing literature, and to identify gaps in this literature and future opportunities.

The framework maps a series of conceptually distinct factors that are arranged to represent, from left to right, the spectrum of upstream, distal (or fundamental) causes of health (see Link and Phelan, 1995), to intermediate causes of health at the level of social and personal resources, to a series of mechanisms more proximate to health and disease. Although this sequence of influences corresponds broadly to an underlying temporal or causal model of social and individual-level influences on health, it is likely that the actual causal processes involve a greater degree of complexity than this framework suggests. The figure is designed to underscore the broader social and biological context in which social and personal resources are related to health (House, 1987; Pearlin, 1985).

Although we will classify the resources reviewed in this chapter on the basis of their "social" or "personal" nature, the boundaries between these two sets of resources are somewhat artificial. Social resources, categorized here into social and community networks, emphasize the social or structural nature of the asset. These assets may be considered a resource because they provide the potential conduits through which personal resources are accessed or activated. Personal resources, on the other hand, encompass assets that place primary emphasis on the individual, even if the asset has an inherent social dependency. This chapter will focus on two types of personal resources, social engagement and social support.

It is important to note that our conceptualization of social and personal resources is somewhat restrictive, and that there are other such resources with important health benefits. For example, assets attributable to social class or social position, such as political and economic assets, are important personal resources associated with significant health disparities. The role of such socioeconomic resources in ethnic disparities in late-life health is reviewed in Chapter 9. Personal resources may also be conceptualized in terms of psychological attributes that have been linked with health outcomes. Their role is reviewed in further detail in Chapter 13. Although we will briefly discuss the influence of neighborhood characteristics in late-life health, a more extensive discussion of this topic can be found in Chapter 11. The remainder of this chapter will focus on differences in the patterning of social and personal resources as already defined across race and ethnic groups, as well as their differential impact on late-life health.

A Comment on the Term "Race"

Much has been written about the use and misuse of the concepts of race and ethnicity in health research (Kaufman and Cooper, 2001; Muntaner,

Nieto, and O'Campo, 1996; Witzig, 1996). In the context of this chapter, these concepts are used as an indicator of a "social" reality, rather than pertaining to some underlying biological dimension (Goodman, 2000; Williams, Lavizzo-Mourey, and Warren, 1994). When addressing racial/ethnic disparities in health, one is usually presented with the inevitable dilemma of selecting one group to serve as a reference for comparisons between persons of differing racial/ethnic backgrounds. In most of the literature on this topic, that group is the dominant or majority sub-population of non-Hispanic whites. While this choice may have important scientific and social ramifications, for the purpose of convenience, we will adopt the same approach in this chapter.

The remainder of the chapter is divided into three sections. In the second section, we will review the evidence regarding the differential distribution of social and personal resources by race and ethnicity. In the third section, we will examine the degree to which racial/ethnic differences in social and personal resources may contribute to disparities in late-life health. In the final section, we will briefly describe some of the mechanisms that have been postulated to link these resources to health processes, and present some information on possible intervention strategies. Next, we will identify important gaps in our understanding of the role of social and personal resources in ethnic disparities in late-life health, and discuss some of main methodological challenges that have hampered progress in this field. We will conclude with an overall summary of the findings, and an agenda for future research.

DIFFERENCES IN SOCIAL AND PERSONAL RESOURCES AMONG OLDER ADULTS OF DIFFERENT RACIAL OR ETHNIC BACKGROUNDS

Consideration of differences in the distribution of social resources across subpopulations defined by race or ethnicity is a first step toward a better understanding of the role of these resources in disparities in late-life health. For the purpose of this discussion, we will first review the evidence regarding racial/ethnic differences in the structural and compositional arrangements of the social and community networks of older adults. Next, we will turn our attention to the differential distribution by race/ethnicity of personal resources. These resources are further classified into social engagement, defined as participation in meaningful social activity, and social support. Social engagement itself is a relatively broad construct that consists of various forms of behavior that take place in a social context, including religious involvement, social activity, and productive activity (activities that produce goods and services with economic value). Religious involvement will be defined based on both participation in organized religious activities and personal religiousness or spirituality.

Social Networks

Social networks refer to the matrix of social relationships to which individuals are tied (Fischer, 1982). This matrix has structural and functional characteristics that constitute the social parameters of available resources. Social networks are generally characterized in terms of several categories, including the availability of ties (number, proximity, and accessibility of ties), the structural characteristics of those ties (density, multiplexity, and other factors), the composition of ties (with kin versus nonkin, friendships, and ties gained through formal organizational linkages), and the efficacy of those ties, or the ability of ties to facilitate the transfer of resources. At a community level, following the theoretical work of Wandersman and Nation (1998) and Glass and Balfour (2003), we differentiate three aspects of community networks (or neighborhoods and complex organizations) that are analytically distinct and appear to play a role in shaping the availability and effectiveness of personal resources. These include the physical characteristics of communities (e.g., graffiti, lighting, noise); the mediating institutions such as houses of worship, schools, and neighborhood organizations that link individuals to the larger social context (Berger and Neuhaus, 1977); the services available (both municipal and commercial); and the social organization of those communities (disorder, violence, crime, social capital, social cohesion).

The exact effects of aging on changes in social networks in late life remain somewhat unclear. Some evidence indicates that networks tend to shrink due to loss of network members who have died (Antonucci and Akiyama, 1987; Morgan, 1988). These losses affect mostly peripheral members of the social network, resulting in smaller but denser social networks (Antonucci and Akiyama, 1987; Carstensen, 1995). However, some of these losses may be counterbalanced by replacement with new relationships, or by intensification of existing relationships (Martire, Schulz, Mittelmark, and Newsom, 1999; van Tilburg, 1998). For example, some have suggested that older adults tend to draw increasingly close to network members that are most likely to satisfy their emotional and tangible needs—usually their children or children-in-law, siblings, or other close kin (Carstensen, 1995; Field and Minkler, 1988; van Tilburg, 1998). In sum, there may be considerable stability in the overall size of social networks among older adults, even if the composition of network members changes as people age.

Earlier gerontologic work suggested that older African Americans tend to have larger social networks compared with whites (Ball, Warheit, Vandiver, and Holzer, 1980; Taylor and Chatters, 1986a; Vaux, 1985).

Most of the racial differences in network size are due to older blacks having more children and being more integrated with extended family members (Gibson and Jackson, 1987; Johnson and Barer, 1990; Taylor, Chatters, Tucker, and Lewis, 1990). More recent studies have been less consistent in reporting differences in overall network size between blacks and whites, with some studies even reporting smaller networks for older blacks. For example, in a study of a biracial population in the Piedmont region of North Carolina, there were no differences in network size between blacks and whites, but blacks had slightly larger networks of children and relatives, whereas whites had larger networks of friends (Mendes de Leon, Gold, Glass, Kaplan, and George, 2001). A slightly larger children network was also noted among older blacks in the New Haven Established Populations for Epidemiological Studies of the Elderly (EPESE) Study, but no racial differences in overall network size were noted between blacks and whites (Glass, Mendes de Leon, Seeman, and Berkman, 1997).

Data from the Cardiovascular Health Study revealed smaller networks of family and friends for blacks compared with whites, although the proportion of blacks in this study was very small (Martire et al., 1999). A similar pattern was found in a population-based study of older adults in Detroit. In that study, older blacks reported smaller networks, but more frequent contact with network members, closer proximity, and a greater proportion of close kin compared with whites (Ajrouch, Antonucci, and Janevic, 2001). There were also no substantial racial differences in the availability of informal caregivers. However, blacks tend to draw from a larger pool of more distant relatives when they are disabled than do whites (Burton et al., 1995; Thorton, White-Means, and Choi, 1993). Based on the available evidence, the overall pattern is that older blacks have similarly sized or slightly smaller social networks, but that these networks are more likely to include extended family and fictive kin (Ajrouch et al., 2001).

These racial patterns in network size are further borne out by examining differences in living arrangements by race. Coresidence serves as an indicator of the proximity of social network ties. As shown in Table 10-1, among all persons aged 65 and over, blacks are much less likely to be living in the same household with their spouse than whites. Only 24.3 percent of black women and 53.5 percent of black men live with their spouse, compared with 42.4 percent and 74.3 percent respectively among whites. On the other hand, older blacks are more likely to live with other relatives or nonrelatives compared with whites. The net result is that black women are very comparable to white women in terms of living alone, at 40.8 percent and 41.3 percent respectively. On the other hand, older black men (24.9 percent) are slightly more likely to live alone compared to white men.

Much less is known about the social network characteristics of other ethnic groups. Baxter and colleagues (1998) report no differences in net-

TABLE 10-1 Living Arrangements of Persons Aged 65 and Older, 1998

Sex and Living Arrangements	All Ethnicities	White	Black	Hispanic	Asian or Pacific Islander
Women					
With spouse	40.7	42.4	24.3	36.9	41.3
With other relatives	16.8	14.8	32.2	33.8	36.7
With nonrelatives	1.7	1.6	2.7	1.8	0.8
Alone	40.8	41.3	40.8	27.4	21.2
Men					
With spouse	72.6	74.3	53.5	66.8	72.0
With other relatives	7.0	6.0	14.8	15.0	20.8
With nonrelatives	3.0	2.7	6.8	4.3	0.6
Alone	17.3	17.0	24.9	14.0	6.6

SOURCE: Federal Interagency Forum on Aging Related Statistics (2000). Older Americans 2000: Key Indicators of Well-Being.

work size between older Hispanics and non-Hispanic whites who live in a mostly rural area. However, older Hispanics living in New York City reported more children and close relatives in their social networks compared to either blacks or whites, but significantly fewer distant relatives, friends, and other social contacts (Cantor, 1975; Cantor, Brennan, and Sainz, 1994).

Table 10-1 provides some additional data on the living arrangements of older Hispanics and other ethnic groups. Both older Hispanics and Asian or Pacific Islanders are somewhat less likely to be living alone compared with whites and blacks. This is primarily because they are more likely to share a household with relatives other than a spouse. Thus, these data suggest that in terms of the most proximate social ties, older Hispanics and Asian and Pacific Islanders appear to have larger networks than either blacks or whites. However, there are insufficient data on other types of social relationships, particularly more discretionary types of ties that do not involve close kin. Thus, it is too early to make more conclusive inferences about differences in the size and composition of social network structures between these ethnic groups.

Neighborhood Characteristics

The availability of social and personal resources across racial/ethnic groups is partly conditioned by the stark differences that exist in the neighborhoods in which these ethnic groups live. Early studies by Lawton and Byerts (1973) demonstrate that older adults meet most of their social and daily needs within a six-block radius. Thus the features of the immediate neighborhood environment are important determinants of personal resources at the individual level. It is fairly clear that residential segregation by race/ethnicity is a common pattern in the United States that leads to stark differences in the social characteristics of neighborhoods in which various ethnic groups reside (LaVeist, 1993; Massey and Eggers, 1990). Residential segregation leads to differential forms of social organization that in turn are associated with variations in health status. For example, blacks tend to live in neighborhoods with higher rates of female-headed households, a characteristic that has been linked to higher rates of heart disease in women (LeClere, Rogers, and Peters, 1998). Ethnic minority elders tend to live in neighborhoods that also have higher crime and poverty rates, a finding that has important implications for both the need for and the availability of resources (Massey and Eggers, 1990). Differences in the character of neighborhoods where minority groups live have been used to explain some of the disparities in the health status of these groups (Kawachi and Kennedy, 1997; Waitzman and Smith, 1998).

Social Engagement

Research on the activity patterns of elderly persons shows considerable variation, with a substantial proportion of older persons remaining active well into their later years. Postretirement age has become widely accepted as a stage of continued engagement and personal growth (Glass, in press; Glass, Seeman, Herzog, Kahn, and Berkman, 1995; Ryff and Singer, 1998). Some studies suggest that older blacks are more actively involved in their networks compared with whites. For example, older blacks report more frequent contacts with network members (Ajrouch et al., 2001), particularly children and other relatives (Johnson and Barer, 1990; Mendes de Leon et al., 2001), which may be a function of their higher level of integration into family networks. Older blacks also are believed to engage in a more active flow of resources among network members. For example, several studies report that older blacks provide more support and assistance to others in their network compared with whites (Lee, Peek, and Coward, 1998; Miner, 1995). Other evidence suggests, however, that greater levels of social engagement among older blacks is not uniform. Using data from the National Survey of Family and Households (NSFH), Silverstein and Waite (1993) found that black adults are slightly less likely to be providers of instrumental support than whites, although these differences were somewhat attenuated in older ages. Hispanic adults were also less likely to be support providers compared with whites (Silverstein and Waite, 1993). Others have found no evidence that either blacks or Hispanics were more active agents of assistance and support in their respective networks (Cantor et al., 1994; Pugliesi and Shook, 1998). Both blacks and Hispanics have also been observed to be less involved in volunteer work compared with older whites (Baxter et al., 1998; Kincade et al., 1996).

An important aspect of social engagement among older adults is participation in productive activity. Gerontologic research on productive activity has challenged long-held beliefs, suggesting a substantial proportion of older persons remaining productive well into their later years. Herzog and colleagues (1987) found that productive activity declines on average with increasing age, but that controls for health status and education sharply reduce the magnitude of these age-related declines. In part, declines in productivity in older age result from the cessation of paid work and child care, while older adults remain as active as their younger counterparts in unpaid work, volunteerism, and informal help to others (Cutler, 1977; Herzog and Morgan, 1989; Herzog, Kahn, Morgan, Jackson, and Antonucci, 1989).

A number of studies have pointed to the importance of race/ethnicity and gender as critical contexts in which to understand productivity among older adults (Danigelis and McIntosh, 1993; Herzog and Morgan, 1992). A recent systematic review of this topic was undertaken by Jackson (2001), who argues that engagement in productive activity is affected over the life course by both blocked opportunities and economic necessity. From that standpoint, racial and ethnic heterogeneity in patterns of participation in productive activity is to be reasonably expected. Among the findings from this literature is the importance of considering productive activities that fall outside traditional definitions of economic activity such as paid work and volunteering. Failure to do so risks underestimating the true economic value of those activities that nonwhite ethnic groups tend to participate in to greater extents, including caregiving (Chatters, Taylor, and Jackson, 1985; Taylor and Chatters, 1986a; Taylor and Taylor, 1982) and bartering (Stack, 1974). Given that participation in primary and secondary labor markets throughout the life course is less satisfactory to disadvantaged groups, it appears clear that continued participation in productive activity must be seen in a larger context. Studies that have attempted to include measures of activity participation that include informal and social forms of productivity generally have observed that blacks and whites demonstrate comparable degrees of continuity in late life (Antonucci, Jackson, Gibson, and Herzog, 1989; Glass et al., 1995; Jackson, 2001). Participation in productive activities may play an especially important role in maintaining identity in persons in disadvantaged groups because they perceive that their activities help to meet community needs (Deimling, Harel, and Noelker, 1983).

Caregiving is another form of productive activity that is relatively common among the elderly. In a community-based study of older adults, blacks were 30 percent more likely to report caregiving compared with whites, after controlling for age, sex, marital status, and education (McCann et al., 2000). However, data from the National Survey of Self-Care and Aging did not show any racial differences in caregiving, although blacks were more likely to provide emotional support (Kincade et al., 1996). Data on caregiving in other ethnic groups is largely absent.

Another area of social engagement that has received considerable attention is participation in formal and informal organizations, especially those centered around religious activity. Participation in religious activity typically presents an opportunity for social interaction with others who are likely to have similar beliefs and values. In addition, it may provide an important conduit through which both personal and social resources are activated and maintained (Levin, Taylor, and Chatters, 1994). The importance of the church has long been a topic of particular interest in the unique history and social conditions of blacks (Chatters and Taylor, 1994). The seminal work by Taylor and Chatters has further underscored the centrality of church-related activity and religiosity in older black adults (Taylor, 1986; Taylor and Chatters, 1986a). This research has highlighted the significance of the church in black communities as a resource to adapt to the adverse life conditions and social disadvantage, and to provide opportunities for personal and spiritual growth and well-being (Chatters, 2000).

Levin and colleagues (1994) undertook a systematic quantitative analysis of racial differences in church attendance and other indicators of religious engagement. They found only minor differences between older blacks and whites in levels of religious affiliation, as church membership was nearly 100 percent in both groups; however, blacks reported slightly higher levels of church attendance than whites. There were more pronounced racial differences in nonorganizational religious activity and subjective religiosity. For example, blacks were much more likely to read religious books and to listen to religious radio programs. They also rated their religion as being more important to them than older whites did. Other studies also have shown that older blacks tend to have higher levels of religious involvement than whites (Johnson and Barer, 1990; Kim and McKenry, 1998). In contrast, participation in other types of social or work-related organizations tends to be lower among blacks (Cutler and Hendricks, 2000; Miner and Tolnay, 1998).

Fewer data are available on church-related activity and other forms of social engagement for other ethnic groups. A study of a rural Hispanic population showed patterns of engagement similar to those of older blacks. Participation in church-related groups was found to be higher, but involvement in other social groups and organizations was lower, among older Hispanics relative to non-Hispanic whites (Baxter et al., 1998).

Social Support

The social support needs of adults are likely to change as they enter the postretirement years. The need for financial assistance, for help with daily tasks as health declines, and for emotional support may all increase (Carstensen, 1995; Silverstein and Waite, 1993). Older adults of all racial/

ethnic groups tend to rely heavily on family members as the primary source of both instrumental and emotional support. Even so, help and assistance from immediate family or next of kin is thought to be more common among older blacks than older whites (Lee et al., 1998; Mutran, 1985). Cantor and colleagues (1994) report that both black and Hispanic children are more likely to provide practical and informational types of support to their aged parents than do white children. This could be partly because of the greater care needs of older blacks and Hispanics, who may be in poorer health. However, other research suggests that underlying differentials in health are not a sufficient explanation for the greater use of support among older blacks and other minority elders (Tennstedt and Chang, 1998). Instead, it has been suggested that older disabled whites tend to replace informal support with formal support services in times of poor health, whereas older blacks may acquire formal services in addition to the informal assistance they receive from family and friends (Miner, 1995).

Overall, a picture has emerged of elderly blacks and Hispanics being more likely to benefit from cross-generational exchanges of supportive resources (Mutran, 1985). Similar patterns of intergenerational support also have been described for older Asian Americans, although there is considerable diversity in family relationships and support structures among Asian populations, depending on the country of origin. For example, elderly Koreans seem to rely more on their children for assistance and emotional support than do elderly Chinese or Japanese (Ishii-Kuntz, 1997).

Several other studies, however, are less consistent with important ethnic/racial differences in social support among the elderly. For example, in the NSFH data, older blacks and Hispanic men were no more likely to receive instrumental or emotional support than non-Hispanics, while Hispanic women were significantly less likely to receive these two types of support (Silverstein and Waite, 1993). In another population-based study of older adults living in the Piedmont area of North Carolina, blacks reported slightly higher levels of instrumental support than whites, but there were no differences in emotional support (Mendes de Leon et al., 2001). In one of the few longitudinal investigations of social support changes in older adults, Martire and colleagues (1999) found no black-white differences in emotional, instrumental, or informational support, although blacks showed somewhat higher declines in informational support over time than whites.

In conclusion, this review suggests there is little evidence for substantial differences by race or ethnicity in social and personal resources in older adults. In general, minority elders may have somewhat closer knit family networks compared to non-Hispanic whites, but possibly a smaller overall network, particularly with regard to more discretionary types of ties, such as friends. A similar pattern is apparent for social engagement. Overall, elderly whites appear somewhat more socially active, especially with regard to volunteer activities and membership in formal or informal social organizations. On the other hand, most data indicate that minority elders are more involved in church-based organizations and activities.

SOCIAL AND PERSONAL RESOURCES AND HEALTH DISPARITIES IN LATE LIFE

The first part of this section provides an overview of the research examining the association of social and personal resources with health outcomes, with an emphasis on research in elderly populations. This review focuses mostly on studies of mortality, physical disability, and cognitive decline, as these health outcomes have particular relevance for elderly populations and have been the most widely studied. Later in this section, we will discuss the literature that has begun to examine the role of social and personal resources in ethnic disparities in late-life health.

Social Networks and Late-Life Health

The health benefits of social and personal resources have been a major theme in social epidemiology since the 1970s. One of the first seminal papers in this area was a study by Berkman and Syme (1979) based on data from 4,500 community-dwelling residents of Alameda County, California. Participants in this study reported on four types of social ties, including marriage, network size (number of relatives and friends seen frequently), church membership, and participation in formal or informal groups. A summary measure of these four ties was called the "Social Network Index." Those who scored low on this index were estimated to have a twofold increased mortality risk independent of other predictors of mortality, such as low SES, poor health habits, and self-reported poor physical health status (Berkman and Syme, 1979). This finding was later replicated in a variety of other cohort studies, such as the Tecumseh Community Health Study (House, Robbins, and Metzner, 1982), the Evans County, Georgia, study (Schoenbach, Kaplan, Fredman, and Kleinbaum, 1986), a study in Durham County, North Carolina (Blazer, 1982), a study of male health professionals (Kawachi et al., 1996), and studies in Sweden and Finland (Kaplan, Seeman, Cohen, Knudsen, and Guralnik, 1987; Orth-Gomer and Johnson, 1987). In summarizing this literature, House and colleagues concluded that social relationships, or some aspects of social involvement, confer a remarkably consistent survival benefit that cannot be attributed to other determinants of physical health (House, Landis, and Umberson, 1988).

The survival benefits of social network ties have been found to extend into older adulthood. For example, in a follow-up analysis of data from the Alameda County study, Seeman and colleagues investigated the relationship of social network ties, as measured by the Social Network Index, with overall mortality in four age groups ranging from ages 38 to 40 to ages 70 and up. They found that this index was independently predictive of 17-year mortality across all age groups, even if the magnitude of the benefit was somewhat attenuated in the older age groups compared with middle-aged adults (Seeman, Kaplan, Knudsen, Cohen, and Guralnik, 1987). This finding was later replicated in three population-based cohort studies (in New Haven, East Boston, and Iowa, respectively) of older adults that were part of the EPESE program. After rigorous control for other determinants of mortality, low social ties was associated with approximately a twofold increased risk of mortality among New Haven men and women and Iowa women. The effects in the other groups (Iowa men and East Boston men and women) were predictive of mortality after adjustment for age only, but somewhat weaker and no longer statistically significant in the fully adjusted models (Seeman et al., 1993a). A number of other prospective studies have provided additional evidence for the protective effect of social relationships and social involvement more generally with regard to risk of death among the elderly (Jylha and Aro, 1989; Shye, Mullooly, Freeborn, and Pope, 1995; Steinbach, 1992).

An important limitation of the research on social network ties and survival is that most studies have relied on relatively crude measures of social network ties, which often lack a specific theoretical foundation (Glass et al., 1997). For example, the Social Network Index includes information on network size (number of friends and relatives seen at least monthly), organizational membership (membership in religious and other groups), and marital status (a specific kind of social tie). Similar "composite" measures of social networks and social engagement have also been used in studies of dementia and cognitive decline. In the Swedish Kungsholmen Project, a summary social network measure was constructed on the basis of being married and living with someone, having regular and satisfying contacts with children (friends or relatives). This index was found to be significantly predictive of 3-year incidence of dementia after adjustment for age, sex, education, baseline cognitive status, and depression. The risk for dementia was 60 percent higher at lower social network levels compared with higher levels (Fratiglioni, Wang, Ericsson, Maytan, and Winblad, 2000). Using longitudinal data from the New Haven EPESE study, Bassuk and colleagues constructed a composite index that combined information on indicators of personal ties, group membership, and social engagement. This index was found to be significantly predictive of incident cognitive decline, independent of a series of demographic, lifestyle, and health-related control variables. Those with lower scores on this index had approximately a twofold higher risk of showing cognitive decline during follow-up than those with the highest scores (Bassuk, Glass, and Berkman, 1999; Boult, Kane, Louis, Boult, and McCaffrey, 1994). They further commented that none of the individual social network or engagement indicators were as predictive of incident cognitive decline as the combined index, suggesting that the effect was not due to any particular feature of personal networks, group membership, or social activity.

Other studies have started to examine whether social network ties confer a protective effect against age-related physical disabilities. An analysis of the 4-year follow-up data from the Longitudinal Study on Aging revealed that adults aged 70 and up who reported no social contacts were more than twice as likely to either die or become physically disabled (Boult et al., 1994). A similar effect was found in the Alameda County study, where having five or more close personal relationships was significantly associated with the likelihood of "successful aging," defined as lack of physical disability (Strawbridge, Cohen, Shema, and Kaplan, 1996; Unger, McAvay, Bruce, Berkman, and Seeman, 1999). This is further corroborated by findings from the MacArthur Studies of Successful Aging, a cohort study of a group of high-functioning elderly. These studies were specifically designed to examine factors associated with high function, or lack of disability, and maintenance of high function over time. An analysis of the MacArthur data showed that a greater number of social ties was protective of increases in physical disability during follow-up (Unger et al., 1999). However, a few other studies have failed to find clear evidence for such a relationship (Harris, Kovar, Suzman, Kleinman, and Feldman, 1989; Seeman et al., 1995).

Most of the work on social network ties and disability is based on simple counts of available network contacts, without differentiation with regard to the composition or the structure of ties. More recent studies suggest that the beneficial effect of social network ties is not uniform across different types of social relationships. For example, a series of longitudinal analyses of the EPESE data have shown that ties with relatives and friends appear to provide protective effects against disability and to promote recovery from disability. Ties with children, on the other hand, were found to be unrelated to disability risks (Mendes de Leon et al., 1999, 2001). However, these results further indicated that the exact causal relationships between social resources and disability remain somewhat unclear. Although findings in this literature are often interpreted as though greater availability of social ties is causally involved in the prevention of functional decline and disability, the actual interrelationships may be more complex. While older adults with larger social networks on average report significantly less disability, it may also be true that the absence of disability is directly related to the magnitude of one's social network that one is able to maintain (Mendes de Leon et al., 2001).

Community Networks and Late-Life Health

There is an emerging literature on the health effects of broader social structures, which are often defined at the level of community or neighborhood. To some extent, this work is based on the notion that characteristics at the neighborhood level, such as a Census tract area, have an important influence on population health (Kaplan, 1996; Macintyre, Maciver, and Sooman, 1993; Robert, 1999). Although most studies in this area have focused on aggregate-level indicators of socioeconomic status, most pertinent to the discussion in this chapter is research on specific community resources, or the absence or threats to those types of resources, and their impact on late-life health.

One example of this research is an analysis of the Alameda County Study data in which individual-level data were combined with data at the neighborhood level to predict 11-year mortality risk. A neighborhood social environment score was constructed on the basis of information at the level of Census tracts on population socioeconomic status (e.g., per capita income, residential crowding), availability of commercial resources (e.g., pharmacies, supermarkets), and characteristics of environment/housing (e.g., percentage renters, percentage single-family dwellings). Persons living in neighborhoods with lower social environment scores were found to have about 50 percent increased odds of dying during follow-up, compared to those living in neighborhoods with higher social environment scores. This association persisted after adjustment for individual-level indicators of socioeconomic status and poor health habits (Yen and Kaplan, 1999).

In another study using the Alameda County study data, Balfour and Kaplan used self-reported information on six specific neighborhood problems (e.g., crime, traffic) in a prospective analysis of change in physical function. Persons reporting two or more neighborhood problems were at a more than twofold increased risk of a loss in physical function, after adjustment for a range of sociodemographic, socioeconomic, and health-related variables (Balfour and Kaplan, 2002). Neighborhood problems most strongly associated with loss in physical function included heavy traffic, excessive noise, poor access to public transportation, and inadequate street lighting.

Overall, most of the empirical evidence suggests that structural and contextual aspects of the social environment are related to important health outcomes in late life. Although the exact nature of this role is still poorly understood, most research to date has produced relatively consistent and robust findings, especially with regard to all-cause mortality and, to a lesser degree, changes in physical and cognitive function. It is important to note that most studies in this area included statistical controls for other determinants of these age-related health outcomes. Thus, it appears that the rela-

tionships between social networks and late-life health are mostly independent of other important influences such as socioeconomic status, lifestyle
habits, and poor physical health status.

Social Engagement and Late-Life Health

An emerging body of research has begun to evaluate the health benefits
of various forms of social engagement in older populations. A well-established finding in the epidemiological literature is that activity confers an
important survival advantage, and significantly reduces risk for heart disease and other age-related disability outcomes (Kampert, Blair, Barlow, and
Kohl, 1996; Kaplan, Strawbridge, Cohen, and Hungerford, 1996;
Paffenbarger, Hyde, Wing, and Hsieh, 1986; Vita, Terry, Hubert, and Fries,
1998). Activity is usually assessed strictly in terms of physical activity, and
its benefit is believed to be mostly from improved cardiopulmonary fitness
(Blair et al., 1996).

One of the first studies to directly challenge this idea was performed by
Glass and colleagues, who tested the survival benefits of other, nonphysical,
forms of activity (Glass, Mendes de Leon, Marottoli, and Berkman, 1999).
They used data from the New Haven EPESE study to construct separate
measures for three types of activity: social activity (e.g., playing cards; visits
to cinema, restaurants, or sporting events), productive activity (e.g., gardening, shopping, paid or unpaid community work), and fitness activity
(e.g., swimming, walking). Summary measures of each of these types of
activity were found to have a significant and gradient effect on 13-year
mortality. A multivariate survival analysis adjusting for the main sets of
risk factors for mortality showed that each type of activity was independently associated with reduced mortality. Comparing the highest to lowest
quarter of activity, social activity was associated with a 19 percent risk
reduction (Hazard Ratio [HR] = 0.81; 95 percent Confidence Intervals
[CIs] 0.74-0.89), fitness activity with a 15 percent risk reduction (HR =
0.85; 95 percent CIs 0.77-0.95), and productive activity with a 23 percent
risk reduction (HR = 0.77; 95 percent CIs 0.71-0.85).

Other studies have reported similar survival benefits due to social engagement in the general adult population (Bygren, Konlaan, and Johansson,
1996; Welin et al., 1985) as well as among residents of long-term care
facilities (Kiely, Simon, Jones, and Morris, 2000; Stones, Dornan, and
Kozma, 1989). Another form of social engagement, volunteering, also has
been linked with specific health benefits. Using data from a nationally
representative sample of older adults, Musick and colleagues found that
volunteering was associated with a reduced risk of mortality, after adjustment for sociodemographic, socioeconomic, health-related, and social integration variables (Musick, Herzog, and House, 1999). The beneficial effect

appeared to be confined to moderate levels of volunteering in this study, as higher levels of volunteering were unrelated to survival.

Not all studies, however, have found survival benefits due to social or productive activity. Data from a recent cohort study in Sweden showed no association between either social or productive activity with mortality risk (Lennartsson and Silverstein, 2001). The only one type of activity related to prolonged survival was solitary-active activities, such as hobbies and gardening. Of note is that in this cohort, church attendance was also found to be unrelated to survival. This is in contrast to most studies in American populations, where relatively clear survival advantages have been found for church attendance (to be discussed).

Other research has focused on the role of social engagement in physical disability, cognitive decline, and dementia, as well as overall well-being. For example, in a cross-sectional analysis of data from a convenience sample of older adults, social activity (e.g., traveling, attending parties, attending church) was found to be significantly correlated with a global measure of physical functioning after adjustment for age, gender, marital status, and income. Other forms of activity, such as high-demand leisure activity (physical activity) and low-demand leisure activity (cognitive activity), were also significantly associated with physical functioning (Everard, Lach, Fisher, and Baum, 2000).

To examine this relationship prospectively, Mendes de Leon and colleagues used nine waves of data from the New Haven EPESE study to relate baseline social engagement to changes in disability status during follow-up. They found that older adults with higher levels of social engagement had a significantly better functional status (less disability) on three separate indices of disability. However, it did not appear that higher levels of social engagement at baseline were associated with less functional decline over time. Instead, older adults with high levels of social engagement had a substantial disability advantage at baseline, which decreased slightly over time, although this decrease was too small to compensate for the initial advantage in function (Mendes de Leon, Glass, and Berkman, 2003). This kind of relationship may allude to a pattern of causation characterized by reciprocal influences, whereby declining physical or cognitive function reduces social engagement, which, in turn, accelerates losses in physical and cognitive function. This pattern of association might also be explained as a "use-it-or-lose-it" mechanism (Hultsch, Hertzog, Small, and Dixon, 1999; Mendes de Leon et al., 2001).

As already described, composite measures that include information on social engagement have been found to be associated with a reduced risk of cognitive decline and dementia (Bassuk et al., 1999; Fratiglioni et al., 2000). Fabrigoule and colleagues (1995) have reported on a more specific analysis of social engagement and risk of dementia using data from a cohort study in a French population. In this study, a number of different forms of social and leisure activity were inversely related to dementia risk, although only a few—traveling, gardening, or odd jobs or knitting—remained significantly associated with this outcome after controlling for age and baseline cognitive status.

Other studies have found significant positive associations between markers of social engagement and overall well-being (Herzog. Franks, Markus, and Holmberg, 1998; Menec and Chipperfield, 1997; Michael, Berkman, Colditz, and Kawachi, 2001; Van Willigen, 2000). Herzog and colleagues used data from a representative sample of adults aged 65 and over from the Detroit metropolitan area to examine the relationship between activity and well-being. They found that both social (leisure) and productive activity were significantly associated with physical health and depressive symptoms, although the effects due to productive activity were mostly indirect (Herzog et al., 1998). Using data from a Canadian sample of older adults, Menec and Chipperfield reported a significant positive cross-sectional association of overall social and productive activity with concurrent life satisfaction and self-rated health. The same activity index was also prospectively related to an increase in life satisfaction over a 7-year period (Menec and Chipperfield, 1997). Van Willigen used data from the American Changing Lives study to compare the health effects of volunteering in younger (age <60 years old) and older (age ≥60) adults. She found that volunteering was associated prospectively with an increase in both life satisfaction and self-rated health during follow-up, and that these effects were stronger among older adults than middle-aged adults (Van Willigen, 2000). Four-year follow-up data from the Nurses Health Study have also shown a positive effect of social engagement on changes in mental health and quality of life, particularly among those middle-aged women who were living alone (Michael et al., 2001).

As has been indicated before, one of the problems in evaluating these results is substantial variability across studies in definitions and assessment of social engagement and its components. For example, there is little consensus on which forms of engagement should be considered (mostly) physical, social, or cognitive, and often these forms of activity are combined into single summary measures (Hultsch, Hammer, and Small, 1993). Recent evidence clearly suggests that cognitive forms of activity protect against risk of cognitive decline and Alzheimer's disease (Friedland et al., 2001; Hultsch et al., 1999; Wilson et al., 2002). Is cognitive activity a form of social engagement? Or could some cognitive activities be considered forms of social engagement? For the purpose of this discussion, we focus primarily on forms of activity that take place in the context of a social environment, that is, activity that involves other persons, or groups or communities of other persons. In this light, we will review studies that have addressed the health effects of other specific forms of social engagement, including volunteering and religious activity. Clearly, these forms of activity can often be defined in both their social and cognitive content or purpose.

Over the past 20 years, there has been an increasing interest in the effect of religious involvement on health (Ellison and Levin, 1998; Levin, 1996). The most recent studies in this area suggest that church attendance confers an important protective effect against overall mortality (Hummer, Rogers, Nam, and Ellison, 1999; Koenig et al., 1999; Krause, 1998; Oman and Reed, 1998; Strawbridge, Cohen, Shema, and Kaplan, 1997). They suggest further that this protective effect is not entirely attributable to other factors that may be related to both church attendance and mortality, such as socioeconomic status, lifestyle variables, and initial physical health status. For example, Hummer and colleagues used data from a nationally representative supplement of the 1987 National Health Interview Survey, which includes the general U.S. adult population (aged 21 years and over) and contains information on frequency of church attendance and relevant covariates. Respondents were linked to the National Death Index to generate 8-year mortality follow-up data. Analysis of these data revealed a clear gradient relationship between church attendance and risk of death, after adjustment for a comprehensive set of potential confounders, including sociodemographic, health-related, and psychosocial variables. Net of all these factors, adults who reported never attending church had a 50 percent increased risk of death (HR = 1.50, p < 0.01) compared with those who attended church more than once a week. Mortality risks among those attending less often than weekly (HR = 1.24, p < 0.05) and attending weekly (HR = 1.21, p < 0.05) were also elevated compared with those who attended more than once a week (Hummer et al., 1999).

Several other studies have reported a protective effect of church attendance on mortality, most of them with remarkably similar effect sizes as those reported by Hummer and colleagues (Koenig et al., 1999; Oman and Reed, 1998; Strawbridge et al., 1997). Moreover, the survival benefits of church attendance have also been documented specifically for elderly populations. Using 6-year follow-up data from the North Carolina EPESE study, Koenig and colleagues showed that frequent church attendance was an adjusted mortality risk of HR = 0.72 (95 percent CI 0.64-0.81), a reduction of 36 percent compared to infrequent attenders (Koenig et al., 1999). An additional analysis of the same data suggested that private religious activity, such as prayer and bible reading, was not independently associated with prolonged survival. There was a suggestion, however, that private religiosity has a positive effect among nondisabled older persons (Helm, Hays, Flint, Koenig, and Blazer, 2000).

Religious involvement has also been studied in relation to health outcomes other than mortality, particularly physical disability, overall health status, and well-being. In the most rigorous study of religious involvement and physical disability to date, Idler and Kasl compared the long-term effects of church attendance and subjective religiosity using yearly follow-up data from the New Haven EPESE cohort study. Subjective religiosity was measured by questions assessing how deeply religious a person feels, and how much strength and comfort they received from their religion. They found that church attendance was prospectively associated with change in disability status over a 12-year follow-up period. This effect proved to be independent of a comprehensive set of other predictors of disability, and relatively constant throughout follow-up. On the other hand, subjective religiosity was unrelated to changes in disability status over time (Idler and Kasl, 1997).

Levin and Chatters (1998) examined the effect of religious involvement on both subjective (self-rated) health status and psychological well-being using cross-sectional data from three national data sets of older adults. The strongest and most consistent associations were found for organizational religiosity (church attendance) and subjective health. There were less consistent associations for the effect of organizational religiosity and subjective religiosity on psychological well-being. The cross-sectional relationship between church attendance and subjective health seems to be congruent with the findings regarding mortality risk and disability. However, when this association was examined prospectively, the effect of church attendance on change in subjective health was almost entirely accounted for by differences in physical health status between frequent and infrequent church attenders (Musick, 1996). Private religiosity, however, did seem to be positively associated with changes in subjective health, such that those reporting more private religious practices tended to improve in subjective health status over a 3-year follow-up period, after adjustment for other sociodemographic, lifestyle, and physical health status variables.

Whereas these findings suggest a positive health effect for private religiosity, another study reported that adult blacks and whites with higher levels of private religiosity also reported more depressive symptoms. However, this finding pertains to a cross-sectional analysis, in which causal order cannot be determined. In other words, it is possible that persons who feel depressed (e.g., because of stressful circumstances) may turn to private religiosity as a means of coping, rather than that their private religiosity "caused" the negative emotions. Church attendance was inversely related to depressive symptoms in this study, but this protective effect was observed among whites only (Ellison, 1995).

Overall, the most consistent health effects for religious involvement have been found for church attendance, particularly in relation to overall survival. Other evidence suggests that church attendance is also related to long-term changes in physical disability, whereas little empirical evidence is yet available with regard to its effect on cognitive changes or risk for dementia. Finally, most studies suggest that religion possibly plays an important if somewhat limited role in the mental health and well-being of older adults, although much of these associations are still poorly understood (Ellison and Levin, 1998).

Social Support and Late-Life Health

Social support is typically regarded as a key resource that is exchanged between members of personal and community networks. Therefore, it is often postulated as a critical component of the health benefits that accrue to those who have higher levels of social integration and who are more socially engaged. Nonetheless, most empirical evidence suggests that social support affects health and well-being in ways that differ substantially from the mechanisms that link other aspects of social and personal resources with health.

Few epidemiologic studies to date have focused on specific indices of social support in relation to mortality risk. In an earlier study in this area, Blazer (1982) examined the effect of various indicators of social networks and support on 30-month mortality in a sample of older adults. He found that impaired perceived social support was associated with a more than threefold increased mortality risk, after adjustment for a series of socio-demographic and health-related control variables. Another significant risk factor for mortality was a low level of social interaction, which was associated with an almost twofold increased mortality risk (Blazer, 1982).

In a more recent, population-based study of adults aged > 55 years from the Netherlands, emotional support was found to be significantly associated with decreased mortality risk over a 29-month follow-up period, after careful adjustment for sociodemographic and lifestyle variables, as well as self-reported physical health status (Penninx et al., 1997). However, there was no clear gradient effect between emotional support and mortality risk. Compared with low emotional support, a moderate level of emotional support was associated with about a 50 percent decrease in odds of dying (Odds Ratio [OR] = 0.49, 95 percent CI 0.33-0.72), whereas a high level of support was associated with 32 percent decreased odds of dying (OR = 0.68, 95 percent CI 0.47-0.98). In the same study, loneliness, which was used as a marker of lack of perceived social support, was also found to have a significant association with mortality risk (Penninx et al., 1997). Although these results suggest that social support has a protective effect against mortality, the durations of the follow-up periods were relatively short compared to studies of social networks or social engagement and mortality reviewed previously in this chapter.

Other studies have begun to investigate the role of social support in physical disability and cognitive decline in older populations. These relationships have been prospectively examined in several large, population-based studies of older adults, such as the New Haven and North Carolina EPESE studies and the MacArthur Studies of Successful Aging. For example, using 2.5-year follow-up data from the MacArthur Studies of Successful Aging, Seeman and colleagues found that availability of emotional social support attenuated age-related declines in physical function as measured by a series of standard performance tests of function, such as chair stands and walking. However, this effect was only apparent among those with low levels of instrumental support. In fact, perceived adequacy of support, another marker of social support, was significantly associated with an *increased* risk for decline in physical function (Seeman et al., 1995). Emotional social support has also failed to show an association with self-reported disability status both cross-sectionally (Everard et al., 2000) and longitudinally (Mendes de Leon et al., 1999, 2001; Seeman, Bruce, and McAvay, 1996; Unger et al., 1999).

The degree to which social support affects cognitive decline in older adults remains mostly unclear. A longitudinal analysis from the New Haven EPESE data suggests that emotional support is unrelated to cognitive decline over 3- to 12-year follow-up periods (Bassuk et al., 1999). However, emotional support was the only social variable that was predictive of changes in cognitive function in the MacArthur Studies of Successful Aging cohort. Emotional support was found to be associated with a significant protective effect against cognitive decline over a 7.5-year follow-up period (Seeman, Lusignolo, Albert, and Berkman, 2001a).

The other type of social support that has received systematic attention in the epidemiologic literature is instrumental support, usually defined as the availability and/or adequacy of assistance with daily chores, such as shopping or meal preparation. Overall, the available evidence indicates that this form of support tends to have a detrimental effect on various health outcomes. For example, in the Dutch study described by Penninx and colleagues, it was found that persons who reported high levels of instrumental support had a 74 percent increased odds of dying (OR = 1.74, 95 percent CI 1.12-2.69), after adjustment for a comprehensive set of other risk factors for mortality (Penninx et al., 1997). Equally adverse effects due to instrumental social support have been obtained in prospective studies of disability. In both the New Haven and North Carolina EPESE studies, instrumental support was found to increase risk for self-reported disability over 9- and 6-year follow-up periods (Mendes de Leon et al., 1999, 2001). Similar adverse effects on disability due to instrumental support have been reported for the MacArthur Studies of Successful Aging (Seeman et al., 1996).

The negative effect of instrumental support on long-term changes in health is possibly because the use of practical assistance with everyday tasks may be an indication of declining health, even if such a decline has not manifested itself yet in overt clinical signs and symptoms, or disability. Alternatively, the use or availability of instrumental support may foster greater dependence, which may lead to an acceleration of functional decline. Such an explanation would suggest that some of these relationships may be more complex than unidirectional causal effect one way or the other, and may reflect reciprocal patterns of association. In other words, the "use-it-or-lose-it" mechanism may apply to the relationship between personal resources and late-life health more generally, whereby initial declines in health lead to less engagement and more assistance, in turn leading to further health declines.

The discussion so far suggests that social support shows either a mixed pattern of association with age-related health outcomes, or has an adverse effect on such outcomes, depending on the type of support. However, other research raises the possibility that social support plays a more important role in other health processes that have particular relevance to older adults. One example is the literature on recovery from acute illness episodes. There is considerable evidence that patients with higher levels of social support have better outcomes after acute clinical events than those who report lower levels of support (Berkman, Leo-Summers, and Horwitz, 1992; Glass and Maddox, 1992; Glass, Matchar, Belyea, and Feussner, 1993; Jenkins, Stanton, and Jono, 1994; Mutran, Reitzes, Mossey, and Fernandez, 1996; Oxman and Hull, 1997; Wilcox, Kasl, and Berkman, 1994). For example, Glass and colleagues studied the effect of social support on functional recovery following a first stroke. They found that high levels of perceived social support were prospectively associated with more rapid rate of recovery and greater overall improvement in functioning after 6 months (Glass et al., 1993). Further analysis revealed that there was a gradient effect for emotional support, such that more support was associated with better outcomes. For instrumental support, however, moderate levels appeared to be most effective in promoting recovery (Glass and Maddox, 1992). The latter finding suggests that instrumental assistance, while beneficial in moderate amounts in times of a medical crisis, may also create greater dependency and lead to negative long-term consequences. Such an interpretation would be consistent with the adverse long-term health effects of instrumental support described previously in this section.

Social support has also been studied extensively in patient populations with acute or subacute heart disease. In a large clinical trial of male patients with myocardial infarction (MI), lack of social support (social isolation) was highly predictive of subsequent mortality, especially in the context of high levels of general life stress (Ruberman, Weinblatt, Goldberg, and Chaudhary, 1984). While this study did not specify the type of social support, other studies have focused more specifically on emotional support in recovery from heart disease. For example, Berkman and colleagues found that MI patients who reported no source of emotional support had a more than twofold increased chance of dying during the first 6 months following an MI than those reporting one or more sources of emotional support. This effect became even stronger after adjustment for sociodemographic characteristics, clinical severity, co-morbidity, and functional status (Berkman et al., 1992).

Similarly robust associations have been found between lack of social support or social isolation and outcomes in other studies of patients with heart disease or heart failure (Case, Moss, Case, McDermott, and Eberly, 1992; Gorkin et al., 1993; Jenkins et al., 1994; Krumholz et al., 1998; Oxman and Hull, 1997; Williams et al., 1992). Most of these studies have been based on large patient samples, with some sample sizes exceeding 1,000 patients (Case et al., 1992; Gorkin et al., 1993; Williams et al., 1992), and some have examined these issues specifically in older populations (Berkman et al., 1992; Krumholz et al., 1998; Oxman and Hull, 1997). It is important to note that most of these studies included careful control for important potential confounders, in particular clinical severity and co-morbidity or other markers of preevent health status. Thus, the use of rigorous methods lends further confidence in the validity of a causal effect of social support, particularly emotional support, on recovery outcomes after acute medical events.

Another key area of inquiry has focused on the role of social support on mental well-being. Although this topic is reviewed in more detail elsewhere in this volume (see Chapter 13), it is generally assumed that social support has a positive impact on overall mental health and well-being among older adults, although the magnitude of this effect tends to be modest (Ingersoll-Dayton, Morgan, and Antonucci, 1997; Krause, 1986; Krause, Liang, and Keith, 1990; Liang, Krause, and Bennett, 2001; Matt and Dean, 1993; Silverstein and Bengtson, 1994). Additional studies have shown that social support may be especially important for older adults who are faced with adverse or stressful situations in their lives. For example, emotional support has been shown to buffer the deleterious influences of a variety of stressors, such as economic strain (Atienza, Collins, and King, 2001; Krause, 1987, 1997), caregiver stress (Atienza et al., 2001; Li, Seltzer, and Greenberg, 1997; Ostwald, Hepburn, Caron, Burns, and Mantell, 1999; Suitor and Pillemer, 1996), bereavement (Silverstein and Bengtson, 1994), and poor health (Krause, 1990). At the same time, there is some suggestion that social support may not always have unequivocally beneficial effects. Several studies have found that older adults suffer psychologically when receiving support, particularly in situations of an imbalance between the amount of support received and support provided to others (Liang et al., 2001; Newsom and Schulz, 1998). This may be especially the case when the type of support received is mostly in the form of assistance with daily chores, rather than emotional support (Davey and Eggebeen, 1998), mirroring the adverse health effects of instrumental support described earlier for other health outcomes.

Although most social support research has been conceptualized from the perspective of the support recipient, a limited number of studies have started to examine the health effects of providing support to others. Generally, this work shows that lending assistance to others is associated with increased well-being (Krause, Herzog, and Baker, 1992; Liang et al., 2001; Silverstein, Chen, and Heller, 1996). For example, using cross-sectional data from the American Changing Lives Study, Krause and colleagues reported that providing informal assistance to others, mostly in the form of instrumental support, is associated with lower levels of depressive symptoms, primarily by enhancing feelings of personal control (Krause et al., 1992). This is not to suggest that providing support to others may not sometimes come at a psychological, if not physical, cost, as the well-documented harmful effects of caregiver burden clearly suggest (Ory, Hoffman, Yee, Tennstedt, and Schulz, 1999; Schulz, O'Brien, Bookwala, and Fleissner, 1995).

Finally, some evidence is emerging that not only does actual exchange of resources between network members possibly influence health and well-being among older adults, but that the nature of the social interactions have a health impact in their own right. For example, Ingersoll-Dayton and colleagues examined the effect of social exchanges on psychological well-being in a representative sample of middle-aged and older adults. Positive social exchanges included interactions of confiding, reassurance, and getting respect, and negative exchanges included interactions that were considered demanding or conveyed a lack of understanding. They showed that positive exchanges are essentially associated with greater positive affect, and negative exchanges with greater negative affect (Ingersoll-Dayton et al., 1997). These findings are corroborated by a more recent study, which showed that negative interactions were significantly associated with higher levels of depressive symptoms among older adults (Liang et al., 2001). However, other research suggests that positive social interactions are a more important determinant of feelings of depression and general distress than are negative social interactions (Okun and Keith, 1998). It is likely that there are complex interactions between the nature of social exchanges and the actual content of those exchanges and their effects on mental health and well-being, and only a few studies have begun to specifically address these complexities (Liang et al., 2001). Although little is known about whether negative social interactions have consequences for physical health outcomes, disability, and cognitive decline, evidence in favor of this view is growing (Rook, 1984). Some studies have found that negative interactions are more powerful predictors of mental health outcomes than are positive interactions and ties (Finch, Okun, Barrera, Zautra, and Reich, 1989; Finch and Zautra, 1992). Negative interactions and burdensome obligations are more strongly associated with family ties (Morgan, 1989), suggesting that racial/ethnic groups that have a higher proportion of kinship-based ties may experience more negative interactions.

Role of Social and Personal Resources in Health Disparities in the Elderly

The evidence reviewed thus far suggests that social and personal resources play an important if still poorly understood role in the health and well-being of older adults. Compared to the considerable interest this topic has generated, remarkably little effort has been directed at exploring the degree to which these resources contribute to ethnic disparities in late-life health. There may be two reasons for this relative lack of interest. First, most investigations have been focused on the differential distributions in socioeconomic resources as a primary determinant of ethnic differences in late-life health (e.g., Guralnik, Land, Blazer, Fillenbaum, and Branch, 1993; Peek, Coward, Henretta, Duncan, and Dougherty, 1997). In other words, it is often believed that socioeconomic resources are a sufficient explanation for ethnic disparities in health, which may have suppressed attempts to identify additional explanations for racial/ethnic disparities in health. Second, the lack of clear evidence for substantial differences in resources between racial and ethnic subpopulations may have discouraged researchers from examining their role in ethnic disparities in late-life health.

Investigation of the role of social and personal resources to health disparities may be formulated in two ways. One approach would consist of testing the degree to which resources that are less available among those at a health disadvantage account for such health disparities. A second approach would be to test the degree to which resources affect health outcomes differentially across racial/ethnic groups, regardless of differences in distribution. That is, some resources may confer fewer health benefits in subpopulations that are at greater health risks, and hence contribute to observed health disparities between groups. Perhaps partly due to the lack of clear differences in resources among racial/ethnic groups, most studies have followed the second approach by examining the relative health effects of particular social or personal resources in different racial/ethnic groups.

A number of studies have focused on the differential role of religious involvement across racial/ethnic subpopulations, particularly African Americans and non-Hispanic whites. In an 8-year follow-up study of a nationally representative sample of the U.S. adult population, Hummer and colleagues found that blacks had a more than 50 percent higher risk of dying compared with nonblacks, after accounting for church attendance and basic sociodemographic variables (Hummer et al., 1999). No data for mortality risk among blacks before adjustment for church attendance were given, so the degree to which church attendance accounted for any excess risk among blacks is unclear. The same analysis does reveal, however, that crude measures of social networks and social engagement did not alter the estimated relative mortality risk among blacks, suggesting that these resources do not account for any excess risk in the black adult population.

Another study focused on the beneficial health effects of private religiosity, and found that this aspect of religious involvement was associated with significantly reduced blood pressure levels among African Americans, but not among whites (Steffen, Hinderliter, Blumenthal, and Sherwood, 2001). However, other studies show a more complex picture for the differential health benefits of religious involvement across race. For example, using data from the North Carolina EPESE study, Ellison found that lack of a formal religious affiliation was associated with more depression among blacks, but not whites. This is consistent with the notion that religious involvement may have greater health benefits for blacks than whites. However, he also found that public religiosity, or church attendance, attenuated levels of depression among whites, but not among blacks. Furthermore, private religiosity was associated with higher levels of depression in both racial groups (Ellison, 1995). This latter finding appears inconsistent with an analysis from the same data set, which showed that private religiosity was positively associated with self-rated health. This effect was stronger among blacks than whites, although the difference in effect was not statistically significant (Musick, 1996). Musick also reported from the same study that public religiosity was associated prospectively with a decrease in depressive symptoms among blacks with cancer, but not whites (Musick, Koenig, Hays, and Cohen, 1998).

Taken together, some of this research is consistent with the possibility that religious involvement may confer greater health benefits for older blacks than whites. However, given the paucity of studies in this area, and some of the conflicting findings, it would be premature to state that religious involvement plays an important role in racial/ethnic disparities in late-life health. Moreover, the literature summarized earlier in this chapter suggests that older blacks have higher levels of religious involvement. Thus, to the degree that this resource is protective against adverse health outcomes, it might, if anything, suppress health differences between blacks and whites that otherwise would have been even larger.

Data from several other studies allow for some inferences regarding the role of other social factors and personal resources in racial/ethnic disparities among the elderly. In their study of living arrangements and health, Waite and Hughes showed that the health disadvantages among older Hispanics and blacks were reduced after accounting for a series of indicators representing socioeconomic resources and personal network ties (Waite and Hughes, 1999). The combined influence of these indicators appeared to account for more of the health disadvantages among Hispanics than blacks. In addition, these factors were less strongly associated with health differentials in self-rated health, mobility, and cognitive status than they were for emotional health and depression. It was unclear from their analysis whether most of the reduction in health differentials was due to the influence of socioeconomic resources, of network ties, or a combination of the two. Another study suggests, however, that socioeconomic resources may be more important, as racial differences in distress were eliminated after accounting for SES-related variables, whereas social support did not seem to mediate this relationship (Kubzansky, Berkman, and Seeman, 2000).

Other studies have focused on the relative potency of the health benefits of social supports across different racial/ethnic groups. For example, in the Evans County study, Blazer and colleagues noted that social integration had a much stronger protective effect with regard to 3-year mortality risk among whites compared with blacks (Blazer, 1982). In contrast, no such differential effect by race was found for social network ties in a longitudinal analysis of changes in disability in the North Carolina EPESE cohort. There was a suggestion, however, that the adverse effect of instrumental support, described previously in this chapter, was weaker among older blacks than it was among whites. A possible interpretation for this finding is that receiving assistance with daily chores might be more normative in black families and communities, and may therefore be less an indication of dependency (Mendes de Leon et al., 2001).

Data from the New Haven and North Carolina EPESE studies afford another opportunity to evaluate the effect of personal resources on racial differences in late-life health. In this analysis, we examine the effect of social engagement on racial differences in physical disability. Disability is often used as an indicator of overall health status in populations over the age of 65. Previous analyses of these data have noted important differences in disability between blacks and whites (Mendes de Leon et al., 1995, 1997). Each study contains slightly different measures of social engagement. In the New Haven EPESE study, assessment of social engagement is based on a series of questions about social and productive activities that are common among older people, such as doing volunteer work, going to museums or concerts, or going on overnight trips (see Glass et al., 1999). In the North Carolina EPESE study, a measure of social engagement is constructed based on either visual or telephone contact with friends and relatives, as well as participation in formal or informal groups/organizations (see Mendes de Leon et al., 2001). Two measures of physical disability are used in the analysis. The first measure is an index based on six Activities of Daily Living (ADLs), representing the number of basic ADL tasks (dressing, bathing, walking across a room) a person can do without help from another person or device (Jette and Branch, 1981). The second is a three-item measure of overall mobility and strength (walking stairs, walking half a mile, and doing heavy household work), based on the work by Rosow and Breslau (1966). For both measures, higher scores mean better function, or less disability. A total of nine waves of yearly disability data were available in the New Haven EPESE cohort, and seven waves in the North Carolina EPESE cohort. Generalized Estimating Equations were fitted to model disability data across follow-up, using a logistic link function and binomial error structure. For the purpose of this analysis, we compare the influence of social engagement and of socioeconomic status on racial differences in disability, controlling for the effects of age, sex, and follow-up time. Socioeconomic status is represented by indicators of education (years of formal schooling) and income level.

As shown in Table 10-2, blacks had significantly higher disability levels, as indicated by the negative regression coefficients, on each measure of disability. This effect represents the difference in disability level between blacks and whites averaged across all yearly assessments in each data set. The effect was consistent across the two sites, although racial differences in ADL disability were only marginally significant in the North Carolina data. Social engagement accounted for part of the racial heterogeneity in disability in the New Haven cohort, reducing the size of racial differences in disability by about 30 percent. No further reduction was seen after adjustment for indicators of SES in this population. In the North Carolina cohort, social engagement appeared to account for only a small part of the racial heterogeneity in disability which proves to be due mostly to factors related

TABLE 10-2 Black-White Differences in ADL and Mobility/Strength Disability: The New Haven and North Carolina EPESE Studies

	ADL Disability		Mobility/Strength Disability	
	New Haven	EPESE		
	Beta[a] (se)	p-value	Beta (se)	p-value
Main race effect	−0.44 (0.16)	0.007	−0.41 (0.12)	0.001
Race effect modified by:				
Social engagement	−0.32 (0.15)	0.04	−0.27 (0.11)	0.02
Social engagement and SES	−0.32 (0.15)	0.04	−0.18 (0.11)	0.11
	North Carolina	EPESE		
Main race effect	−0.16 (0.08)	0.06	−0.26 (0.05)	0.001
Race effect modified by:				
Social engagement	−0.13 (0.08)	0.13	−0.24 (0.06)	0.001
Social engagement and SES	0.10 (0.09)	0.24	0.15 (0.06)	0.02

[a]All betas adjusted for the effects of age, sex, and follow-up time.

to socioeconomic status in this population. The inconsistency in findings across these two studies may be partly because of differences in social engagement measures. Overall, however, these findings raise the possibility that differential distribution of social resources contribute to black-white differences in disability among older adults, although the magnitude of this contribution may vary across geographically defined populations.

FUTURE DIRECTIONS: TOWARD ELIMINATION OF RACIAL/ETHNIC DISPARITIES RELATED TO SOCIAL AND PERSONAL RESOURCES

Possible Mechanisms Linking Social and Personal Resources to Late-Life Health

The mechanisms through which personal and social resources affect health and well-being in older adults are complex and, for the most part still poorly understood. Increasingly, the field has moved away from documenting racial and ethnic disparities in health outcomes to a search for a deeper level of understanding of these mechanisms. In the conceptual model presented earlier, we argue in favor of several possible mechanisms that might account for the relationships of interest. We will summarize briefly the empirical research that supports these arguments.

One of the ways in which social resources may influence health is through multiple system activation, or "use-it-or-lose-it." The positive health consequences of physical activity are beyond dispute. Many studies show that blacks engage in lower levels of physical exercise compared with whites (for a review, see King et al., 1992). However, it is equally clear that individual predictors of levels of physical activity are unable to explain patterns of activity across racial groups and across the life course. The consistent finding across many studies that blacks report lower levels of exercise independent of education and earnings suggests that race is not an adequate control variable for the association between socioeconomic status and physical activity. Other factors such as availability of family support (Rakowski, Julius, Hickey, and Halter, 1987), neighborhood physical barriers (Ross, 1993, 2000), and low mastery (Emery and Gatz, 1990; Glass et al., 1995) must be considered.

Several psychosocial mechanisms appear to be important. For example, self-efficacy beliefs have been shown to be associated with a variety of health and functional outcomes in older adults (Grembowski et al., 1993; McAuley, 1993; Mendes de Leon, Seeman, Baker, Richardson, and Tinetti, 1996; Seeman, Rodin, and Albert, 1993b; Tinetti and Powell, 1993). The association between social networks and health-promoting behavior such as exercise also has been shown to be mediated through self-efficacy (Duncan and McAuley, 1993). Work by McAvay, Seeman, and Rodin

(1996) suggests that ongoing social network contact has a reciprocal influence on the maintenance of self-efficacy. In addition, evidence suggests that social support promotes functional and adaptive coping styles (Holahan and Moos, 1987; Wolf et al., 1991). An influential study by Dunkel-Schetter, Folkman, and Lazarus (1987) has shown, however, that these relationships are also likely to be reciprocal. Their evidence suggests that in stressful situations, different coping styles elicit different responses from the social environment.

Social and personal resources may additionally operate by affecting life stress, which in turn has been shown to affect emotion, mood, and perceived well-being. Numerous studies have shown that social support alters the consequences of life stress on mental health outcomes (Bowling and Browne, 1991; Holahan, Moos, Holahan, and Brennan, 1995, 1997; Lin and Dean, 1984; Matt and Dean, 1993; Morris, Robinson, Raphael, and Bishop, 1991). As mentioned previously, social support, especially perceived emotional support, may buffer the deleterious influences of stressful life events on depression (Lin, Dean, and Ensel, 1986; Paykel, 1994; Vilhjalmsson, 1993). Social support has also been shown to buffer life stress and cardiovascular reactivity in minority groups (Kamarck et al., 1998; Strogatz et al., 1997).

Lin and Ensel have completed a series of important studies of two sets of personal resources, personal (e.g., mastery and self-esteem) and social (e.g., integration and social support) resources and how these factors modulate stress over the life course (Ensel and Lin, 1991). This model builds a compelling case that the mechanisms that we list in our conceptual model interact in important and synergistic ways over the life course. In more recent work, Ensel and colleagues (1996) have extended their life stress paradigm to late life, finding evidence that distal or lagged stressors (15 years) show persistent effects on physical symptoms and that social and psychological resources tend to mediate these associations.

Important advances also have been made in our understanding of the physiological mechanisms that mediate the effect of social structural conditions and personal resources on health outcomes. For example, there is reasonable evidence that lack of social support and disruptive social relationships may be linked to altered or maladaptive responses in a variety of physiological systems, including the cardiovascular system, immune system, and endocrine function (Seeman and McEwen, 1996; Seeman, Berkman, Blazer, and Rowe, 1994; Uchino, Cacioppo, and Keicolt-Glaser, 1996). More recent work has started to focus on allostatic load as a marker of the cumulative physiological burden due to the stress resulting from the organism's efforts to adapt to external challenges. Allostatic load is believed to consist of ten individual biological markers reflecting functioning of the hypothalamic-pituitary axis (HPA), the sympathetic nervous system, the cardiovascular system, and metabolic processes (McEwen, 1998; Seeman, McEwen, Rowe, and Singer, 2001b). Allostatic load has been found to be significantly predictive of a variety of health outcomes among the elderly, including overall mortality, incident cardiovascular disease, and change in physical and cognitive function (Seeman and McEwen, 1996; Seeman et al., 2001b). Based on these initial results, allostatic load, or some of its individual components, may provide an opportunity to more directly examine the stress-related pathways by which deprivation in social and personal resources causes physiological responses that increase vulnerability to disease and death.

In addition to personal networks, the characteristics of community networks (or in urban settings, neighborhood characteristics) have received some attention. Glass and Balfour (2003) recently reviewed the literature on neighborhood influences on aging and found increasing evidence that various contextual factors are associated with risk of disability (Balfour and Kaplan, 2002; Clark and Davies, 1990), fear of crime (Ferraro, 1995; Jeffords, 1983; Joseph, 1997; Perkins, Meeks, and Taylor, 1992; Ross and Jang, 2000), and general well-being (Krause, 1996; Malmstrom, Sundquist, and Johansson, 1999; Robert and Li, 2001; Ross and Mirowsky, 2001). The mechanisms through which neighborhood features affect health in older adults are not yet clear. However, evidence suggests that much of the deleterious effect of neighborhood disorder may be mediated by fear of crime (LaGrange, Ferraro, and Supancic, 1992; Ross and Jang, 2000; Ross and Mirowsky, 2001). This provides an important clue because older persons who perceive barriers to venturing outside the home may suffer the effects of disuse atrophy disproportionately. Grzywacz and Marks (2001) present data from the National Survey of Midlife Development in the U.S., showing that a variety of contextual factors, including living in an unsafe neighborhood, explained differential participation in regular physical exercise. Neighborhood safety predicted exercise behavior independent of individual health and SES, and helped to explain the persistent pattern of lower levels of exercise in blacks compared to nonblacks. It is too early to know if higher rates of physical disability in minority groups are a function of living in more unsafe or disordered neighborhoods, but fear of crime is clearly an important mediator.

Social disorganization in the environment can increase the chances of negative behaviors and can undermine the protective effects of personal resources. For example, Boardman, Finch, Ellison, Williams, and Jackson (2001) found that social stress increases the likelihood of drug use, and that this association is further mediated by neighborhood disadvantage. To the extent that stress and distress mediate the association between neighborhood factors and risky behaviors, the differential patterns of substance abuse in minority groups may be rooted in the social ecology of life stress.

Evidence Regarding Interventions

Intervention approaches to boost or enhance social and personal resources are just beginning to be developed and tested. In a review of the literature on psychosocial intervention, Glass (2000) identified 15 randomized trials of interventions designed to modify or improve some aspect of social integration (social support, social networks, or social cohesion). Conceptual models and intervention methodologies to optimize personal and psychosocial resources have been developed by Gottlieb (1985, 1988, 1992). These approaches emphasize the mobilization of mutual aid and self-help within naturally occurring networks that can optimize psychosocial resources brought to bear to solve particular adaptive challenges. This approach has led to intervention models designed to improve access to transportation (Glasgow, 2000), Alzheimer's disease (Pillemer, Suitor, Landreneau, Henderson, and Brangman, 2000), and recovery from stroke (Glass et al., 2000). In practice, however, this type of research is exceptionally difficult to undertake. The majority of these studies have failed to find evidence that interventions targeting social integration lead to health improvements. What has been demonstrated repeatedly is that adding a social support component to health education interventions leads to enhanced benefits on a variety of outcomes (Evans, Matlock, Bishop, Stranahan, and Pederson, 1988; Gilden, Hendryx, Clar, Casia, and Singh, 1992).

There have been few social support interventions specifically targeted at older adults. Several studies have focused on caregivers of patients with Alzheimer's disease, with the objective of developing strategies to improve social resources available to caregivers and patients (Bourgeois, Schultz, and Burgio, 1996; Pillemer et al., 2000). There are also a series of "friendly-neighbor-visitation" interventions based on a combined peer-support and social network approach (Biegel, Shore, and Gordon, 1984). Interventions such as these that approach social resources from an ecological viewpoint are even more rare. A welcome and noteworthy exception is the Cornell Retirees Volunteering in Service Program (Moen, Fields, Meador, and Rosenblatt, 2000). That model shows how interventions designed to improve personal resources can be framed within a life-course developmental perspective in which purposeful and productive activity is the goal of the intervention (rather than provision of services to address the "needs" of older persons) and health promotion is a secondary consequence.

Important Gaps and Methodological Challenges

A number of important limitations in the extant literature prevent a better understanding of the potential role of social and personal resources with regard to racial/ethnic disparities in late-life health. One limitation is that the nature and magnitude of the racial and ethnic differences in social and personal resources in older populations remain poorly understood. This may be due in part to the frequent use of brief, atheoretical measures, especially in epidemiologic research (Glass et al., 1997). Related to this issue is that measures of social and personal resources are often not sufficiently informed by the race- or ethnicity-specific contexts in which these social structures and resources exist. In other words, standardized measures may fail to adequately capture aspects of these resources that may have particular relevance for specific minority groups. For example, there may be important differences in terms of the cultural or familial expectations for assistance and care when persons are disabled (Lee et al., 1998; Tennstedt and Chang, 1998), and the particular meaning that is attached to the receipt of such assistance within different ethnic/racial communities (Groger and Kunkel, 1995).

Another important limitation is the lack of information on the social and personal resources in racial and ethnic groups other than non-Hispanic white and African American. There is an emerging literature on the social network and support structures of the Hispanic (Baxter et al., 1998) and Asian (Ishii-Kuntz, 1997) elderly, but clearly, more efforts are needed to describe the resources available to older adults in these and other minority populations. In addition, only recently have studies begun to explore the neighborhood social contexts of older adults. One issue that has challenged this research is that it remains unclear whether it is best to study the objective characteristics of places, such as those reflected in census data, or to study resident perceptions of the ecological conditions. The best available data on this question come from Perkins and Taylor (1996), who assessed three methods of measuring community disorder (resident surveys, on-site trained observers, and news media) and concluded that each was equally predictive of fear of crime. Many other critical issues remain untapped with regard to neighborhood contexts. For example, how should neighborhood areas be defined, and what are the essential physical and social characteristics of neighborhoods that affect the daily lives of older adults? An equally important issue is to examine the degree to which neighborhood contexts and personal social networks are interlinked, and to explore the processes by which they, in conjunction with one another, facilitate access to personal resources of particular relevance to older adults. Furthermore, do these linkages and processes show differences among various racial/ethnic groups?

Another issue that deserves further inquiry is the mechanisms by which social and personal resources affect late-life health. A potentially fruitful area in this regard is the extent to which minority health is related to higher levels of life stress. However, few studies have addressed the question of whether life stress is associated with accelerated aging in minority groups.

Animal research provides clues that it might be so. The work of Shively and colleagues (Shively, 1998; Shively and Clarkson, 1994; Shively, Laber-Laird, and Anton, 1997) on social stress and cardiovascular disease in cynomolgus monkeys has demonstrated conclusively that subordination among social primates pays a considerable price on the organism. This finding is suggested also by Sapolsky, Alberts, and Altman (1997) in their studies of wild baboons. Both sets of investigations lay the groundwork for the study of life stress as a consequence of subordination to dominant groups as well as the potential role of social resources in buffering the deleterious effects of that stress. To date, few studies have looked specifically at this issue in older adults (for exceptions, see Jackson et al., 1996).

In addition, more work is needed to increase our understanding of the physiological processes by which social and personal resources affect health. While initial studies in this area suggest that these resources may be linked with neuroendocrine regulation and allostatic load in the elderly (Seeman and McEwan, 1996; Seeman et al., 2001b), few studies to date have specifically sought to assess the impact of social and personal resources on these physiological processes. Even less is known about the degree to which these mechanisms differ across racial or ethnic groups. One question of potential relevance in this regard would be to examine whether certain minority groups show greater adverse responses in neuroendocrine function or allostatic load due to deprivation in social and personal resources, possibly because the burden of lacking adequate resources has accumulated to a much greater degree during the life course than in more advantaged population groups.

A number of methodological challenges also need to be addressed in order to overcome some of the limitations of previous studies in this area. One of the limitations in this research is that much of the information has come from epidemiologic studies of defined cohorts, usually defined on the basis of geographic location. Examples of such research include the EPESE and Alameda County studies. Such studies offer certain methodological advantages that allow for frequent and intense follow-up, as well as the collection of more detailed health information, which often requires the collection of data from multiple sources such as individual participants, hospitals, and nursing homes. However, these advantages are partly offset by the fact that they focus on very local populations, whose experience may be unique to a small geographic area and not representative of that of the national population. Thus, future research would do well to address the role of social and personal resources in ethnic disparities in late-life health at a national level, perhaps by linking more detailed and sensitive social and/or health information into ongoing panel studies of nationally representative samples. Similarly, it might prove fruitful to coordinate such studies across nations, for example, by matching, where possible, designs and measures in studies conducted in different countries.

There is also an urgent need for more studies with longitudinal or panel designs for several other reasons. First of all, many age-related health outcomes, such as changes in physical function and disability and cognitive decline, tend to progress slowly over time. Only longitudinal study designs with repeated assessments across longer periods of time will enable researchers to characterize these changes with sufficient precision to differentiate the variable trajectories of decline and/or improvement among older adults. Moreover, studies using such designs suggest that the interrelationships between personal resources and late-life health are more complex than simple, unidirectional causal effects, and likely involve reciprocal mechanisms of causation (Mendes de Leon et al., 2001; Verbrugge, Reoma, and Gruber-Baldini, 1994). Such patterns of association are also more consistent with some of the processes that have been proposed to explain the relationship between social and personal resources and late-life health, such as the "use-it-or-lose-it" mechanism. A better understanding of these processes and pathways will depend on studies that move away from more traditional analytic methods that are based primarily on modeling incident outcome events, and rather use approaches that begin to describe the complex interplays between these processes as they evolve over time.

Another issue of concern is that little information is available on how the observed health benefits due to social and personal resources can be translated into more effective interventions. As summarized in the previous section, there has been limited systematic study of the efficacy of interventions aimed at bolstering these resources. In fact, an argument can be made that the "technology" to produce change in these areas is still largely absent. Some recent developments, especially those targeted at caregivers of patients with Alzheimer's disease, have shown some promise. It is likely, however, that a combination of public policy strategies and interventions targeted at individuals is going to be required to maximize the availability and health efficacy of social and personal resources among older adults.

Finally, a better understanding of the role of social and personal resources in racial/ethnic disparities in late-life health will require more attention to a life-course approach. Most health disparities are clearly present at the time adults enter old age. In fact, it may be that for some health outcomes such as mortality and physical disability, health disparities do not continue to increase in old age, usually defined as beginning at age 65 (Corti et al., 1999; Mendes de Leon et al., 1997; Sorlie, Backlund, and Keller, 1995). This raises the possibility that the actual contribution of social and personal resources to racial/ethnic disparities in health is materialized mostly before adults reach the age of 65. Evidence in support of this notion comes from work on the influence of socioeconomic deprivation during childhood and adulthood on late-life health outcomes (Kaplan et al., 2001; Lynch, Kaplan, and Shema, 1997; Turrell et al., 2002). Other studies point to the fact that measures of social and community cohesion, as well as the availability of social support at the individual level, are unequally distributed across different socioeconomic strata (Kawachi, Kennedy, Lochner, and Prothrow-Stith, 1997; Kawachi, Kennedy, and Glass, 1999; Sampson, Raudenbush, and Earls, 1997; Turner and Marino, 1994; Turrell et al., 2002).

Taken together, these findings suggest that differences in social and personal resources over the life course, rather than old age itself, may be responsible in part for the racial/ethnic disparities in health observed among the elderly. In fact, communities may construct or organize social structures and personal resources among members partly in response to health disadvantages accumulated throughout life. Some evidence indicates that the church plays such a role in African-American communities (Taylor and Chatters, 1986a, 1986b). Perhaps a similar argument applies to the denser family and intergenerational support networks that have been observed in groups with greater health disparities (Ajrouch et al., 2001; Baxter et al., 1998).

SUMMARY AND CONCLUSIONS

As described in Chapter 2, health disparities in the American society continue into old age, and affect minority populations across a variety of health outcomes that have particular relevance for older adults. In this chapter, we considered the role of social and personal resources and their contribution to health disparities among the elderly. Toward that end, we first presented a framework to describe the substantial gerontologic and social-epidemiologic literature on the availability of these resources among older adults, and the empirical evidence concerning their relationship to late-life health. Overall, the research in this area has produced a number of key findings that have led to important gains in our understanding of the role of these resources in late-life health.

First, the social resources of older persons show important linkages with health and well-being. There is now reasonably consistent evidence that social ties are associated with prolonged survival, and a decreased risk for physical disability and cognitive decline. Much of the evidence in support of these relationships comes from rigorous, longitudinal studies, with careful control for the potentially confounding influences of age, socioeconomic status, and health-related and lifestyle factors. While the health benefits of social networks have been recognized previously for the overall adult population (House et al., 1988), it has now become clear that these benefits also apply to the oldest segments of the adult population. Although less well established, initial studies of community networks suggest that they may be involved in long-term changes in late-life health as well. In view of this evidence, more recent research has begun to explore the complex behavioral, psychological, and neuroimmunological pathways that may mediate the relationship between social networks and health outcomes. It is possible that some of the health benefits due to social networks are not merely the result of having larger social networks, but may include the effect of social engagement as well, due to the use of composite measures of social networks and engagement in epidemiologic research. More recent evidence suggests, however, that various forms of social engagement, such as social activity, productive activity, and religious participation provide long-term health benefits to older adults in their own right, given their prospective associations with mortality, physical disability, and cognitive decline.

Second, most evidence indicates that social support confers a health benefit that is quite distinct from the benefits due to social network ties and social engagement. Social support does not seem to provide a long-term health advantage. In fact, some forms of social support, particularly instrumental support, may increase health risks among the elderly. On the other hand, social support has been shown to provide a clear benefit to older adults recovering from episodes of acute illness. There is a suggestion, however, that large amounts of support may not be any better, and may be worse, during recovery than moderate amounts of support. Social support is also thought to lead to improved mental health and well-being, although recent work has begun to uncover some of the complexities involved in the psychological effects of receiving and providing support, as well as the effects of positive and negative social interactions more generally.

Third, the evidence to date indicates that the distribution of social and personal resources does not differ substantially by racial/ethnic groups. Although the composition of the social networks among minority elders tends to favor extended family ties compared with older whites, there are few differences in actual availability of ties between groups. There may be more important racial/ethnic differences in community networks, although few data are available that specifically focus on these types of networks in the elderly. Similarly, there appear to be few differences in personal resources between older adults of various subpopulations, although again, the actual forms of social engagement, and social support may differ from one group to the other. Reasonably solid evidence suggests that older blacks engage more in religious activity, whereas older whites may be more actively involved in other formal organizations and volunteering. In addition, there may be more active and more frequent exchanges in supportive resources in black communities than in white communities.

Finally, there is little evidence to date that these resources play a major role in producing health disparities in older age. However, this conclusion must be tempered by the fact that there has been little systematic research of this issue. Although a few studies suggest that these factors contribute to health disparities in the elderly, the overall findings have been very mixed. Few consistent patterns have emerged from either previously published studies or our own analysis of this issue. As mentioned previously in this chapter, the lack of more systematic research may be due to either the emphasis on socioeconomic resources as major determinants of ethnic/racial disparities in late-life health, or the lack of clearer differences in social and personal resources across racial/ethnic groups of older adults.

We have also identified new directions that may lead to a better understanding of the contribution of social and personal resources in racial/ethnic disparities in late-life health. A potentially fruitful area of investigation in this regard includes a greater emphasis on a life-course approach, examining the dynamics and ecology of the social structures and personal resources as they evolve in specific racial and ethnic populations throughout adulthood, and possibly even earlier. In addition, more effort is needed to describe the role of social and personal resources in health disparities at the national and international levels. This should also include a better representation of subpopulations that have received relatively little attention thus far. Finally, we advocate that more serious consideration is given to the complexity of the interrelationships between resources and age-related changes in health, instead of the relatively crude causal mechanisms in which the health effects of these resources are usually conceptualized. Clearly, such research has to be informed by continuing efforts to identify the psychological, behavioral, and physiological mechanisms that link personal resources to health and well-being. Such an agenda may provide the foundation necessary to achieve more progress toward the elimination of racial/ethnic disparities in late-life health.

ACKNOWLEDGMENT

Work on this chapter was supported by the National Institute of Environmental Health Sciences grant R01-ES10902.

REFERENCES

Ajrouch, K.J., Antonucci, T.C., and Janevic, M.R. (2001). Social networks among blacks and whites: The interaction between race and age. *Journal of Gerontology: Series B: Psychological Sciences and Social Sciences, 56,* 112-128.

Antonucci, T., and Akiyama, H. (1987). Social networks in adult life and a preliminary examination of the convoy model. *Journal of Gerontology, 42,* 519-527.

Antonucci, T.C., Jackson, J.S., Gibson, R.C., and Herzog, A.R. (1989). *Age, gender, race, and productive activity across the life span.* Muncie, IN: Ball State University.

Atienza, A.A., Collins, R., and King, A.C. (2001). The mediating effects of situational control on social support and mood following a stressor: A prospective study of dementia caregivers in their natural environments. *Journal of Gerontology: Series B: Psychological Sciences and Social Sciences, 56,* S129-S139.

Balfour, J.L., and Kaplan, G.A. (2002). Neighborhood environment and loss of physical function in older adults: Prospective evidence from the Alameda County Study. *American Journal of Epidemiology, 155,* 507-515.

Ball, R., Warheit, G., Vandiver, J., and Holzer, C. (1980). Friendship networks: More supportive of low income black women? *Ethnicity, 7,* 70-77.

Baltes, M.M., and Lang, F.R. (1997). Everyday functioning and successful aging: The impact of resources. *Psychology and Aging, 12,* 433-443.

Bassuk, S.S., Glass, T.A., and Berkman, L.F. (1999). Social disengagement and incident cognitive decline in community-dwelling elderly persons. *Annals of Internal Medicine, 131,* 165-173.

Baxter, J., Shetterly, S.M., Eby, C., Mason, L., Cortese, C.F., and Hamman, R.F. (1998). Social network factors associated with perceived quality of life. *Journal of Aging and Health, 10,* 287-310.

Berger, P., and Neuhaus, R. (1977). *To empower people: The role of mediating institutions.* Washington, DC: American Enterprise Institute for Public Policy Research.

Berkman, L.F., and Syme, S.L. (1979). Social networks, host resistance, and mortality: A nine-year follow-up study of Alameda County residents. *American Journal of Epidemiology, 109,* 186-204.

Berkman, L.F., Leo-Summers, L., and Horwitz, R.I. (1992). Emotional support and survival after myocardial infarction: A prospective, population-based study of the elderly. *Annals of Internal Medicine, 117,* 1003-1009.

Biegel, D.E., Shore, B.K., and Gordon, E. (1984). *Building support networks for the elderly: Theory and applications.* Beverly Hills, CA: Sage.

Blair, S.N., Kampert, J.B., Kohl, H.W., III, Barlow, C.E., Macera, C.A., Paffenbarger, R.S., Jr., et al. (1996). Influences of cardiorespiratory fitness and other precursors on cardiovascular disease and all-cause mortality in men and women. *Journal of American Medical Association, 276,* 205-210.

Blazer, D.G. (1982). Social support and mortality in an elderly community population. *American Journal of Epidemiology, 115,* 684-694.

Boardman, J.D., Finch, B.K., Ellison, C.G., Williams, D.R., and Jackson, J.S. (2001). Neighborhood disadvantage, stress, and drug use among adults. *Journal of Health and Social Behavior, 42,* 151-165.

Boult, C., Kane, R.L., Louis, T.A., Boult, L., and McCaffrey, D. (1994). Chronic conditions that lead to functional limitation in the elderly. *Journal of Gerontology, 49,* M28-M36.

Bourgeois, M.S., Schulz, R., and Burgio, L. (1996). Interventions for caregivers of patients with Alzheimer's disease: A review and analysis of content, process, and outcomes. *International Journal of Aging and Human Development, 43,* 35-92.

Bowling, A., and Browne, P.D. (1991). Social networks, health, and emotional well-being among the oldest old in London. *Journal of Gerontology, 46,* S20-S32.

Burton, L., Kasper, J., Shore, A., Cagney, K., LaVeist, T., Cubbin, C., et al. (1995). The structure of informal care: Are there differences by race? *The Gerontologist, 35,* 744-752.

Bygren, L.O., Konlaan, B.B., and Johansson, S.E. (1996). Attendance at cultural events, reading books or periodicals, and making music or singing in a choir as determinants for survival: Swedish interview survey of living conditions. *British Medical Journal, 313,* 1577-1580.

Cantor, M.H. (1975). Life space and the social support system of the inner-city elderly of New York. *Gerontologist, 15,* 23-26.

Cantor, M.H., Brennan, M., and Sainz, A. (1994). The importance of ethnicity in the social support systems of older New Yorkers: A longitudinal perspective (1970-1990). *Journal of Gerontological Social Work, 22,* 95-128.

Carstensen, L.L. (1995). Evidence for a life-span theory of socioemotional selectivity. *Current Directions in Psychological Science, 4,* 151-156.

Case, R.B., Moss, A.J., Case, N., McDermott, M., and Eberly, S. (1992). Living alone after myocardial infarction: Impact on prognosis. *Journal of American Medical Association, 267,* 515-519.

Chatters, L.M. (2000). Religion and health: Public health research and practice. *Annual Review of Public Health, 21,* 335-367.

Chatters, L.M., and Taylor, R.J. (1994). Religious involvement among older African Americans. In J.S. Levin (Ed.), *Religion in aging and health: Theoretical foundations and methodological frontiers* (pp. 196-230). Thousand Oaks, CA: Sage.

Chatters, L.M., Taylor, R.J., and Jackson, J.S. (1985). Aged black's nominations to an informal helper network. *Journal of Gerontology, 41,* 94-100.

Clark, W.A., and Davies, S. (1990). Elderly mobility and mobility outcomes: Households in the later stage of the life course. *Research on Aging, 12,* 430-462.

Corti, M.C., Guralnik, J.M., Ferrucci, L., Izmirlian, G., Leveille, S.G., Pahor, M., et al. (1999). Evidence for a black-white crossover in all-cause and coronary heart disease mortality in an older population: The North Carolina EPESE. *American Journal of Public Health, 89,* 308-314.

Cutler, S.J. (1977). Aging and voluntary association participation. *Journal of Gerontology, 32,* 470-479.

Cutler, S.J., and Hendricks, J. (2000). Age differences in voluntary association memberships: Fact or artifact. *Journals of Gerontology: Series B: Psychological Sciences and Social Sciences, 55,* 98-107.

Danigelis, N.L., and McIntosh, B.R. (1993). Resources and the productive activity of elders: Race and gender as contexts. *Journal of Gerontology, 48,* S192-S203.

Davey, A., and Eggebeen, D.J. (1998). Patterns of intergenerational exchange and mental health. *Journals of Gerontology: Series B: Psychological Sciences and Social Sciences, 53,* 86-95.

Deimling, G., Harel, Z., and Noelker, L. (1983). Racial differences in social integration and life satisfaction among aged public housing residents. *International Journal of Aging and Human Development, 17,* 203-12.

Duncan, T.E., and McAuley, E. (1993). Social support and efficacy cognitions in exercise adherence–latent growth curve analysis. *Journal of Behavioral Medicine, 16,* 199-218.

Dunkel-Schetter, C., Folkman, S., and Lazarus, R.S. (1987). Correlates of social support receipt. *Journal of Personality and Social Psychology, 53,* 71-80.

Ellison, C.G. (1995). Race, religious involvement and depressive symptomatology in a southeastern U.S. community. *Social Science and Medicine, 40,* 1561-1572.

Ellison, C.G., and Levin, J.S. (1998). The religion-health connection: Evidence, theory, and future directions. *Health Education and Behavior, 25,* 700-720.

Emery, C.F., and Gatz, M. (1990). Psychological and cognitive effects of an exercise program for community-residing older adults. *Gerontologist, 30,* 184-188.

Ensel, W.M., and Lin, N. (1991). The life stress paradigm and psychological distress. *Journal of Health and Social Behavior, 32,* 321-341.

Ensel, W.M., Peek, M.K., Lin, N., and Lai, G. (1996). Stress in the life course: A life history approach. *Journal of Aging and Health, 8,* 389-416.

Evans, R.L., Matlock, A.-L., Bishop, D.S., Stranahan, S., and Pederson, C. (1988). Family intervention after stroke: Does counseling or education help? *Stroke, 19,* 1243-1249.

Everard, K.M., Lach, H.W., Fisher, E.B., and Baum, M.C. (2000). Relationship of activity and social support to the functional health of older adults. *Journals of Gerontology: Series B: Psychological Sciences and Social Sciences, 55,* S208-S212.

Fabrigoule, C., Letenneur, L., Dartigues, J.F., Zarrouk, M., Commenges, D., and Barberger-Gateau, P. (1995). Social and leisure activities and risk of dementia: A prospective longitudinal study. *Journal of the American Geriatrics Society, 43,* 485-490.

Ferraro, K.F. (1995). *Fear of crime: Interpreting victimization risk.* Albany: State University of New York Press.

Ferraro, K.F., and Farmer, M.M. (1996). Double jeopardy to health hypothesis for African Americans: Analysis and critique. *Journal of Health and Social Behavior, 37,* 27-43.

Field, D., and Minkler, M. (1988). Continuity and change in social support between young-old and old-old or very-old age. *Journal of Gerontology, 43,* 100-106.

Fillenbaum, G.G., Heyman, A., Huber, M.S., Woodbury, M.A., Leiss, J., Schmader, K.E., et al. (1998). The prevalence and 3-year incidence of dementia in older black and white community residents. *Journal of Clinical Epidemiology, 51,* 587-595.

Finch, J., Okun, M., Barrera, M., Jr., Zautra, A., and Reich, J. (1989). Positive and negative social ties among older adults: Measurement models and the prediction of psychological distress and well-being. *American Journal of Community Psychology, 17,* 585-605.

Finch, J.F., and Zautra, A.J. (1992). Testing latent longitudinal models of social ties and depression among the elderly: A comparison of distribution-free and maximum likelihood estimates with nonnormal data. *Psychology and Aging, 7,* 107-118.

Fischer, C.S. (1982). *To dwell among friends: Personal networks in town and city.* Chicago: University of Chicago Press.

Fratiglioni, L., Wang, H.X., Ericsson, K., Maytan, M., and Winblad, B. (2000). Influence of social network on occurrence of dementia: A community-based longitudinal study. *Lancet, 355,* 1315-1319.

Friedland, R.P., Fritsch, T., Smyth, K.A., Koss, E., Lerner, A.J., Chen, C.H., et al., (2001). Patients with Alzheimer's disease have reduced activities in midlife compared with healthy control-group members. *Proceedings of the National Academy of Sciences USA, 98,* 3440-3445.

Froehlich, T.E., Bogardus, S.T., Jr., and Inouye, S.K. (2001). Dementia and race: Are there differences between African Americans and Caucasians? *Journal of the American Geriatrics Society, 49,* 477-484.

Gibson, R., and Jackson, J. (1987). The health, physical functioning, and informal supports of the black elderly. *The Milbank Quarterly, 65*(Suppl. 2), 421-454.

Gilden, J.L., Hendryx, M.S., Clar, S., Casia, C., and Singh, S.P. (1992). Diabetes support groups improve health care of older diabetic patients. *Journal of the American Geriatric Society, 40,* 147-150.

Glasgow, N. (2000). An intervention to improve transportation arrangements. In K. Pillemer, P. Moen, E. Wethington, and N. Glasgow (Eds.), *Social integration in the second half of life* (pp. 231-246). Baltimore: Johns Hopkins University Press.

Glass, T.A. (2000). Psychosocial interventions. In L.F. Berkman and I. Kawachi (Eds.), *Social epidemiology* (pp. 267-305). New York: Oxford University Press.

Glass, T.A. (in press). Successful aging. In R. Tallis and H. Fillit (Eds.), *Brocklehurst's textbook of geriatric medicine and gerontology.* London: Harcourt Health Sciences.

Glass, T.A., and Balfour, J.L. (2003). Neighborhood effects on the health of the elderly. In I. Kawachi and L.F. Berkman (Eds.), *Neighborhoods and health* (pp. 303-334). New York: Oxford University Press.

Glass, T.A., and Maddox, G.L. (1992). The quality and quantity of social support: Stroke recovery as psycho-social transition. *Social Science and Medicine, 34,* 1249-1261.

Glass, T.A., Matchar, D.B., Belyea, M., and Feussner, J.R. (1993). Impact of social support on outcome in first stroke. *Stroke, 24,* 64-70.

Glass, T.A., Seeman, T.E., Herzog, A.R., Kahn, R., and Berkman, L.F. (1995). Change in productive activity in late adulthood: MacArthur Studies of Successful Aging. *Journal of Gerontology: Social Sciences, 50B,* S65-S76.

Glass, T.A., Mendes de Leon, C.F., Seeman, T.E., and Berkman, L.F. (1997). Beyond single indicators of social networks: A LISREL analysis of social ties among the elderly. *Social Science Medicine, 44,* 1503-1517.

Glass, T.A., Mendes de Leon, C.F., Marottoli, R.A., and Berkman, L.F. (1999). Population based study of social and productive activities as predictors of survival among elderly Americans. *British Medical Journal, 319,* 478-483.

Glass, T.A., Dym, B., Greenberg, S., Rintell, D., Roesch, C., and Berkman, L.F. (2000). Psychosocial intervention in stroke: The Families in Recovery from Stroke Trial (FIRST). *American Journal of Orthopsychiatry, 70,* 169-181.

Goodman, A.H. (2000). Why genes don't count (for racial differences in health). *American Journal of Public Health, 90,* 1699-1702.

Gorkin, L., Schron, E., Brooks, M., Wiklund, I., Kellen, J., Verter, J., et al. (1993). Psychosocial Predictors of Mortality in the Cardiac Arrhythmia Suppression Trial-1 (CAST-1). *American Journal of Cardiology, 71,* 263-267.

Gottlieb, B. (1985). Theory into practice: Issues that surface in planning interventions which mobilize support. In I.G. Sarason and B.R. Sarason (Eds.), *Social support: Theory, research, and application* (pp. 417-437). The Hague, Netherlands: Martinus Nijhoff.

Gottlieb, B.H. (1988). *Marshalling social support.* Beverly Hills, CA: Sage.

Gottlieb, B.H. (1992). Quandaries in translating support concepts to intervention. In H.O.F. Veiel and U. Baumann (Eds.), *The meaning and measurement of social support* (pp. 293-309). New York: Hemisphere.

Grembowski, D., Patrick, D., Diehr, P., Durham, M., Beresford, S., Kay, E., et al. (1993). Self-efficacy and health behavior among older adults. *Journal of Health and Social Behavior, 34,* 89-104.

Groger, L., and Kunkel, S. (1995). Aging and exchange: Differences between black and white elders. *Journal of Cross-Cultural Gerontology, 10,* 269-287.

Grzywacz, J.G., and Marks, N.F. (2001). Social inequalities and exercise during adulthood: Toward an ecological perspective. *Journal of Health and Social Behavior, 42,* 202-220.

Guralnik, J., Land, K., Blazer, D., Fillenbaum, G., and Branch, L. (1993). Educational status and active life expectancy among older blacks and whites. *New England Journal of Medicine, 329,* 110-116.

Harris, T., Kovar, M.G., Suzman, R., Kleinman, J.C., and Feldman, J.J. (1989). Longitudinal study of physical ability in the oldest-old. *American Journal of Public Health, 79,* 698-702.

Helm, H.M., Hays, J.C., Flint, E.P., Koenig, H.G., and Blazer, D.G. (2000). Does private religious activity prolong survival? A six-year follow-up study of 3,851 older adults. *Journals of Gerontology: Series A: Biological Sciences and Medical Sciences, 55,* 400-405.

Herzog, A.R., and Morgan, J.N. (1989). *Factors related to productive involvement.* Unpublished manuscript.

Herzog, A.R., and Morgan, J.N. (1992). Age and gender differences in the value of productive activities: Four different approaches. *Research on Aging, 14,* 169-198.

Herzog, A.R., Antonucci, T.C., Jackson, J.S., Kahn, R.L., and Morgan, J.N. (1987, February 14-18). *Productive activities and health over the life course.* Paper presented at the annual meeting of the American Association for the Advancement of Science, Chicago, Illinois.

Herzog, A.R., Kahn, R.L., Morgan, J.N., Jackson, J.S., and Antonucci, T.C. (1989). Age differences in productive activities. *Journal of Gerontology: Social Sciences, 44,* S129-S138.

Herzog, A.R., Franks, M.M., Markus, H.R., and Holmberg, D. (1998). Activities and well-being in older age: Effects of self-concept and educational attainment. *Psychology and Aging, 13,* 179-185.

Holahan, C.J., and Moos, R.H. (1987). Personal and contextual determinants of coping strategies. *Journal of Personality and Social Psychology, 52,* 946-955.

Holahan, C.J., Moos, R.H., Holahan, C.K., and Brennan, P.L. (1995). Social support, coping, and depressive symptoms in a late-middle-aged sample of patients reporting cardiac illness. *Health Psychology, 14,* 152-163.

Holahan, C.J., Moos, R.H., Holahan, C.K., and Brennan, P.L. (1997). Social context, coping strategies, and depressive symptoms: An expanded model with cardiac patients. *Journal of Personality and Social Psychology, 72,* 918-928.

House, J., Robbins, C., and Metzner, H. (1982). The association of social relationships and activities with mortality: Prospective evidence from the Tecumseh Community Health Study. *American Journal of Epidemiology, 116,* 123-140.

House, J., Landis, K., and Umberson, D. (1988). Social relationships and health. *Science, 241,* 540-545.

House, J.S. (1987). Social support and social structure. *Sociological Forum, 2,* 135-146.

Hultsch, D.F., Hammer, M., and Small, B.J. (1993). Age differences in cognitive performance in later life: Relationships to self-reported health and activity life style. *Journal of Gerontology, 48,* 1-11.

Hultsch, D.F., Hertzog, C., Small, B.J., and Dixon, R.A. (1999). Use it or lose it: Engaged lifestyle as a buffer of cognitive decline in aging? *Psychology of Aging, 14,* 245-263.

Hummer, R.A. (1996). Black-white differences in health and mortality: A review and conceptual model. *Sociological Quarterly, 37,* 105-125.

Hummer, R.A., Rogers, R.G., Nam, C.B., and Ellison, C.G. (1999). Religious involvement and U.S. adult mortality. *Demography, 36,* 273-285.

Idler, E.L., and Kasl, S.V. (1997). Religion among disabled and nondisabled persons: Attendance at religious services as a predictor of the course of disability. *Journals of Gerontology: Series B: Psychological Sciences and Social Sciences, 52,* 306-316.

Ingersoll-Dayton, B., Morgan, D., and Antonucci, T. (1997). The effects of positive and negative social exchanges on aging adults. *Journals of Gerontology: Series B: Psychological Sciences and Social Sciences, 52,* 190-199.

Ishii-Kuntz, M. (1997). Intergenerational relationships among Chinese, Japanese, and Korean Americans. *Family Relations: Interdisciplinary Journal of Applied Family Studies, 46,* 23-32.

Jackson, J.S. (2001). Changes over the life course in productive activities. In N. Morrow-Howell, J. Hinterlong, and M. Sherraden (Eds.), *Productive aging: Concepts and challenges* (pp. 214-241). Baltimore: Johns Hopkins University Press.

Jackson, J.S., Brown, T.N., Williams, D.R., Torres, M., Sellers, S.L., and Brown, K. (1996). Racism and the physical and mental health status of African Americans: A thirteen year national panel study. *Ethnicity and Disease, 6,* 132-147.

Jeffords, C.R. (1983). The situational relationship between age and the fear of crime. *International Journal of Aging and Human Development, 17,* 103-111.

Jenkins, C.D., Stanton, B.A., and Jono, R.T. (1994). Quantifying and predicting recovery after heart surgery. *Psychosomatic Medicine, 56,* 203-212.

Jette, A., and Branch, L. (1981). The Framingham Disability Study: Physical disability among the aging. *American Journal of Public Health, 71,* 1211-1216.

Johnson, C., and Barer, B. (1990). Families and networks among older inner-city blacks. *The Gerontologist, 30,* 726-733.

Joseph, J. (1997). Fear of crime among black elderly. *Journal of Black Studies, 27,* 698-717.

Jylha, M., and Aro, S. (1989). Social ties and survival among the elderly in Tampere, Finland. *International Journal of Epidemiology, 18,* 158-164.

Kamarck, T.W., Shiffman, S.M., Smithline, L., Goodie, J.L., Paty, J.A., Gnys, M., et al. (1998). Effects of task strain, social conflict, and emotional activation on ambulatory cardiovascular activity: Daily life consequences of recurring stress in a multiethnic adult sample. *Health Psychology, 17,* 17-29.

Kampert, J.B., Blair, S.N., Barlow, C.E., and Kohl, H.W., III. (1996). Physical activity, physical fitness, and all-cause and cancer mortality: A prospective study of men and women. *Annuals of Epidemiology, 6,* 452-457.

Kaplan, G.A. (1996). People and places: Contrasting perspectives on the association between social class and health. *International Journal of Health Services, 26,* 507-519.

Kaplan, G.A., Seeman, T.E., Cohen, R.D., Knudsen, L.P., and Guralnik, J. (1987). Mortality among the elderly in the Alameda County Study: Behavioral and demographic risk factors. *American Journal of Public Health, 77,* 307-312.

Kaplan, G.A., Strawbridge, W., Cohen, R., and Hungerford, L. (1996). Natural history of leisure-time physical activity and its correlates: Associations with mortality from all causes and cardiovascular disease over 28 years. *American Journal of Epidemiology, 144,* 793-797.

Kaplan, G.A., Turrell, G., Lynch, J.W., Everson, S.A., Helkala, E.L., and Salonen, J.T. (2001). Childhood socioeconomic position and cognitive function in adulthood. *International Journal of Epidemiology, 30,* 256-263.

Kaufman, J.S., and Cooper, R.S. (2001). Commentary: Considerations for use of racial/ethnic classification in etiologic research. *American Journal of Epidemiology, 154,* 291-298.

Kawachi, I., and Kennedy, B.P. (1997). Health and social cohesion: Why care about income inequality? *British Medical Journal, 314,* 1037-1040.

Kawachi, I., Colditz, G., Ascherio, A., Rimm, E., Giovanucci, E., Stampfer, M., et al. (1996). A prospective study of social networks in relation to total mortality and cardiovascular disease in men in the USA. *Journal of Epidemiology and Community Health, 50,* 245-251.

Kawachi, I., Kennedy, B.P., Lochner, K., and Prothrow-Stith, D. (1997). Social capital, income inequality, and mortality. *American Journal of Public Health, 87,* 1491-1498.

Kawachi, I., Kennedy, B.P., and Glass, R. (1999). Social capital and self-rated health: A contextual analysis. *American Journal of Public Health, 89,* 1187-1193.

Kiely, D.K., Simon, S.E., Jones, R.N., and Morris, J.N. (2000). The protective effect of social engagement on mortality in long-term care. *Journal of American Geriatric Society, 48,* 1367-1372.

Kim, H.K., and McKenry, P.C. (1998). Social networks and support: A comparison of African Americans, Asian Americans, Caucasians, and Hispanics. *Journal of Comparative Family Studies, 29,* 313-314.

Kincade, J.E., Rabiner, D.J., Bernard, S.L., Woomert, A., Konrad, T.R., DeFriese, G.H., et al. (1996). Older adults as a community resource: Results from the National Survey of Self-Care and Aging. *Gerontologist, 36,* 474-482.

King, A.C., Blair, S.N., Bild, D.E., Dishman, R.K., Dubbert, P.M., Marcus, B.H., et al. (1992). Determinants of physical activity and interventions in adults. *Medical Science and Sports Exercise, 24,* S221-S236.

Koenig, H.G., Hays, J.C., Larson, D.B., George, L.K., Cohen, H.J., McCullough, M.E., et al. (1999). Does religious attendance prolong survival? A six-year follow-up study of 3,968 older adults. *Journals of Gerontology: Series A: Biological Sciences and Medical Sciences, 54,* 370-376.

Krause, N. (1986). Social support, stress, and well-being among older adults. *Journal of Gerontology, 41,* 512-519.

Krause, N. (1987). Chronic financial strain, social support, and depressive symptoms among older adults. *Psychology and Aging, 2,* 185-192.

Krause, N. (1990). Perceived health problems, formal/informal support, and life satisfaction among older adults. *Journal of Gerontology, 45*, S193-S205.

Krause, N. (1996). Neighborhood deterioration and self-rated health in later life. *Psychology and Aging, 11*, 342-352.

Krause, N. (1997). Anticipated support, received support, and economic stress among older adults. *Journal of Gerontology: Series B: Psychological Sciences and Social Sciences, 52*, 284-293.

Krause, N. (1998). Stressors in highly valued roles, religious coping, and mortality. *Psychology and Aging, 13*, 242-255.

Krause, N., Liang, J., and Keith, V. (1990). Personality, social support, and psychological distress in later life. *Psychology and Aging, 5*, 315-326.

Krause, N., Herzog, A.R., and Baker, E. (1992). Providing support to others and well-being in later life. *Journal of Gerontology, 47*, 300-311.

Krumholz, H.M., Butler, J., Miller, J., Vaccarino, V., Williams, C.S., Mendes de Leon, C.F., et al. (1998). Prognostic importance of emotional support for elderly patients hospitalized with heart failure. *Circulation, 97*, 958-964.

Kubzansky, L.D., Berkman, L.F., and Seeman, T.E. (2000). Social conditions and distress in elderly persons: Findings from the MacArthur Studies of Successful Aging. *Journal of Gerontology: Series B: Psychological Sciences and Social Sciences, 55*, 238-246.

LaGrange, R.L., Ferraro, K.F., and Supancic, M. (1992). Perceived risk and fear of crime—role of social and physical incivilities. *Journal of Research in Crime and Delinquency, 29*, 311-334.

Lang, F.R. (2001). Regulation of social relationships in later adulthood. *Journal of Gerontology: Series B: Psychological Sciences and Social Sciences, 56*, 321-326.

Lang, F.R., Featherman, D.L., and Nesselroade, J.R. (1997). Social self-efficacy and short-term variability in social relationships: The MacArthur successful aging studies. *Psychology and Aging, 12*, 657-666.

LaVeist, T.A. (1993). Segregation, poverty, and empowerment: Health consequences for African Americans. *Milbank Quarterly, 71*, 41-64.

Lawton, M.P., and Byerts, T. (1973). *Community planning for the elderly*. Washington, DC: U.S. Department of Housing and Urban Development.

LeClere, F.B., Rogers, R.G., and Peters, K. (1998). Neighborhood social context and racial differences in women's heart disease mortality. *Journal of Health and Social Behavior, 39*, 91-107.

Lee, G.R., Peek, C.W., and Coward, R.T. (1998). Race differences in filial responsibility expectations among older parents. *Journal of Marriage and the Family, 60*, 404-412.

Lennartsson, C., and Silverstein, M. (2001). Does engagement with life enhance survival of elderly people in Sweden? The role of social and leisure activities. *Journal of Gerontology: Series B: Psychological Sciences and Social Sciences, 56*, S335-S342.

Levin, J.S. (1996). How religion influences morbidity and health: Reflections on natural history, salutogenesis and host resistance. *Social Science and Medicine, 43*, 849-864.

Levin, J.S., and Chatters, L.M. (1998). Religion, health, and psychological well-being in older adults: Findings from three national surveys. *Journal of Aging and Health, 10*, 504-531.

Levin, J.S., Taylor, R.J., and Chatters, L.M. (1994). Race and gender differences in religiosity among older adults: Findings from four national surveys. *Journal of Gerontology, 49*, S137-S145.

Li, L.W., Seltzer, M.M., and Greenberg, J.S. (1997). Social support and depressive symptoms: Differential patterns in wife and daughter caregivers. *Journal of Gerontology: Series B: Psychological Sciences and Social Sciences, 52*, S200-S211.

Liang, J., Krause, N.M., and Bennett, J.M. (2001). Social exchange and well-being: Is giving better than receiving? *Psychology and Aging, 16*, 511-523.

Lin, N., and Dean, A. (1984). Social support and depression: A panel study. *Social Psychiatry, 19,* 83-91.

Lin, N., Dean, A., and Ensel, W.M. (1986). *Social support, life events, and depression.* New York: Academic Press.

Link, B.G., and Phelan, J. (1995). Social conditions as fundamental causes of disease. *Journal of Health and Social Behavior,* (Extra Issue), 80-94.

Lynch, J.W., Kaplan, G.A., and Shema, S.J. (1997). Cumulative impact of sustained economic hardship on physical, cognitive, psychological, and social functioning. *New England Journal of Medicine, 337,* 1889-1895.

Macintyre, S., Maciver, S., and Sooman, A. (1993). Area, class and health: Should we be focusing on places or on people? *Journal of Social Policy, 22,* 213-234.

Malmstrom, M., Sundquist, J., and Johansson, S.E. (1999). Neighborhood environment and self-reported health status: A multilevel analysis. *American Journal of Public Health, 89,* 1181-1186.

Martire, L.M., Schulz, R., Mittelmark, M.B., and Newsom, J.T. (1999). Stability and change in older adults' social contact and social support: The Cardiovascular Health Study. *Journals of Gerontology: Series B: Psychological Sciences and Social Sciences, 54,* S302-S311.

Massey, D.S., and Eggers, M.L. (1990). The ecology of inequality—minorities and the concentration of poverty, 1970-1980. *American Journal of Sociology, 95,* 1153-1188.

Matt, G.E., and Dean, A. (1993). Social support from friends and psychological distress among elderly persons: Moderator effects of age. *Journal of Health and Social Behavior, 34,* 187-200.

McAuley, E. (1993). Self-efficacy, physical activity, and aging. In J.R. Kelly (Ed.), *Activity and aging: Staying involved in later life* (pp. 187-206). Newbury Park, CA: Sage.

McAvay, G.J., Seeman, T.E., and Rodin, J. (1996). A longitudinal study of change in domain-specific self-efficacy among older adults. *Journals of Gerontology: Series B: Psychological Sciences and Social Sciences, 51,* 243-253.

McCann, J.J., Hebert, L.E., Beckett, L.A., Morris, M.C., Scherr, P.A., and Evans, D.A. (2000). Comparison of informal caregiving by black and white older adults in a community population. *Journal of American Geriatrics Society, 48,* 1612-1617.

McEwen, B.S. (1998). Protective and damaging effects of stress mediators. *New England Journal of Medicine, 338,* 171-179.

Mendes de Leon, C.F., Fillenbaum, G.G., Williams, C.S., Brock, D.B., Beckett, L.A., and Berkman, L.F. (1995). Functional disability among elderly blacks and whites in two diverse areas: The New Haven and North Carolina EPESE (Established Populations for the Epidemiologic Studies of the Elderly). *American Journal of Public Health, 85,* 994-998.

Mendes de Leon, C.F., Seeman, T.E., Baker, D.I., Richardson, E.D., and Tinetti, M.E. (1996). Self-efficacy, physical decline, and change in functioning in community-living elders: A prospective study. *Journals of Gerontology: Series B: Psychological Sciences and Social Sciences, 51,* S183-S190.

Mendes de Leon, C.F., Beckett, L.A., Fillenbaum, G.G., Brock, D.B., Branch, L.G., Evans, D.A., et al. (1997). Black-white differences in risk of becoming disabled and recovering from disability in old age: A longitudinal analysis of two EPESE populations. *American Journal of Epidemiology, 145,* 488-497.

Mendes de Leon, C.F., Glass, T.A., Beckett, L.A., Seeman, T.E., Evans, D.A., and Berkman, L.F. (1999). Social networks and disability transitions across eight intervals of yearly data in the New Haven EPESE. *Journals of Gerontology: Series B: Psychological Sciences and Social Sciences, 54,* 162-172.

Mendes de Leon, C.F., Gold, D.T., Glass, T.A., Kaplan, L., and George, L.K. (2001). Disability as a function of social networks and support in elderly African Americans and whites: The Duke EPESE 1986-1992. *Journals of Gerontology: Series B: Psychological Sciences and Social Sciences, 56,* S179-S190.

Mendes de Leon, C.F., Glass, T.A., and Berkman, L.F. (2003). Social engagement and disability in a community population of older adults: The New Haven EPESE. *American Journal of Epidemiology, 157,* 633-642.

Menec, V.H., and Chipperfield, J.G. (1997). Remaining active in later life. *Journal of Aging and Health, 9,* 105-125.

Michael, Y.L., Berkman, L.F., Colditz, G.A., and Kawachi, I. (2001). Living arrangements, social integration, and change in functional health status. *American Journal of Epidemiology, 153,* 123-131.

Miner, S. (1995). Racial differences in family support and formal service utilization among older persons: A nonrecursive model. *Journals of Gerontology: Series B: Psychological Sciences and Social Sciences, 50,* S143-S153.

Miner, S., and Tolnay, S. (1998). Barriers to voluntary organization membership: An examination of race and cohort differences. *Journals of Gerontology: Series B: Psychological Sciences and Social Sciences, 53,* 241-248.

Moen, P., Fields, V., Meador, R., and Rosenblatt, H. (2000). Fostering integration: A case study of the Cornell Retirees Volunteering in Service (CRVIS) program. In K. Pillemer, P. Moen, E. Wethington, and N. Glasgow (Eds.), *Social integration in the second half of life* (pp. 247-264). Baltimore: Johns Hopkins University Press.

Morgan, D. (1989). Adjusting to widowhood: Do social networks really make it easier? *The Gerontologist, 29,* 101-107.

Morgan, D.L. (1988). Age differences in social network participation. *Journal of Gerontology, 43,* 129-137.

Morris, P.L., Robinson, R.G., Raphael, B., and Bishop, D. (1991). The relationship between the perception of social support and post-stroke depression in hospitalized patients. *Psychiatry, 54,* 306-316.

Muntaner, C., Nieto, F.J., and O'Campo, P. (1996). The Bell Curve: On race, social class, and epidemiologic research. *American Journal of Epidemiology, 144,* 531-536.

Musick, M.A. (1996). Religion and subjective health among black and white elders. *Journal of Health Social Behavior, 37,* 221-237.

Musick, M.A., Koenig, H.G., Hays, J.C., and Cohen, H.J. (1998). Religious activity and depression among community-dwelling elderly persons with cancer: The moderating effect of race. *Journals of Gerontology: Series B: Psychological Sciences and Social Sciences, 53,* 218-227.

Musick, M.A., Herzog, A.R., and House, J.S. (1999). Volunteering and mortality among older adults: Findings from a national sample. *Journals of Gerontology: Series B: Psychological Sciences and Social Sciences, 54,* 173-180.

Mutran, E. (1985). Intergenerational family support among blacks and whites: Response to culture or to socioeconomic differences. *Journal of Gerontology, 40,* 382-389.

Mutran, E., Reitzes, D., Mossey, J., and Fernandez, M. (1996). Social support, depression, and recovery of walking ability following hip fracture surgery. *Journal of Gerontology and Social Sciences, 51B,* 354-361.

National Research Council. (1997). *Racial and ethnic differences in the health of older Americans.* L.G. Martin and B.J. Soldo (eds.), Committee on Population, Commission on Behavioral and Social Sciences and Education. Washington, DC: National Academy Press.

Newsom, J.T., and Schulz, R. (1998). Caregiving from the recipient's perspective: Negative reactions to being helped. *Health Psychology, 17,* 172-181.

Okun, M.A., and Keith, V.M. (1998). Effects of positive and negative social exchanges with various sources on depressive symptoms in younger and older adults. *Journals of Gerontology: Series B: Psychological Sciences and Social Sciences, 53,* 4-20.

Oman, D., and Reed, D. (1998). Religion and mortality among the community-dwelling elderly. *American Journal of Public Health, 88,* 1469-1475.

Orth-Gomer, K., and Johnson, J.V. (1987). Social network interaction and mortality: A six year follow-up study of a random sample of the Swedish population. *Social Science and Medicine, 33*(10), 1189-1195.

Ory, M.G., Hoffman, R.R., III, Yee, J.L., Tennstedt, S., and Schulz, R. (1999). Prevalence and impact of caregiving: A detailed comparison between dementia and nondementia caregivers. *The Gerontologist, 39,* 177-185.

Ostwald, S.K., Hepburn, K.W., Caron, W., Burns, T., and Mantell, R. (1999). Reducing caregiver burden: A randomized psychoeducational intervention for caregivers of persons with dementia. *The Gerontologist, 39,* 299-309.

Oxman, T.E., and Hull, J.G. (1997). Social support, depression, and activities of daily living in older heart surgery patients. *Journals of Gerontology: Series B: Psychological Sciences and Social Sciences, 52,* 1-14.

Paffenbarger, R.S., Jr., Hyde, R.T., Wing, A.L., and Hsieh, C.C. (1986). Physical activity, all-cause mortality, and longevity of college alumni. *New England Journal of Medicine, 314,* 605-613.

Paykel, E.S. (1994). Life events, social support and depression. *Acta Psychiatrica Scandinavica, 377*(Suppl.), 50-58.

Pearlin, L.I. (1985). Social structure and processes of social support. In S. Cohen and S.L. Syme (Eds.), *Social support and health* (pp. 43-60). Orlando, FL: Academic Press.

Peek, C.W., Coward, R.T., Henretta, J.C., Duncan, R.P., and Dougherty, M.C. (1997). Differences by race in the decline of health over time. *Journals of Gerontology: Series B: Psychological Sciences and Social Sciences, 52,* 336-344.

Penninx, B.W., van Tilburg, T., Kriegsman, D.M., Deeg, D.J., Boeke, A., and van Eijk, J.T. (1997). Effects of social support and personal coping resources on mortality in older age: The Longitudinal Aging Study Amsterdam. *American Journal of Epidemiology, 146,* 510-519.

Perkins, D.D., and Taylor, R.B. (1996). Ecological assessments of community disorder: Their relationship to fear of crime and theoretical implications. *American Journal of Community Psychology, 24,* 63-107.

Perkins, D.D., Meeks, J.W., and Taylor, R.B. (1992). The physical environment of street blocks and resident perceptions of crime and disorder: Implications for theory and measurement. *Journal of Environmental Psychology, 12,* 21-34.

Pillemer, K., Suitor, J.J., Landreneau, L.T., Henderson, C.R., and Brangman, S. (2000). Peer support for Alzheimer's caregivers: Lessons from an intervention study. In K. Pillemer, P. Moen, E. Wethington, and N. Glasgow (Eds.), *Social integration in the second half of life* (pp. 265-286). Baltimore: Johns Hopkins University Press.

Pugliesi, K., and Shook, S.L. (1998). Gender, ethnicity, and network characteristics: Variation in social support resources. *Sex Roles, 38,* 215-238.

Rakowski, W., Julius, M., Hickey, T., and Halter, J.B. (1987). Correlates of preventive health behavior in late-life. *Research on Aging, 9,* 331-355.

Robert, S.A. (1999). Neighborhood socioeconomic context and adult health: The mediating role of individual health behaviors and psychosocial factors. *Annals of the New York Academy of Sciences, 896,* 465-468.

Robert, S.A., and Li, L.W. (2001). Age variation in the relationship between community socioeconomic status and adult health. *Research on Aging, 32,* 233-258.

Rook, K.S. (1984). The negative side of social interaction: Impact on psychological well-being. *Journal of Personality and Social Psychology, 46,* 1097-1108.

Rosow, I., and Breslau, N. (1966). A Guttman health scale for the aged. *Journal of Gerontology, 21,* 556-559.

Ross, C.E. (1993). Fear of victimization and health. *Journal of Quantitative Criminology, 9,* 159-175.

Ross, C.E. (2000). Walking, exercising, and smoking: Does neighborhood matter? *Social Science and Medicine, 51,* 265-274.

Ross, C.E., and Jang, S.J. (2000). Neighborhood disorder, fear, and mistrust: The buffering role of social ties with neighbors. *American Journal of Community Psychology, 28,* 401-420.

Ross, C.E., and Mirowsky, J. (2001). Neighborhood disadvantage, disorder, and health. *Journal of Health and Social Behavior, 42,* 258-276.

Ruberman, W., Weinblatt, E., Goldberg, J., and Chaudhary, B. (1984). Psychosocial influences on mortality after myocardial infarction. *New England Journal of Medicine, 311,* 552-559.

Ryff, C.D. (1991). Possible selves in adulthood and old age: A tale of shifting horizons. *Psychology and Aging, 6,* 286-295.

Ryff, C.D., and Singer, B. (1998). The role of purpose in life and personal growth in positive human health. In P.T.P. Wong and P.S. Frey (Eds.), *The human quest for meaning* (pp. 213-235). Mahwah, NJ: Lawrence Erlbaum Associates.

Sampson, R., Raudenbush, S.W., and Earls, F. (1997). Neighborhoods and violent crime: A multilevel study of collective efficacy. *Science, 277,* 918-924.

Sapolsky, R.M., Alberts, S.C., and Altmann, J. (1997). Hypercortisolism associated with social subordinance or social isolation among wild baboons. *Archives of General Psychiatry, 54,* 1137-1143.

Schoenbach, V., Kaplan, B., Fredman, L., and Kleinbaum, D. (1986). Social ties and mortality in Evans County, Georgia. *American Journal of Epidemiology, 123,* 577-591.

Schulz, R., O'Brien, A.T., Bookwala, J., and Fleissner, K. (1995). Psychiatric and physical morbidity effects of dementia caregiving: Prevalence, correlates, and causes. *Gerontologist, 35,* 771-791.

Seeman, T.E., and McEwen, B.S. (1996). Impact of social environment characteristics on neuroendocrine regulation. *Psychosomatic Medicine, 58,* 459-471.

Seeman, T.E., Kaplan, G.A., Knudsen, L., Cohen, R., and Guralnik, J. (1987). Social network ties and mortality among the elderly in the Alameda County Study. *American Journal of Epidemiology, 126,* 714-723.

Seeman, T.E., Berkman, L.F., Kohout, F., LaCroix, A., Glynn, R., and Blazer, D. (1993a). Intercommunity variations in the association between social ties and mortality in the elderly. A comparative analysis of three communities. *Annals of Epidemiology, 3,* 325-335.

Seeman, T.E., Rodin, J., and Albert, M. (1993b). Self-efficacy and cognitive performance in high-functioning older individuals: MacArthur studies of successful aging. *Journal of Aging and Health, 5,* 455-474.

Seeman, T.E., Berkman, L., Blazer, D., and Rowe, J.W. (1994). Social ties and support and neuroendocrine function: The MacArthur studies of successful aging. *Annals of Behavioral Medicine, 16,* 95-106.

Seeman, T.E., Berkman, L.F., Charpentier, P.A., Blazer, D.G., Albert, M.S., and Tinetti, M.E. (1995). Behavioral and psychosocial predictors of physical performance: MacArthur studies of successful aging. *Journals of Gerontology: Series A: Biological Sciences and Medical Sciences, 50,* M177-M183.

Seeman, T.E., Bruce, M.L., and McAvay, G.J. (1996). Social network characteristics and onset of ADL disability: MacArthur studies of successful aging. *Journals of Gerontology: Series B: Psychological Sciences and Social Sciences, 51,* 191-200.

Seeman, T.E., Lusignolo, T.M., Albert, M., and Berkman, L. (2001a). Social relationships, social support, and patterns of cognitive aging in healthy, high-functioning older adults: MacArthur studies of successful aging. *Health Psychology, 20,* 243-255.

Seeman, T.E., McEwen, B.S., Rowe, J.W., and Singer, B.H. (2001b). Allostatic load as a marker of cumulative biological risk: MacArthur studies of successful aging. *Proceedings of the National Academy of Sciences of the United States of America, 98*, 4770-4775.

Shively, C.A. (1998). Social subordination stress, behavior, and central monoaminergic function in female cynomolgus monkeys. *Biological Psychiatry, 44*, 882-891.

Shively, C.A., and Clarkson, T.B. (1994). Social status and coronary artery atherosclerosis in female monkeys. *Arteriosclerosis Thrombosis, 14*, 721-726.

Shively, C.A., Laber-Laird, K., and Anton, R. F. (1997). Behavior and physiology of social stress and depression in female cynomolgus monkeys. *Biological Psychiatry, 41*, 871-882.

Shye, D., Mullooly, J.P., Freeborn, D.K., and Pope, C.R. (1995). Gender differences in the relationship between social network support and mortality: A longitudinal study of an elderly cohort. *Social Science and Medicine, 41*, 935-947.

Silverstein, M., and Bengtson, V.L. (1994). Does intergenerational social support influence the psychological well-being of older parents? The contingencies of declining health and widowhood. *Social Science and Medicine, 38*, 943-957.

Silverstein, M., and Waite, L.J. (1993). Are blacks more likely than whites to receive and provide social support in middle and old age? Yes, no, and maybe so. *Journal of Gerontology, 48*, S212-S222.

Silverstein, M., Chen, X., and Heller, K. (1996). Too much of a good thing? Intergenerational social support and the psychological well-being of older parents. *Journal of Marriage and the Family, 58*, 970-982.

Sorlie, P.D., Backlund, E., and Keller, J.B. (1995). US mortality by economic, demographic, and social characteristics: The National Longitudinal Mortality Study. *American Journal of Public Health, 85*, 949-956.

Stack, C. (1974). *All our kin.* New York: Harper and Row.

Steffen, P.R., Hinderliter, A.L., Blumenthal, J.A., and Sherwood, A. (2001). Religious coping, ethnicity, and ambulatory blood pressure. *Psychosomatic Medicine, 63*, 523-530.

Steinbach, U. (1992). Social networks, institutionalization, and mortality among elderly people in the United States. *Journal of Gerontology, 47*, S183-S190.

Stones, M., Dornan, B., and Kozma, A. (1989). The prediction of mortality in elderly institution residents. *Journal of Gerontology: Series B: Psychological Sciences and Social Sciences, 44*, 72-79.

Strawbridge, W.J., Cohen, R.D., Shema, S.J., and Kaplan, G.A. (1996). Successful aging: Predictors and associated activities. *American Journal of Epidemiology, 144*, 135-141.

Strawbridge, W.J., Cohen, R.D., Shema, S.J., and Kaplan, G.A. (1997). Frequent attendance at religious services and mortality over 28 years. *American Journal of Public Health, 87*, 957-961.

Strogatz, D.S., Croft, J.B., James, S.A., Keenan, N.L., Browning, S.R., Garrett, J.M., et al. (1997). Social support, stress, and blood pressure in black adults. *Epidemiology, 8*, 482-487.

Suitor, J., and Pillemer, K. (1996). Sources of support and interpersonal stress in the networks of married caregiving daughters: Findings from a 2-year longitudinal study. *Journal of Gerontology: Series B: Psychological Sciences and Social Sciences, 51B*, S297-S306.

Tang, M.X., Stern, Y., Marder, K., Bell, K., Gurland, B., Lantigua, R., et al. (1998). The APOE-epsilon4 allele and the risk of Alzheimer disease among African Americans, whites, and Hispanics. *Journal of American Medical Association, 279*, 751-755.

Taylor, R.J. (1986). Religious participation among elderly blacks. *Gerontologist, 26*, 630-636.

Taylor, R.J., and Chatters, L.M. (1986a). Church-based informal support networks among elderly blacks. *The Gerontologist, 26*, 637-642.

Taylor, R.J., and Chatters, L.M. (1986b). Patterns of informal support to elderly black adults: Family, friends, and church members. *Social Work, 31,* 432-438.

Taylor, R.J., and Taylor, W.H. (1982). The social and economic status of the black elderly. *Phylon, 43,* 295-306.

Taylor, R.J., Chatters, L.M., Tucker, M.B., and Lewis, E. (1990). Developments in research in black families: A decade review. *Journal of Marriage and the Family, 52,* 993-1014.

Tennstedt, S., and Chang, B.H. (1998). The relative contribution of ethnicity versus socioeconomic status in explaining differences in disability and receipt of informal care. *Journal of Gerontology: Series B: Psychological Sciences and Social Sciences, 53,* S61-S70.

Thorton, N.C., White-Means, S.I., and Choi, H.K. (1993). Sociodemographic correlates of the size and composition of informal caregiver networks among frail ethnic elderly. *Journal of Comparative Family Studies, 24,* 235-250.

Tinetti, M.E., and Powell, L. (1993). Fear of falling and low self-efficacy: A case of dependence in elderly persons. *Journal of Gerontology, 48*(Special Issue), 35-38.

Turner, R.J., and Marino, F. (1994). Social support and social structure: A descriptive epidemiology. *Journal of Health and Social Behavior, 35,* 193-212.

Turrell, G., Lynch, J.W., Kaplan, G.A., Everson, S.A., Helkala, E.L., Kauhanen, J., et al. (2002). Socioeconomic position across the lifecourse and cognitive function in late middle age. *Journal of Gerontology: Series B: Psychological Sciences and Social Sciences, 57,* S43-S51.

Uchino, B.N., Cacioppo, J.T., and Keicolt-Glaser, J.K. (1996). The relationship between social support and physiological processes: A review with emphasis on underlying mechanisms and implications for health. *Psychological Bulletin, 119,* 488-531.

Unger, J.B., McAvay, G., Bruce, M.L., Berkman, L., and Seeman, T. (1999). Variation in the impact of social network characteristics on physical functioning in elderly persons: MacArthur Studies of Successful Aging. *Journals of Gerontology: Series B: Psychological Sciences and Social Sciences, 54,* 245-251.

van Tilburg, T. (1998). Losing and gaining in old age: Changes in personal network size and social support in a four-year longitudinal study. *Journals of Gerontology: Series B: Psychological Sciences and Social Sciences, 53,* 313-323.

Van Willigen, M. (2000). Differential benefits of volunteering across the life course. *Journal of Gerontology: Series B: Psychological Sciences and Social Sciences, 55,* S308-S318.

Vaux, A. (1985). Variations in social support associated with gender, ethnicity and age. *Journal of Social Issues, 41,* 89-110.

Verbrugge, L.M., and Jette, A.M. (1994). The disablement process. *Social Science and Medicine, 38,* 1-14.

Verbrugge, L.M., Reoma, J.M., and Gruber-Baldini, A.L. (1994). Short-term dynamics of disability and well-being. *Journal of Health Social Behavior, 35,* 97-117.

Vilhjalmsson, R. (1993). Life stress, social support and clinical depression: A reanalysis of the literature. *Social Science and Medicine, 37,* 331-342.

Vita, A.J., Terry, R.B., Hubert, H.B., and Fries, J.F. (1998). Aging, health risks, and cumulative disability. *New England Journal of Medicine, 338,* 1035-1041.

Waite, L.J., and Hughes, M.E. (1999). At risk on the cusp of old age: Living arrangements and functional status among black, white and Hispanic adults. *Journals of Gerontology: Series B: Psychological Sciences and Social Sciences, 54,* 136-144.

Waitzman, N.J., and Smith, K.R. (1998). Separate but lethal: The effects of economic segregation on mortality in metropolitan America. *Milbank Quarterly, 76,* 341-373.

Wandersman, A., and Nation, M. (1998). Urban neighborhoods and mental health: Psychological contributions to understanding toxicity, resilience, and interventions. *American Psychologist, 53,* 647-656.

Welin, L., Tibblin, G., Svardsudd, K., Tibblin, B., Ander-Peciva, S., Larsson, B., et al. (1985). Prospective study of social influences on mortality: The study of men born in 1913 and 1923. *Lancet, 60*(22), 915-918.

Wilcox, V., Kasl, S., and Berkman, L. (1994). Social support and physical disability in older people after hospitalization: A prospective study. *Health Psychology, 13,* 170-179.

Williams, D.R., Lavizzo-Mourey, R., and Warren, R.C. (1994). The concept of race and health status in America. *Public Health Reports, 109,* 26-41.

Williams, R.B., Barefoot, J.C., Califf, RM., Haney, T.L., Saunders, W.B., Pryor, D.B., et al. (1992). Prognostic importance of social and economic resources among medically treated patients with angiographically documented coronary artery disease [published erratum appears in *JAMA, 268*(19), 2652]. *Journal of the American Medical Association, 267,* 520-524.

Wilson, R.S., Mendes de Leon, C.F., Barnes, L.L., Schneider, J.A., Bienias, J.L., Evans, D.A., et al. (2002). Participation in cognitively stimulating activities and risk of incident Alzheimer disease. *Journal of the American Medical Association, 287,* 742-748.

Witzig, R. (1996). The medicalization of race: Scientific legitimization of a flawed social construct. *Annals of International Medicine, 125,* 675-679.

Wolf, T.M., Balson, P.M., Morse, E.V., Simon, P.M., Gaumer, R.H., Dralle, P.W., et al. (1991). Relationship of coping style to affective state and perceived social support in asymptomatic and symptomatic HIV-infected persons: Implications for clinical management. *Journal of Clinical Psychiatry, 52,* 171-173.

Yen, I.H., and Kaplan, G.A. (1999). Neighborhood social environment and risk of death: Multilevel evidence from the Alameda County Study. *American Journal of Epidemiology, 149,* 898-907.

11

What Makes a Place Healthy? Neighborhood Influences on Racial/ Ethnic Disparities in Health over the Life Course

Jeffrey D. Morenoff and John W. Lynch

Our main purpose in this chapter is to suggest a conceptual framework for better understanding how characteristics of neighborhoods can affect racial/ethnic differences in health, with a special emphasis on health in aging populations. At the outset we should recognize that the specific studies in this field are sparse. However, we will try to draw from the more diverse sociological and epidemiological literature on neighborhoods and health to illustrate the potential for certain characteristics of neighborhoods to affect racial/ethnic health differences in aging.

In recent years, epidemiologists and sociologists have become increasingly interested in studying the effects of local context on individual health and well-being. Although a long history of research shows that health status varies strongly across local, state, regional, and national settings (Murray, Michaud, McKenna, and Marks, 1998), what distinguishes the new generation of research on neighborhoods and health is its attention to investigating the multilevel causation of these differences. The basic premise is that both individual and contextual characteristics play a role in health. This concern is captured by the search for so-called "neighborhood effects," which generally refers to the study of how local context influences the health and well-being of individuals in a way that cannot be reduced to the properties of the individuals themselves.

Most of the research on neighborhood effects has focused on social and behavioral outcomes, including child cognitive and behavioral development, school dropout, educational attainment, crime and delinquency, substance use, sexual activity, contraceptive use, childbearing, income, and labor force participation (see recent reviews by Gephart, 1997; Leventhal and Brooks-Gunn, 2000; Sampson, Morenoff, and Gannon-Rowley, 2002). Until recently, health outcomes had been noticeably absent from this list, but multilevel studies are becoming increasingly popular in health research. This new multilevel research on local social context and health has garnered wide attention in social epidemiology, as evidenced by the publication of four reviews of this literature in the past 3 years (Diez-Roux, 2002; Ellen, Mijanovich, and Dillman, 2001; Pickett and Pearl, 2001; Robert, 1999).

One of the reasons that public health scientists have become so interested in local context is to better understand the striking and persistent racial and ethnic differences across a range of health outcomes that have eluded most efforts to explain them using data at the individual level (Krieger, 1994; Williams and Collins, 1995a). There are large racial/ethnic differences across many causes of morbidity and mortality, and even through casual observation it seems obvious that perhaps some of this health inequality is related to the different types of contexts, or "ecological niches," into which different racial/ethnic groups are born, and within which they grow up, live, and work. As research on residential segregation demonstrates (Acevedo-Garcia, 2000; Cooper et al., 2001; Ellen, 2000; LaVeist and Wallace, 2000; Massey and Denton, 1993; Polednak, 1996) place-based disparities are of central importance to understanding race-based health disparities in the United States. Moreover, a better understanding of why place and context matter also promises to yield new insights and intervention strategies for addressing racial/ethnic inequalities in health. Thus, the potential of place-based research to inform health intervention strategies that target places as well as people has given further impetus to this research in public health (Macintyre, MacIver, and Sooman, 1993; Sooman, Macintyre, and Anderson, 1993).

At this point, research on local context and health remains somewhat disengaged from recent theoretical and methodological developments in the sociological literature on neighborhoods. For example, whereas the sociological literature on neighborhood effects has taken a "process turn" in recent years and begun to focus more on the mechanisms that explain *why* neighborhoods matter (Sampson et al., 2002), most research on the neighborhood context of health is still attempting to establish *that* context matters. This is partly because most health research is framed in a paradigm where individual-level proximal influences—such as behaviors or biomarkers of pathogenic processes—take precedence over contextual factors (Krieger, 1994; Palloni and Morenoff, 2001; Schwartz, Susser, and Susser, 1999; Susser, 1998).[1]

To some extent neighborhood effects research on health remains mired in a "poverty paradigm" (Rowley et al., 1993) focusing mostly on the association between Census-based indicators of community socioeconomic position and individual health outcomes, with a heavy emphasis on the deleterious effects of concentrated poverty and other forms of disadvantage. The main thrust of such studies has been to show that poorer places are associated with worse health outcomes, above and beyond the characteristics of the individuals who live there (Robert, 1999). This emphasis on disadvantage, to the exclusion of other facets of neighborhood environments, is partly the result of a lack of appropriate data, but we argue that it also reflects a paucity theory that can inform questions about how neighborhoods may affect specific types of health outcomes.

In this chapter we discuss both the promises and shortcomings of this growing literature on local context and health. In doing so, we bring together epidemiological perspectives concerned with exposure measurement and mechanisms—what are the measurable characteristics of neighborhoods (exposures) that can plausibly influence different types of health-related outcomes (specific causal pathways)—with sociological concerns about how to conceptualize and analyze neighborhoods. Rather than engaging in a comprehensive literature review—excellent reviews already exist (e.g., Diez-Roux, 2001; Ellen et al., 2001; Pickett and Pearl, 2001; Robert, 1999; Yen and Syme, 1999)—in this chapter we will focus on issues relating to the current state of research on neighborhoods and health, the dimensions of neighborhood environments that may be related to health, the pathways through which neighborhoods translate into specific types of health outcomes, how neighborhood effects intersect with the study of aging and the life course, and selection processes relating to the sorting of individuals into neighborhoods. We also present an empirical analysis of the neighborhood context of mortality in Chicago neighborhoods and conclude by suggesting new directions for neighborhood research on health.

THE CONCEPT OF NEIGHBORHOOD

Robert Park and Ernest Burgess laid the foundation for urban sociology by defining local communities as "natural areas" that developed as a result of competition between businesses for land use and between population groups for affordable housing. A neighborhood, according to this view, is a subsection of a larger community—a collection of both people and institutions occupying a spatially defined area influenced by ecological, cultural, and sometimes political forces (Park, 1916). Suttles (1972) later refined this view by recognizing that local communities do not form their identities only as the result of free-market competition. Instead, some communities have their identity and boundaries imposed on them by outsiders. Suttles also argued that the local community is best thought of not as a single entity, but rather as a hierarchy of progressively more inclusive residential groupings. In this sense, we can think of neighborhoods as ecological units nested within successively larger communities.

In practice, most social scientists and virtually all studies we assess rely on "statistical" neighborhoods that depend on geographic boundaries defined by the Census Bureau or other administrative agencies (e.g., school districts, police districts). Although administratively defined units such as Census tracts and block groups are reasonably consistent with the notion of overlapping and nested ecological structures, they offer imperfect operational definitions of neighborhoods for research and policy. However, the term "neighborhood" has been defined quite broadly in health research, encompassing units as small as block groups and as large as counties. Thus far there has been little systematic research into how geographic scale affects contextual estimates, although there is some evidence that estimates of place effects are stronger when using smaller geographic areas (Boyle and Willms, 1999).

Increasingly, researchers have become interested in new methods that might help define neighborhoods in such a way that is more respectful of the logic of street patterns and possibly more reflective of the social networks of "neighboring" behavior (Coulton, Korbin, Chan, and Su, 2001; Grannis, 1998). One important avenue for future research is to explore whether and how such neighboring patterns vary across demographic subgroups. For example, children and the elderly may both face more geographical constraints on the range of social networks and routine activity patterns that could make the more proximate neighborhood environment more consequential in their daily lives (Booth, Owen, Bauman, Clavisi, and Leslie, 2000; Carstensen, Isaacowitz, and Charles, 1999). Race/ethnicity may also play a role in shaping the geographic reach of routine activities and social networks. Understanding how the concept of neighborhood varies across these demographic groups is critical in advancing research on neighborhood environments as sources of group disparities in health.

WHAT DO WE KNOW ABOUT NEIGHBORHOODS AND HEALTH?

One of the hallmarks of neighborhood effects research is its attention to the potentially confounding influences of individual-level attributes in making neighborhood-level inferences, either through the use of multilevel research designs and statistical methods, or through randomized experimental designs. Investigations in this field have attempted to unravel the extent to which characteristics of neighborhoods (contextual effects) influence health outcomes after accounting for the fact that neighborhoods are composed of people with different individual characteristics (compositional effects), who in some cases choose to live in different types of neighborhoods, or more likely are sorted into them by economic, political, and other social processes. As we will discuss later, this beguilingly simple framing of the research objective raises important conceptual problems as to what should be considered a contextual or compositional effect. For example, at any one point in time an individual may "possess" a certain level of education, which could be considered an individual-level predictor of that person's health status. Yet educational attainment is also the complex product of prior influences of the individual (e.g., innate characteristics), family (e.g., educational expectations), and social context (e.g., quality of schooling). Thus, the association between individual educational attainment and health could, in part, reflect the effects of prior social context, and yet its effect on health typically would be attributed to compositional rather than contextual factors. Thus, the line between compositional and contextual is conceptually very fuzzy, and is simultaneously a problem of not having appropriate data, appropriate methodology, and perhaps most importantly, appropriate sociological and epidemiological theory.

The literature on neighborhood effects and health is expanding rapidly. One recent review (Pickett and Pearl, 2001) identified 25 multilevel studies of neighborhood effects on health, 23 of which reported significant associations between health and at least one measure of neighborhood socioeconomic status. Even in the 2 years since the publication of that review, the literature has grown substantially. We have identified more than 60 multilevel studies of health that encompass the following array of outcomes:

- *Mortality:* Specific outcomes include *all-cause* mortality (Anderson, Sorlie, Backlund, Johnson, and Kaplan, 1997; Bond Huie, Hummer, and Rogers, 2002; Bosma, van de Mheen, Borsboom, and MacKenbach, 2001; Ecob and Jones, 1998; Haan, Kaplan, and Camacho, 1987; Kaplan, 1996; LeClere, Rogers, and Peters, 1997; Malmstrom, Johansson, and Sundquist, 2001; Sloggett and Joshi, 1994, 1998; Veugelers, Yip, and Kephart, 2001; Waitzman and Smith, 1998a; Yen and Kaplan, 1999) and mortality due to specific causes, including *heart disease, cancer, kidney disease,* and *injury* (Alter, Naylor, Austin, and Tu, 1999; Cubbin, LeClere, and Smith, 2000; Garg, Diener-West, and Powe, 2001; LeClere et al., 1998; Waitzman and Smith, 1998a).
- *Adult physical health status:* This category includes studies of *blood pressure* (Davey Smith, Hart, Watt, Hole, and Hawthorne, 1998; Diez-Roux et al., 1997; Krieger, 1992; Merlo et al., 2001; Wilson, Kliewer, Plybon, and Sica , 2000), *cholesterol* (Davey Smith et al., 1998; Diez-Roux et al., 1997), *coronary heart disease* (Diez-Roux et al., 1997; Lee and Cubbin, 2002), *respiratory function* (Ecob, 1996; Humphreys and Carr-Hill, 1991), *height and waist-hip ratio* (Ecob, 1996; Krieger, 1992), indicators of *obesity* (Davey Smith et al., 1998; Ecob, 1996; Marmot et al., 1998; Robert, 1998; Sundquist, Malmstrom, and Johansson, 1999), *lead expo-*

sure among older adults (Elreedy et al., 1999), and survey-reported conditions such as *functional limitations, chronic conditions,* and *self-rated health* (Balfour and Kaplan, 2002; Chandola, 2001; Ecob, 1996; Humphreys and Carr-Hill, 1991; Malmstrom et al., 2001; Malmstrom, Sundquist, and Johansson, 1999; Shouls, Congdon, and Curtis, 1996; Stafford, Bartley, Mitchell, and Marmot, 2001).

- *Infant and child health:* Most of these studies are of *birthweight* (Buka, Brennan, Rich-Edwards, Raudenbush, and Earls, 2003; Ellen, 2000; Gorman, 1999; Morenoff, 2003; O'Campo, Xue, and Wang, 1997; Pearl, Braveman, and Abrams, 2001; Rauh, Andrews, and Garfinkel, 2001; Roberts, 1997; Sloggett and Joshi, 1998), but there are also some on *infant mortality* (Matteson, Burr, and Marshall, 1998), *childhood asthma and respiratory illness* (Morgan and Chinn, 1983), *accidental injuries* (Reading, Langford, Haynes, and Lovett, 1999), and *emotional and behavioral problems* (Caspi, Taylor, Moffitt, and Plomin, 2000; Kalff et al., 2001) among young children.

- *Mental health:* This category includes measures of *depression, anxiety*, and various other outcomes (Aneshensel and Sucoff, 1996; Katz, Kling, and Liebman, 2001; Marmot et al., 1998; Reijneveld and Schene, 1998; Ross and Jang, 2000; Schulz et al., 2000).

- *Health behaviors:* Outcomes in this group include *substance use* (Boardman et al., 2001; Diehr et al., 1993; Diez-Roux et al., 1997; Duncan, Jones, and Moon, 1998; Ecob and Macintyre, 2000; Finch, Vega, and Kolody, 2001; Ganz, 2000; Hart, Ecob, and Smith, 1997; Kleinschmidt, Hills, and Elliott, 1995; Krieger, 1992; Lee and Cubbin, 2002; Reijneveld and Schene, 1998; Robert, 1998; Schroeder et al., 2001; Sundquist et al., 1999), *dietary practices* (Diehr et al., 1993; Ecob and Macintyre 2000; Hart et al., 1997; Karvonen and Rimpela, 1996; Lee and Cubbin, 2002), and *physical activity* (Ecob and Macintyre, 2000; Lee and Cubbin, 2002; Robert, 1998; Ross, 2000b; Sundquist et al., 1999).

- *Health services:* Some studies use multilevel data to examine neighborhood differences in the availability of health services, including *cardiopulmonary resuscitation* (Iwashyna, Christakis, and Becker, 1999), *cardiac procedures* (Alter et al., 1999), and *kidney transplants* (Garg et al., 2001).

With only a few exceptions (e.g., Sloggett and Joshi, 1994; Veugelers et al., 2001), nearly all of the multilevel studies we reviewed found that after controlling for individual-level characteristics, there is still an association between neighborhood environments and health outcomes. However, these studies varied widely in the way they operationalized the concept of neighborhood and measured neighborhood characteristics, making it difficult to reach a conclusion about the magnitude and substantive importance of these effects.

The vast majority of the studies we reviewed focus on the deleterious effects of socioeconomic disadvantage using Census-based measures of local area socioeconomic composition. The most common way to measure neighborhood socioeconomic status (SES) is through an index of socioeconomic deprivation/disadvantage (e.g., Boardman et al., 2001; Bosma et al., 2001; Caspi et al., 2000; Cubbin et al., 2000; Diez-Roux et al., 1997; Duncan et al., 1998; Ecob, 1996; Ecob and Jones, 1998; Ecob and Macintyre, 2000; Hart et al., 1997; Hart, Hole, and Smith, 2000; Malmstrom et al., 1999; Marmot et al., 1998; Morgan and Chinn, 1983; Reading et al., 1999; Reijneveld and Schene, 1998; Roberts, 1997; Sloggett and Joshi, 1994, 1998; Stafford et al., 2001; Sundquist et al., 1999; Wilson et al., 2000; Yen and Kaplan, 1999). However, some studies eschew the single index approach in favor of using single- or multiple-item indicators of neighborhood disadvantage, such as measures based on income, poverty, unemployment, public assistance, education, and occupational status (e.g., Ganz, 2000; Humphreys and Carr-Hill, 1991; Kaplan, 1996; Karvonen and Rimpela, 1996, 1997; LeClere et al., 1998; LeClere, Rogers, and Peters, 1997; Lee and Cubbin, 2002; O'Campo et al., 1997; Pearl et al., 2001; Robert, 1998; Ross, 2000a; Veugelers et al., 2001). Other studies take a categorical approach to measuring neighborhood disadvantage by constructing neighborhood typologies, such as the distinction between "poverty" and "nonpoverty" areas (Geis and Ross, 1998; Haan et al., 1987; Humphreys and Carr-Hill, 1991; Waitzman and Smith, 1998a).

A smaller number of studies have analyzed other neighborhood compositional/structural factors such as racial/ethnic composition (Bond Huie et al., 2002; Cubbin et al., 2000; LeClere et al., 1997, 1998; Lee and Cubbin, 2002; Roberts, 1997), family structure (Cubbin et al., 2000; LeClere et al., 1997, 1998; Lee and Cubbin, 2002; Ross, 2000a; Veugelers et al., 2001), residential stability (Cubbin et al., 2000; Kaplan, 1996; Lee and Cubbin, 2002; Roberts, 1997; Ross, Reynolds, and Geis, 2000), population density/urbanization (Cubbin et al., 2000; Iwashyna et al., 1999; Lee and Cubbin, 2002), and housing condition/owner occupancy (Kaplan, 1996; Karvonen and Rimpela, 1997; Lee and Cubbin, 2002; O'Campo et al., 1997; Roberts, 1997; Stafford et al., 2001). However, the evidence on how these factors affect health is much less consistent across studies.

Neighborhood Context and Racial/Ethnic Disparities in Aging Health

Given that race/ethnic minority groups are disproportionately exposed to disadvantaged social environments, it is not surprising that many researchers have looked to neighborhood environmental factors, such as residential segregation and the concentration of poverty, as potential explanations for racial/ethnic disparities in health (e.g., Williams and Collins, 1995b). To this point, however, only a few studies have explicitly made this connection. Two such studies track the mortality of respondents to the

National Health Interview Survey (NHIS) using the National Death Index (NDI). In the first of these studies, LeClere and colleagues (1997) used tract-level contextual data from the 1990 Census to explain racial/ethnic disparities in all-cause mortality among NHIS respondents from 1986 to 1990. The authors found that after adjusting for individual-level indicators of SES (i.e., income, education, and marital status), neighborhood characteristics fully explain the remaining mortality differential between African Americans and non-Hispanic whites, but not the mortality differential between Mexicans and whites. (Mexicans had lower mortality rates than whites, and neighborhood characteristics do not explain Mexicans' mortality advantage.) In this study, the main contextual factor driving the convergence in the mortality differential between African Americans and whites was neighborhood racial/ethnic composition.

In a follow-up study, Bond Huie and colleagues (2002) modified the NHIS-NDI data set by expanding the number of years of NHIS respondents (1986-1997), adding more individual-level control variables, and changing the definition of neighborhood from Census tracts to very small areas (VSAs). They found that the introduction of contextual variables reduced the mortality risk for African Americans and Puerto Ricans by 12 and 14 percent, respectively, but significant mortality disparities remained even after adjusting for neighborhood characteristics. As was the case in the study by LeClere and colleagues (1997), neighborhood characteristics explained fewer of the mortality disparities between whites and either Mexicans or other Hispanics.[2] Although differences in model specification make it difficult to compare the results of the two NHIS-NDI studies, it does appear that neighborhood characteristics contribute substantially to the explanation of black-white mortality disparities in both studies, but less so to Mexican-white mortality differences.

Another issue that has also received relatively little attention is whether neighborhood context is more predictive of health outcomes for certain age groups. Most of the available evidence on this topic also comes from multilevel studies of mortality. Two of these studies (Haan et al., 1987; Waitzman and Smith, 1998a) show that residence in a poverty area is more predictive of mortality among younger age groups than older age groups. Using data from the National Health and Nutrition Examination Survey (1971-1974), Waitzman and Smith (1998a) found that poverty area residence is associated with elevated mortality risk among 25- to 54-year-olds, but reduced mortality risk among 55- to 74-year-olds. The authors attribute the counterintuitive effect of poverty in the older age group to a "crossover" effect in which elderly survivors living in poverty areas may be selectively less frail than their counterparts in nonpoverty areas. In another study showing that neighborhood effects on mortality may be less pronounced among the elderly, LeClere and colleagues (1997) found that contextual characteristics account for a greater reduction in racial/ethnic mortality disparities within younger age groups (18 to 44 and 45 to 64) than within the oldest group (65 and over). However, this study does not report the results of age-specific regression coefficients for neighborhood covariates, so it is not clear whether the neighborhood effects themselves are stronger among the younger groups.

Other mortality studies using the NHIS-NDI data set have failed to replicate the finding that neighborhood effects on mortality are weaker among the elderly. In one of these, Waitzman and Smith (1998b) showed that the metropolitan area-level concentration of poverty was associated with an elevated risk of mortality among respondents to the 1986-1994 NHIS in both the 30 to 44 and 65 and over age groups. In a more recent study using smaller geographic units to measure contextual effects (VSAs) and a longer time series of respondents to the NHIS (1986-1997), Bond Huie and colleagues (2002) found that most contextual covariates have slightly larger effects among the older age group (45 to 64) compared to the younger group (18 to 44). They also found interactions between age and some neighborhood covariates, such as immigrant composition, which is protective against mortality for the older group, but a risk factor for the younger group. Thus, the empirical evidence is mixed on the question of how contextual effects on mortality vary by age.

The view that neighborhood context may be more salient for the elderly is corroborated by multilevel research focusing on health outcomes other than mortality. For example, Balfour and Kaplan (2002) found that self-reported neighborhood problems, such as excessive noise, inadequate lighting, and heavy traffic, were strongly associated with functional loss among participants aged 55 and over in their sample of adults from Alameda County, California. In perhaps the most extensive investigation of age variation in neighborhood effects thus far, Robert and Li (2001) hypothesize that neighborhood effects should actually be stronger among older adults because they may be more vulnerable to negative exposures such as pollution, crime, and weak social and medical services. In keeping with this hypothesis, their findings show that the association between neighborhood socioeconomic characteristics and health (survey reports of self-rated health and the number of chronic conditions) is weakest in young adulthood, but becomes progressively stronger in successively older age groups, peaks between ages 60 and 69, then gets weaker again at ages 70 and older.

In sum, although there is relatively little research on how the relation between neighborhood environments and health may vary across demographic subgroups, the available evidence suggests that racial/ethnic differences in neighborhood context may account for a large proportion of racial/ethnic disparities in health (focusing primarily on mortality), but there is more disagreement on whether and how neighborhood effects vary across age groups. A common limitation of the studies that have analyzed the connection between neighborhood environments and racial/ethnic health disparities is that they do not consider interactions between race/ethnicity and age. This is especially problematic in the case of mortality, where a large number of studies have found a black-white crossover in mortality curves at older ages (Hummer, Rogers, and Eberstein, 1998), implying that racial/ethnic disparities are not fixed entities, but moving targets that vary depending on which age groups are being compared. We will consider such interactions in an analysis of racial/ethnic disparities in mortality using multilevel data on all-cause mortality in Chicago neighborhoods.

UNDERSTANDING WHY NEIGHBORHOODS MATTER

Most of the previous research on neighborhood environments and health has been concerned with the question of *whether* neighborhoods, and specifically socioeconomic characteristics of neighborhoods, matter for the health of individuals. The overwhelming majority of these studies indicate that lower neighborhood socioeconomic status does appear to be related to poor health, net of individual characteristics. Without neglecting the importance of this question, we believe that research should begin to pay more attention to the question of *why* neighborhoods matter—what does the association between area socioeconomic status and individual health, even net of all other individual-level factors, mean? One way to answer this question is to explore interactions between neighborhood- and individual-level factors that might explain the individual circumstances under which neighborhoods influence individual health—or, considered another way, the neighborhood conditions under which individual-level factors influence health. Some studies have explored such "cross-level" interactions (e.g., Diez-Roux et al., 1997; Ecob and Macintyre, 2000; O'Campo et al., 1997; Rauh et al., 2001). Another strategy is to directly measure the neighborhood "mechanisms" that might explain the relationship between neighborhood SES and health (Morenoff, Sampson, and Raudenbush, 2001; Sampson et al., 2002). This calls for an infusion of new theory and new data.

One problem with the current state of this research is that neighborhood characteristics are used somewhat interchangeably and with little theoretical justification in the search for neighborhood effects. Whereas many frameworks have been proposed for organizing individual-level predictors of health status into conceptual categories and for determining the order in which they should be entered into statistical models, health researchers are much less accustomed to thinking about neighborhood-level mechanisms and how they are interrelated. We propose a conceptual framework, consistent with a stress and adaptation perspective on how social environments come to affect health (House, 2002; Lin and Ensel, 1989), that highlights the importance of stressful neighborhood conditions that may deleteriously affect health and the availability of resources from social relations that may counteract or buffer the impact of contextual stressors on health.

Structural/Physical Environment

Structural characteristics refer to properties of a neighborhood's population composition that are typically measured as aggregations of individual-level attributes. In the health literature, the most commonly studied structural measures are indicators of socioeconomic and racial/ethnic composition. In the case of socioeconomic composition, concentrated poverty may be a marker of institutional abandonment. For example, poor neighborhoods may lack access to quality health services, nutritional food, and well-maintained recreational areas (Sooman et al., 1993). Disadvantaged neighborhoods may also expose residents to more dilapidated housing, pollutants, and sources of stress that include crime, violence, and overcrowding. In contrast, affluent areas may offer access to better health care, stores with nutritional food, recreational areas, and other institutional resources that promote good health. Thus, measures of socioeconomic composition could be proxies for a bundle of health risks associated with the concentration of disadvantage and protective factors associated with the concentration of affluence.

The relationship between neighborhood racial/ethnic composition and health is more complex. On the one hand, measures of racial/ethnic composition are markers for residential segregation, and previous research demonstrates that segregation imposes multiple health risks on members of poor minority areas (Cooper et al., 2001; Ellen, 2000; LaVeist, 1993; Massey and Denton, 1993; Polednak, 1996). The health consequences of segregation are likely to overlap with those of concentrated disadvantage, but segregation could impose additional risks. For example, individuals who face barriers to residential mobility because of their race could face psychological risks associated with discrimination (Williams and Collins, 1995b). Moreover, studies have shown that African-American neighborhoods are more likely to suffer from institutional risk factors such as the proliferation of liquor stores and insufficient supplies of prescription drugs at local pharmacies (LaVeist and Wallace, 2000; Morrison, Wallenstein, Natale, Senzel, and Huang, 2000). On the other hand, ethnically homogeneous neighborhoods could also be havens for group resources. For example, some scholars have argued that Mexican culture emphasizes strong family support and reinforces healthy behaviors (Balcazar, Aoyama, and Cai, 1991; Scribner, 1996). Mexican women may be more likely to adhere to traditional cultural practices when living in neighborhoods with higher concentrations of Mexicans. Thus, the expected association between racial/ ethnic composition and health is ambiguous—more homogeneous minority neighborhoods may present health risks associated with segregation, yet they also may produce important group resources through shared cultural experiences.

A testament to the power of structural characteristics to affect health can be seen in recent historical examples, where geographic distributions of poverty are overlaid on geographic distributions of health (Murray et al., 1998). For example, in London, neighborhoods identified as having high poverty and poorer health in 1900 were in almost exactly the same situation in 1999 (Dorling, Mitchell, Shaw, Orford, and Smith, 2000). The geographic pattern of economic and health disadvantage had changed little in 100 years—despite that fact that four or five generations of individuals had moved through those neighborhoods. The same processes can be seen in some U.S. cities (Sampson and Morenoff, 2001).

A closely related group of neighborhood characteristics includes physical and geographic features of the local environment, such as natural amenities, street layout, and pollution. The importance of local toxic environmental exposures for health is clear. There is evidence of negative health effects from a variety of such exposures, including diesel exhaust, lead, and water quality—PCBs, toxic waste dumps, chemical releases, and airborne particulates (Bjorksten, 1999; Burns, Baghurst, Sawyer, McMichael, and Tong, 1999; Eggleston et al., 1999; Howel, Darnell, and Pless-Mulloli, 2001; Northridge et al., 1999; Pandya, Solomon, Kinner, and Balmes, 2002). By their very nature, some of these exposures are inherently "local" and thus are potentially important sources of racial/ethnic differences in health. Balanced against this is the fact that some of the more extreme exposures are quite rare and so are unlikely to aid in explaining the systematic and wide-ranging differences in health across race/ethnic groups. However, we also need to consider that it may not only be the independent effects of the relatively more common exposures—such as geographically specific poor air quality—but their capacity to interact with other exposures to produce poorer health. For example, environmental exposures involved in the pathogenesis of asthma may interact with lack of adequate medical management of the disease to exacerbate its effects. These are clearly important areas for research on context effects on racial/ethnic differences in certain outcomes.

Mounting evidence also exists that physical characteristics of neighborhoods can be crucial determinants of health behaviors. Humpel, Owen, and Leslie (2002) show that accessibility to bicycle paths, parks, walkways, and even local shopping facilities all positively affect deliberate and incidental physical activity. Recent research also suggests that certain physical characteristics of neighborhoods promote outdoor activity and may also afford opportunities for social interaction among area residents (Balfour and Kaplan, 2002; Humpel et al., 2002). Neighborhood characteristics that discourage residents from leaving their homes to interact with neighbors may be especially relevant to the elderly in light of recent evidence showing that diverse social interactions are crucial to maintaining cognitive functioning among the elderly (Fratiglioni, Wang, Ericsson, Maytan, and Winblad, 2000). Thus, it is possible that the physical characteristics of neighborhoods affect cognitive decline among the elderly.

Stressful Social Conditions

One of the main reasons that lower SES neighborhoods may be unhealthy places to live is that they expose residents to stressful conditions, such as violent crime. Repeated exposure to stress fosters a condition known as allostatic load, which refers to the physiological costs of chronic overactivity or underactivity of systems within the body (e.g., the hypothalamic-pituitary-adrenal axis or the autonomic nervous system) that fluctuate to meet demands of repeated exposure to environmental stressors (McEwen, 1998). Geronimus (1992) argues that prolonged exposure to high-stress neighborhood environments can take a cumulative toll on maternal health in the form of "weathering."

Although there is relatively little research on crime and health, some evidence shows that fear of crime may be a key mechanism in explaining the effects of neighborhood structural characteristics on self-rated health and mental health (Aneshensel and Sucoff, 1996; Chandola, 2001; Cutrona, Russell, Hessling, Adama Brown, and Murray, 2000; Geis and Ross, 1998; Ross and Jang, 2000; Ross et al., 2000) and that higher neighborhood crime is associated with a greater risk of low birthweight (Collins and David, 1997; Morenoff, 2003; Zapata, Rebolledo, Atalah, Newman, and King, 1992). There are also strong theoretical reasons to believe that violent crime is a primary source of stress in many urban neighborhoods. First, research on the fear of crime shows that people tend to perceive crime largely in geographic terms (Warr, 1994), which makes the neighborhood environment a particularly salient context for generating fear, and hence stress. Moreover, neighborhood crime can be stressful not only for people who perceive high personal risks of victimization, but also for those who fear for the safety of family members and friends, which Warr and Ellison (2000) call "altruistic fear."

Second, research shows that people who perceive more crime and disorder in their neighborhoods have a higher risk of mental health problems related to stress, such as anxiety, depression, powerlessness, fear, and mistrust (Aneshensel and Sucoff, 1996; Cutrona et al., 2000; Geis and Ross,

1998; Ross and Jang, 2000; Ross et al., 2000). By promoting distrust of others, neighborhood crime can also lead to social isolation from close social relationships (Krause, 1991), which in turn has been linked to adverse physical health outcomes (Berkman and Glass, 2000; House, Landis, and Umberson, 1988).

Third, research on exposure to violence among children and adolescents has linked repeated encounters with violence (both direct and indirect) to the development of emotional problems, posttraumatic stress syndrome, substance use, and increasing pessimism in one's own ability, and that of health professionals, to improve health (Fick and Thomas, 1995; Margolin and Gordis, 2000; Selner-O'Hagan, Kindlon, and Buka, 1998).

Finally, some scholars suggest that in addition to fostering stress, neighborhood crime also promotes risky behaviors, such as substance use, because residents of crime-ridden neighborhoods perceive themselves to have relatively short life expectancies, leaving them less concerned with the long-term health consequences of their actions (Ellen et al., 2001; Ganz, 2000).

Social Relations/Engagement

How people adapt to stressful environments depends, in part, on their access to informal resources such as those produced through social relationships and institutions (i.e., social capital). In places where neighbors are more engaged in the social life of their community, residents are more likely to generate informal resources by assisting one another with favors; providing each other with health-related advice and other information; aiding one another with everyday tasks, such as childcare; monitoring each others' property; and participating in local voluntary associations, such as block clubs, tenants' associations, and religious organizations (Morenoff, 2003).

Thus far, most of the research on social relations/engagement and health has focused on individual-level measures of social ties and social support. A major finding from this research is that social isolation—the relative lack of social relationships—is a risk factor for mortality, with a relative risk ratio comparable to that of cigarette smoking (Berkman and Glass, 2000; House et al., 1988; Singer and Ryff, 2001). A related line of research finds that participation in voluntary organizations, a form of social engagement, may promote both physical and mental health (Wilson and Musick, 1999).

Relatively few studies have analyzed the connection between neighborhood-level measures of social relations/engagement and health. Those that have focus mainly on mental health (Aneshensel and Sucoff, 1996; Cutrona et al., 2000; Geis and Ross, 1998; Ross and Jang, 2000; Ross et al., 2000), and most of these studies characterize neighborhood social processes by relying on only a single individual's report of what happens in his or her neighborhood. A more reliable approach to measuring neighborhood social processes is to aggregate the reports of multiple respondents living in the same neighborhood (Raudenbush and Sampson, 1999; Sampson et al., 2002), but this strategy has not been used in many health studies (for an exception, see Cutrona et al., 2000).

Sampson and colleagues use such an approach to measure neighborhood "collective efficacy," defined as the shared willingness of residents to actively cooperate in pursuit of commonly held goals (Sampson, Morenoff, and Earls, 1999; Sampson, Raudenbush, and Earls, 1997), but most of their research focuses on crime-related outcomes, not health.[3] This research shows that neighborhoods with higher levels of collective efficacy have lower levels of violent crime (Morenoff et al., 2001; Sampson et al., 1997) and disorder (Sampson and Raudenbush, 1999), and that collective efficacy—as well as other social processes, such as reciprocal exchange—is predicted by structural factors, such as concentrated disadvantage and residential stability (Morenoff et al., 2001; Sampson et al., 1999). In related work, Morenoff (2003) found that the neighborhoods with higher levels of reciprocal exchange among neighbors and participation in local voluntary associations are protective against the risk of low birthweight, even after adjusting for a large set of sociodemographic, behavioral, and biomedical individual-level risk factors. A recent study of middle-aged women in Sweden shows that greater levels of neighborhood social participation also increases the use of hormone replacement therapy (HRT) net of individual socioeconomic, behavioral, and other risk factors (Merlo et al., 2001). The authors speculate that greater social participation in neighborhoods may reflect communication processes whereby women living in neighborhoods with higher levels of social participation influence each other's use of HRT or unmeasured characteristics such as different prescribing patterns of physicians in those neighborhoods.

Influences from Outside the Neighborhood

The social environment and context in which individuals live their lives comprises not only their own immediate neighborhood, but also surrounding neighborhoods in which people work, shop, attend school, visit with friends, travel, and conduct other activities in the course of their daily lives. Most previous research on neighborhoods and health focuses exclusively on the "internal" properties of neighborhoods, but does not consider the possible influences that the wider social environment surrounding a given neighborhood may have on the health of its residents. The tendency to abstract the idea of "neighborhood" from its broader spatial context runs counter to the long theoretical tradition in urban sociology, dating back to the Chicago School, that views neighborhoods as spatially interrelated parts of a broader social system that Park, Burgess, and McKenzie (1967, p. 54) characterized as a "moving equilibrium of social order." Thus far, only a few studies have explored the wider spatial context of neighborhood effects (e.g., Baller, Anselin, and Messner, 2001; Morenoff and Sampson, 1997; Morenoff et al., 2001; Sampson et al., 1999; Smith, Frazee, and Davison, 2000), and most of these are ecological-level studies that do not control for characteristics of individuals. However, in his study of birthweight in Chicago neighborhoods, Morenoff (2003) found that after adjusting for potentially confounding covariates at both the individual and neighborhood levels, there was strong spatial autocorrelation in birthweight such that the incidence of low birthweight in a given neighborhood was correlated .69 with the rate of low birthweight in adjacent neighborhoods.

A key issue in spatial analysis is how to conceptualize and model the spatial process under study (Anselin, 2001). Some outcomes diffuse over space, such as acts of violence in one neighborhood that instigate retaliatory acts in nearby neighborhoods or an infectious disease that is spread from one area to another through social networks (Cohen and Tita, 1999). Such diffusion processes apply to the case of infectious disease, but noninfectious health outcomes do not diffuse over space in the sense that the occurrence of the event/disease in one neighborhood does not directly affect the likelihood of a similar outcome occurring in a geographically proximate area. In the case of noninfectious health outcomes, spatial dependence can still arise as a result of "spillover" effects from nearby neighborhoods, also known as spatial externalities. For example, crime in nearby areas may provoke fear in a given neighborhood, regardless of the level of crime in that neighborhood (Morenoff and Sampson, 1997). Likewise, informal social resources generated through social relations and collective engagement may accrue not just to the residents of a particular neighborhood, but potentially to residents in adjacent areas as well (Sampson et al., 1999). The general point is that neighborhood conditions may be reinforced, exacerbated, moderated, or counteracted by the characteristics of adjacent and proximate neighborhoods.

PATHWAYS TO HEALTH: SPECIFICITY, NATURAL HISTORY, AND LIFE COURSE

We now consider how future research could improve our understanding of the pathways through which neighborhoods come to affect health by proposing three related ideas that we believe are useful for better understanding how neighborhoods might affect racial/ethnic disparities in aging and health: (1) why we need to think about specific outcomes related to neighborhood effects on health, (2) how the timing of neighborhood exposures intersects with the natural history of health outcomes, and (3) how neighborhood effects may vary over the life course.

Neighborhood Effects and the Specificity of Health Outcomes

The first idea involves conceptualizing "health." Obviously health is multidimensional and cannot be captured in a single outcome, although there are many useful summary measures of health, such as overall mortality and life expectancy, and measures that tap into disease burden as well as death, such as disability-adjusted life years (DALY) and quality-adjusted life years (QALY). In considering how neighborhoods may affect aging, we are concerned with the major chronic disease conditions and their sequelae, such as heart disease, diabetes, stroke, cancer, and respiratory disease. We are also concerned with mental health; aspects of physical, social, emotional, and cognitive functioning; and health-related behaviors, such as exercise, diet, and medication and health care utilization. This list is not intended to be exhaustive or exclusive. Rather, it serves to illustrate our first principle, that in thinking about how neighborhood processes could affect health outcomes, we need to think about how specific types of neighborhood processes link to specific types of health outcomes.

For example, the proximal neighborhood exposures causing falls among the elderly, such as uneven or broken pavements, are not the same causal exposures implicated in respiratory disease. Although sometimes we may be forced to pragmatically use a count of uneven or broken pavements as a surrogate for the causal exposures for respiratory disease that are present in a neighborhood—indeed, tallies of dilapidated buildings and broken windows have been used as surrogate measures of neighborhood environment linked to certain health outcomes (Cohen et al., 2000)—it is important nevertheless to be clear on what the relevant causal exposures are for each type of health outcome. Broken windows do not cause heart disease, unless they contribute to a complicated miasma of "stressful environment" that affects heart disease risk through cognitively mediated psychoneuroendocrine and immunologic processes. On the other hand, general aspects of the appearance of the environment may be important for mental health. The point is that unless we attempt to study specific outcomes, it will be difficult to know which neighborhood characteristics are important for which outcomes.

As another example of this specificity criterion, it is relatively easy to understand how "collective efficacy" might be associated with outcomes such as juvenile delinquency, violent behavior, or perhaps even behaviors such as smoking. It is less clear how the same neighborhood-level exposure might affect the pathogenesis of breast cancer or depression among the elderly. In fact, one of the strengths of the concept of collective efficacy is that it was formulated as a task-specific construct, meaning that what constitutes collective efficacy may differ depending on the outcome or age group in question (Sampson et al., 1999). This specific outcome/mechanism approach is, in our opinion, one way forward and needs to be applied more rigorously across a range of potential health outcomes relevant to disparities in aging. Such a recognition may also mean that general health outcomes such as self-rated health or functional health indicators that mix physical, psychological, and functional morbidity are potentially of less interest in regard to understanding the specific mechanisms of health-related neighborhood processes, simply because there are so many potential pathways to individuals rating their general state of health. This is not meant to imply that such investigations are uninformative—instead they are limited in the extent to which they can provide clues to the ways in which specific neighborhood processes affect different health outcomes.

We do not wish to appear as overly reductionist, and we hold open the possibility that some neighborhood factors may be implicated in a range of outcomes. For example, it would not be a surprise to find that neighborhood poverty was associated with higher infant mortality, homicide, and heart disease—three disparate outcomes, with biologically different causal mechanisms, primarily affecting different age groups in the population. We would all recognize that poverty is a multidimensional construct that implicates a variety of more specific exposures such as poor housing, pollution, lack of education, unemployment, inadequate diet, and so on. The fact that these specific exposures cluster in certain geographic spaces—and so appear to be empirically associated with all the outcomes—should not be confused with the idea that they all have specific, proximal mechanistic pathways to different health outcomes. It simply means that neighborhoods that have poor-quality housing are also more likely to have more pollution, unsafe playgrounds, and no places to buy fresh fruit and vegetables. Thus, poverty is a convenient marker of many more specific damaging neighborhood exposures of which we are either ignorant or unable to measure directly. We should also be aware of the potential for such clusters of exposures to interact in producing disease, so that it is the spatial aggregation of a series of negative neighborhood forces that act synergistically to magnify the total exposure load and/or increase susceptibility to certain outcomes. However, the general principle of moving toward a search for greater conceptual and mechanistic specificity—in both social and biological domains—of neighborhood influences on health remains important.

Neighborhood Effects and the Natural History of Different Health Outcomes

The second and related principle is to consider the natural history of different types of health outcomes and at which stage in the natural history of an outcome neighborhood environments might be most relevant. For many health outcomes, especially chronic disease outcomes, there is a natural history, which may begin with exposure to certain risk factors such as high-fat diet or smoking, metabolic or hemostatic changes, and the appearance of subclinical manifestations that increase susceptibility, such as asymptomatic atherosclerosis or elevated blood pressure. Then some triggering mechanism may come that leads to a clinically defined event (such as a heart attack), and assuming survival, the consequences of the disease where afflicted individuals learn to live on a day-to-day basis with any physical, social, behavioral, and psychological limitations imposed by their condition. It seems likely that different aspects of neighborhoods could affect these processes differently depending on which stage of the natural history of the particular disease is of concern. For example, it is possible that neighborhood characteristics may play little immediate role in the pathogenesis of stroke, but neighborhood factors may be very important in the quality of life and access to resources of people who have survived stroke and are living with some of the functional limitations that can impose.

Our point here is to suggest that there is no single pathway to health and thus no unique set of neighborhood characteristics that will be universally important for all health outcomes or at all stages of the outcomes. While this may be seen as lurching toward reductionism, we think it is an appropriate recognition of potential complexity. These two principles are important in guiding the next phase of research on health-related neighborhood effects, and this recognition is motivated by the overwhelming body of knowledge that suggests that there are indeed different pathways to different types and stages of health outcomes. Our specific topic here is to better understand racial/ethnic differences in health and aging. This clearly implicates disparities in a large array of different health outcomes and implicates different mechanisms.

Neighborhood Effects and the Life Course

The third principle also relates to the first two and involves considering life-course processes (Kuh and Ben Shlomo, 1997). If research on neighborhoods is to fulfill its promise for better understanding racial/ethnic disparities in major aging outcomes such as chronic disease, then it may be misleading to look for "explanations" of these disparities based on contemporaneous neighborhood exposures. As we have discussed, chronic diseases have latency periods, which implies that exposures from across the life course may be important in the pathogenesis and progression of these diseases (Barker, 1998; Davey Smith, Gunnell, and Ben Shlomo, 2000; Davey Smith et al., 1998; Hertzman, Power, Matthews, and Manor, 2001; Leon, 2001b; Leon and Davey Smith, 2000).

One way that research on neighborhoods and health could move forward is to better conceptualize how measured exposures to neighborhood conditions match up with the temporal logic of the stage of the outcome. In simple terms this means that we should start thinking about the potential effects of neighborhoods through a life-course perspective. It is possible that exposure to current neighborhood conditions per se has little to do with the current distribution of disparities in the incidence of chronic disease outcomes, such as rates of heart disease or cancer. Rather, these probably reflect neighborhood and individual influences from earlier in the life course. This recognition means that both individual and neighborhood life-course exposures are of interest in better understanding contemporary racial/ethnic differentials in some outcomes such as heart disease, cancer, chronic lung disease, and diabetes.

In its broadest conceptualization, a life-course approach recognizes that:

- exposures in early life can have both direct and indirect long-term effects on health;
- there may be genetic, biological, and social intergenerational inheritance of risk factors;
- biological and social exposures coevolve over the life course, so that contextual exposures at one point of the life course may be literally "embodied"; and
- the effects of exposures can accumulate over time.

Space limitations constrain our discussion of these principles here, but they have been well elaborated in previous work (Aboderin et al., 2002; Davey Smith, Ben-Shlomo, and Lynch, 2002; Davey Smith, Gunnell, and Ben Shlomo, 2000; Harding, 2001; Kuh and Ben Shlomo, 1997; Leon, 2001a).

Consider the example of neighborhood effects on coronary heart disease (CHD). CHD is a major cause of morbidity and mortality in the United States, and there are large and potentially widening racial/ethnic disparities in heart disease (Barnett and Halverson, 2001; Schalick, Hadden, Pamuk, Navarro, and Pappas, 2000). The long incubation period for CHD has been recognized for many years, and a life-course approach to its etiology is a natural extension of this view. Most of the important risk factors identified for CHD are socially patterned. Davey Smith and Lynch (2002) have detailed the risk factors for incident coronary heart disease according to stages of the life course:

- Maternal health, development, and diet before and during pregnancy
- Parental history of CHD

- Low birthweight
- Socioeconomic deprivation from childhood onward
- Stress from childhood onward
- Poor growth in childhood
- Short leg length in childhood
- Obesity in childhood
- Certain infections acquired in childhood
- Poor diet from childhood onward
- High blood pressure in late adolescence
- High serum cholesterol in late adolescence
- Smoking from late adolescence onward
- Little physical activity from late adolescence onward
- High blood pressure in adulthood
- High serum cholesterol in adulthood
- Obesity in adulthood
- Job insecurity and unemployment in adulthood
- Short stature in adulthood
- Binge alcohol drinking in adulthood
- Diabetes and components of syndrome X in adulthood
- Elevated fibrinogen and other acute phase reactants in adulthood
- Certain infections acquired in adulthood

This list summarizes factors that are putative CHD risk factors and of particular interest from a life-course perspective, according to their period of influence. It is clear that CHD can be considered the archetype of diseases whose determinants should be sought across the entire life course— from conditions existing at the time of conception and during intrauterine development, through nutrition, growth, and health in childhood, to social conditions, occupation, diet, physical activity, and smoking throughout adult life. Applied to the potential for neighborhood characteristics to affect CHD, it is obvious that many of the factors listed are influenced by the contexts in which people have lived and that these contextual influences may be expressed at many stages of the life course.

Even greater complexity is added when we consider that these contextual effects may differ by birth cohort. The life-course conditions and exposures of individuals born into a poor neighborhood in Detroit in the 1940s may be very different from those born into the same conditions in the same city today. Poor neighborhoods in the 1940s may have implied greater exposure to environmental conditions conducive to undernutrition, while today they may be more likely to increase the risk of obesity. Yet it is the health of that cohort born in the 1940s that we are now beginning to observe in population health statistics. So, to explain current racial/ethnic disparities in health, we may need—depending on the outcome—to consider the complex coevolution of individual and neighborhood processes over time that may in some cases be specific to birth cohort and the outcome being studied.

If we consider the schema presented in Figure 11-1 as a representation of some of the factors involved in the natural history of CHD across the life course, we could ask many questions about the potential for neighborhood processes to affect CHD at one or more points in time. Neighborhood effects on CHD are likely to be stronger at some stages than others. For example, we could hypothesize that neighborhood factors may be very important in dealing with the functional consequences of CHD.

Although our specific focus here is on neighborhood processes, we should also remember that neighborhoods might not be the relevant dimension of context for all stages of all health outcomes. For example, families, peers, schools, and workplaces may be more relevant dimensions of context than neighborhoods when considering the adoption, maintenance, and extinction of known behavioral CHD risk factors such as smoking. Nevertheless, neighborhoods lacking the infrastructure for healthy eating and exercise may impact the development of health behaviors, metabolic changes, and the subclinical development of atherosclerosis. Neighborhoods with high levels of crime and social stress could help trigger a heart attack. Neighborhoods with inadequate health care infrastructure probably affect

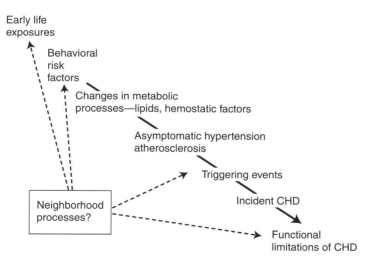

FIGURE 11-1 Neighborhood effects and the natural history of coronary heart disease.

access to emergency services, and the proper and timely diagnosis and immediate management of the condition. Finally, it is conceivable that neighborhoods also differ in their capacity—through such factors as housing, social networks, and transport—to foster adequate levels of physical and social functioning of individuals living with various degrees of CHD-induced disability. This approach raises more questions than it answers, but it does suggest a framework within which to examine such issues.

The life-course approach to chronic diseases such as CHD in adulthood—and therefore the life-course approach to disparities in the distribution of chronic diseases in adulthood—attempts to move beyond an epidemiology that concentrates on individual-level risk factors acting in a relatively instantaneous and supposedly independent manner. This search for instantaneous and independent contributors to risk is partly an outcome of the underlying model of disease causation, captured in the well-known metaphor of the "web of causation." Although the idea of a complex web of causal components—even a web of multilevel contextual causal components—is certainly useful, it does not explicitly include a temporal component and masks the fact that what we observe at any point in time as an array of adult risk factors for CHD is the result of interlacing multilevel chains of biological and social exposures that have coevolved over time. Many of these risk factors have come from previous contextual exposures. In this way the life-course approach addresses the recent debate regarding the individualistic focus of much epidemiology, which concentrates on the lifestyles or physiological risk factor profiles of people abstracted from their social and temporal contexts (Krieger, 1999; Pearce, 1996; Susser, 1998; Weed, 1998). The many weaknesses of epidemiological approaches, which fail to locate exposure-disease associations within their historical, political, and social contexts, have been convincingly elaborated elsewhere (Koopman and Lynch, 1999; Leon, 2001a; McMichael, 1999; Palloni and Morenoff, 2001; Schwartz et al., 1999).

A life-course approach attempts not to abstract individual life trajectories from their contexts; indeed the long-term and sometimes irreversible outcomes of social circumstances at different stages of life can be seen as becoming literally embodied. Human bodies and minds in different social locations become crystallized reflections of the social experiences within which they have developed. Such biological and psychosocial development occurs within contexts of families, peers, and schools and thus also implies the potential for neighborhood influences.

The socially patterned nutritional, health, and environmental experiences of parents influence birthweight, height, weight, and lung function of their children, what are in turn important indicators of future health prospects. The life-course approach to health disparities views the physical and the social as being mutually constitutive, because aspects of bodily form can influence social trajectory in the same way as social experiences become embodied. Low birthweight, growth patterns through childhood into adulthood, persistent infections acquired in early life (such as *Helicobacter pylori*) or the failure to acquire certain infections (leading to immunological programming and increased risk of atopy), lung function, degree of adiposity, and a habitus that embraces particular dispositional characteristics (including attitudes, health-related behaviors, and mood) and ways of dealing with misfortune may seem to fall within different categories, but they are all essential components of life trajectories that influence health. These trajectories are subject to the influence of context.

Better understanding racial/ethnic health disparities means we have to consider both contextual and individual processes acting over the life course of particular birth cohorts to affect racial/ethnic differences in particular outcomes. This implies a potentially important role for neighborhood influences on these processes over time and raises several methodological problems in studying the effects of contemporary indicators of neighborhood on outcomes that we know develop over time. For example, how should we interpret cross-sectional studies that show "small" effects of current neighborhood conditions on chronic disease or mortality after adjusting for individual factors such as behaviors and health indicators? It is precisely these "individual" risk factors that may be partly the result of a complex dynamic of life trajectories influenced by contexts that are now embodied as high lipid levels, obesity, or a positive history of hypertension. For example, evidence shows that individual dietary patterns are determined, at least in part, early in life and may be related to aspects of the neighborhoods in which individuals were raised. Thus, a study of obesity may find no evidence of contemporaneous neighborhood effects after controlling for individual dietary patterns, but these dietary patterns may carry with them the indirect effects of prior exposure to neighborhoods in which fresh fruit and vegetables were not widely available and dietary norms promoted less healthy nutritional practices.

SELECTION PROCESSES

Tilly (2002) argues that all empirical social research rests on two types of theories: one theory that explains the substantive phenomenon under study and a second theory that explains the generation of evidence concerning that phenomenon. Thus far our discussion of neighborhood environments and health has focused solely on the first type of theory—substantive explanations for how neighborhood environments may be related to health and well-being.[4] Both sociologists and epidemiologists who study neighborhoods and health have been far less attentive to Tilly's second type of theory—one that focuses on the processes that generate the empirical data, which in this case means how individuals get sorted into neighborhoods. Such explanations generally fall under the rubric of selection arguments because they seek to understand how individuals and/or neighborhoods are "selected" into certain environmental contexts.

In fact, one of the major critiques of research on "neighborhood effects," generally made by economists (e.g., Ludwig, 2002; Manski, 1993), is that it ignores potentially important selection processes that could generate empirical associations between neighborhood properties and individual health outcomes that are mere artifacts of individual-level causal processes. For example, individual-level health status may play an important role in determining how individuals sort themselves (or are sorted by broader macrosocial forces) into neighborhoods, such that less healthy people are selectively sorted into more disadvantaged neighborhood environments. As a result, the apparent associations between ecological properties of neighborhood environments, such as socioeconomic disadvantage, and individual-level health outcomes could be mere reflections of individual-level factors that are causally related to both health outcomes and sorting into residential neighborhood of residence. In other words, the correlation between disadvantaged neighborhoods and worse health outcomes could reflect compositional differences between neighborhoods rather than true contextual effects.

A recent body of research has taken up this issue directly by examining an ongoing housing program in five major cities across the United States (Boston, Baltimore, New York, Chicago, and Los Angeles) called the Moving to Opportunity program (Katz et al., 2001; Ludwig, Duncan, and Hirschfield, 2001). Participants were randomly assigned to one of two treatment groups—both groups received housing vouchers, but one group could use the voucher only to move to a neighborhood that had a sufficiently low poverty rate, while the other group could use the voucher to move to any neighborhood—or a control group, which received no voucher. Although this experimental design does not eliminate all sources of selection (for example, there is still selection in who takes up the treatment), issues of selective neighborhood sorting are much less of a concern because of the random assignment to treatment and control groups. Results from the Boston study reveal that adults in the experimental group (those who were given vouchers to move to more affluent neighborhoods) experienced improvements in self-rated health and mental health after they moved, and children in these families experienced fewer injuries and a lower probability of having an asthma attack (Katz et al., 2001).

In the following section we consider how selection processes may distort estimates of neighborhood effects and racial/ethnic health disparities in nonexperimental research through a case study of mortality in Chicago neighborhoods. Surprising patterns of racial/ethnic mortality disparities across neighborhood contexts defined by socioeconomic disadvantage suggest that neighborhood selection processes may be more complex than commonly believed. In addition to the possibility that less healthy people are selectively sorted into the most disadvantaged neighborhood environments, we argue that in some contexts it is equally possible that less healthy people may be selectively sorted into more *affluent* neighborhood environments.

A Case Study of Mortality in Chicago Neighborhoods

In this section we present the results of a multilevel analysis on mortality in Chicago neighborhoods to illustrate the connection between neighborhood environments and racial/ethnic disparities in mortality, and also to suggest how attending to selection processes may be critical to advancing our understanding of these disparities. Our data set consists of vital statistics on all deaths in Chicago during 1990 and aggregate Census data from the same year. One obstacle to performing a multilevel analysis with vital statistics data is that there is no variation on the dependent variable because the records only include information on individuals who died, not survivors. However, by combining the vital statistics with Census data from the same year, we obtain information on cases of both mortality and survival within 144 sociodemographic strata, defined through a cross-classification of age (18 categories, as presented in Table 11-1), race/ethnicity (4 categories), and gender (2 categories).[5] We can thus perform a two-level analysis of mortality rates for the age-, race-, and sex-specific demographic strata, which, in turn, are nested within 342 neighborhood clusters (aggregates of Census tracts).[6] Henceforth we refer to the characteristics of each stratum (age, race/ethnicity, and sex) as "individual-level" covariates in our analysis.

Descriptive statistics on population and death counts by race/ethnicity, age, and gender are reported in Table 11-1. Whites are the largest racial/ethnic group in the sample, accounting for just over 35 percent of the population and 50 percent of all deaths, followed by African Americans. The crude death rate is higher for whites than any other group, which, in part, is attributable to a higher number of whites at older, high-mortality risk ages. The age distributions for each racial/ethnic group are displayed in Table 11-2. Whites have the oldest age structure of all racial/ethnic groups, while Hispanics have the youngest.

Table 11-3 presents the results of our multilevel analysis of mortality. The first model contains only individual-level covariates for race/ethnicity (whites are the reference group), age (linear, squared, and cubed), and gender (males are the reference group).[7] The results show that mortality is significantly higher among African Americans compared to whites, while

TABLE 11-1 Descriptive Statistics on Population and Deaths by Race/
Ethnicity, Age, and Gender

	Population Frequency	(%)	Death Frequency	(%)	Crude Death Rate (per 1,000)
N	4,013,165		27,630		
Race/ethnicity					
White	1,407,925	(35.08)	14,078	(50.95)	10.00
African American	1,271,609	(31.69)	11,345	(41.06)	8.92
Hispanic	720,535	(17.95)	1,894	(6.85)	2.63
Other race	613,096	(15.28)	313	(1.13)	0.51
Age					
<5	312,822	(7.79)	806	(2.92)	2.58
5-9	296,656	(7.39)	232	(0.84)	0.78
10-14	287,105	(7.15)	159	(0.58)	0.55
15-19	291,709	(7.27)	350	(1.27)	1.20
20-24	324,459	(8.08)	383	(1.39)	1.18
25-29	345,344	(8.61)	513	(1.86)	1.49
30-34	344,237	(8.58)	693	(2.51)	2.01
35-39	294,651	(7.34)	809	(2.93)	2.75
40-44	244,601	(6.09)	821	(2.97)	3.36
45-49	202,636	(5.05)	918	(3.32)	4.53
50-54	184,359	(4.59)	1,137	(4.12)	6.17
55-59	166,311	(4.14)	1,488	(5.39)	8.95
60-64	167,392	(4.17)	2,289	(8.28)	13.67
65-69	155,348	(3.87)	2,883	(10.43)	18.56
70-74	131,579	(3.28)	3,205	(11.60)	24.36
75-79	110,305	(2.75)	3,403	(12.32)	30.85
80-84	82,818	(2.06)	3,217	(11.64)	38.84
85+	70,833	(1.77)	4,324	(15.65)	61.04
Gender					
Male	1,960,974	(48.86)	14,888	(5,388.35)	7.59
Female	2,052,191	(51.14)	12,742	(4,611.65)	6.21

SOURCE: Chicago Vital Statistics and Census (1990).

Hispanics and members of other races have significantly lower mortality rates than whites. In model 2, we introduce three neighborhood-level covariates, which are based on a principal components analysis (with a varimax rotation) of ten Census variables. These factor scores have been used in previous research on Chicago neighborhoods and the details of the principal components analysis are reported elsewhere (Sampson et al., 1997). The first neighborhood covariate represents the concentration of disadvantage and racial segregation (variables loading highly onto this factor include the percentage of poor families, families on public assistance, female-headed families, individuals in the labor force who are unemployed, individuals under the age of 18, and individuals who are African American). It has a significant positive effect on mortality, indicating that after controlling for age, race/ethnicity, and gender, the risk of mortality is still higher in

TABLE 11-2 Age Distribution of Chicago Population by Race/Ethnicity

Age	Relative Frequency (%)			
	White	African American	Hispanic	Other
<5	5.9	8.3	9.4	8.2
5-9	5.4	8.0	8.9	8.0
10-14	5.0	8.1	8.5	7.8
15-19	5.2	8.2	8.3	8.1
20-24	7.6	7.4	8.9	8.8
25-29	8.3	8.0	9.1	8.9
30-34	8.9	8.0	8.3	8.4
35-39	7.8	6.9	7.0	7.1
40-44	6.5	5.9	5.6	5.9
45-49	5.4	5.1	4.6	4.9
50-54	5.0	4.9	4.0	4.2
55-59	4.8	4.3	3.5	3.7
60-64	5.2	4.3	3.2	3.4
65-69	5.2	3.8	2.7	3.1
70-74	4.8	3.0	2.2	2.6
75-79	4.1	2.4	2.1	2.4
80-84	2.9	1.8	1.9	2.3
85+	2.3	1.6	1.9	2.1

SOURCE: Chicago Vital Statistics and Census (1990).

disadvantaged neighborhoods. The second variable represents the concentration of Hispanic and immigrant populations, which is significantly protective against the risk of mortality in model 2. The third variable represents residential stability (based on the percentage of individuals who lived in the same house in 1985 and the percentage of homes that are owner occupied), and it also has a significant protective effect. Adding the three neighborhood-level covariates in model 2 reduces the estimated risk of being African American compared to white (as represented by the individual-level coefficient) by 79 percent, making it statistically nonsignificant, but it does not significantly change the protective effects associated with being Hispanic or belonging to another race.

In model 3, we allow racial/ethnic status to interact with age, gender, and neighborhood characteristics. Because race/ethnicity is now fully interacted with the other characteristics in the model, the racial/ethnic group coefficients in model 3 are no longer comparable to those in models 1 and 2. We focus our discussion of these results on the association between neighborhood disadvantage and mortality, and its implications for racial/ethnic mortality disparities, because concentrated disadvantage is such a pivotal construct in neighborhood health research. An important result from model 3 is that the effect of neighborhood disadvantage varies signifi-

TABLE 11-3 Individual- and Neighborhood-Level Coefficients from Hierarchical Poisson Regressions of Mortality

Variable	(1) Coefficient	T-ratio	(2) Coefficient	T-ratio	(3) Coefficient	T-ratio
Individual level						
African American	0.20	(701.16)	0.04	(0.95)	0.55	(8.15)
Hispanic	-0.95	(-1,722.91)	-0.95	(-21.12)	0.02	(0.32)
Other race	-2.70	(-2,124.74)	-2.72	(-27.56)	-2.22	(-16.37)
Age	0.07	(4,502.69)	0.07	(64.65)	0.08	(82.77)
African American					-0.02	(-22.03)
Hispanic					-0.03	(-23.22)
Other					-0.01	(-2.81)
Age squared[a]	0.39	(1,586.70)	0.38	(17.57)	0.49	(17.34)
African American					-0.27	(-6.78)
Hispanic					-0.40	(-8.17)
Other[a]					-0.36	(-3.16)
Age cubed	-0.01	(-1,084.13)	-0.01	(-17.50)	-0.01	(-19.39)
Female	-0.44	(-1,621.79)	-0.45	(-30.32)	-0.47	(-26.44)
African American					-0.07	(-2.53)
Hispanic					0.02	(0.46)
Other					0.07	(0.76)
Neighborhood level						
Concentrated disadvantage			0.06	(3.76)	-0.5	(-10.38)
African American					0.89	(15.68)
Hispanic					0.66	(11.93)
Other					0.02	(0.25)
Hispanic immigrant concentration			-0.11	(-6.89)	0.25	(8.26)
African American					-0.71	(-10.83)
Hispanic					-0.14	(-3.20)
Other					-0.38	(-4.97)
Residential stability			-0.04	(-2.37)	-0.07	(-2.20)
African American					-0.02	(-0.37)
Hispanic					-0.03	(-0.76)
Other					-0.50	(-6.50)
Intercept	-4.88	(-16,266.80)	-4.83	(-193.61)	-5.60	(-101.67)

[a] Coefficients have been multiplied by 1,000.

SOURCE: Chicago Vital Statistics and Census (1990).

cantly across racial/ethnic groups. Among whites (the reference group), concentrated disadvantage is negatively related to mortality, which means that white mortality rates are actually higher in less disadvantaged (i.e., more affluent) neighborhoods—a very counterintuitive result that we will attempt to explain. However, for African Americans and Hispanics, concentrated disadvantage is associated with higher levels of mortality, a result that would be expected based on previous research.

To better illustrate what the results in model 3 imply about the neighborhood context of racial/ethnic disparities in mortality, we graph the age-mortality hazard curves by race/ethnicity and levels of neighborhood disadvantage in Figure 11-2. The main point of Figure 11-2 is that racial/ethnic mortality disparities vary as a function of both individual age and neighborhood disadvantage. As is the case in previous mortality research, we observe a black-white crossover in the mortality hazard curves, but with a distinctive twist involving the level of neighborhood disadvantage. At younger ages, African Americans living in highly disadvantaged neighborhoods (75th percentile of disadvantage) have the highest risk of mortality, but at about age 67, this risk is surpassed by whites living in low-disadvantage

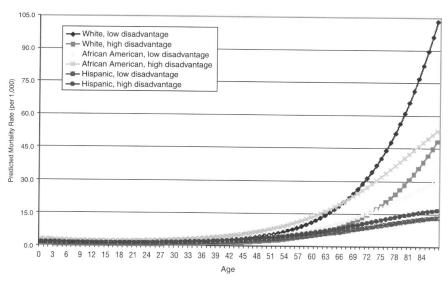

FIGURE 11-2 Model-based mortality rates by race/ethnicity and neighborhood disadvantage.
SOURCE: Chicago Vital Statistics and Census (1990).

neighborhoods (25th percentile of disadvantage), and these low-disadvantage whites continue to display the highest mortality rates at successively older ages. Waitzman and Smith (1998a) report a similar finding that mortality risk is lower in the 65-and-over age group for residents of poverty areas, except that they did not report interactions between poverty area residence and race, so it is not clear whether this effect is driven largely by older whites, as it is in our sample.

Needless to say, the finding that whites living in more affluent neighborhoods have the highest risk of mortality at older ages is somewhat counterintuitive, but at the same time it suggests some intriguing hypotheses about possible selection processes that could account for such results. Most speculation about the direction of selection bias in research on neighborhood effects and health presumes that estimates of their association may be overstated because of the potential for less healthy individuals to selectively reside in more disadvantaged neighborhoods. In other words, the correlation between disadvantaged neighborhoods and worse health outcomes could reflect compositional differences between neighborhoods rather than true contextual effects.

Our findings suggest that it may be equally important to consider selection processes through which less healthy individuals, particularly at older ages, are selected into more *affluent* neighborhood environments. For example, it is possible that nursing homes in Chicago and other cities may be located predominantly in more affluent neighborhoods, attracting a selectively frail older age population to these neighborhoods that is reflected in a higher risk of mortality. At the same time, those who survive to older ages in more disadvantaged neighborhoods may be selectively less frail because they have had to overcome greater ecological risks. These are examples of selection processes that would result in the counterintuitive greater mortality risk in affluent compared to disadvantaged neighborhood environments. Such processes could also vary across racial/ethnic groups if, for example, there is selective out-migration of healthier whites away from the city, particularly at older ages, but less out-migration for African Americans due to the constraints of a segregated housing market. In sum, there are plausible reasons why the surviving population of whites at older ages in more affluent neighborhoods may be selectively more frail than similarly situated African Americans. Ironically, the net effect of such adverse forms of selection among elderly residents of affluent neighborhoods could be to *understate* the risk associated with disadvantaged neighborhood environments.

We present this case study not only to underscore the importance of selection bias in neighborhood research, but also to suggest that much remains to be learned about the direction of this bias and its consequences for causal inferences about neighborhoods. Our analysis raises questions about selection bias that we are admittedly not equipped to answer with our current data set, but it also poses a challenge for future research to better understand the ways in which health status may play a role in the processes through which individuals are sorted into neighborhoods. In short, research on neighborhoods and health could benefit from further development of Tilly's second type of theory.

CONCLUSION

The recent explosion of studies on neighborhood environments and health has provided strong initial evidence that characteristics of neighborhood environments, particularly those relating to the concentration of disadvantage and segregation, are associated with a wide array of health outcomes and may also be implicated in explaining why there are persisting racial/ethnic disparities in so many health outcomes even after controlling for sociodemographic and behavioral characteristics of individuals. Yet much remains to be learned in this area of research. We now conclude with several suggestions on avenues for future research that require the most attention:

- *Collecting data on neighborhood mechanisms for health:* One of the top priorities is to better understand the specific exposures that neighborhood environments offer and how they may be related to health. Socioeconomic disadvantage and segregation are undoubtedly key dimensions of neighborhood life, but researchers need to better understand how they are connected to social processes, institutions, sources of stress, and characteristics of the physical environment that may be more directly relevant to health. Some of the most notable advances in neighborhood research in recent years have been the development of research designs and methods that enable researchers to measure neighborhood social and institutional processes either through surveys or systematic social observation (Raudenbush and Sampson, 1999). This research has shown that community-based surveys can indeed yield reliable and valid measures of neighborhood characteristics when surveying multiple respondents living in the same ecological areas and using their collective assessment to build neighborhood indicators (e.g., Cook, Shagle, and Degirmencioglu, 1997; Elliott et al., 1996; Sampson et al., 1997), as opposed to a strategy of constructing neighborhood indicators based on a single individual's report of his or her neighborhood. Another trend in this direction is the recent advance in collecting observational data on the physical and social features of neighborhood environments. This strategy, known as "systematic social observation" (Sampson and Raudenbush, 1999), is important for health research because it more directly captures the sights, sounds, and feel of neighborhood environments that may be important for some health outcomes, particularly among children and the elderly, whose routine activity patterns may depend heavily on the microlevel conditions of the blocks in and around where they live. By observing block faces (one side of a street within a block), data can be aggregated to any level of analysis desired (e.g., block, block group, housing project, or neighborhood) to characterize social and physical characteristics. Such data can be exploited to build new measures of "microneighborhood" contexts.

• *Age- and race/ethnic-specific effects:* By and large, most research on neighborhood context and health has focused on the main effects of neighborhood characteristics. Only a few studies have considered interactions between neighborhood characteristics and individual-level race/ethnicity (Pearl et al., 2001) and age (Bond Huie et al., 2002; Haan et al., 1987; LeClere et al., 1997, 1998; Rauh et al., 2001; Robert and Li, 2001; Waitzman and Smith, 1998a, 1998b). In our analysis of mortality, interactions revealed that racial/ethnic disparities in mortality vary as a function of both neighborhood characteristics and age. More research on how neighborhood effects vary across demographic subgroups could yield new insights into the connection between neighborhood environments and racial/ethnic disparities in health and aging.

• *Selection processes and life-course perspectives:* The issue of selection bias should be understood not only as a threat to causal inference, but also an opportunity to better understand important socioeconomic processes that may underlie racial/ethnic disparities in health (Palloni and Morenoff, 2001), such as the sorting of individuals into neighborhoods. Our multilevel analysis of mortality produced results that appeared to be counterintuitive until they were cast in the light of possible selection processes that could operate in some contexts to channel less healthy people from older age groups into more affluent urban neighborhoods and other forms of selection that may produce a selectively more healthy stock of survivors in poor urban environments. Researchers should thus attempt not only to control for selection, but also to study such processes more directly by collecting information on residential histories and integrating this analysis into the study of neighborhood effects on health. Understanding residential histories would also address concerns we have raised about the life course and timing of an individual's exposure to neighborhood environments. Some sociologists have begun to consider the enduring effects of childhood community context and independent effects of adult community context on health-related outcomes (Axinn and Yabiku, 2001). This is precisely the kind of research that promises to yield a richer understanding of the multiple developmental influences that neighborhood environments may have across the life course. Investigating neighborhood effects on health from a life-course perspective requires the collection of longitudinal data on both individuals and their neighborhoods. Some existing data sets offer these possibilities, including national studies, such as the Panel Study of Income Dynamics (http://www.isr.umich.edu/src/psid/), and local area studies, such as the Project on Human Development in Chicago Neighborhoods (http://phdcn.harvard.edu/).

• *Spatial perspectives on health:* To gain a fuller appreciation of contextual effects on health it is also necessary to widen the geographic lens beyond the often arbitrary boundaries of statistically defined neighborhoods. A wider spatial perspective on health may also shed new light on racial/ethnic health disparities. For example, if African-American neighborhoods are embedded in more disadvantaged environments than are similarly endowed white neighborhoods, then the consequences of racial segregation may be greater and more systemic than previously thought (Morenoff et al., 2001). Patillo-McCoy's (1999) ethnographic study of "Groveland," a community in Chicago, suggests that black middle-class families face such a spatial (and structural) disadvantage. Despite networks of social control, she found that black middle-class families must constantly struggle to escape the problems of drugs, violence, and disorder that spill over from neighboring communities. Finally, from a public health viewpoint, understanding how and why spatial externalities occur may be critical in designing community intervention strategies. These findings carry with them both a caution that treating neighborhoods as "islands unto themselves" for the purposes of intervention is potentially misguided, but also the promise that if interventions can foster protective factors, such as social resources, they may spawn positive spatial externalities and thus benefit a wider geographic area.

ENDNOTES

1. Some public health researchers also use neighborhood variables, such as Census tract income, as proxies for unmeasured characteristics at the individual level, such as socioeconomic status (Alter et al., 1999; Geronimus and Bound, 1998; Krieger, 1992).

2. In the Bond Huie et al. study (2002), Mexicans have significantly higher mortality than non-Hispanic whites in all models, while other Hispanics have significantly lower mortality than non-Hispanic whites.

3. There are, however, two studies from the Project on Human Development in Chicago Neighborhoods (PHDCN) researchers relating neighborhood social processes to health (Buka et al., 2003; Morenoff, 2003).

4. The idea of using Tilly's (2002) classification theories to illustrate the theoretical importance of selection processes comes from Winship (2002), who refers to Tilly's first type of theory as "substantive theory" and his second type as "methodological theory."

5. By merging the vital statistics data from death certificates with population data from the Census, we encounter several sources of measurement error. First, because the vital statistics data track death over the entire year, 1990, it is possible that some people who died were not recorded in the Census population counts, which represent a snapshot at one point in

time. It is also possible that some people who were recorded in the Census population data may have died during 1990, but their deaths were not recorded in the vital statistics data. Empirically, we found that in several sociodemographic strata there were more deaths than population. Therefore it was necessary to add a constant of 15 people to each of the strata so that the numerator never exceeded the denominator. However, adding fictional people to the denominator necessarily lowers the mortality rate of each stratum. To check how this may have affected our results, we reran the models by adding higher numbers of people to the denominator (20, 25, and 30). We found that our findings were robust to all specifications, but that the magnitude of the mortality rates was sensitive to the number of people we added to the denominator. Thus we caution against making generalizations based on the absolute levels of mortality represented in our data.

6. The project team cluster analyzed 1990 Census data in order to determine which tracts could be combined to form relatively homogeneous neighborhood clusters (NCs) with respect to distributions of racial/ethnic mix, SES, housing density, and family structure. Then they fine-tuned these combinations to ensure that the final NC boundaries would be consistent with major ecological barriers (e.g., railroad tracts, parks, and main thoroughfares) and local knowledge of neighborhood borders. The average NC contains 7,950 people. In comparison, the average Census tract contains 3,156 people, while the Local Community Area, another commonly used geographic unit in Chicago that is aggregated from Census tracts, has an average of 35,415 people. More details about the PHDCN sample design are available in previous publications (e.g., Sampson et al., 1997). Although the vital statistics data were geocoded to the level of the Census tract, we chose to use the somewhat larger neighborhood clusters in order to obtain more stable estimates of mortality within each neighborhood.

7. We also ran models where age was specified with dummy variables for 17 of the 18 categories, and this yielded very similar findings. We present the linear, quadratic, and cubic specifications in the interest of parsimony.

REFERENCES

Aboderin, I., Kalache, A., Ben-Shlomo, Y., Lynch, J.W., Yajnik, C.S., and Kuh, D. (2002). *Life course perspectives on coronary heart disease, stroke and diabetes. The evidence and implications for policy and research.* Geneva, Switzerland: World Health Organization.

Acevedo-Garcia, D. (2000). Residential segregation and the epidemiology of infectious diseases. *Social Science and Medicine, 6*(1), 45-72.

Alter, D.A., Naylor, C.D., Austin, P., and Tu, J.V. (1999). Effects of socioeconomic status on access to invasive cardiac procedures and on mortality after acute myocardial infarction. *New England Journal of Medicine, 341,* 1359-1367.

Anderson, R.T., Sorlie, P., Backlund, E., Johnson, N., and Kaplan, G.A. (1997). Mortality effects of community socioeconomic status. *Epidemiology, 8,* 42-47.

Aneshensel, C.S., and Sucoff, C.A. (1996). The neighborhood context of adolescent mental health. *Journal of Health and Social Behavior, 37,* 293-310.

Anselin, L. (2001). Spatial externalities, spatial multipliers, and spatial econometrics. Unpublished manuscript, University of Illinois, Urbana-Champaign.

Axinn, W.G., and Yabiku, S.T. (2001). Social change, the social organization of families, and fertility limitation. *American Journal of Sociology, 106,* 1219-1261.

Balcazar, H., Aoyama, C., and Cai, X. (1991). Interpretive views on Hispanics' perinatal problems of low birth weight and prenatal care. *Public Health Reports, 106,* 420-426.

Balfour, J.L., and Kaplan, G.A. (2002). Neighborhood environment and loss of physical function in older adults: Evidence from the Alameda County study. *American Journal of Epidemiology, 155,* 507-515.

Baller, R.D., Anselin, L., and Messner, S.F. (2001). Structural covariates of U.S. county homicide rates: Incorporating spatial effects. *Criminology, 39,* 561-590.

Barker, D.J.P. (1998). *Mothers, babies, and health in later life.* Edinburgh, Scotland: Churchill Livingstone.

Barnett, E., and Halverson, J. (2001). Local increases in coronary heart disease mortality among blacks and whites in the United States, 1985-1995. *American Journal of Public Health, 91,* 1499-1506.

Berkman, L.F., and Glass, T. (2000). Social integration, social networks, social support, and health. In I. Kawachi (Ed.), *Social epidemiology* (pp. 137-173). Oxford, England: Oxford University Press.

Bjorksten, B. (1999). The environmental influence on childhood asthma. *Allergy, 54,* 17-23.

Boardman, J.D., Finch, B.K., Ellison, C.G., Williams, D.R., and Jackson, J.S. (2001). Neighborhood disadvantage, stress, and drug use among adults. *Journal of Health and Social Behavior, 42,* 151-165.

Bond Huie, S.A., Hummer, R.A., and Rogers, R.G. (2002). Individual and contextual risk factors of death among race and ethnic groups in the United States. *Journal of Health and Social Behavior, 43,* 359-381.

Booth, M.L., Owen, N., Bauman, A., Clavisi, O., and Leslie, E. (2000). Social-cognitive and perceived environment influences associated with physical activity in older Australians. *Preventive Medicine, 31,* 15-22.

Bosma, H., van de Mheen, H.D., Borsboom, G.J. and Mackenbach, J.P. (2001). Neighborhood socioeconomic status and all-cause mortality. *American Journal of Epidemiology, 153*(4), 363-371.

Boyle, M.H., and Willms, J.D. (1999). Place effects for areas defined by administrative boundaries. *American Journal of Epidemiology, 149,* 577-585.

Buka, S.L., Brennan, R.T., Rich-Edwards, J.W., Raudenbush, S.W., and Earls, F. (2003). Neighborhood support and the birth weight of urban infants. *American Journal of Epidemiology, 157*(1), 1-8.

Burns, J.M., Baghurst, P.A., Sawyer, M.G., McMichael, A.J., and Tong, S.L. (1999). Lifetime low-level exposure to environmental lead and children's emotional and behavioral development at ages 11-13 years: The Port Pirie Cohort Study. *American Journal of Epidemiology, 149,* 740-749.

Carstensen, L.L., Isaacowitz, D.M., and Charles, S.T. (1999). Taking time seriously: A theory of socioemotional selectivity. *American Psychologist, 54,* 165-181.

Caspi, A., Taylor, A., Moffitt, T.E., and Plomin, R. (2000). Neighborhood deprivation affects children's mental health: Environmental risks identified in a genetic design. *Psychological Science, 11,* 338-342.

Chandola, T. (2001). The fear of crime and area differences in health. *Health and Place, 7,* 105-116.

Cohen, D., Spear, S., Scribner, R., Kissinger, P., Mason, K., and Wildgen, J. (2000). "Broken windows" and the risk of gonorrhea. *American Journal of Public Health, 90,* 230-236.

Cohen, J., and Tita, G. (1999). Diffusion in homicide: Exploring a general method for detecting spatial diffusion processes. *Journal of Quantitative Criminology, 15,* 451-493.

Collins, J.W., Jr., and David, R.J. (1997). Urban violence and African-American pregnancy outcome: An ecologic study. *Ethnicity and Disease, 7,* 184-190.

Cook, T.D., Shagle, S.C., and Degirmencioglu, S.M. (1997). Capturing social process for testing mediational models of neighborhood effects. In J. Brooks-Gunn, G.J. Duncan, and J. L. Aber (Eds.), *Neighborhood poverty: Policy implications in studying neighborhoods* (pp. 94-119). New York: Russell Sage Foundation.

Cooper, R.S., Kennelly, J.F., Durazo-Arvizu, R., Oh, H., Kaplan, G., and Lynch, J. (2001). Relationship between premature mortality and socioeconomic factors in black and white populations of US metropolitan areas. *Public Health Reports, 116,* 464-474.

Coulton, C.J., Korbin, J., Chan, T., and Su, M. (2001). Mapping residents' perceptions of neighborhood boundaries: A methodological note. *American Journal of Community Psychology, 29,* 371-383.

Cubbin, C., LeClere, F.B., and Smith, G.S. (2000). Socioeconomic status and injury mortality: Individual and neighbourhood determinants. *Journal of Epidemiology and Community Health, 54,* 517-524.

Cutrona, C.E., Russell, D.W., Hessling, R.M., Adama Brown, P., and Murry, V. (2000). Personality processes and individual differences—direct and moderating effects of community context on the psychological well-being of African American women. *Journal of Personality and Social Psychology, 79,* 1088-1101.

Davey Smith, G., and Lynch, J.W. (2002). Socioeconomic differentials. In D. Kuh and Y. Ben-Shlomo (Eds.), *A life course approach to chronic disease epidemiology.* Oxford, England: Oxford University Press.

Davey Smith, G., Hart, C., Watt, G., Hole, D., and Hawthorne, V. (1998). Individual social class, area-based deprivation, cardiovascular disease risk factors, and mortality: The Renfrew and Paisley study. *Journal of Epidemiology and Community Health, 52,* 399.

Davey Smith, G., Gunnell, D., and Ben Shlomo, Y. (2000). Life course approaches to socio-economic differentials in cause-specific adult mortality. In D. Leon and G. Walt (Eds.), *Poverty, inequality and health* (pp. 88-124). Oxford, England: Oxford University Press.

Davey Smith, G., Ben-Shlomo, Y., and Lynch, J.W. (2002). Life course approaches to in-equalities in coronary heart disease risk. In S. Stansfeld and M. Marmot (Eds.), *Stress and the heart: Psychosocial pathways to coronary heart disease* (pp. 20-49). London: British Medical Journal Books.

Diehr, P., Koepsell, T., Cheadle, A., Psaty, B.M., Wagner, E., and Curry, S. (1993). Do communities differ in health behaviors? *Journal of Clinical Epidemiology, 46,* 1141-1149.

Diez-Roux, A.V. (2001). Investigating neighborhood and area effects on health. *American Journal of Public Health, 91,* 1783-1789.

Diez-Roux, A.V. (2002). Invited commentary: Places, people, and health. *American Journal of Epidemiology, 155,* 516-519.

Diez-Roux, A.V., Nieto, F.J., Muntaner, C., Tyroler, H.A., Comstock, G.W., Shahar, E., Cooper, L.S., Watson, R.L., and Szklo, M. (1997). Neighborhood environments and coronary heart disease: A multilevel analysis. *American Journal of Epidemiology, 146,* 48-63.

Dorling, D., Mitchell, R., Shaw, M., Orford, S., and Smith, G.D. (2000). The ghost of Christmas past: Health effects of poverty in London in 1896 and 1991. *British Medical Journal, 321,* 1547-1551.

Duncan, C., Jones, K., and Moon, G. (1998). Smoking and deprivation: Are there neighbourhood effects? *Social Science and Medicine, 48*(4), 497-507.

Ecob, R. (1996). A multilevel modelling approach to examining the effects of area of residence on health and functioning. *Journal of the Royal Statistical Society, Series A (General), 159,* 61.

Ecob, R., and Jones, K. (1998). Mortality variations in England and Wales between types of place: An analysis of the ONS longitudinal study. *Social Science and Medicine, 47*(12), 2055-2067.

Ecob, R., and Macintyre, S. (2000). Small area variations in health related behaviours: Do these depend on the behaviour itself, its measurement, or on personal characteristics? *Health and Place, 6,* 261-274.

Eggleston, P.A., Buckley, T.J., Breysse, P.N., Wills-Karp, M., Kleeberger, S.R., and Jaakkola, J.J. (1999). The environment and asthma in U.S. inner cities. *Environmental Health Perspectives, 107,* 439-450.

Ellen, I.G. (2000). Is segregation really bad for your health? The case of low birthweight. *Brookings-Wharton Papers on Urban Affairs, 1*, 203-229.

Ellen, I.G., Mijanovich, T., and Dillman, K.-N. (2001). Neighborhood effects on health: Exploring the links and assessing the evidence. *Journal of Urban Affairs, 23*, 391-408.

Elliott, D.S., Wilson, W.J., Huizinga, D., Sampson, R.J., Elliott, A., and Rankin, B. (1996). The effects of neighborhood disadvantage on adolescent development. *Journal of Research in Crime and Delinquency, 33*, 389-427.

Elreedy, S., Krieger, N., Ryan, P.B., Sparrow, D., Weiss, S.T., and Hu, H. (1999). Relations between individual and neighborhood-based measures of socioeconomic position and bone lead concentrations among community-exposed men: The Normative Aging Study. *American Journal of Epidemiology, 150*, 129-141.

Fick, A.C., and Thomas, S.M. (1995). Growing up in a violent environment: Relationship to health-related beliefs and behaviors. *Youth and Society, 27*(2), 136-148.

Finch, B.K., Vega, W.A., and Kolody, B. (2001). Substance use during pregnancy in the state of California, USA. *Social Science and Medicine, 52*, 571-583.

Fratiglioni, L., Wang, H.X., Ericsson, K., Maytan, M., and Winblad, B. (2000). Influence of social network on occurrence of dementia: A community-based longitudinal study. *Lancet, 355*, 1315-1319.

Ganz, M.L. (2000). The relationship between external threats and smoking in central Harlem. *American Journal of Public Health, 90*, 367-371.

Garg, P.P., Diener-West, M., and Powe, N.R. (2001). Income-based disparities in outcomes for patients with chronic kidney disease. *Seminars in Nephrology, 21*, 377-385.

Geis, K.J., and Ross, C.E. (1998). A new look at urban alienation: The effect of neighborhood disorder on perceived powerlessness. *Social Psychology Quarterly, 61*, 232-246.

Gephart, M.A. (1997). Neighborhoods and communities as contexts for development. In J. Brooks-Gunn, G.J. Duncan, and J.L. Aber (Eds.), *Neighborhood poverty: Volume II. Context and consequences for children* (pp. 1-43). New York: Russell Sage Foundation.

Geronimus, A.T. (1992). The weathering hypothesis and the health of African-American women and infants: Evidence and speculations. *Ethnicity and Disease, 2*, 207-221.

Geronimus, A., and Bound, J. (1998). Use of Census-based aggregate variables to proxy for socioeconomic group: Evidence from national samples. *American Journal of Epidemiology, 148*, 475-486.

Gorman, B.K. (1999). Racial and ethnic variation in low birthweight in the United States: Individual and contextual determinants. *Health and Place, 5*, 195-207.

Grannis, R. (1998). The importance of trivial streets: Residential streets and residential segregation. *American Journal of Sociology, 103*, 1530-1564.

Haan, M., Kaplan, G.A., and Camacho, T. (1987). Poverty and health: Prospective evidence from the Alameda County study. *American Journal of Epidemiology, 125*, 989-998.

Harding, J.E. (2001). The nutritional basis of the fetal origins of adult disease. *International Journal of Epidemiology, 30*, 15-23.

Hart, C., Ecob, R., and Smith, G.D. (1997). People, places and coronary heart disease risk factors: A multilevel analysis of the Scottish Heart Health Study archive. *Social Science and Medicine, 45*, 893-902.

Hart, C.L., Hole, D.J., and Smith, G.D. (2000). Influence of socioeconomic circumstances in early and later life on stroke risk among men in a Scottish cohort study. *Stroke, 31*, 2093-2097.

Hertzman, C., Power, C., Matthews, S., and Manor, O. (2001). Using an interactive framework of society and life course to explain self-rated health in early adulthood. *Social Science and Medicine, 53*, 1575-1585.

House, J.S. (2002). Understanding social factors and inequalities in health: 20th century progress and 21st century prospects. *Journal of Health and Social Behavior, 43*, 125-143.

House, J.S., Landis, K.R., and Umberson, D. (1988). Social relationships and health. *Science, 241*, 540-554.

Howel, D., Darnell, R., and Pless-Mulloli, T. (2001). Children's respiratory health and daily particulate levels in 10 nonurban communities. *Environmental Research, 87*, 1-9.

Hummer, R.A., Rogers, R.G., and Eberstein, I.W. (1998). Sociodemographic differentials in adult mortality: A review of analytic approaches. *Population and Development Review, 24*(3), 553-578.

Humpel, N., Owen, N., and Leslie, E. (2002). Environmental factors associated with adults' participation in physical activity: A review. *American Journal of Preventive Medicine, 22*, 188-199.

Humphreys, K., and Carr-Hill, R. (1991). Area variations in health outcomes: Artifact or ecology. *International Journal of Epidemiology, 20*, 251-258.

Iwashyna, T.J., Christakis, N.A., and Becker, L.B. (1999). Neighborhoods matter: A population-based study of provision of cardiopulmonary resuscitation. *Annals of Emergency Medicine, 34*, 459-468.

Kalff, A.C., Kroes, M., Vles, J.S., Hendriksen, J.G., Feron, F.J., Steyaert, J., van Zeben, T.M., Jolles, J., and van Os, J. (2001). Neighbourhood level and individual level SES effects on child problem behaviour: A multilevel analysis. *Journal of Epidemiology and Community Health, 55*, 246-250.

Kaplan, G.A. (1996). People and places: Contrasting perspectives on the association between social class and health. *International Journal of Health Services, 26*, 507-521.

Karvonen, S., and Rimpela, A. (1996). Socio-regional context as a determinant of adolescents' health behaviour in Finland. *Social Science and Medicine, 43*, 1467-1474.

Karvonen, S., and Rimpela, A.H. (1997). Urban small area variation in adolescents' health behaviour. *Social Science and Medicine, 45*, 1089-1098.

Katz, L.F., Kling, J.R., and Liebman, J.B. (2001). Moving to opportunity in Boston: Early results of a randomized mobility experiment. *Quarterly Journal of Economics, 116*, 607-654.

Kleinschmidt, I., Hills, M., and Elliott, P. (1995). Smoking behavior can be predicted by neighborhood deprivation measures. *Journal of Epidemiology and Community Health, 49*, S72-S77.

Koopman, J.S., and Lynch, J.W. (1999). Individual causal models and population system models in epidemiology. *American Journal of Public Health, 89*, 1170-1174.

Krause, N. (1991). Stress and isolation from close ties in later life. *Journals of Gerontology, 46*, S183-S194.

Krieger, N. (1992). Overcoming the absence of socioeconomic data in medical records: Validation and application of a Census-based methodology. *American Journal of Public Health, 82*, 703-710.

Krieger, N. (1994). Epidemiology and the web of causation: Has anyone seen the spider? *Social Science and Medicine, 39*, 887-903.

Krieger, N. (1999). Sticky webs, hungry spiders, buzzing flies, and fractal metaphors: On the misleading juxtaposition of "risk factor" versus "social" epidemiology. *Journal of Epidemiology and Community Health, 53*, 678-680.

Kuh, D., and Ben Shlomo, Y. (1997). *A life course approach to chronic disease epidemiology.* Oxford, England: Oxford University Press.

LaVeist, T.A. (1993). Segregation, poverty, and empowerment: Health consequences for African Americans. *Milbank Quarterly, 71*, 41-64.

LaVeist, T.A., and Wallace, J.M., Jr. (2000). Health risk and inequitable distribution of liquor stores in African American neighborhoods. *Social Science and Medicine, 51*, 613-617.

LeClere, F.B., Rogers, R.G., and Peters, K.D. (1997). Ethnicity and mortality in the United States: Individual and community correlates. *Social Forces, 76,* 169-198.

LeClere, F.B., Rogers, R.G., and Peters, K. (1998). Neighborhood social context and racial differences in women's heart disease mortality. *Journal of Health and Social Behavior, 39,* 91-108.

Lee, R.E., and Cubbin, C. (2002). Neighborhood context and youth cardiovascular health behaviors. *American Journal of Public Health, 92,* 428-436.

Leon, D. (2001a). Common threads: Underlying components of inequalities in mortality between and within countries. In D. Leon and G. Walt (Eds.), *Poverty, inequality and health* (pp. 58-87). Oxford, England: Oxford University Press.

Leon, D.A. (2001b). Commentary: Getting to grips with fetal programming—aspects of a rapidly evolving agenda. *International Journal of Epidemiology, 30,* 96-98.

Leon, D.A., and Davey Smith, G. (2000). Infant mortality, stomach cancer, stroke, and coronary heart disease: Ecological analysis. *British Medical Journal, 320,* 1705-1706.

Leventhal, T., and Brooks-Gunn, J. (2000). The neighborhoods they live in: The effects of neighborhood residence on child and adolescent outcomes. *Psychological Bulletin, 126*(2), 309-337.

Lin, N., and Ensel, W.M. (1989). Life stress and health: Stressors and resources. *American Sociological Review, 54,* 382-399.

Ludwig, J. (2002). *Neighborhood effects and self-selection.* Unpublished manuscript, Georgetown Public Policy Institute.

Ludwig, J., Duncan, G.J., and Hirschfield, P. (2001). Urban poverty and juvenile crime: Evidence from a randomized housing-mobility experiment. *Quarterly Journal of Economics, 116,* 655-679.

Macintyre, S., MacIver, S., and Sooman, A. (1993). Area, class and health: Should we be focusing on places or people? *Journal of Social Policy, 22,* 213-234.

Malmstrom, M., Sundquist, J., and Johansson, S.E. (1999). Neighborhood environment and self-reported health status: A multilevel analysis. *American Journal of Public Health, 89,* 1181-1186.

Malmstrom, M., Johansson, S., and Sundquist, J. (2001). A hierarchical analysis of long-term illness and mortality in socially deprived areas. *Social Science and Medicine, 53*(3), 265-277.

Manski, C.F. (1993). Identification of endogenous social effects—the reflection problem. *Review of Economic Studies, 60,* 531-542.

Margolin, G., and Gordis, E.B. (2000). The effects of family and community violence on children. *Annual Review of Psychology, 51,* 445-479.

Marmot, M.G., Fuhrer, R., Ettner, S.L., Marks, N.F., Bumpass, L.L., and Ryff, C.D. (1998). Contribution of psychosocial factors to socioeconomic differences in health. *Milbank Quarterly, 76,* 403-448.

Massey, D.S., and Denton, N.A. (1993). *American apartheid: Segregation and the making of the underclass.* Cambridge, MA: Harvard University Press.

Matteson, D., Burr, J., and Marshall, J. (1998). Infant mortality: A multi-level analysis of individual and community risk factors. *Social Science and Medicine, 47,* 1841-1854.

McEwen, B.S. (1998). Protective and damaging effects of stress mediators. *New England Journal of Medicine, 338,* 171-179.

McMichael, A.J. (1999). Prisoners of the proximate: Loosening the constraints on epidemiology in an age of change. *American Journal of Epidemiology, 149,* 887-897.

Merlo, J., Ostergren, P.O., Hagberg, O., Lindstrom, M., Lindgren, A., Melander, A., Rastam, L., and Berglund, G. (2001). Diastolic blood pressure and area of residence: Multilevel versus ecological analysis of social inequity. *Journal of Epidemiology and Community Health, 55,* 791-798.

Morenoff, J.D. (2003). Neighborhood mechanisms and the spatial dynamics of birthweight. *American Journal of Sociology, 108,* 976-1017.

Morenoff, J.D., and Sampson, R.J. (1997). Violent crime and the spatial dynamics of neighborhood transition: Chicago, 1970-1990. *Social Forces, 76,* 31-64.

Morenoff, J.D., Sampson, R.J., and Raudenbush, S.W. (2001). Neighborhood inequality, collective efficacy, and the spatial dynamics of urban violence. *Criminology, 39,* 517-559.

Morgan, M., and Chinn, S. (1983). ACORN group, social class, and child health. *Journal of Epidemiology and Community Health, 37,* 196-203.

Morrison, R.S., Wallenstein, S., Natale, D.K., Senzel, R.S., and Huang, L.L. (2000). "We don't carry that"—Failure of pharmacies in predominantly nonwhite neighborhoods to stock opioid analgesics. *New England Journal of Medicine, 342,* 1023-1026.

Murray, C.J.L., Michaud, C.M., McKenna, M.T., and Marks, J.S. (1998). U.S. patterns of mortality by county and race: 1965-1994. *Harvard Center for Population and Development Studies* (Monograph Series). Cambridge, MA.

Northridge, M.E., Yankura, J., Kinney, P.L., Santella, R.M., Shepard, P., Riojas, Y., Aggarwal, M., and Strickland, P. (1999). Diesel exhaust exposure among adolescents in Harlem: A community-driven study. *American Journal of Public Health, 89,* 998-1002.

O'Campo, P., Xue, X., and Wang, M.C. (1997). Neighborhood risk factors for low birthweight in Baltimore: A multilevel analysis. *American Journal of Public Health, 87,* 1113-1118.

Palloni, A., and Morenoff, J.D. (2001). Interpreting the paradoxical in the Hispanic paradox: Demographic and epidemiologic approaches. *Annals of the New York Academy of Sciences, 954,* 140-175.

Pandya, R.J., Solomon, G., Kinner, A., and Balmes, J.R. (2002). Diesel exhaust and asthma: Hypotheses and molecular mechanisms of action. *Environmental Health Perspectives, 110,* 103-112.

Park, R. (1916). Suggestions for the investigations of human behavior in the urban environment. *American Journal of Sociology, 20,* 577-612.

Park, R.E., Burgess, E.W., and McKenzie, R.D. (1967). *The city.* Chicago: University of Chicago Press.

Patillo-McCoy, M. (1999). *Black picket fences: Privilege and peril among the black middle class.* Chicago: University of Chicago Press.

Pearce, N. (1996). Traditional epidemiology, modern epidemiology, and public health. *American Journal of Public Health, 86,* 678-683.

Pearl, M., Braveman, P., and Abrams, B. (2001). The relationship of neighborhood socioeconomic characteristics to birthweight among 5 ethnic groups in California. *American Journal of Public Health, 91,* 1808-1814.

Pickett, K.E., and Pearl, M. (2001). Multilevel analyses of neighbourhood socioeconomic context and health outcomes: A critical review. *Journal of Epidemiology and Community Health, 55,* 111-122.

Polednak, A.P. (1996). Trends in US urban black infant mortality, by degree of residential segregation. *American Journal of Public Health, 86,* 723-726.

Raudenbush, S.W., and Sampson, R.J. (1999). Ecometrics: Toward a science of assessing ecological settings, with application to the systematic social observation of neighborhoods. *Sociological Methodology, 29,* 1-41.

Rauh, V.A., Andrews, H.F., and Garfinkel, R.S. (2001). The contribution of maternal age to racial disparities in birthweight: A multilevel perspective. *American Journal of Public Health, 91,* 1815-1824.

Reading, R., Langford, I.H., Haynes, R., and Lovett, A. (1999). Accidents to preschool children: Comparing family and neighbourhood risk factors. *Social Science and Medicine, 48,* 321-330.

Reijneveld, S.A., and Schene, A.H. (1998). Higher prevalence of mental disorders in socioeconomically deprived urban areas in The Netherlands: Community or personal disadvantage? *Journal of Epidemiology and Community Health, 52*, 2-7.

Robert, S.A. (1998). Community-level socioeconomic status effects on adult health. *Journal of Health and Social Behavior, 39*, 18-38.

Robert, S.A. (1999). Socioeconomic position and health: The independent contribution of community socioeconomic context. *Annual Review of Sociology, 25*, 489-516.

Robert, S.A., and Li, L.W. (2001). Age variation in the relationship between community socioeconomic status and adult health. *Research on Aging, 23*(2), 234-259.

Roberts, E.M. (1997). Neighborhood social environments and the distribution of low birthweight in Chicago. *American Journal of Public Health, 87*, 597-603.

Ross, C.E. (2000a). Neighborhood disadvantage and adult depression. *Journal of Health and Social Behavior, 41*, 177-187.

Ross, C.E. (2000b). Walking, exercising, and smoking: Does neighborhood matter? *Social Science and Medicine, 51*, 265-274.

Ross, C.E., and Jang, S.J. (2000). Neighborhood disorder, fear, and mistrust: The buffering role of social ties with neighbors. *American Journal of Community Psychology, 28*, 401-420.

Ross, C.E., Reynolds, J.R., and Geis, K.J . (2000). The contingent meaning of neighborhood stability for residents' psychological well-being. *American Sociological Review, 65*, 581-597.

Rowley, D.L., Hogue, C.J.R., Blackmore, C.A., Ferre, C.D., Hatfield-Timajchy, K., Branch, P., and Atrash, H.K. (1993). Preterm delivery among African-American women: A research strategy. *American Journal of Preventive Medicine, 9*, 1-6.

Sampson, R.J., and Morenoff, J.D. (2001, July). *Durable inequality: Spatial dynamics, social processes, and the persistence of poverty in Chicago neighborhoods.* Paper presented at "Poverty Traps" Conference, Santa Fe Institute, CA.

Sampson, R.J., and Raudenbush, S.W. (1999). Systematic social observation of public spaces: A new look at disorder in urban neighborhoods. *American Journal of Sociology, 105*, 603-651.

Sampson, R.J., Raudenbush, S.W., and Earls, F. (1997). Neighborhoods and violent crime: A multilevel study of collective efficacy. *Science, 277*, 918-924.

Sampson, R.J., Morenoff, J.D., and Earls, F. (1999). Beyond social capital: Spatial dynamics of collective efficacy for children. *American Sociological Review, 64*, 633-660.

Sampson, R.J., Morenoff, J.D., and Gannon-Rowley, T. (2002). Assessing "neighborhood effects": Social processes and new directions in research. *Annual Review of Sociology, 28*, 443-478.

Schalick, L.M., Hadden, W.C., Pamuk, E., Navarro, V., and Pappas, G. (2000). The widening gap in death rates among income groups in the United States from 1967 to 1986. *International Journal of Health Services, 30*, 13-26.

Schroeder, J.R., Latkin, C.A., Hoover, D.R., Curry, A.D., Knowlton, A.R., and Celentano, D.D. (2001). Illicit drug use in one's social network and in one's neighborhood predicts individual heroin and cocaine use. *Annals of Epidemiology, 11*, 389-394.

Schulz, A., Williams, D., Israel, B., Becker, A., Parker, E., James, S.A., and Jackson, J. (2000). Unfair treatment, neighborhood effects, and mental health in the Detroit metropolitan area. *Journal of Health and Social Behavior, 41*, 314-332.

Schwartz, S., Susser, E., and Susser, M. (1999). A future for epidemiology? *Annual Review of Public Health, 20*, 15-35.

Scribner, R. (1996). Editorial: Paradox as paradigm—the health outcomes of Mexican Americans. *American Journal of Public Health, 86*, 303-305.

Selner-O'Hagan, M.B., Kindlon, D.J., and Buka, S.L. (1998). Assessing exposure to violence in urban youth. *The Journal of Child Psychology and Psychiatry and Allied Disciplines, 39*, 215-224.

Shouls, S., Congdon, P., and Curtis, S. (1996). Modelling inequality in reported long term illness in the UK: Combining individual and area characteristics. *Journal of Epidemiology and Community Health, 50,* 66-76.

Singer, B.H., and Ryff, C.D. (Eds.). (2001). *New horizons in health: An integrative approach.* Washington, DC: National Academy Press.

Sloggett, A., and Joshi, H. (1994). Higher mortality in deprived areas: Community or personal disadvantage? *British Medical Journal, 309,* 1470-1474.

Sloggett, A., and Joshi, H. (1998). Deprivation indicators as predictors of life events 1981-1992 based on the UK ONS Longitudinal Study. *Journal of Epidemiology and Community Health, 52,* 228-233.

Smith, W.R., Frazee, S.G., and Davison, E.L. (2000). Furthering the integration of routine activity and social disorganization theories: Small units of analysis and the study of street robbery as a diffusion process. *Criminology, 38,* 489-523.

Sooman, A., Macintyre, S., and Anderson, A. (1993). Scotland's health—a more difficult challenge for some? The price and availability of healthy foods in socially contrasting localities in the west of Scotland. *Health Bulletin, 51,* 276-284.

Stafford, M., Bartley, M., Mitchell, R., and Marmot, M. (2001). Characteristics of individuals and characteristics of areas: Investigating their influence on health in the Whitehall II study. *Health and Place, 7,* 117-129.

Sundquist, J., Malmstrom, M., and Johansson, S.E. (1999). Cardiovascular risk factors and the neighbourhood environment: A multilevel analysis. *International Journal of Epidemiology, 28,* 841-845.

Susser, M. (1998). Does risk factor epidemiology put epidemiology at risk? Peering into the future. *Journal of Epidemiology of Community Health, 52,* 608-611.

Suttles, G.D. (1972). *The social construction of communities.* Chicago: University of Chicago Press.

Tilly, C. (2002). Event catalogs as theories. *Sociological Theory, 20,* 248-254.

Veugelers, P.J., Yip, A.M., and Kephart, G. (2001). Proximate and contextual socioeconomic determinants of mortality: Multilevel approaches in a setting with universal health care coverage. *American Journal of Epidemiology, 154,* 725-732.

Waitzman, N.J., and Smith, K.R. (1998a). Phantom of the area: Poverty-area residence and mortality in the United States. *American Journal of Public Health, 88,* 973-976.

Waitzman, N.J., and Smith, K.R. (1998b). Separate but lethal: The effects of economic segregation on mortality in metropolitan America. *Milbank Quarterly, 76,* 341-373.

Warr, M. (1994). Public perceptions and reactions to violent offending and victimization. In A.J. Reiss, Jr., and J.A. Roth (Eds.), *Understanding and preventing violence. Vol. 4: Consequences and control* (pp. 1-66). Washington, DC: National Academy Press.

Warr, M., and Ellison, C.G. (2000). Rethinking social reactions to crime: Personal and altruistic fear in family households. *American Journal of Sociology, 106,* 551-578.

Weed, D.L. (1998). Beyond black box epidemiology. *American Journal of Public Health, 88,* 12-14.

Williams, D.R., and Collins, C. (1995a). US socioeconomic and racial differences in health: Patterns and explanations. *Annual Review of Sociology, 21,* 349-386.

Williams, D.R., and Collins, C. (1995b). Racial residential segregation: A fundamental cause of racial disparities in health. *Public Health Reports, 116,* 404-416.

Wilson, D.K., Kliewer, W., Plybon, L., and Sica, D.A. (2000). Socioeconomic status and blood pressure reactivity in healthy black adolescents. *Hypertension, 35,* 496-500.

Wilson, J., and Musick, M. (1999). The effects of volunteering on the volunteer. *Law and Contemporary Problems, 62*(4), 141-168.

Winship, C. (2002, July). *Counterfactual models of causal inference: Useful or useless?* Presentation made at University of Michigan, Department of Sociology Colloquium.

Yen, I.H., and Kaplan, G.A. (1999). Neighborhood social environment and risk of death: Multilevel evidence from the Alameda County study. *American Journal of Epidemiology, 149,* 898-907.

Yen, I.H., and Syme, S.L. (1999). The social environment and health: A discussion of the epidemiologic literature. *Annual Review of Public Health, 20,* 287-308.

Zapata, B.C., Rebolledo, A., Atalah, E., Newman, B., and King, M.C. (1992). The influence of social and political violence on the risk of pregnancy complications. *American Journal of Public Health, 82,* 685-690.

12

Racial/Ethnic Disparities in Health Behaviors: A Challenge to Current Assumptions

Marilyn A. Winkleby and Catherine Cubbin

One of the primary goals of *Healthy People 2010* is "eliminating health disparities" among all population subgroups. This replaces the policy in earlier Healthy People Objectives of setting differential health goals by race/ethnicity, age, gender, and indicators of socioeconomic status (SES). These new objectives acknowledge the need to eliminate, rather than merely reduce, social inequalities in order to achieve a parity of health.

This chapter has two goals that contribute to our understanding of health disparities. First, we examine racial/ethnic disparities in a comprehensive set of health behaviors related to chronic diseases to evaluate the extent to which disparities differ across health behaviors, age groups, and gender. Second, we assess the extent to which racial/ethnic disparities in health behaviors are related to underlying differences in indicators of SES. In addressing these goals, we challenge conventional assumptions about racial/ethnic disparities in health behaviors, especially the assumptions that populations of color have less healthy behaviors than white populations, and that racial/ethnic groups are internally homogeneous. We conclude that for some health behaviors, white populations have less healthy behaviors than do black and/or Hispanic populations, and for other health behaviors, the opposite is true. Furthermore, we conclude that disparities exist *within* each racial/ethnic group by important sociodemographic indicators, including age, gender, educational attainment, household income, and for Mexican Americans, country of birth and language spoken.

We focus on the following health behaviors and risk factors, all of which are related to chronic diseases: smoking, obesity, physical inactivity, poor diet, high alcohol consumption, and inadequate cancer screening practices. We selected these factors because of their effect on other chronic disease risk factors (hypertension, high cholesterol, diabetes) and important chronic disease outcomes (heart disease, stroke, cancer). While the underlying causes of these behaviors are not yet fully understood, they are all preventable, and change at any age can result in improved health.

In this chapter, we argue that fundamental explanations for racial/ethnic disparities in health behaviors are largely socioeconomic in nature. Despite a consensus that race and ethnicity are sociopolitical constructs, as opposed to biological categories (Muntaner, Nieto, and O'Campo, 1996; Williams, 1996), some researchers and policy makers have interpreted racial/ethnic disparities in health behaviors, either implicitly or explicitly, as reflecting inherent genetically based differences (for a critique of this approach, see Krieger, 2001). Rather, racial/ethnic disparities may reflect the consequences of a historical pattern of discrimination, by individuals as well as institutions (Geronimus, 1992; Lynch, Kaplan, and Shema, 1997). The consequences of discrimination are expressed through a variety of mechanisms, including differences in population-level SES (Jones, 2000) (e.g., blacks and Hispanics in the United States are far more likely to be poor than whites) and residential environments (e.g., blacks and Hispanics in the United States are far more likely to live in poor communities than whites). Such differences in SES and residential environments have been shown repeatedly to be associated with unhealthy behaviors for whites as well as populations of color (Conference of Socioeconomic Status and Cardiovascular Health and Disease, 1995; Cubbin, Hadden, and Winkleby, 2001; Kaplan and Keil, 1993; Marmot and Elliot, 1992; Winkleby, Kraemer, Ahn, and Varady, 1998). Racial/ethnic disparities in health behaviors may also reflect differences in cultural norms and values. This interpretation may be particularly relevant for groups who have recently immigrated to the United States; for example, foreign-born Mexican Americans may have healthier diets and exercise patterns than those who are born in the United States.

We present data for the three largest racial/ethnic groups in the United States: white non-Hispanics, black non-Hispanics, and Hispanics (with a focus on Mexican Americans when possible). We do not present data on other racial/ethnic groups because data are limited from nationally representative samples across broad age groups. We base our main observations on data from two national data sets, the 1988-1994 Third National Health and Nutrition Examination Survey (NHANES III) and the 2000 Behavioral Risk Factor Surveillance System (BRFSS).

In the first section of this chapter, we (1) present population projections from Census data for selected racial/ethnic and age groups in the United States for the next 50 years; (2) review selected scientific literature on racial/

ethnic disparities in chronic disease outcomes and health behaviors; and (3) evaluate the importance of considering socioeconomic status, residential environments, and acculturation in studies on racial/ethnic disparities in health behaviors. In the second section of this chapter, we present new findings from analyses of racial/ethnic disparities in health behaviors and practices across a broad range of age groups using data from a national sample of white, black, and Hispanic women and men. In the third section we discuss the implications of our findings, and in the final section, we provide conclusions from our analyses.

POPULATION PROJECTIONS

Dramatic changes in the racial/ethnic and age distributions of the U.S. population over the next 50 years will have a significant impact on chronic diseases, most which manifest in later life. Figure 12-1 presents population projections from the U.S. Census for the years 2000, 2010, and 2050 for white, black, and Hispanic adult women and men by age group (U.S. Census Bureau, 2001). Population sizes are given in thousands. There will be large increases in the Hispanic total adult population and to a lesser

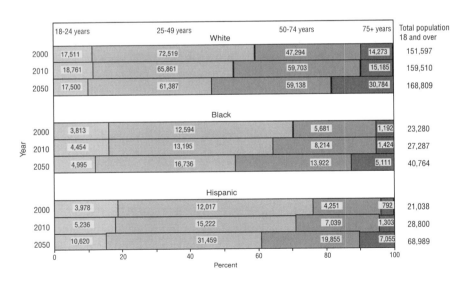

FIGURE 12-1 Population projections in thousands for the years 2000, 2010, and 2050 for white, black, and Hispanic adults, 18 and older, by age group. Population in thousands.
SOURCE: U.S. Census Bureau (2001).

degree in the black population. In 2000, Hispanics and blacks accounted for 11 percent and 12 percent, respectively, of the three racial/ethnic groups aged 18 and over shown in Figure 12-1. By 2050, Hispanics and blacks will account for 25 percent and 15 percent, respectively. There will be even larger changes in the elderly population. By 2050, the elderly white population (aged 75 and older) will increase twofold, the elderly black population will increase fivefold, and the elderly Hispanic population will increase ninefold. For example, while the elderly Hispanic population in 2000 numbered under 1 million (792,000), it is projected to increase to more than 7 million people (7,055,000) by 2050. Given these projections, ethnic minority populations will bear an increased share of chronic diseases.

RACIAL/ETHNIC DISPARITIES IN CHRONIC DISEASE INCIDENCE AND MORTALITY

The leading causes of death for all racial/ethnic groups in the United States are from heart disease (30 percent of all deaths), cancer (23 percent), and stroke (7 percent) (Jemal, Thomas, Murray, and Thun, 2002). These chronic diseases account for nearly three-fourths of all deaths among women and men during some of the most productive years of their lives (25 to 64 years of age). Furthermore, they account for more than $300 billion in direct medical costs each year (Institute of Medicine, 1991).

Although the majority of deaths for all racial/ethnic groups occur from chronic diseases, death rates vary considerably across racial/ethnic groups. Black women and men have higher age-standardized death rates from cardiovascular disease (CVD) than white women and men, regardless of income (Singh, Kochanek, and McDonan, 1996). This includes their strikingly higher death rates from stroke. Higher death rates for blacks from CVD begin in early ages and continue until age 65 (Pamuk, Makue, Heck, Reuben, and Lochner, 1998). After age 65, black-white differences in CVD death rates are smaller, with rates converging or crossing over at the oldest ages (Hollman, 1993). Although there have been large declines in U.S. death rates from CVD since the mid-1960s, the declines since the mid-1980s have been slower for blacks than for whites, producing larger black-white disparities (Singh et al., 1996; Tyroler, Wing, and Knowles, 1993).

Blacks also have higher incidence rates for cancer and higher death rates following diagnosis than whites or Hispanics (Jemal et al., 2002). Death rates for all cancer sites are approximately 33 percent higher for blacks than for whites, and more than twice as high as for Hispanics. In the past decade, black men have shown the largest declines in cancer incidence and mortality of all racial/ethnic and gender-specific groups (Jemal et al., 2002), a change most likely related to a combination of risk factor reduction and better treatment and access to care.

In contrast to blacks, past studies have shown that Hispanics have lower age-standardized death rates from all causes, CVD, and cancer than whites (Aguirre-Molina, Molina, and Zambrana, 2001; Elo and Preston, 1997; Goff et al., 1997; National Cancer Institute, 2001; Sorlie, Backlund, Johnson, and Rogot, 1993; Vega and Amaro, 1994). These rates are consistent for women and men, and for all Hispanic groups, including Mexican-Americans, Cuban Americans, and mainland Puerto Ricans. There are several exceptions to the cancer rates—— Hispanics have higher incidence and/or mortality rates of stomach, liver, cervical, and gallbladder cancer than whites (Gutierrez-Ramirez, Valdez, and Carter-Pokras, 1994; Sorlie et al., 1993). The overall mortality advantage for Hispanics has been termed the "Hispanic paradox" because Hispanics have higher rates of diabetes and obesity and lower socioeconomic status than whites. However, the Hispanic paradox has recently been called into question. Investigators from the Corpus Christi Heart Project reported a greater incidence of hospitalized myocardial infarction among both Mexican-American women and men than among non-Hispanic whites, concluding that the finding was congruent with the risk factor patterns observed in the Mexican-American population (Goff et al., 1997). More recently, investigators from the San Antonio Heart Study reported greater all-cause, CVD, and coronary heart disease mortality among Mexican Americans than non-Hispanic whites (Hunt et al., 2003). These new findings point out the need for studies of larger populations as well as studies that examine possible bias in mortality rates. For example, studies are needed to determine the extent to which Hispanic mortality rates are underestimated because of factors including selective immigration, return of terminally ill persons to their country of birth, age misreporting at older ages, and record linkage issues (Elo and Preston, 1997; Stephen, Foote, Hendershot, and Schoenborn, 1994).

Are Disparities in Mortality Explained by Differences in Health Behaviors?

Given the racial/ethnic disparities in chronic disease mortality, investigators have explored whether differences in health behaviors and risk factors (e.g., smoking, dietary habits, exercise, alcohol consumption) explain these disparities (Lynch, Kaplan, Cohen, Tuomilehto, and Salonen, 1996; Smith, Neaton, Wentworth, Stamler, and Stamler, 1996). Otten and colleagues, Teutsch, Williamson, and Marks (1990), used data for black and white adults from the NHANES Epidemiologic Follow-Up Survey to evaluate whether black-white differences in all-cause mortality (of which chronic diseases are major contributors) were explained by differences in health behaviors and risk factors (cigarette smoking, systolic blood pressure, cholesterol level, body mass index, alcohol intake, and diabetes mellitus). The black-white mortality ratio for women and men aged 35 to 54 was 2.3 without adjustment for health behaviors and risk factors. This decreased to 1.9 when the six factors were taken into account, and to 1.4 when family income was also considered. The authors concluded that 31 percent of the black-white differences in all-cause mortality could be accounted for by the six health behaviors and risk factors and an additional 38 percent by family income (Otten et al., 1990). The remaining differences in mortality, unexplained by known health behaviors, risk factors, and/or SES, suggest that other mechanisms contribute to racial/ethnic disparities in mortality. However, in this study, as well as in others, adjustment for SES was most likely incomplete.

Racial/Ethnic Disparities in Health Behaviors Among Adults

Many studies have examined racial/ethnic disparities in health behaviors among adults, although most have not used representative samples or had adequate sample sizes to assess differences by gender, age, and/or SES. Studies on smoking show that white women, particularly those with lower SES, are more likely to smoke and to smoke more heavily than black or Hispanic women, especially Mexican-American women (U.S. Department of Health and Human Services, 2001). Although some studies show that white men are more likely to smoke than black and Hispanic men, this finding varies according to the age of the study population, the composition of the Hispanic sample, and the consideration of SES in the analysis (Haynes, Harvey, Montes, Nickens, and Cohen, 1990). Studies that have examined smoking among men from the three main Hispanic populations in the United States (Mexican Americans, mainland Puerto Ricans, and Cuban Americans) have found that Cuban-American men smoke the most and Mexican-American men smoke the least (Rogers, 1991).

In contrast to studies on smoking, other studies consistently show that black women have higher prevalences of excess weight and physical inactivity and poorer diets than white women; differences between black and white men are less consistent and generally of lower magnitude (Burke et al., 1992; DiPietro, Williamson, Caspersen, and Eaker, 1993; Duelberg, 1992; Folsom et al., 1991; Gidding et al., 1996; Kumanyika, Wilson, Guilford-Davenport, 1993). Other studies, with some inconsistencies, show that Mexican-American women have higher prevalences of excess weight and physical inactivity than white women (Balcazar and Cobas, 1993; Diehl and Stern, 1989; Haffner et al., 1986; Kuczmarski, Flegal, Campbell, and Johnson, 1994; Mitchell, Stern, Haffner, Hazuda, and Patterson, 1990; Winkleby, Fortmann, and Rockhill, 1993; Winkleby et al., 1998). Again, findings are less consistent for men (Winkleby et al., 1993; Winkleby, Cubbin, Ann, and Kraemer, 1999a; Elder et al., 1991).

In general, these studies show much higher prevalences among those with lower SES.

Most studies of alcohol consumption show few or no differences between black and white populations. Some groups of Hispanic men show heavier alcohol consumption than white men. Mexican-American and Puerto Rican men show heavy use in younger ages, with decreasing use in older ages (Markides, Ray, Stroup-Benham, and Trevino, 1990; Rogers, 1991). As with smoking, alcohol consumption is low for Hispanic women, especially those of Mexican origin; however, rates appear to increase with level of acculturation (Black and Markides, 1993). Heavy alcohol consumption is much more likely in men than in women for all racial/ethnic groups, and has shown inverse associations with SES.

Recent studies of racial/ethnic differences in health behaviors have had the opportunity to include data on representative samples of women and men from the largest racial/ethnic groups in the United States. Given the large sample sizes, these studies have been able to evaluate the influence of SES as well as age. One of the largest national surveys to include multiple racial/ethnic groups, with clinical examination, is NHANES III (National Center for Health Statistics, 1994b). This national survey was conducted from 1988 to 1994 at 89 sites to assess the health and nutrition status of the U.S. population aged 2 months and older. It is noteworthy because it included an oversampling of black and Mexican-American women and men who represent a wide range of SES levels.

In a previous analysis, Winkleby and Cubbin used NHANES III data to examine racial/ethnic differences in health behaviors among 3,229 black, 3,025 Mexican-American, and 3,775 white (non-Hispanic) women and men, ages 25 to 64 (Winkleby et al., 1999a). This analysis evaluated differences in three factors related to chronic disease health behaviors: smoking, obesity, and leisure-time physical inactivity. The results showed that race/ethnicity was independently associated with health behaviors after adjustment for educational attainment and family income divided by family size. Black and Mexican-American women had significantly higher odds of obesity and physical inactivity than white women (odds ratios 1.5 to 2.3, p values <0.01). Black men had higher odds of smoking and physical inactivity than white men (odds ratios 1.3 and 1.4 respectively, p values <.05). In contrast, both Mexican-American women and men had lower odds of smoking than white women and men (odds ratios 0.19 and 0.37 respectively, p values <0.001). The magnitude of the racial/ethnic differences was large for many comparisons (Winkleby et al., 1998). For example, black women were, on average, 16.8 pounds heavier than white women of comparable education and age. While these analyses of NHANES III data adjusted for age, differences across age groups were not examined.

Racial/Ethnic Disparities in Health Behavior Among Children and Young Adults

A number of studies have examined racial/ethnic differences in health behaviors among children and young adults (Anderson, Crespo, Bartlett, Cheskin, and Pratt, 1998; Belcher et al., 1993; Berenson et al., 1998; The Bogalusa Heart Study, 1995; Dwyer et al., 1998; Folsom et al., 1989; McNutt et al., 1997, Srinivasan, Bao, Wattigney, and Berenson, 1996; Tortolero et al., 1997). Using NHANES III data, Winkleby et al., examined racial/ethnic differences in health behaviors in a sample of 2,769 black, 2,854 Mexican-American, and 2,063 white children and young adults, aged 6 to 24 years (Winkleby, Robinson, Sundquist, and Kraemer, 1999b). The analysis evaluated the age groups at which racial/ethnic differences were first apparent and whether differences remained after accounting for educational attainment of the head of the household and family income divided by family size. Whites, especially those from less educated households, had the highest prevalences of smoking; 77 percent of young white men and 61 percent of young white women, aged 18 to 24 years, from lower educated households were current smokers. In contrast, black and Mexican-American girls had significantly higher levels of body mass index (BMI) and percentages of energy from dietary fat than white girls. The racial/ethnic differences for BMI were evident by 6 to 9 years of age (a difference of approximately 0.5 BMI units) and widened thereafter (a difference of more than 2 BMI units among 18- to 24-year-olds). Black boys had higher levels of dietary fat energy intake than white boys. All racial/ethnic differences remained significant after adjusting for age and education of the head of the household. Adjusting for family income showed similar results.

Racial/Ethnic Disparities in Health Behaviors Among the Elderly

Few studies have examined racial/ethnic differences in health behaviors among elderly populations, especially using nationally representative samples. The initial studies in this area show that: (1) older white women and men are more likely to have ever smoked, but are also more likely to have quit smoking than older black women and men; and (2) older black women and men are more obese and physically inactive, but are less likely to have high alcohol consumption than older white women and men (National Research Council, 1997).

Sundquist and colleagues used data from NHANES III to examine whether racial/ethnic differences in health behaviors shown for younger women and men in NHANES III persisted for elderly women and men (Sundquist, Winkleby, and Pudaric, 2001). His analysis included 700 black,

628 Mexican-American, and 2,192 white women and men aged 65 to 84 years. The health behaviors examined were cigarette smoking, abdominal obesity, and leisure-time physical inactivity. No significant racial/ethnic differences were found for smoking. However, black women were significantly more likely to be obese and physically inactive than white women after accounting for age and years of education (odds ratios 1.8 and 2.6 respectively). Black men were significantly more likely to be physically inactive than white men (odds ratio 1.9). No significant differences were found between Mexican Americans and whites for the three health behaviors. The racial/ethnic differences documented by this study may be underestimated because of survival bias. The study population represents an age cohort born between 1904 and 1929 who survived to 1988 to 1994, the dates of the NHANES III assessments. Therefore, people in this age cohort who survived to 1988 to 1994 may represent those with healthier behaviors. Underestimation may be especially true for the black-white differences because of the substantially higher rates of early death from chronic diseases and injuries for black compared with white women and men (Corti et al., 1999; Ventura, Peters, Martin, and Maurer, 1997).

Health Behaviors Across Age Groups

Despite the strong associations between age and chronic disease outcomes, few studies have examined racial/ethnic disparities in health behaviors across a broad range of age groups. Some studies indicate that disparities in health behaviors are larger for younger and middle-aged adults than for older adults; however, most studies have lacked sufficient sample sizes within racial/ethnic subgroups to provide definitive answers. Because chronic diseases reflect a progressive process that begins early in the life course and initiation of unhealthy behaviors often occurs in early adolescence, it is important to include young populations in analyses of racial/ethnic disparities in health behaviors. It is also important to include populations across a broad age range to examine when disparities are first apparent and whether disparities differ across age groups. This can provide insight about causal pathways and the timing, focus, and content of primary, secondary, and tertiary prevention programs and policies (Lowry, Kahn, Collins, and Kolbe, 1996; Smith, Hart, Watt, Hole, and Hawthorne, 1998; Winkleby et al., 1999a).

The Role of Socioeconomic Status

Racial/ethnic disparities in health behaviors most likely result from complex relationships, with SES, residential environments, and cultural characteristics each playing a role. SES, however measured, has shown strong, consistent associations with chronic disease outcomes and health behaviors for decades (Adler, Boyce, Chesney, Folkman, and Syme, 1993; Conference of Socioeconomic Status and Cardiovascular Health and Disease, 1995; Kaplan and Keil, 1993; Marmot and Elliot, 1992). Studies on racial/ethnic disparities in health that assess SES should ideally measure multiple dimensions of SES (e.g., measuring power, status, and economic class) at multiple levels (individual, household, neighborhood, community). However, because of its complexity, measuring SES fully is exceedingly difficult. In addition, there are issues of bias because SES measures such as education and income may not be commensurate across racial/ethnic groups. Thus it is likely that residual confounding by SES exists in any study that investigates racial/ethnic disparities even after "adjusting" for multiple measures of SES (Braveman, Cubbin, Marchi, Egerter, and Chavez, 2001; Kaufman, Cooper, and McGee, 1997; Winkleby and Cubbin, 2003).

Individual-level education, income, and occupational status have most commonly been used as indicators of SES in studies of health behaviors. Each measure has limitations (Smith and Kington, 1997); some are related to general measurement bias and others are particularly relevant to investigations of how racial/ethnic disparities vary across age groups.

The measurement of education in the United States is compromised because measures of educational attainment (e.g., years of education or credentials) do not account for large inequalities in quality of schooling, especially for those from certain racial/ethnic groups and those from the current generation of elderly people. Furthermore, the same level of educational attainment does not convey the same meaning when examining differences in health behaviors across age groups; for example, a high school degree for an elderly population may confer the same status and prestige as a college degree for a younger population. Finally, the measurement of education is difficult to interpret when sample populations include people who have been educated in countries outside the United States.

Measurement of income and occupation/employment status present additional challenges in studies of racial/ethnic differences in health behaviors. Current income may not reflect earnings over one's lifetime and does not reflect wealth (e.g., investment income), especially among the retired. This is particularly problematic in that racial/ethnic differences in wealth are far greater than differences in income (Eller, 1994). Occupational status is also complicated in analyses across age groups because the same occupational category may reflect different exposures, experiences, and/or status across racial/ethnic groups. In addition, standard occupational categories in the United States combine a broad range of occupations and are based on types of work rather than social class theory, limiting their use as a socioeconomic measure (Krieger, Williams, and Moss, 1997).

THE ROLE OF RESIDENTIAL ENVIRONMENTS

In recent years there has been an increasing interest in contextual studies that combine characteristics of both individuals and residential environments to investigate their joint association on individual-level health outcomes (Diez-Roux, 1998; Pickett and Pearl, 2001). A number of investigators have proposed that racial/ethnic differences in health behaviors may be explained in part by factors beyond the individual, such as neighborhood-level influences.

There is a growing consensus that the residential environment that encompasses the immediate physical surroundings, social relationships, and cultural milieus within which people function and interact may influence both the SES and health of their residents. This includes the built infrastructure; industrial and occupational structure; labor markets; social and economic processes; wealth; social, human, and health services; government; race relations; cultural practices; religious institutions and practices; and beliefs about place and community (Macintyre, Ellaway, and Cummins, 2002; Winkleby and Cubbin, 2003). Differences in these residential environments can translate into differences in access to tobacco, alcohol, healthy food choices, safe places to exercise, and preventive health care, all of which can promote or impede healthy behaviors.

Racial/ethnic groups in the United States are highly segregated, resulting in populations of color being far more likely to live in disadvantaged places. Thus, taking into account the characteristics of residential environments may partly explain racial/ethnic disparities in health, after accounting for differences in individual-level demographic and socioeconomic characteristics.

A growing body of research supports the independent association of neighborhood socioeconomic characteristics on chronic disease morbidity and mortality, risk factors, and health behaviors. Residence in a socioeconomically disadvantaged area has been found to be independently associated with heart disease morbidity (Diez-Roux et al., 1997, 2001; Jones, 2000; Smith et al., 1998) and mortality (LeClere, Rogers, and Peters, 1998; Smith et al., 1998; Winkleby and Cubbin, 2003), and CVD risk factors and health behaviors (Cubbin et al., 2001; Diez-Roux et al., 1997, 1999; Duncan, Jones, and Moon, 1996; Ellaway, Anderson, and Macintyre, 1997; Hart, Ecob, and Smith, 1997; Lee and Cubbin, 2002; Smith et al., 1998; Sundquist, Malmstrom, and Johansson, 1999; Yen and Kaplan, 1998). For example, living in a low-SES neighborhood has been independently associated with lower physical activity (Yen and Kaplan, 1998), higher body mass index (Cubbin et al., 2001; Ellaway et al., 1997; Smith et al., 1998), higher prevalence of smoking (Cubbin et al., 2001; Diez-Roux et al., 1997; Smith et al., 1998; Sundquist et al., 1999), and less healthy dietary habits in adults (Diez-Roux et al., 1999) as well as youth (Lee and Cubbin, 2002).

The Role of Acculturation

The role of cultural characteristics in racial/ethnic disparities in health behaviors has been examined using various indicators of acculturation (Aguirre-Molina et al., 2001; Hazuda, Stern, and Haffner, 1988). Acculturation is defined as the degree to which a person participates in the language, values, and practices of his or her ethnic community compared with those in the dominant culture (Padilla, 1980). Some studies that have examined the influence of acculturation on health behaviors suggest that health behaviors may worsen as populations become more acculturated (Espino, Burge, and Moreno, 1991). Other studies suggest that a healthy immigrant effect may bias studies on acculturation (e.g., those who immigrate to the United States have healthier behaviors than those who do not immigrate) (Jasso, Massey, Rosenzweig, and Smith, 2000). Although we could not assess a healthy immigrant effect, we were able to examine the association between level of acculturation and unhealthy behaviors across a wide range of age groups using data from the NHANES III sample of Mexican-American women and men aged 18 to 74. We stratified the Mexican-American sample by two frequently used indicators of acculturation: country of birth (born in the United States or in Mexico) and primary language spoken at home (English or Spanish). We examined differences in four health behaviors and risk factors related to chronic disease:

- *Cigarette smoking* (smoked at least 100 cigarettes in entire life and currently smoking cigarettes everyday).
- *Obesity* (body mass index ≥30 units).
- *Low vegetable and/or fruit consumption* (<3 servings of vegetables and/or fruits per day in the past month).
- *High alcohol consumption* (≥5 alcoholic drinks on ≥1 occasion in the past month and/or an average of ≥2 drinks per day for women and ≥3 drinks per day for men among those who drank alcoholic beverages in the past month). The analysis used predicted values from linear models, adjusted for education (in years) and family income.

In general, we found that women and men born in the United States had notably higher predicted prevalences of unhealthy behaviors than those born in Mexico, after adjustment for education and income (Figure 12-2). The relationships were remarkably consistent across health behaviors and gender, and across most age groups. The largest differences were seen for younger women and older men for smoking, younger women and younger men for vegetable and/or fruit consumption, and younger women for high alcohol consumption; adjusted prevalences were two to three times higher for those born in the United States compared with those born in Mexico.

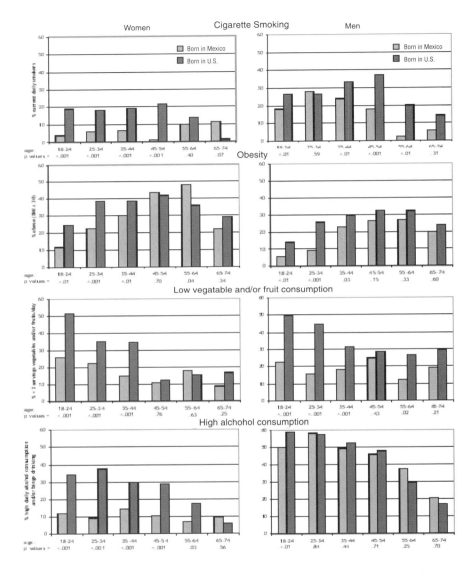

FIGURE 12-2 Unhealthy behaviors among Mexican-American women and men, ages 18-74, by country of birth and age group, adjusted for education and family income. Percentages were calculated with normalized sample weights.
SOURCE: National Health and Nutrition Examination Survey III, 1988-1994.

There was little change in these findings when the analysis was not adjusted for education and income. We found similar associations for language spoken; after adjustment for education and income, those who spoke English had higher predicted prevalences of unhealthy behaviors than those who spoke Spanish.

Analyses of the BRFSS

In the following analyses, we build on the results of previous studies to further our knowledge of racial/ethnic differences in health behaviors across a wide range of age groups. We use data from the Behavioral Risk Factor Surveillance System, a national cross-sectional survey that has standardized definitions and assessments of health behaviors in women and men aged 18 and over from multiple racial/ethnic groups. This analysis provides a picture of racial/ethnic disparities in a comprehensive set of health behaviors across age groups, with consideration of the role of SES. Data are presented for white, black, and Hispanic women and men aged 18 to 74.

The main questions addressed in these analyses are: (1) To what extent do racial/ethnic disparities differ across health behaviors and age groups? (2) To what extent are racial/ethnic disparities in health behaviors accounted for by differences in individual-level indicators of SES?

Background of the BRFSS

The BRFSS is a continuous, state-based telephone survey conducted by state health departments in collaboration with the Centers for Disease Control and Prevention to assess the health of the civilian adult population ages 18 and older (http://www.cdc.gov/nccdphp/brfss). The survey methodology is based on a stratified sampling design whereby eligible individuals are randomly selected within households that have working telephone numbers. Trained interviewers use Computer Assisted Telephone Interview (CATI) software to complete more than 150,000 surveys each year. The BRFSS includes questions on health behaviors, demographic characteristics, socioeconomic status, health status, and health insurance; these are organized as core questions, rotating modules, and state-added questions. The BRFSS thus provides some of the most recent national estimates of health behaviors and screening known to affect chronic disease. The sample for this analysis included 114,325 white (non-Hispanic), 11,938 black (non-Hispanic), and 13,088 Hispanic women and men aged 18 to 74 years who were interviewed for the 2000 BRFSS and were not missing information on educational attainment or household income. Data were not collected for separate groups of Hispanics in the 2000 BRFSS.

Statistical analysis. We carried out our primary statistical analyses, based on linear models, using SUDAAN, a program that adjusts for the complex BRFSS sample design for calculating variance estimates (Shah, Barnwell, Hunt, Nileen, and LaVange, 1991). All analyses incorporated sampling weights that adjusted for unequal probabilities of selection. We used SAS to calculate weighted prevalences. We used multiple linear regression models to calculate odds ratios, unadjusted and adjusted for educational attainment and household income. The dependent variables in our models were seven health behaviors and risk factors and two cancer screening tests (to be defined). The independent variables in the adjusted models were race/ethnicity (black and Hispanic women and men compared separately to white women and men), educational attainment, and household income (to be defined). Because of multiple outcome variables, we selected a conservative level of statistical significance of $P < 0.01$, two-tailed.

Defining Race/Ethnicity and SES

In the BRFSS analyses, we employ the term race/ethnicity to refer to the three social groups in our sample: white, black, and Hispanic adults. We recognize that SES is a multidimensional construct, and choose educational attainment and household income as indicators of SES. We consider both measures as indicators of prestige, economic resources, and/or power, the dimensions of social class under Weber's framework (Runciman, 1978). We defined race/ethnicity and SES as follows:

Race/ethnicity: Self-reported race/ethnicity as white (not of Spanish or Hispanic origin), black (not of Spanish or Hispanic origin), and Hispanic (of Spanish or Hispanic origin).

Educational attainment: Highest grade or year of school completed (none or elementary school, some middle or high school, high school graduate, some college or technical school, college graduate).

Household income: Annual household income from all sources (<$15,000, $15,000 to <$25,000, $25,000 to <$50,000, $50,000 to <$75,000, ≥$75,000). Respondents who did not report income (12 percent of the sample) were excluded from the analysis. These respondents were more likely to be women, older, and Hispanic, and to have completed less education compared to those who reported income.

The seven health behaviors and risk factors we analyzed were defined as follows:

Current cigarette smoker: Smoked at least 100 cigarettes in entire life and currently smoking cigarettes every day or some days.

Secondhand smoke exposure: Lived in a home where anyone, including the respondent, had smoked cigarettes, cigars, or pipes in the past 30 days.

Failure to quit smoking: Among those who ever smoked cigarettes, those currently smoking cigarettes.

Obesity: BMI ≥30 units, calculated as weight in kg/height in m².

No leisure-time physical activity: Questions adapted from the 1985 National Health Interview Survey (National Center for Health Statistics, 1994a). No leisure-time physical activity in the past month, including exercises, sports, or physically active hobbies.

Low vegetable and/or fruit intake: <3 servings of vegetables and/or fruits (green salad, carrots, nonfried potatoes, other vegetables, fruit, fruit juices) per day.

High alcohol consumption: ≥5 alcoholic drinks on ≥1 occasion in the past month and/or an average of ≥2 drinks per day for women and ≥3 drinks per day for men among those who drank alcoholic beverages in the past month.

We chose two screening tests that reflect health behaviors related to breast and cervical cancer, both of which have shown racial/ethnic differences in survival (Ragland, Selvin, and Merrill, 1991).

Pap test screening: No Pap test within the past 2 years.

Mammography screening: No mammogram within the past 2 years (among women aged 45 to 74).

Although the 2000 BRFSS included colorectal cancer screening questions, these questions were asked only in four states and therefore are not included.

Results of BRFSS Analysis

Table 12-1 presents the prevalences of unhealthy behaviors for white, black, and Hispanic women and men by age group. Because the main focus of this analysis is on the relationship of race/ethnicity and SES, these prevalences are presented for background information only.

Table 12-2 presents the associations between race/ethnicity and health behaviors by gender and age group. We initially examined differences by 10-year age groups, but then combined the data into 20-year age groups for 25- to 44-year-olds and 45- to 64-year-olds because no substantial differences existed between these 10-year age groups. Odds ratios are presented for each health behavior for black and Hispanic women and men, with white women and men as the reference group. Odds ratios greater than 1.00 indicate higher odds of unhealthy behaviors for black and/or Hispanic

TABLE 12-1 Prevalences of Unhealthy Behaviors for White, Black, and Hispanic Women and Men by Age Group: BRFSS, 2000[a]

Women, Unadjusted Prevalence	18-24	25-44	45-64	65-74
Cigarette smoking				
White, non-Hispanic	34.0	28.2	21.2	12.7
Black, non-Hispanic	13.0	20.9	22.7	8.3
Hispanic	21.2	16.6	12.3	9.8
Secondhand smoke exposure[b]				
White, non-Hispanic	39.7	31.0	30.5	20.6
Black, non-Hispanic	30.4	30.1	34.3	23.9
Hispanic	22.1	20.4	23.8	8.7
Failure to quit smoking[c]				
White, non-Hispanic	75.3	60.4	42.8	26.4
Black, non-Hispanic	75.7	68.9	50.6	21.6
Hispanic	77.8	60.3	42.5	36.9
Obesity (BMI ≥30)				
White, non-Hispanic	9.4	17.0	23.2	22.2
Black, non-Hispanic	20.1	34.4	41.3	37.5
Hispanic	12.6	24.4	33.1	28.6
No leisure-time physical activity				
White, non-Hispanic	17.5	22.4	26.3	31.6
Black, non-Hispanic	33.5	35.3	38.6	45.5
Hispanic	36.4	44.5	42.1	41.4
Low vegetable and/or fruit intake				
White, non-Hispanic	43.4	36.7	28.1	19.4
Black, non-Hispanic	50.1	44.0	36.2	30.3
Hispanic	44.9	38.6	36.1	29.3
High alcohol consumption[d]				
White, non-Hispanic	30.9	14.0	5.2	2.2
Black, non-Hispanic	7.7	9.2	5.6	0.0
Hispanic	13.8	10.6	5.2	0.6
No Pap test past 2 years				
White, non-Hispanic	17.3	13.4	19.9	33.0
Black, non-Hispanic	17.2	9.4	17.2	35.7
Hispanic	29.7	17.3	20.5	25.8
No mammogram past 2 years (women 45-74)				
White, non-Hispanic	—	—	19.8	19.2
Black, non-Hispanic	—	—	18.3	19.4
Hispanic	—	—	21.1	15.6

women and men compared with white women and men. To assess the extent to which racial/ethnic disparities in health behaviors were accounted for by differences in SES, the odds ratios are first presented unadjusted, and then adjusted for two indicators of SES—educational attainment and household income.

Black and Hispanic women and men had substantially lower odds of smoking than white women and men in nearly every age group

TABLE 12-1 (continued)[a]

Men, Unadjusted Prevalence	18-24	25-44	45-64	65-74
Cigarette smoking				
White, non-Hispanic	34.9	28.4	23.7	11.6
Black, non-Hispanic	22.0	26.1	30.3	19.3
Hispanic	23.7	24.8	24.0	8.4
Secondhand smoke exposure[b]				
White, non-Hispanic	41.7	29.4	29.3	23.2
Black, non-Hispanic	43.7	36.0	36.9	25.2
Hispanic	29.8	22.7	18.9	16.6
Failure to quit smoking[c]				
White, non-Hispanic	76.2	59.6	37.5	16.8
Black, non-Hispanic	82.3	69.0	47.1	35.7
Hispanic	70.7	57.7	45.2	13.0
Obesity (BMI ≥30)				
White, non-Hispanic	11.7	20.5	25.6	19.7
Black, non-Hispanic	11.7	28.4	28.5	23.9
Hispanic	15.2	26.0	29.2	22.5
No leisure-time physical activity				
White, non-Hispanic	12.1	19.1	25.2	26.2
Black, non-Hispanic	14.8	23.9	32.5	28.1
Hispanic	22.5	39.6	45.6	35.7
Low vegetable and/or fruit intake				
White, non-Hispanic	49.0	48.7	39.0	29.0
Black, non-Hispanic	47.0	49.4	43.2	39.3
Hispanic	44.7	50.7	45.7	33.3
High alcohol consumption[d]				
White, non-Hispanic	47.0	36.8	18.3	8.0
Black, non-Hispanic	28.7	18.1	17.0	0.0
Hispanic	43.7	41.4	23.4	7.9

[a] BRFSS indicates Behavioral Risk Factor Surveillance System.
[b] Based on data from 20 states.
[c] Among those who ever smoked.
[d] Based on data from 12 states.

(Table 12-2). The differences in smoking were large and fairly consistent across age groups, and most remained significant after adjustment for education and income. In general, adjustment for education and income increased the racial/ethnic differences in smoking; in some cases, comparisons that were not significant in the unadjusted analysis became significant after adjustment (e.g., the black/white comparisons for women aged 65 to 74). After adjustment, black and Hispanic women had approximately a quarter to half the odds of smoking than white women. The black/white odds of smoking for men showed similar patterns, although the racial/ethnic disparities were not generally as large as those for women.

TABLE 12-2 Odds Ratios for Unhealthy Behaviors for White, Black, and Hispanic Women and Men by Age Group, Unadjusted and Adjusted for Education and Family Income: BRFSS, 2000[a]

Women	18-24		25-44		45-64		65-74	
	Un-adjusted	Adjusted[b]	Un-adjusted	Adjusted	Un-adjusted	Adjusted	Un-adjusted	Adjusted
Cigarette smoking								
White, non-Hispanic	1.00	1.00	1.00	1.00	1.00	1.00	1.00	1.00
Black, non-Hispanic	0.29*	0.24*[c]	0.67*	0.45*	1.10	0.82	0.63	0.53*
Hispanic	0.52*	0.41*	0.51*	0.30*	0.52*	0.37*	0.75	0.56
Secondhand smoke exposure[d]								
White, non-Hispanic	1.00	1.00	1.00	1.00	1.00	1.00	1.00	1.00
Black, non-Hispanic	0.66	0.56*	0.95	0.63*	1.19	0.90	1.21	0.93
Hispanic	0.43*	0.33*	0.57*	0.36*	0.71	0.51*	0.36	0.30
Failure to quit smoking[e]								
White, non-Hispanic	1.00	1.00	1.00	1.00	1.00	1.00	1.00	1.00
Black, non-Hispanic	1.02	0.92	1.46*	1.07	1.37*	1.03	0.77	0.67
Hispanic	1.15	1.03	1.00	0.69*	0.98	0.74	1.63	1.29
Obesity (BMI ≥30)								
White, non-Hispanic	1.00	1.00	1.00	1.00	1.00	1.00	1.00	1.00
Black, non-Hispanic	2.42*	2.09*	2.56*	2.02*	2.34*	1.90*	2.10*	1.78*
Hispanic	1.39	1.14	1.58*	1.09	1.64*	1.19	1.40	0.9
No leisure-time physical activity								
White, non-Hispanic	1.00	1.00	1.00	1.00	1.00	1.00	1.00	1.00
Black, non-Hispanic	2.38*	2.00*	1.89*	1.50*	1.76*	1.29*	1.81*	1.48
Hispanic	2.70*	1.96	2.79*	1.75*	2.03*	1.27	1.53	0.96
Low vegetable and/or fruit intake								
White, non-Hispanic	1.00	1.00	1.00	1.00	1.00	1.00	1.00	1.00
Black, non-Hispanic	1.31	1.23	1.36*	1.16*	1.45*	1.22	1.81*	1.49
Hispanic	1.06	1.01	1.08	0.89	1.44*	1.13	1.72*	1.10

	18-24		25-44		45-64		65-74	
	Un-adjusted	Adjusted[b]	Un-adjusted	Adjusted	Un-adjusted	Adjusted	Un-adjusted	Adjusted
High alcohol consumption[f]								
White, non-Hispanic	1.00	1.00	1.00	1.00	1.00	1.00	1.00	1.00
Black, non-Hispanic	0.19*	0.18*	0.62	0.57*	1.07	1.11	N/A[g]	N/A
Hispanic	0.36*	0.35*	0.73	0.79	1.00	1.14	0.26	0.48
No Pap test past 2 years								
White, non-Hispanic	1.00	1.00	1.00	1.00	1.00	1.00	1.00	1.00
Black, non-Hispanic	0.99	0.94	0.67*	0.50*	0.84	0.61*	1.12	0.96
Hispanic	2.02*	1.86*	1.36	0.89	1.04	0.66*	0.70	0.51*
No mammogram past 2 years(women 45-74)								
White, non-Hispanic	—	—	—	—	1.00	1.00	1.00	1.00
Black, non-Hispanic	—	—	—	—	0.91	0.66*	1.01	0.81
Hispanic	—	—	—	—	1.09	0.66*	0.78	0.49*
Men	Un-adjusted	Adjusted[b]	Un-adjusted	Adjusted	Un-adjusted	Adjusted	Un-adjusted	Adjusted
Cigarette smoking								
White, non-Hispanic	1.00	1.00	1.00	1.00	1.00	1.00	1.00	1.00
Black, non-Hispanic	0.53*	0.44*[c]	0.89	0.68*	1.41*	1.04	1.83*	1.24
Hispanic	0.58*	0.46*	0.83	0.47*	1.02	0.70	0.70	0.35*
Secondhand smoke exposure[d]								
White, non-Hispanic	1.00	1.00	1.00	1.00	1.00	1.00	1.00	1.00
Black, non-Hispanic	1.09	1.03	1.35*	1.01	1.41*	1.05	1.12	0.91
Hispanic	0.59	0.47*	0.71	0.40*	0.56*	0.38*	0.66	0.55
Failure to quit smoking[e]								
White, non-Hispanic	1.00	1.00	1.00	1.00	1.00	1.00	1.00	1.00
Black, non-Hispanic	1.45	1.23	1.51*	1.27	1.48*	1.13	2.74*	1.98*
Hispanic	0.76	0.66	0.92	0.70*	1.37	1.06	0.74	0.41

TABLE 12-2 (continued)

Men	18-24		25-44		45-64		65-74	
	Un-adjusted	Adjusted	Un-adjusted	Adjusted	Un-adjusted	Adjusted	Un-adjusted	Adjusted
Obesity (BMI ≥30)								
White, non-Hispanic	1.00	1.00	1.00	1.00	1.00	1.00	1.00	1.00
Black, non-Hispanic	1.00	0.96	1.54*	**1.44***	1.16	1.07	1.29	1.22
Hispanic	1.35	1.43	1.36*	1.18	1.20	1.02	1.19	1.09
No leisure-time physical activity								
White, non-Hispanic	1.00	1.00	1.00	1.00	1.00	1.00	1.00	1.00
Black, non-Hispanic	1.26	1.02	1.33*	1.04	1.43*	1.02	1.10	0.75
Hispanic	2.11*	1.47	2.77*	**1.46***	2.49*	**1.45***	1.56	0.87
Low fruit and/or vegetable intake								
White, non-Hispanic	1.00	1.00	1.00	1.00	1.00	1.00	1.00	1.00
Black, non-Hispanic	0.92	0.86	1.03	0.95	1.19	1.03	1.58	1.29
Hispanic	0.84	0.85	1.09	0.93	1.31	1.02	1.22	0.87
High alcohol consumption[f]								
White, non-Hispanic	1.00	1.00	1.00	1.00	1.00	1.00	1.00	1.00
Black, non-Hispanic	0.45	0.47	0.38*	**0.38***	0.91	0.85	N/A[g]	N/A
Hispanic	0.88	0.87	1.22	1.17	1.37	1.44	0.99	0.77

[a] BRFSS indicates Behavioral Risk Factor Surveillance System.

White women and men are the reference group for black and Hispanic women and men.

Odds ratios of > 1.00 indicate higher odds of adverse health behaviors for black and/or Hispanic women and men compared to white women and men.

[a] An asterisk indicates a p value of < 0.01.

[b] Adjusted for education and household income.

[c] Bold indicates significance at p < 0.01 with adjustment for education and family income.

[d] Based on data from 20 states.

[e] Among those who ever smoked.

[f] Based on data from 12 states.

[g] N/A = zero prevalence.

Black and Hispanic women also had lower odds of exposure to second-hand smoke than white women, especially in the younger age groups. Hispanic men compared with white men showed similar differences. After adjustment, no differences were found between black and white men.

Few significant racial/ethnic differences were found for failure to quit smoking after adjustment among those who had ever smoked. There were two exceptions. Hispanic women and men aged 25 to 44 were more likely to quit smoking than white women and men of the same ages. In contrast, black men aged 65 to 74 were much less likely to quit smoking than white men aged 65 to 74. This is reflected in the cigarette smoking prevalence rates of black men compared with white men that are lower or similar across younger ages, but then cross over and become higher from ages 45 on (see Table 12-1).

In contrast to smoking, black women had substantially higher odds of obesity and leisure-time physical inactivity than white women after adjusting for education and income. The odds of obesity were approximately twice as high for black women compared with white women at every age group, after adjustment. Hispanic women aged 25 to 44 had higher odds of physical inactivity than white and black women. The patterns for men after SES adjustment were different. Black men had similar odds of obesity and physical inactivity compared with white men (with the exception of higher odds of obesity for black men aged 25 to 44) and Hispanic men (aged 25-64) had higher odds of physical inactivity than white men. Few significant racial/ethnic disparities in low vegetable and/or fruit intake were found for either women or men.

While few racial/ethnic differences were observed for high alcohol consumption, there were several important exceptions. Black and Hispanic women aged 18 to 24, and black women and men aged 25 to 44, had significantly lower odds of alcohol consumption than white women or men in the same age groups after adjustment for education and income.

Black women aged 25-64 were more likely to report having a recent Pap test than white women after adjustment for education and income. The adjusted results for Hispanic women compared with white women were mixed; Hispanic women were less likely to be screened at ages 18 to 24 and more likely to be screened at ages 45 to 74. Black and Hispanic women aged 45 to 64 and Hispanic women aged 65 to 74 were significantly more likely to report a recent mammogram than white women in the same age groups. However, none of the odds for mammography screening were significant when unadjusted for education and income.

Although not the focus of this chapter, we also examined the separate influence of SES on health behaviors. As shown in many past analyses, we found strong, inverse associations between educational attainment and income at almost every age group for each health behavior, except for high alcohol consumption, where education and income were generally not statistically significant. For all other health behaviors, women and men with lower educations and/or lower incomes had higher odds of unhealthy behaviors compared to those with higher educations and/or incomes, after adjusting for race/ethnicity (data not shown).

In addition to adjusted analyses, stratified analyses offer insight about racial/ethnic disparities in health behaviors. From our previous work (Winkleby et al., 1998, 1999b; Winkleby, Schooler, Kraemer, Lin, and Fortmann, 1995), we were aware of the large differences in unhealthy behaviors by educational attainment and household income, especially within black and white racial/ethnic groups. To examine these relationships across age groups, we stratified the BRFSS data for white, black, and Hispanic women and men by age group and educational attainment (<12 and ≥12 years of education) and annual household income (<$25,000 and ≥$25,000). We are aware that the categorization of education and income into two levels introduces assumptions regarding residual confounding (Kaufman et al., 1997); however, more than two levels of categories for three racial/ethnic groups are cumbersome to present.

We found large differences in unhealthy behaviors by both level of education and income for black and white adults that persisted across age groups. The differences were apparent for all of the seven health behaviors and risk factors and two cancer screening tests, with the exception of alcohol consumption. The differences by education for Hispanic women and men were generally much weaker or not apparent, except for obesity for both women and men, and cancer screening for women. Selected findings for cigarette smoking by level of education and obesity by household income are shown in Figures 12-3 and 12-4. The solid lines represent those having lower educational and lower income levels. For smoking, large disparities are seen by education for both black and white women and men, and to a lesser degree for Hispanic women. For obesity, the largest disparities by income are seen for women.

IMPLICATIONS OF OUR FINDINGS

Like the answers to many scientific questions, our findings yield a complex picture. We demonstrate that the pattern of racial/ethnic differences in health behaviors varies by health behavior and for subgroups defined by indicators of SES, gender, and age. In setting the goals for this chapter, we challenged the often-held assumption that populations of color have poorer indicators of health behaviors than white populations. We found that unhealthy behaviors are not limited to any one racial/ethnic group. While whites had unhealthier behaviors than blacks and Hispanics for some behaviors, the reverse was true for other health behaviors. In

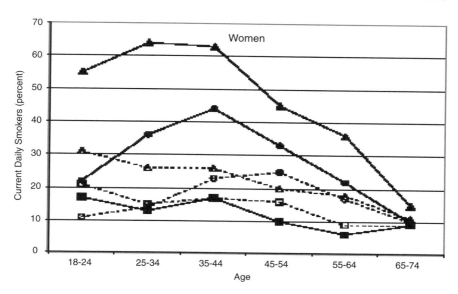

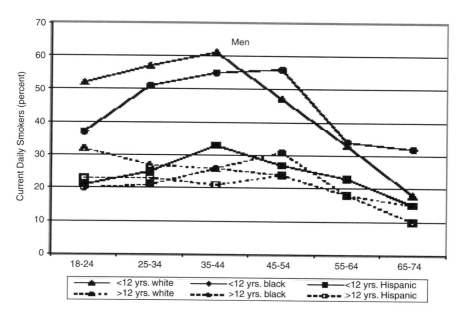

FIGURE 12-3 Prevalence of cigarette smoking at each age group by level of education for white, black, and Hispanic women and men, ages 18-74.
SOURCE: Behavioral Risk Factor Surveillance System (2000).

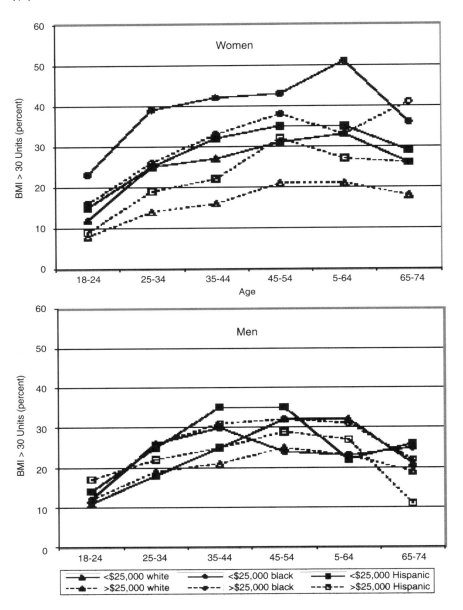

FIGURE 12-4 Prevalence of obesity at each age group by household income for white, black, and Hispanic women and men, ages 18-74.
SOURCE: Behavioral Risk Factor Surveillance System (2000).

general, racial/ethnic disparities were substantially influenced by education and income, were stronger for women than for men, and were stronger for younger and middle-aged adults than for older adults. Levels of unhealthy behaviors varied within racial/ethnic groups by level of education, household income, and, for Mexican Americans, by country of birth and language spoken.

Racial/Ethnic Disparities in Smoking

In our stratified analysis of BRFSS data, we found that SES greatly influenced smoking among white and black women and men. White women and men with lower SES (indicated by either educational attainment or income) at almost every age group had the highest prevalences of cigarette smoking compared to any other group. Lower SES black men, and to a lesser degree lower SES black women, had higher prevalences of smoking than their higher SES counterparts. In general, white women and men also had the highest probability of exposure to secondhand smoke. Hispanic women at every age group had lower odds of smoking compared with white women. The stratified analysis showed that lower SES white and black women and men (especially older black men) were the most likely to fail to quit smoking.

These findings are consistent with earlier findings from the National Health Interview Survey (NHIS) (Pamuk et al., 1998), which showed that smoking was highest for women and men with less than 12 years of education. In the NHIS, lower educated women and men, unlike higher educated women and men, showed almost no declines in smoking over the past 20 years, from 1974 to 1995 (Pamuk et al., 1998). This has produced a steeper SES gradient in smoking prevalence over time. Although black women and Hispanic women and men in the NHIS were less likely to smoke than their white counterparts, they also showed a gradient in smoking by SES.

Smoking is a particularly important health behavior because it is the leading cause of preventable death and disability in the United States and is a risk factor for heart disease, lung cancer, and other chronic diseases. It is critical to address the exceptionally high rates of smoking in lower educated white and black adults. Smoking prevention programs are needed that focus on white and black youth before they begin smoking and reach those who are at particular risk, such as those who attend continuation high schools and those who are not in school (Winkleby et al., 2004). Because many youth continue smoking into adulthood and other people begin smoking during adulthood, programs that encourage quit attempts and smoking cessation also must be available later in life, with a special focus on those with few financial resources. Given the influence of the tobacco industry, smoking programs and strategies must address the social context of smoking, such as the restriction of tobacco advertising, promotion of low-cost cigarettes, and sponsorship of sports events (Winkleby et al., 2004). In addition, smoking cessation programs, free or low-cost nicotine patches or gum, and support groups on weight and stress reduction are needed (Davis, 1987; Englander, 1986; Ernster, 1991; Pierce, Choi, Gilpin, Farkes, and Berry, 1998). Finally, the lower smoking among Hispanic women and men, and the more successful patterns of quitting for Hispanic women, should be reinforced, especially given that smoking levels are higher among those with longer "exposure" to the U.S. environment.

Racial/Ethnic Disparities in Obesity, Physical Inactivity, and Diet

We found that black women at every age group (with one exception) had significantly higher odds of obesity and physical inactivity than white women after adjustment for education and income. Black women also showed lower vegetable and/or fruit intake than white women at every age group, although these findings were not statistically significant, except for women aged 25 to 44. Black men aged 25 to 44 had significantly higher odds of obesity than white men. Some age groups of Hispanic women and men showed higher odds of leisure-time physical inactivity than white women and men. While neither Hispanic women nor men showed higher odds of obesity than white women and men after adjustment for income and education, there is some recent evidence that even Hispanic populations who work in blue-collar jobs have high prevalences of overweight; a 1999 random sample of 971 Hispanic farm workers from seven California communities found high levels of obesity among men (28 percent) and women (37 percent) during clinical examinations (Villarejo et al., 2000).

Our obesity findings for black women are consistent with the NHIS, NHANES III, and other surveys that show higher odds of obesity for black compared with white women (Kumanyika et al., 1993; Flegal et al., 1998). Our findings for Hispanic women are inconsistent with NHANES III data (Winkleby et al., 1999a) that show odds ratios for obesity for Mexican-American women that are intermediate between black and white women (odds ratios of 1.92 for black women and 1.48 for Mexican-American women with white women as the reference, p values < 0.01). Unlike our finding of higher odds of obesity for black compared with white men (ages 25 to 44), NHANES showed no higher odds of obesity for black men; however the men in the NHANES analysis were ages 25 to 64 (Winkleby et al., 1999a). These differences may be due to measurement differences (self-report versus clinical exam), definitions of race/ethnicity (Mexican American versus Hispanic), our stratification by age groups in the BRFSS, and/or variables used to adjust for SES.

Our findings for physical inactivity are consistent with past studies that have found that black adults (especially women) engage in less leisure-time physical activity than whites (Burke et al., 1992), that these differences remain after accounting for SES (Duelberg, 1992; Winkleby et al., 1998), and that the largest differences are among those with less than a high school education (Folsom et al., 1991). In the NHIS, black and Hispanic women and men aged 18 and older had higher prevalences of leisure-time inactivity than white women and men, with strong gradients evident by family income (Pamuk et al., 1998).

The health and medical care consequences of the current obesity epidemic in the United States are enormous. Overweight contributes to hypertension, diabetes, and other health conditions that are major risk factors for chronic diseases (Pi-Sunyer, 1993). It is well established that proper body weight, regular physical activity, and a diet high in vegetables and fruits can reduce related risk factors and chronic disease outcomes (National Heart, Lung, and Blood Institute, 1998). Given that more than 54 percent of Americans are overweight (an increase of 8 percent in less than 15 years) (Flegal, Carroll, Kuczmarski, and Johnson, 1998), prevention and treatment efforts must include both populationwide and tailored strategies. Of particular concern is the high prevalence of obesity in women, especially black women with lower SES. Because both ethnic minority status and lower SES are related to obesity, tailored treatment programs and behavioral strategies need to be developed that consider economic resources, literacy, culture, and language (Howard-Pitney, Winkleby, Albright, and Bruce, and Fortmann, 1993; Kumanyika et al., 1993). The rapid increases in obesity, physical inactivity, and poor dietary behaviors in the United States in the past decade point to environmental factors as underlying mechanisms and illustrate the need for broad societal changes. These include the availability of affordable, healthy foods in all neighborhoods; policy changes regarding processed and fast food sales; standards for food portion sizes; and safe, convenient places to walk and exercise (French, Story, and Jeffrey, 2001; Jeffery et al., 2000; Young and Nestle, 2002).

Racial/Ethnic Disparities in Alcohol Consumption

We found few racial/ethnic differences in heavy alcohol use in the BRFSS data. There was one notable exception: younger black women and men and younger Hispanic women had a 60 to 80 percent lower likelihood of high alcohol consumption than younger white women and men. The higher heavy alcohol consumption in younger white women and men points to the need for special outreach programs to address their high alcohol intake and/or binge drinking because this health behavior is linked to chronic diseases, injuries, adverse pregnancy outcomes, and other serious health problems.

The Influence of Acculturation

Within the Mexican-American population, we found that those who were born in the United States exhibited less healthy behaviors than those born in Mexico. Some of the largest differences by country of birth were among younger Mexican Americans for smoking (women), low vegetable and/or fruit consumption (women and men), obesity (women), and high alcohol consumption (women). A possible explanation for these findings is that those born in Mexico may have closer ties to the traditional Mexican culture that promotes family and community social support and healthy lifestyles such as nonsmoking, diets high in vegetables and fruits, and physical activity than those born in the United States (Sundquist and Winkleby, 1999).

Racial/Ethnic Disparities in Cervical Cancer and Breast Cancer Screening

We found that white women aged 25 to 64 were less likely to have received recent Pap screening than black women after adjustment for education and income and that Hispanic women aged 18 to 24 were less likely to have received recent Pap screening than white women. White women were also less likely to have received recent mammography screening than black or Hispanic women, although the difference in one age group was not statistically significant. All differences in mammography screening and several for Pap screening would have been missed if results were not adjusted for education and income. As with other health behaviors, the differences by SES were large.

These results for cancer screening are consistent with previous studies. A study of women aged 15 to 44 from the 1995 National Survey of Family Growth found that black women were more likely that any other racial group to be screened for cervical cancer (Hewitt, Devesa, and Breen, 2002). Another study using NHIS data showed that black women aged 50 and older were as likely or more likely than white women to have a mammogram in the past 2 years after controlling for income. NHIS differences were especially apparent for low-income women, with low-income black women being approximately 60 percent more likely than low-income white women to have had a recent mammogram. Low-income Hispanic women in the NHIS were intermediate between black and white women for mammography screening (Pamuk et al., 1998). Other studies have shown that Hispanic women receive Pap and mammography screening as often as white women when screening is covered as part of their health care insurance (Pérez-Stable, Otero-Sabogal, Sabogal, McPhee, and Hiatt, 1994).

Pap and mammography screening are well established as being effective in reducing breast and cervical cancer mortality, especially when the cancers are detected early (Young, 2002). Although we found that black and Hispanic women were more likely to report recent screening for cervical and breast cancer after adjustment for education and income, they are more likely to be diagnosed at later stages and have poorer survival following diagnosis (Miller et al., 1996). Potential explanations for why black and Hispanic women have higher screening rates but later diagnoses and poorer survival include poorer quality of screening tests, barriers to follow-up treatment including inadequate access to health care, and discrimination in the delivery of health services (Institute of Medicine, 1991).

The Influence of SES

Our results confirm the importance of considering socioeconomic factors when assessing racial/ethnic disparities in health behaviors related to chronic diseases. Adjustment for educational attainment and family income had a significant impact on our results, in some instances reducing disparities and in other instances heightening disparities. This has implications for interpreting past studies of racial/ethnic disparities, especially those that have not adjusted for SES.

Socioeconomic factors are important to consider in investigations of health behaviors in any population, but these factors have particular relevance in studies of racial/ethnic disparities. Researchers often adjust for SES using inadequate measures and then conclude that any remaining racial/ethnic disparities are due to cultural and/or innate physiologic or genetic differences. The result is that considerable residual confounding by SES likely exists in studies of racial/ethnic disparities (Kaufman et al., 1997). Because SES is so difficult to measure completely, residual confounding by SES is likely to exist in any study of racial/ethnic disparities, even when multiple measures of SES are used. Care needs to be taken in the interpretation of "independent" effects of race or ethnicity, particularly given the overwhelming evidence that race/ethnicity is not genetically based and in light of recent evidence of the effects of discrimination on health (Krieger, 1999). Furthermore, studies need to emphasize that the variable "race/ethnicity" is likely to capture unmeasured socioeconomic factors, even after adjusting for multiple measures of SES (Braveman et al., 2001). Thus, researchers need to acknowledge the limitations of the socioeconomic measures used to adjust for SES. For example, we were not able to consider a person's past SES, socioeconomic characteristics of her or his residential environment, or other factors such as occupational status or wealth. Based on these limitations, as well general limitations of the measures we used (e.g., no information on the quality of schooling), we believe that residual confounding by SES likely exists; that is, the variable race/ethnicity in our models represents, in part, unmeasured socioeconomic factors.

Based on our conceptual framework and on previous empirical evidence, it is evident that racial/ethnic disparities in health behaviors are complex phenomena and that factors beyond SES are partly responsible for their explanations. For example, while some studies show that Hispanic populations experience better health than would be expected given their socioeconomic characteristics alone (Franzini, Ribble, and Keddie, 2001; Markides and Coreil, 1986), findings from other studies counter these findings (Goff et al., 1997; Hunt et al., 2003). It is likely that acculturation is a primary factor accounting for the Hispanic health advantage in some studies. An important health policy question is whether this advantage will diminish as greater numbers of Mexican Americans (as well as other Hispanic populations) are born in the United States and live here longer.

Limitations of the BRFSS and Opportunities for Future Surveys

Although the BRFSS data have limitations that influence the interpretation of analyses on racial/ethnic differences in health behaviors, the opportunity exists to address these limitations in future surveys. The BRFSS is based on self-reported information on health behaviors collected by telephone interviews. Such data are often subject to bias; examples include the underreporting of weight or cigarette smoking or the overreporting of screening tests. In addition, the BRFSS has limited information on physical activity; it is collected for leisure time only. This misses physical activity during working hours that differentially affects racial/ethnic and socioeconomic groups (e.g., black, Hispanic, and lower SES populations are more likely to work in physically demanding jobs compared with white and higher SES populations). Future surveys should collect a broader array of standardized physical activity questions, including those that encompass activity during both leisure and work time.

A serious limitation of the BRFSS is the aggregation of persons of Hispanic origin into one group, making it impossible to distinguish among different Hispanic subgroups such as Mexican Americans, Puerto Ricans, and Cubans. This is important because of the large differences in prevalences of health behaviors within the Hispanic population (e.g., smoking in Mexican-American versus Cuban men). Future BRFSS surveys should delineate Hispanic subgroups. Emphasis also should be placed on including adequate samples of other major racial/ethnic groups in the United States (e.g., Native Americans and Alaska Natives; Chinese, Japanese, Vietnamese, and Filipinos, and other Asian Americans and Pacific Islanders).

Indicators of SES and acculturation available in the BRFSS are limited and lack specificity. If collected with more refinement, these indicators would allow for a more accurate assessment of the degree to which racial/ethnic disparities are explained by SES. For example, income measures could be collected in such a way as to allow for categories of income in relation to the federal poverty level or could include estimates of childhood socioeconomic factors and adult wealth as is done in the National Longitudinal Survey of Youth. Education could include parental education, country of education, and name of the town or city where a person's highest education was obtained (to provide an indicator of geographic region of education and a surrogate of quality of education). Acculturation measures could include country of birth, language(s) spoken at home, and length of time lived in the United States.

The Next Generation of Chronic Disease Prevention

Chronic diseases, with heart disease ranking first, cancer ranking second, and stroke ranking third, will remain the leading causes of death in the United States for the next 50 years for all major racial/ethnic groups (Cooper et al., 2000). The National Conference on Cardiovascular Disease Prevention, held in 1999, addressed national trends in health behaviors related to CVD and other chronic diseases (Cooper et al., 2000). The conference leaders concluded that little progress has been made recently in addressing smoking, obesity, and physical inactivity despite widespread efforts to promote a populationwide adoption of healthy lifestyles, primary prevention for high-risk groups, and secondary prevention. Furthermore, the conference leaders stressed that wide racial/ethnic disparities in CVD mortality continue and that SES disparities in CVD mortality may be increasing. Their conclusions are supported by findings from other studies that show that the mortality disparity between lower and higher SES groups has widened (Pappas, Queen, Hadden, and Fisher, 1993).

The next generation of chronic disease prevention and control programs and policies must acknowledge and effectively address the social and historical context within which health behaviors are inextricably linked (Green and Kreuter, 1991; Minkler, 1990; Syme, 2004; Wallack and Winkleby, 1987; Wallerstein and Bernstein, 1994). The responsibility for improving health behaviors has been framed too often from an individual perspective that places the main responsibility for change with the individual. The rationale for this approach has been that once individuals are informed of their risk, they will adopt or modify behaviors to lower that risk (Wallack and Winkleby, 1987). Although an individual approach can be effective for addressing health problems (especially at the secondary and tertiary prevention levels), it has had limited success when used in isolation because it (1) places the burden for change on individuals who often are those with the fewest resources (e.g., socioeconomically disadvantaged);

(2) can lead to increases in social disparities in health if those with the most resources and power (i.e., white and higher SES populations) are more able to take advantage of health-promoting programs, information, and policies to change their behaviors; (3) deflects attention away from important factors in the social and physical environment that influence choices regarding health-related behaviors; and (4) does not provide reinforcement of positive health behaviors from the environment in which a person lives and works.

In summary, we support a broad health policy agenda for the prevention of chronic diseases that integrates a focus on race/ethnicity, SES, and the social environment (Anderson, 1995; Williams and Collins, 1995). This is critical given that health behaviors are shaped by the communities in which people live (Syme, 2004). A broad focus on socioeconomic inequalities acknowledges the strong influence of SES on chronic disease outcomes, ensures the inclusion of all low-SES populations in health initiatives and guidelines, and achieves more equitable access to resources. Finally, it creates a more valid scientific ground for research on racial/ethnic disparities in health behaviors that goes beyond individual-level measures, and furthers an understanding that social, economic, and political factors are fundamental causes of health (Link and Phelan, 1995).

CONCLUSIONS

In this chapter we examined racial/ethnic disparities in a comprehensive set of health behaviors to assess the extent to which disparities varied across health behaviors, age groups, and gender, and to evaluate the contribution of indicators of SES to racial/ethnic disparities. We used data from national surveys that have large representative samples that allowed for a stratification of data across a wide range of age groups. We included women and men from the three largest ethnic groups in the United States, delineating Mexican Americans when possible. We focused on smoking, obesity, physical inactivity, poor diet, high alcohol consumption, and cancer screening practices, all of which are related to chronic diseases. Our findings highlight many disparities in health behaviors, none of which are restricted to any gender or age group. Furthermore, the disparities were greatly influenced by education and income.

The main conclusions from our BRFSS and NHANES III analyses are:

• For some health behaviors, white populations have higher levels of unhealthy behaviors than black and/or Hispanic populations (particularly for smoking, secondhand smoke exposure, and inadequate Pap and mammogram screening), and for other health behaviors, the opposite is true (particularly for physical inactivity and obesity, with disparities being larger for blacks than for Hispanics). These disparities remain after adjustment for education and income.

• Health behaviors also differ *within* racial/ethnic groups by important sociodemographic indicators, including age, educational attainment, household income, country of birth, and language spoken. These differences have implications for the timing, focus, and content of primary, secondary, and tertiary prevention programs and policies.

• In general, racial/ethnic disparities in health behaviors are stronger for women than for men, in large part because of the greater disparities for women than for men for smoking, secondhand smoke exposure, physical inactivity, and obesity.

• Racial/ethnic disparities in health behaviors tend to be stronger for younger and middle-aged adults than for older adults. This is apparent for smoking, secondhand smoke exposure, physical inactivity, high alcohol consumption, and inadequate mammography screening.

• Both white and black adults with lower SES (as measured by either educational attainment or household income) have considerably less healthy behaviors than those with higher SES for all seven health behaviors, with the exception of high alcohol consumption. These differences show the importance of considering SES when planning and implementing health promotion and disease prevention programs.

• Hispanic adults have different patterns of results than white and black adults. Few differences in health behaviors are evident between Hispanics and whites after adjustment for education and income. In addition, few differences are evident for Hispanics when stratified by education or income, except for obesity, physical inactivity, and mammography screening. However, large differences in health behaviors exist for Mexican Americans by country of birth; adults who are born in the United States and/or who speak English have higher predicted prevalences of unhealthy behaviors than those who are born in Mexico and/or who speak Spanish.

ACKNOWLEDGMENTS

This work was cofunded by the National Institute of Environmental Sciences and the National Heart, Lung, and Blood Institute: Grant RO1 HL67731 to Dr. Marilyn Winkleby. We thank Dr. David Ahn, Dr. Ying-Chih Chuang, and Dr. Michaela Kiernan for their valuable comments on an earlier draft, and Alana Koehler for her technical assistance in preparing the tables and figures.

REFERENCES

Adler, N.E., Boyce, T., Chesney, M., Folkman, S., and Syme, L. (1993). Socioeconomic inequalities in health: No easy solution. *Journal of the American Medical Association, 269,* 3140-3145.

Aguirre-Molina, M., Molina, C.W., and Zambrana, R.E. (2001). *Health issues in the Latin community.* San Francisco: Jossey-Bass.

Anderson, N.B. (1995). Behavioral and sociocultural perspectives on ethnicity and health. *Health Psychology, 14,* 589-591.

Anderson, R.E., Crespo, C.J., Bartlett, S.J., Cheskin, L.J., and Pratt, M. (1998). Relationship of physical activity and television watching with body weight and level of fatness among children: Results from the Third National Health and Nutrition Examination Survey. *Journal of the American Medical Association, 279,* 938-942.

Balcazar, H., and Cobas, J.A. (1993). Overweight among Mexican-Americans and its relationship to life style behavioral risk factors. *Journal of Community Health, 18,* 55-67.

Belcher, J.D., Ellison, R.C., Shepard, W.E., Bigelow, C., Webber, C.S., Wilmore, J.H., Parcel, G.S., Zucker, D.M., and Luepker, R.V. (1993). Lipid and lipoprotein distributions in children by ethnic group, gender, and geographic location: Preliminary findings of the Child and Adolescent Trial for Cardiovascular Health (CATCH). *Preventive Medicine, 22,* 143-153.

Berenson, G.S., Srinivasan, S.R., Bao, W., Newman, W.P., III, Tracy, R.E., and Wattigney, W.A. (1998). Association between multiple cardiovascular risk factors and atherosclerosis in children and young adults. *New England Journal of Medicine, 338,* 1650-1656.

Black, S.A., and Markides, K.S. (1993). Acculturation and alcohol consumption in Puerto Rican, Cuban-American, and Mexican-American women in the United States. *American Journal of Public Health, 83,* 890-893.

The Bogalusa Heart Study 20th Anniversary Symposium. (1995). *American Journal of the Medical Sciences, 310,* S1-S138.

Braveman, P., Cubbin, C., Marchi, K., Egerter, S., and Chavez, G. (2001). Measuring socioeconomic status/position in studies of racial/ethnic disparities: Maternal and infant health. *Public Health Reports, 116,* 449-463.

Burke, G.L., Savage, P.J., Manolio, T.A., Sprafka, J.M., Wagenknecht, L.E., Sidney, S., Perkins, L.L., Liu, K., and Jacobs, D.R., Jr. (1992). Correlates of obesity in young black and white women: The CARDIA Study. *American Journal of Public Health, 82,* 1621-1625.

Conference of Socioeconomic Status and Cardiovascular Health and Disease. (1995). *Report of the Conference of Socioeconomic Status and Cardiovascular Health and Disease, November 6-7, 1995.* Washington, DC: National Heart, Lung, and Blood Institute.

Cooper, R., Cutler, J., Desvigne-Nickens, P., Fortmann, S.P., Friedman, L., Havlik, R., Hogelin, G., Marler, J., McGovern, P., Morosco, G., Mosca, L., Pearson, T., Stamler, J., Stryer, D., and Thom, T. (2000). Trends and disparities in coronary heart disease, stroke, and other cardiovascular diseases in the United States. Findings of the National Conference on Cardiovascular Disease Prevention. *Circulation, 102,* 3137-3147.

Corti, M.C., Guralnik, J.M., Ferrucci, L., Izmirlian, G., Leveille, S.G., Pahor, M., Cohen, H.J., Pieper, C., and Havlik, R.J. (1999). Evidence for a black-white crossover in all-cause and coronary heart disease mortality in an older population: The North Carolina EPESE. *American Journal of Public Health, 89,* 308-314.

Cubbin, C., Hadden, W.C., and Winkleby, M.A. (2001). Neighborhood context and cardiovascular disease risk factors: The contribution of material deprivation. *Ethnicity and Disease, 11,* 687-700.

Davis, R.M. (1987). Current trends in cigarette advertising and marketing. *New England Journal of Medicine, 316,* 725-732.

Diehl, A.K., and Stern, M.P. (1989). Special health problems of Mexican Americans: Obesity, gallbladder disease, diabetes mellitus, and cardiovascular disease. *Advances in Internal Medicine, 34,* 79-96.

Diez-Roux, A.V. (1998). Bringing context back into epidemiology: Variables and fallacies in multi-level analysis. *American Journal of Public Health, 88,* 216-222.

Diez-Roux, A.V., Nieto, F.J., Muntaner, C., Tyroler, H.A., Comstock, G.W., Shahar, E., Cooper, L.S., Watson, R.L., and Szklo, M. (1997). Neighborhood environments and coronary heart disease: A multilevel analysis. *American Journal of Epidemiology, 146,* 48-63.

Diez-Roux, A.V., Nieto, F.J., Caulfield, L., Tyroler, H.A., Watson, R.L., and Szklo, M. (1999). Neighbourhood differences in diet: The Atherosclerosis Risk in Communities (ARIC) Study. *Journal of Epidemiology and Community Health, 53,* 55-63.

Diez-Roux, A.V., Merkin, S.S., Arnett, D., Chambless, L., Massing, M., Nieto, F.J., Sorlie, P., Szklo, M., Tyroler, H.A., and Watson, R.L. (2001). Neighborhood of residence and incidence of coronary heart disease. *New England Journal of Medicine, 345,* 99-106.

DiPietro, L., Williamson, D.F., Caspersen, C.J., and Eaker, E. (1993). The descriptive epidemiology of selected physical activities and body weight among adults trying to lose weight: The Behavioral Risk Factor Surveillance System survey, 1989. *International Journal of Obesity and Related Metabolic Disorders, 17,* 69-76.

Duelberg, S.I. (1992). Preventive health behavior among black and white women in urban and rural areas. *Social Science and Medicine, 34,* 191-198.

Duncan, C., Jones, K., and Moon, G. (1996). Health-related behaviour in context: A multi-level modelling approach. *Social Science and Medicine, 42,* 817-830.

Dwyer, J.T., Stone, E.J., Yang, M., Feldman, H., Webber, L.S., Must, A., Perry, C.L., Nader, P.R., and Parcel, G.S. (1998). Predictors of overweight and overfatness in a multiethnic pediatric population. Child and Adolescent Trial for Cardiovascular Health Collaborative Research Group. *American Journal of Clinical Nutrition, 67,* 602-610.

Elder, J.P., Castro, F.G., de Moor, C., Mayer, J., Candelaria, J.I., Campbell, N., Talavera, G., and Ware, L.M. (1991). Differences in cancer-risk-related behaviors in Latino and Anglo adults. *Preventive Medicine, 20,* 751-763.

Ellaway, A., Anderson, A., and Macintyre, S. (1997). Does area of residence affect body size and shape? *International Journal of Obesity and Related Metabolic Disorders, 21,* 304-308.

Eller, T.J. (1994). *Household wealth and asset ownership*: 1991 (Current Population Reports No. P70-34. Washington, DC: U.S. Bureau of the Census.

Elo, I.T., and Preston, S.H. (1997). Racial and ethnic differences in mortality at older ages. In L.G. Martin and B.J. Soldo (Eds.), *Racial and ethnic differences in the health of older Americans* (pp. 10-42). Committee on Population, Commission on Behavioral and Social Sciences and Education, National Research Council. Washington, DC: National Academy Press.

Englander, T.J. (1986). Cigarette makers shift and strategies. *United States Tobacco and Candy Journal, 213,* 1-46.

Ernster, V. (1991). How tobacco companies target women. *World Smoking and Health, 16,* 8-11.

Espino, D.V., Burge, S.K., and Moreno, C.A. (1991). The prevalence of selected chronic diseases among the Mexican-American elderly: Data from the 1982-1984 Hispanic Health and Nutrition Examination Survey. *Journal of the American Board of Family Practice, 4,* 217-222.

Flegal, K.M., Carroll, M.D., Kuczmarski, R.J., and Johnson, C.L. (1998). Overweight and obesity in the United States: Prevalence and trends, 1960-1994. *International Journal of Obesity and Related Metabolic Disorders, 22,* 39-47.

Folsom, A.R., Burke, G.L., Ballew, C., Jacobs, D.R., Jr., Haskell, W.L., Donahue, R.P., Liu, K.A., and Hilner, J.E. (1989). Relation of body fatness and its distribution to cardiovascular risk factors in young blacks and whites. The role of insulin. *American Journal of Epidemiology, 130,* 911-924.

Folsom, A.R., Cook, T.C., Sprafka, J.M., Burke, G.L., Norsted, S.W., and Jacobs, D.R., Jr. (1991). Differences in leisure-time physical activity levels between blacks and whites in population-based samples: The Minnesota Heart Survey. *Journal of Behavioral Medicine, 14,* 1-9.

Franzini, L., Ribble, J.C., and Keddie, A.M. (2001). Understanding the Hispanic paradox. *Ethnicity and Disease, 11,* 496-518.

French, S.A., Story, M., and Jeffery, R.W. (2001). Environmental influences on eating and physical activity. *Annual Review of Public Health, 22,* 309-335.

Geronimus, A.T. (1992). The weathering hypothesis and the health of African-American women and infants: Evidence and speculations. *Ethnicity and Disease, 2,* 207-221.

Gidding, S.S., Liu, K., Bild, D.E., Flack, J., Gardin, J., Ruth, K.J., and Oberman, A. (1996). Prevalence and identification of abnormal lipoprotein levels in a biracial population aged 23 to 35 years: The CARDIA Study. *American Journal of Cardiology, 78,* 304-308.

Goff, D.C., Nichaman, M.Z., Chan, W., Ramsey, D.J., Labarthe, D.R., and Ortiz, C. (1997). Greater incidence of hospitalized myocardial infarction among Mexican Americans than non-Hispanic whites: The Corpus Christi Heart Project 1988-1992. *Circulation, 95,* 1433-1440.

Green, L.W., and Kreuter, M.W. (1991). *Health promotion planning: An educational and environmental approach,* (2nd ed.). Mountain View, CA: Mayfield.

Gutierrez-Ramirez, A., Valdez, R.B., and Carter-Pokras, O. (1994). Cancer. In C.W. Molina and M. Aguirre-Molina (Eds.), *Latino health in the U.S.: A growing challenge* (pp. 211-246). Washington, DC: American Public Health Association.

Haffner, S.M., Stern, M.P., Hazuda, H.P., Pugh, J.A., Patterson, J.K., and Malina, R. (1986). Upper body and centralized adiposity in Mexican-Americans and non-Hispanic whites: Relationship to body mass index and other behavioral and demographic variables. *International Journal of Obesity, 10,* 493-502.

Hart, C., Ecob, R., and Smith, G.D. (1997). People, places and coronary heart disease risk factors: A multilevel analysis of the Scottish Heart Health Study archive. *Social Science and Medicine, 45,* 893-902.

Haynes, S.G., Harvey, C., Montes, H., Nickens, H., and Cohen, B.H. (1990). Patterns of cigarette smoking among Hispanics in the United States: Results from HHANES 1982-84. *American Journal of Public Health, 80*(Suppl.), 47-53.

Hazuda, H.P., Stern, M.P., and Haffner, S.M. (1988). Acculturation and assimilation among Mexican Americans: Scales and population-based data. *Social Science Quarterly, 69,* 687-706.

Hewitt, M., Devesa, S., and Breen, N. (2002). Papanicolaou test use among reproductive-age women at high risk for cervical cancer: Analyses of the 1995 National Survey of Family Growth. *American Journal of Public Health, 92,* 666-669.

Hollman, F. (1993). *U.S. population estimates by age, sex, race, and Hispanic origin: 1980 to 1991* (Current Population Reports, Series P-25, No. 1095). Washington, DC: U.S. Bureau of the Census.

Howard-Pitney, B., Winkleby, M.A., Albright, C.L., Bruce, B., and Fortmann, S.P. (1997). The Stanford Nutrition Action Program: A dietary fat intervention for low literate adults. *American Journal of Public Health, 87,* 1971-1976.

Hunt, K.J., Resendez, R.G., Williams, K., Haffner, S.M., Stern, M.P., and Hazuda H.P. (2003). All-cause and cardiovascular mortality among Mexican-American and non-Hispanic white older participants in the San Antonio Heart Study—evidence against the "Hispanic paradox". American Journal of Epidemiology, 158, 1048-1057.

Institute of Medicine. (1991). Disability in America: Toward a national agenda for prevention. Washington, DC: National Academy Press.

Jasso, G., Massey, D.S., Rosenzweig, M.R., and Smith, J.P. (2000). The New Immigrant Survey Pilot (NIS-P): Overview and new findings about U.S. legal immigrants at admission. Demography, 37, 127-138.

Jeffery, R.W., Drewnowski, A., Epstein, L.H., Stunkard, A.J., Wilson, G.T., and Wing, R.R. (2000). Long-term maintenance of weight loss: Current status. Health Psychology, 19, 5-16.

Jemal, A., Thomas, A., Murray, T., and Thun, M. (2002). Cancer statistics, 2002. A Cancer Journal for Clinicians, 52, 23-47.

Jones, C.P. (2000). Levels of racism: a theoretic framework and a gardener's tale. American Journal of Public Health, 90, 1212-1215.

Kaplan, G.A., and Keil, J.E. (1993). Socioeconomic factors and cardiovascular disease: A review of the literature. Circulation, 88, 1973-1998.

Kaufman, J.S., Cooper, R.S., and McGee, D.L. (1997). Socioeconomic status and health in blacks and whites: The problem of residual confounding and the resiliency of race. Epidemiology, 8, 621-628.

Krieger, N. (1999). Embodying inequality: A review of concepts, measures, and methods for studying health consequences of discrimination. International Journal of Health Services, 29, 295-352.

Krieger, N. (2001). A glossary for social epidemiology. Journal of Epidemiology and Community Health, 55, 693-700.

Krieger, N., Williams, D.R., and Moss, N.E. (1997). Measuring social class in U.S. public health research: Concepts, methodologies, and guidelines. Annual Review of Public Health, 18, 341-378.

Kuczmarski, R.J., Flegal, K.M., Campbell, S.M., and Johnson, C.L. (1994). Increasing prevalence of overweight among U.S. adults: The National Health and Nutrition Examination Surveys, 1960 to 1991. Journal of the American Medical Association, 272, 205-211.

Kumanyika, S., Wilson, J.F., and Guilford-Davenport, M. (1993). Weight-related attitudes and behaviors of black women. Journal of the American Dietetic Association, 93, 416-422.

Kumanyika, S.K. (1993). Special issues regarding obesity in minority populations. Annals of Internal Medicine, 119, 650-654.

LeClere, F.B., Rogers, R.G., and Peters, K. (1998). Neighborhood social context and racial differences in women's heart disease mortality. Journal of Health and Social Behavior, 39, 91-107.

Lee, R.E., and Cubbin, C. (2002). Neighborhood context and youth cardiovascular health behaviors. American Journal of Public Health, 92, 428-436.

Link, B.G., and Phelan, J. (1995). Social conditions as fundamental causes of disease. Journal of Health and Social Behavior, 35(Suppl.), 80-94.

Lowry, R., Kann, L., Collins, J.L., and Kolbe, L.J. (1996). The effect of socioeconomic status on chronic disease risk behaviors among US adolescents. Journal of the American Medical Association, 276, 792-797.

Lynch, J.W., Kaplan, G.A., Cohen, R.D., Tuomilehto, J., and Salonen, J.T. (1996). Do cardiovascular risk factors explain the relation between socioeconomic status, risk of all-cause mortality, and acute myocardial infarction? American Journal of Epidemiology, 144, 934-942.

Lynch, J.W., Kaplan, G.A., and Shema, S.J. (1997). Cumulative impact of sustained economic hardship on physical, cognitive, psychological, and social functioning. *New England Journal of Medicine, 337,* 1889-1895.

Macintyre, S., Maciver, S., and Sooman, A. (1993). Area, class and health: Should we be focusing on places or people? *Journal of Society and Politics, 22,* 213-234.

Macintyre, S., Ellaway, A., and Cummins, S. (2002). Place effects on health: How can we conceptualise, operationalise, and measure them? *Social Science and Medicine, 55,* 125-139.

Markides, K.S., and Coreil, J. (1986). The health of Hispanics in the southwestern United States: An epidemiologic paradox. *Public Health Reports, 101,* 253-265.

Markides, K.S., Ray, L.A., Stroup-Benham, C.A., and Trevino, F. (1990). Acculturation and alcohol consumption in the Mexican American population of the southwestern United States: Findings from HHANES 1982-84. *American Journal of Public Health, 80*(Suppl.), 42-46.

Marmot, M., and Elliot, P. (1992). *Coronary heart disease epidemiology from aetiology to public health.* New York: Oxford University Press.

Martin, L.G., and Soldo, B.J. (1997). *Racial and ethnic differences in the health of older Americans.* Washington, DC: National Academy Press.

McNutt, S.W., Hu, Y., Schreiber, G.B., Crawford, P.B., Obarzanek, E., and Mellin, L. (1997). A longitudinal study of the dietary practices of black and white girls 9 and 10 years old at enrollment: The NHLBI Growth and Health Study. *Journal of Adolescent Health, 20,* 27-37.

Miller, B.A., Kolonel, L.N., Bernstein, L., Young Jr., J.L., Swanson, G.M., West, D.W., Key, C.R., Liff, J.M., Glover, C.S., Alexander, G.A., Coyle, L., Hankey, B.F., Gloeckler Ries, L.A., Kosary, C.L., Harras, A., Percy, C., and Edwards, B.K. (1996). *Racial/ethnic patterns of cancer in the United States 1988-1992* (NIH Pub. No. 96-4104). Bethesda, MD: National Cancer Institute.

Minkler, M. (1990). Improving health through community organization, In K. Glanz, F.M. Lewis, and B.K. Rimer (Eds.), *Health behavior and health education: Theory, research and practice* (pp. 257-287). San Francisco: Jossey-Bass.

Mitchell, B.D., Stern, M.P., Haffner, S.M., Hazuda, H.P., and Patterson, J.K. (1990). Risk factors for cardiovascular mortality in Mexican Americans and non-Hispanic whites: The San Antonio Heart Study. *American Journal of Epidemiology, 131,* 423-433.

Muntaner, C., Nieto, F.J., and O'Campo, P. (1996). The Bell Curve: On race, social class, and epidemiologic research. *American Journal of Epidemiology, 144,* 531-535.

National Cancer Institute. (2001). *SEER program public-use data tapes 1973-1998, August 2000 submission.* Bethesda, MD: National Institutes of Health.

National Center for Health Statistics. (1994a). *National Health Interview Survey/Multiple Cause of Death Public Use Data 1986-1990. Diskette and documentation.* Hyattsville, MD: Centers for Disease Control and Prevention.

National Center for Health Statistics. (1994b). Plan and operation of the Third National Health and Nutrition Examination Survey, 1988-1994, series 1: Programs and collection procedures. *Vital Health Statistics, 32,* 1-407.

National Heart, Lung, and Blood Institute. (1998). *Clinical guidelines on the identification, evaluation, and treatment of overweight and obesity in adults: The evidence report* (Rep. No. 98-4083). Bethesda, MD: National Institutes of Health.

National Research Council (1997). *Racial and ethnic differences in the health of older Americans.* L.G. Martin and B.J. Soldo (Eds.), Committee on Population, Commission on Behavioral and Social Sciences and Education. Washington, DC: National Academy Press.

Otten, M.W., Jr., Teutsch, S.M., Williamson, D.F., and Marks, J.S. (1990). The effect of known risk factors on the excess mortality of black adults in the United States. *Journal of the American Medical Association, 263,* 845-850.

Padilla, A.M. (Ed.). (1980). *Acculturation: Theory, models, and some new findings* (AAAS Pub. No. SS(NS)-39 ed.). American Association for the Advancement of Science Boulder, CO: Westview Press.

Pamuk, E., Makuc, D., Heck, K., Reuben, C., and Lochner, K. (1998). *Socioeconomic status and health chartbook: Health, United States, 1998* (Rep. No. 71-641496). Hyattsville, MD: National Center for Health Statistics.

Pappas, G., Queen, S., Hadden, W., and Fisher, G. (1993). The increasing disparity in mortality between socioeconomic groups in the United States, 1960 and 1986. *New England Journal of Medicine, 329,* 103-109.

Pérez-Stable, E.J., Otero-Sabogal, R., Sabogal, F., McPhee, S.J., and Hiatt, R.A. (1994). Self-reported use of cancer screening tests among Latinos and Anglos in a prepaid health plan. *Archives of Internal Medicine, 154,* 1073-1081.

Pi-Sunyer, F.X. (1993). Medical hazards of obesity. *Annals of Internal Medicine, 119,* 655-660.

Pickett, K.E., and Pearl, M. (2001). Multilevel analyses of neighborhood socioeconomic context and health outcomes: A critical review. *Journal of Epidemiology and Community Health, 55,* 111-122.

Pierce, J.P., Choi, W.S., Gilpin, E.A., Farkas, A.J., and Berry, C.C. (1998). Tobacco industry promotion of cigarettes and adolescent smoking. *Journal of the American Medical Association, 279,* 511-515.

Ragland, K., Selvin, S., and Merrill, D. (1991). Black-white differences in stage-specific cancer survival: Analysis of seven selected sites. *American Journal of Epidemiology, 133,* 672-682.

Rogers, R.G. (1991). Health-related lifestyles among Mexican Americans, Puerto Ricans, and Cubans in the United States. In I. Rapsenwaike (Ed.), *Mortality of Hispanic patients* (pp. 145-167). New York: Greenwood Press.

Runciman, W.G. (Ed.). (1978). *Weber: Selections in translation.* Cambridge, England: Cambridge University Press.

Shah, B.V., Barnwell, B.G., Hunt, P.N., Nileen, P., and LaVange, L.M. (1991). *SUDAAN user's manual, release 5.50.* Research Triangle Park, NC: Research Triangle Institute.

Singh, G.K., Kochanek, K.D., and McDonan, M.F. (1996). *Advance report of final mortality statistics, 1994.* Hyattsville, MD: National Center for Health Statistics.

Smith, J.P., and Kington, R.S. (1997). Race, socioeconomic status, and health in late life. In L.G. Martin and B.J. Soldo (Eds.), *Racial and ethnic differences in the health of older Americans* (pp. 106-162). Committee on Population, Commission on Behavioral and Social Sciences and Education, National Research Council. Washington, DC: National Academy Press.

Smith, G.D., Neaton, J.D., Wentworth, D., Stamler, R., and Stamler, J. (1996). Socioeconomic differentials in mortality risk among men screened for the Multiple Risk Factor Intervention Trial: I. White men. *American Journal of Public Health, 86,* 486-496.

Smith, G.D., Hart, C., Watt, G., Hole, D., and Hawthorne, V. (1998). Individual social class, area-based deprivation, cardiovascular disease risk factors, and mortality: The Renfrew and Paisley Study. *Journal of Epidemiology and Community Health, 52,* 399-405.

Sorlie, P.D., Backlund, E., Johnson, N.J., and Rogot, E. (1993). Mortality by Hispanic status in the United States. *Journal of the American Medical Association, 270,* 2464-2468.

Srinivasan, S.R., Bao, W., Wattigney, W.A., and Berenson, G.S. (1996). Adolescent overweight is associated with adult overweight and related multiple cardiovascular risk factors: The Bogalusa Heart Study. *Metabolism: Clinical and Experimental, 45,* 235-240.

Stephen, E.H., Foote, K., Hendershot, G.E., and Schoenborn, C.A. (1994). Health of the foreign-born population: United States, 1989-90. Advance data. *Vital Health Statistics, 241,* 1-12.

Sundquist, J., and Winkleby, M.A. (1999). Cardiovascular risk factors in Mexican American adults: A transcultural analysis of NHANES III, 1988-1994. *American Journal of Public Health, 89,* 723-730.

Sundquist, J., Malmstrom, M., and Johansson, S.E. (1999). Cardiovascular risk factors and the neighbourhood environment: A multilevel analysis. *International Journal of Epidemiology, 28,* 841-845.

Sundquist, J., Winkleby, M.A., and Pudaric, S. (2001). Cardiovascular disease risk factors among older black, Mexican American, and white women and men: An analysis of NHANES III, 1988-1994. *Journal of the American Geriatrics Society, 49,* 109-116.

Syme, S.L. (2004). Social determinants of health: The community as an empowered partner. Available: http://www.cdc.gov/pcd/issues/2004/jan/syme.htm.

Tortolero, S.R., Goff, D.C., Jr., Nichaman, M.Z., Labarthe, D.R., Grunbaum, J.A., and Hanis, C.L. (1997). Cardiovascular risk factors in Mexican-American and non-Hispanic white children: The Corpus Christi Child Heart Study. *Circulation, 96,* 418-423.

Tyroler, H.A., Wing, S., and Knowles, M.G. (1993). Increasing inequality in coronary heart disease mortality in relation to educational achievement: Profile of places of residence, United States, 1962 to 1987. *Annals of Epidemiology, 3*(Suppl.), S51-54.

U.S. Census Bureau. (2001). Population Projections of the United States by Age, Sex, Race, Hispanic Origin, and Nativity: 1999 to 2100. Available: http://www.census.gov/population/projections/nation/detail/np-d1-a.txt [Accessed January 26, 2002].

U.S. Department of Health and Human Services. (2001). *Women and smoking: Report of the Surgeon General.* Washington, DC: National Center for Chronic Disease Prevention and Health Promotion.

Vega, W.A., and Amaro, H. (1994). Latino outlook: Good health, uncertain prognosis. *Annual Reviews in Public Health, 15,* 39-67.

Ventura, S.J., Peters, K.D., Martin, J.A., and Maurer, J.D. (1997). Births and deaths: United States, 1996. *Monthly Vital Statistics Report, 46,* 1-40.

Villarejo, D., Lighthall, D., Williams, D., III, Souter, A., Mines, R., Bade, B., Samuels, S., and McCurdy, S. (2000). *Suffering in silence: A report on the health of California's agricultural workers.* Davis, CA: California Institute for Rural Studies.

Wallack, L., and Winkleby, M. (1987). Primary prevention: A new look at basic concepts. *Social Science and Medicine, 25,* 923-930.

Wallerstein, N., and Bernstein, E. (1994). Introduction to community empowerment, participatory education, and health. *Health Education Quarterly, 21,* 141-148.

Williams, D.R. (1996). Race/ethnicity and socioeconomic status: Measurement and methodological issues. *International Journal of Health Services, 26,* 483-505.

Williams, D.R., and Collins, C. (1995). U.S. socioeconomic and racial differences in health: Patterns and explanations. *Annual Review of Sociology, 21,* 349-386.

Winkleby, M.A., and Cubbin, C. (2003). Influence of individual and neighborhood socioeconomic status on mortality among Black, Mexican-American, and White women and men in the U.S. *Journal of Epidemiology and Community Health, 57,* 444-452.

Winkleby, M.A., Fortmann, S.P., and Rockhill, B. (1993). Health-related risk factors in a sample of Hispanics and whites matched on sociodemographic characteristics: The Stanford Five-City Project. *American Journal of Epidemiology, 137,* 1365-1375.

Winkleby, M.A., Schooler, C., Kraemer, H.C., Lin, J., and Fortmann, S.P. (1995). Hispanic versus white smoking patterns by sex and level of education. *American Journal of Epidemiology, 142,* 410-418.

Winkleby, M.A., Kraemer, H.C., Ahn, D.K., and Varady, A.N. (1998). Ethnic and socioeconomic differences in cardiovascular disease risk factors: Findings for women from the Third National Health and Nutrition Examination Survey, 1988-1994. *Journal of the American Medical Association, 280*, 356-362.

Winkleby, M.A., Cubbin, C., Ahn, D.K., and Kraemer, H.C. (1999a). Pathways by which SES and ethnicity influence cardiovascular disease risk factors. *Annals of the New York Academy of Sciences, 896*, 191-209.

Winkleby, M.A., Robinson, T.N., Sundquist, J., and Kraemer, H.C. (1999b). Ethnic variation in cardiovascular risk factors among children and young adults: Findings from the Third National Health and Nutrition Examination Survey, 1988-1994. *Journal of the American Medical Association, 281*, 1006-1013.

Winkleby, M.A., Feighery, E., Dunn, M., Kole, S., Ahn, D., Killen, J. (2004). Effects of an advocacy intervention to reduce smoking among teenagers. *Archives of Pediatrics and Adolescent Medicine, 158*, 269-275.

Yen, I.H., and Kaplan, G.A. (1998). Poverty area residence and changes in physical activity level: Evidence from the Alameda County Study. *American Journal of Public Health, 88*, 1709-1712.

Young, L.R., and Nestle, M. (2002). The contribution of expanding portion sizes to the U.S. obesity epidemic. *American Journal of Public Health, 92*, 246-249.

Young, R.C. (2002). Cancer statistics, 2002: Progress or cause for concern? *CA: A Cancer Journal for Clinicians, 52*, 6-7.

13

Cumulative Psychosocial Risks and Resilience: A Conceptual Perspective on Ethnic Health Disparities in Late Life

Hector F. Myers and Wei-Chin Hwang

Over the past decade, concern has been growing about society's ability to meet the mental health needs of elderly Americans in certain racial/ethnic groups. This issue has become particularly salient given the rapid increase in the U.S. elderly population. In fact, between the years of 1990 and 2000, the elderly population in the United States increased 12 percent, and elderly Americans currently comprise 12.4 percent of the U.S. population (U.S. Census Bureau, 2001). Moreover, the population of racial/ethnic elderly is estimated to be increasing at a faster rate than that of whites (Ruiz, 1995).

Despite these concerns, relatively little attention have been given to studying the mental health needs of aging ethnic minorities. In this chapter, we review the extant literature on ethnic disparities in mental health in late life, using depression as an illustrative disorder. We discuss methodological and conceptual gaps in the literature, and we review available clinical and epidemiological evidence. Moreover, we provide a conceptual framework for understanding the relationships among ethnicity, age, and well-being for elderly minority populations. Specifically, we present a biopsychosocial model of cumulative psychological and physical vulnerability and resilience in later life in which chronic stress burden and psychosocial resources for coping are hypothesized as playing a significant role in accounting for ethnic disparities in mental health. Implications and suggestions for future research are discussed.

AGING AND DEPRESSION

Because of a number of conceptual, diagnostic, and methodological challenges in studying depression in the elderly, findings from research studies have been mixed, with most studies reporting lower prevalence of depression in the elderly (Regier et al., 1988), and some studies showing higher prevalence (Blazer, Burchett, Service, and George, 1991). Similar trends in low prevalence of mood disorders among ethnic elders also have been reported (Weissman, Bruce, Leaf, Florio, and Holzer, 1991), with no significant overall differences between groups in the Epidemiological Catchment Area (ECA) study (George, Blazer, Winfield-Laird, Leaf, and Fischbach, 1988). It would seem that healthy, functioning older adults are at no greater risk for becoming depressed. Instead, age-related effects may be attributable to physical health problems, functional and cognitive disability, chronic illness, low social support, and financial difficulties (Blazer et al., 1991; Roberts, Kaplan, Shema, and Strawbridge, 1997a).

Nevertheless, a number of methodological limitations may lead to underestimates in rates of depression in community studies. Karel (1997) noted that low prevalence rates of major depression among older adults may reflect (1) invalid measurement of depression in older adults (e.g., diagnostic difficulties, symptoms being misattributed to medical causes, symptom recall, and older adults being viewed as less likely to be functionally impaired by depressive symptoms), (2) sampling bias (e.g., older adults may have died, may be unable to participate due to illness and disability, and may be institutionalized or residing in community dwellings for the elderly), or (3) cohort effects due to sociocultural changes (i.e., rates of depression increase in cohorts born after World War II). Several studies have confirmed that rates of depression are increasing in the United States and worldwide (Cross-National Collaborative Group, 1992).

In examining depression in the elderly, it is also important to distinguish between recurrent illness that began earlier in life and first onset illness that manifests itself in late life. Early onset depression has been associated with a more malignant course (Klein et al., 1999; Lewinsohn, Fenn, Stanton, and Franklin, 1986; Sorenson, Rutter, and Aneshensel, 1991), greater vulnerability to chronic life stress (Hammen, Davila, Brown, Gitlin, and Ellicott, 1992), greater psychiatric comorbidity (Kasch and Klein, 1996; Lewinsohn, Rohde, Seeley, and Fischer, 1991), and greater genetic liability (Klein, Taylor, Harding, and Dickstein, 1988; Lyons et al., 1998). Early disorder onset is also associated with greater family psychiatric burden, neuroticism, and dysfunctional past maternal relationships (Brodaty et al., 2001; Van den Berg et al., 2001). On the other hand, first episode of depression in later life is associated with greater medical disability, and decreased neuropsychological and psychophysiological functioning (Lewinsohn et al., 1991). Therefore, it is important to distinguish between depressive subgroups that may possess different etiological pathways: (1) those with early onset and longstanding psychobiological and familial vulnerability, who carry this risk for recurrence into old age; (2) those who become depressed as seniors, perhaps as a reaction to severe life stress; and (3) those whose depression may be associated with significant medical and vascular dysfunction and disability (Van den Berg et al., 2001).

ETHNIC DISPARITIES IN DEPRESSION

Results from large epidemiological studies on ethnic differences in the prevalence of major depression in the United States are mixed, with African Americans and Asian Americans showing lower rates of major depressive disorder (MDD), and Hispanics showing higher rates than whites (Blazer, Kessler, McGonagle, and Swartz, 1994; Somervell, Leaf, Weissman, Blazer, and Bruce, 1989; Zhang and Snowden, 1999). On the other hand, studies with smaller and less representative community samples report a greater prevalence of depressive symptoms in ethnic minorities (Kuo, 1984; Roberts, Roberts, and Chen, 1997b; Siegel, Aneshensel, Taub, Cantwell, and Driscoll, 1998), and more severe depression among ethnic minorities in treatment (Myers et al., 2002a). There has also been debate about the accuracy of these ethnic group differences, especially given the evidence for possible ethnic differences in symptom expression of depression. Although some studies have found similarities in the core features of major depression in all ethnic groups (Ballenger et al., 2001; Weissman et al., 1996), others have found a greater tendency among racial/ethnic minorities in the United States and nonwhites worldwide to somatize their psychological distress, which may also contribute to underestimates of disease prevalence (Kirmayer and Young, 1998; Kuo, 1984; Myers et al., 2002; Zheng, Lin, Takeuchi, Kurasaki, and Cheung, 1997). Several studies have reported that depressed African-American patients are more likely to report anxiety, anger, hostility, and suspiciousness than white patients (Fabrega, Mezzich, and Ulrich, 1988; Myers et al., 2002; Raskin, Crook, and Herman, 1975).

Cross-national studies reveal different rates of major depression in various countries around the world (Weissman et al., 1996). Although we can speculate that differences in risk factors or cultural differences in expression and/or reporting of symptoms may account for some of the differences, we cannot assume they account for all of the differences. Furthermore, no cross-national studies have specifically compared rates of depression among the elderly, with most including only participants up to age 65.

Findings from the ECA and National Comorbidity Study (NCS), the two largest epidemiological studies in the United States, have been mixed. ECA results indicated that whites and Hispanics evidenced higher rates of lifetime major depression (5.3 percent and 4.6 percent) than Asians and African Americans (3.6 and 3.4 percent) (Zhang and Snowden, 1999). Additionally, Hispanics reported higher rates of dysthymia than the other three groups, who reported comparable rates (4 percent, 2.6 percent, 3.2

percent, and 3 percent, respectively). African-American women between the ages of 18 and 24 were at particularly high risk in five ECA sites, and African-American men ages 18 to 24 were at lower risk compared with white men (Somervell et al., 1989).

The NCS also confirmed the existence of some ethnic and gender differences in the prevalence of MDD (Blazer et al., 1994), with whites and Hispanics evidencing higher current and lifetime rates than African Americans, and women in all ethnic groups evidencing consistently higher rates than men. African-American women between the ages of 35 and 44 were also at particularly high risk for becoming depressed.

Results from the more recent NCS also confirmed the existence of some ethnic and gender differences in the prevalence of MDD (Blazer et al., 1994), with whites and Hispanics evidencing higher lifetime rates of major depression than African Americans, and women in all ethnic groups evidencing consistently higher rates than men (see Table 13-1). Risk also varied by age groups, with African-American women between the ages of 35 and 44 and Hispanic women between the ages of 35 and 54 evidencing

TABLE 13-1 Prevalence of Lifetime Major Depressive Episode, by Race/Ethnicity, Sex, and Age from the National Comorbidity Survey (N = 8,098)

Race/Ethnicity	Males		Females		Total	
	%	SE*	%	SE	%	SE
White (years)						
15-24	11.6	2.1	23.1	2.3	16.9	1.5
25-34	14.0	1.4	19.6	1.5	17.0	1.1
35-44	15.2	2.0	24.2	2.4	19.5	1.8
45-54	12.7	2.0	23.1	2.9	17.9	1.6
Total	13.5	1.0	22.3	1.0	17.9	0.8
Black						
15-24	4.7	2.2	9.2	2.7	7.1	1.8
25-34	9.0	4.1	18.6	4.4	14.5	3.3
35-44	5.9	1.8	21.1	4.5	14.9	3.3
45-54	10.2	6.2	9.0	3.9	9.6	4.1
Total	7.2	1.9	15.5	2.2	11.9	1.6
Hispanic						
15-24	10.8	5.1	22.6	5.7	16.5	3.6
25-34	10.0	3.2	19.8	4.2	15.1	2.2
35-44	17.6	6.7	30.2	9.0	24.2	6.0
45-54	9.3	5.0	30.2	11.7	16.0	6.6
Total	11.7	2.4	23.9	3.6	17.7	1.9

*Standard error.
NOTE: Percentages are weighted to the population.

particularly high risk. Although rates of 30-day current major depression proved to be less stable, they revealed similar trends.

Other studies have found no significant differences in prevalence of depression between African Americans and whites, but have found that depression in African Americans is associated with socioeconomic deprivation, including low urbanization, low education, chronic physical condition, uncertainty, job loss, money problems, and social isolation (Dressler and Badger, 1985), and that race interacts with socioeconomic status (SES) to increase psychological vulnerability among African Americans (Williams, Takeuchi, and Adair, 1992).

Because of methodological difficulties and the high cost of surveying the prevalence of psychiatric disorders among the heterogeneous mix of Asian Americans and Native Americans in the United States, we know less about the actual prevalence rates of depressive disorders in these populations. Studies on Chinese and Chinese Americans report lower prevalence rates for depression and lower treatment utilization rates than whites (Chen et al., 1993; Hwu, Yeh, and Chang, 1989; Snowden and Cheung, 1990; Sue, Fujino, Hu, Takeuchi, and Zane, 1991; Takeuchi et al., 1998). For example, lifetime and one-year prevalence of major depression among Chinese Americans as assessed by the University of Michigan-Composite International Diagnostic Interview was 6.9 percent and 3.4 percent, respectively (Takeuchi et al., 1998). Studies conducted in China and Hong Kong reveal even lower prevalence rates (Chen et al., 1993; Hwu et al., 1989). However, rates of dysthymia among Chinese Americans were comparable to the overall U.S. population (Takeuchi et al., 1998). In addition, some evidence indicates higher prevalence of psychiatric disorders among subgroups such as Southeast Asians who evidence high rates of posttraumatic stress disorder (PTSD) (Nicassio, 1985). Studies have also shown that Asian Americans seek treatment less often than other groups, and are more severely impaired at entry into treatment than whites. Therefore, treatment statistics may severely underestimate the need for mental health services in this population (Takeuchi, Leaf, and Kuo, 1988). In any event, mood disorders are the most prevalent psychiatric problem among Asian Americans and the main reason they seek treatment (Altschuler, Wang, Qi, Wang, and Xia, 1988; Flaskerud and Hu, 1994; Nakane et al., 1991). Moreover, there is evidence that Asians and Asian Americans report more severe distress and depressive symptoms in community and treatment settings (Kuo, 1984; Siegel et al., 1998; Sue and Sue, 1987), and that they tend to have worse treatment outcomes compared to whites (Zane, Enomoto, and Chun, 1994).

Immigrant status and acculturation further complicate risk associated with depression and other health and mental health problems in many ethnic minority groups. Some studies indicate that the risk for more severe depressive symptoms and/or syndromal depression increases as ethnic immigrants become more acculturated (Burnam, Hough, Karno, Escobar, and Telles, 1987; Escobar, 1998; Golding, Karno, and Rutter, 1990; Takeuchi et al., 1998; Vega et al., 1998), and that the age of onset for depression is later for those born outside the United States (Hwang, Chun, Takeuchi, Myers, and Prabha, in press; Sorenson et al., 1991). In addition, there is some evidence that gender differences become more pronounced as immigrants become more acculturated (Swensen, Baxter, Shetterly, Scarbro, and Hamman, 2000; Takeuchi et al., 1998). It is possible that when immigrants come to the United States, the increased stress and burden of adapting to a new place increases risk for becoming depressed, and/or that important cultural protective factors (e.g., large family and friend networks) become attenuated. It is also possible that as immigrant populations assimilate into the United States, they evidence a regression to the normative prevalence rates and age of onset patterns of the general U.S. population (Berry, 1998).

Even fewer studies have assessed the mental health needs of Native Americans. Large-scale epidemiological and community studies have failed to include significant numbers of Native Americans to permit meaningful comparisons, especially when the heterogeneity among Native American tribes is considered. Because of past discrimination and relocation, Native Americans remain plagued with economic disadvantage, poverty, physical and mental disability, and lack of access to care (Manson, 1995). In a study conducted by Kinzie et al. (1992), nearly 70 percent of Native Americans in their community sample had experienced a mental disorder in their lifetime. Among Vietnam veterans participating in the American Indian Vietnam Veterans Project, rates of PTSD among Northern Plains and Southwestern Vietnam vets ranged from 27 to 31 percent (current) and 45 to 57 percent (lifetime) (Beals et al., 2002; National Center for Post-Traumatic Stress Disorder and National Center for American Indian and Alaska Native Mental Health Research Center, 1996). Additionally, rates of current and lifetime alcohol abuse and/or dependence were 70 percent and 80 percent, respectively. These rates of PTSD and alcohol use and/or dependence are much higher than for whites, African Americans, and Japanese Americans.

ETHNIC DIFFERENCES IN DEPRESSION AMONG THE ELDERLY

There is a surprising lack of research available on the psychological well-being of older ethnic minorities. Although the NCS did not include those over 54 years of age, the ECA did survey the prevalence of psychiatric disorders in those 65 years and older. Findings revealed that 25- to 44-year-olds were at highest risk for experiencing a major depressive episode, while those over 65 were at lowest risk (Regier et al., 1988, 1993). Again, women evidenced highest risk for all age groups, and age trends were consistent across ethnic groups (Weissman et al., 1991).

On the other hand, in a community study of African Americans, Brown, Ahmed, Gary, and Milburn (1995) found that the one-year prevalence of major depression was highest among those 20 to 29 years old (5.6 percent), decreased among those 30 to 44 years old (2.2 percent) and 45 to 64 (1.2 percent) years old, but then increased among those over age 65 (3.2 percent). Additionally, the large majority of African Americans with major depression did not seek or receive mental health treatment (over 90 percent). Among elderly inpatient veterans at the Veterans Administration hospital, both African-American and Hispanic elderly evidenced significantly higher rates of psychotic disorders than whites (Kales, Blow, Bingham, Copeland, and Mellow, 2000). Although African-American elderly had significantly higher cognitive disorder and substance abuse rates than white and Hispanic elderly, they evidenced lower rates of mood and anxiety disorders. African-American elderly also have been found to report lower levels of depressive symptoms than whites, but report more functional impairment, unmet needs, losses, and physical illnesses, and fewer formal sources of support (Turnbull and Mui, 1995). Common predictors for both groups included the loss of significant others and the loss of a sense of control. Poor perceived health, physical illnesses, and fewer social contacts were significant predictors for frail white elders, but not for African-American elders. Similarly, poor ego strength and chronic medical problems were associated with greater depressive symptoms among African-American elderly in Tennessee (Husaini et al., 1991). Additionally, females were found to be more reactive to life events and to decreases in social support.

Epidemiological evidence also notes significant black-white differences in rates of suicide among the elderly, with rates in white men and women (33.1 and 4.85 per 100,000, respectively) significantly higher than for African-American men and women (11.7 per 100,000 for men and rates that are too low for women for a reliable estimate) (Centers for Disease Control and Prevention, 2001). The rates of passive and active suicide ideation among African-American elderly are also reported to be equally low, with 2.5 percent and 1.4 percent for men and women respectively (Cook, Pearson, Thompson, Black, and Rabins, 2002).

Among Hispanic elderly, Bastida and Gonzalez (1995) suggested that the stresses of migration, relocation, and adapting to a new cultural environment act as chronic stressors that increase risk for mental health problems. Canino et al. (1987) found that lifetime and 6-month prevalence rates for affective, anxiety, and substance abuse disorders increased with age in Puerto Ricans. However, their study did not examine Puerto Rican elders over age 65. Escobar, Karno, Burnam, Hough, and Golding (1988) also found higher rates of phobic and dysthymic disorders in Mexican women over 40, but again, their study did not include those over age 65. In a study of elderly Hispanics living in the San Luis Valley, no difference in risk of depression was found among men (Swenson et al., 2000). However, Hispanic women evidenced greater depressive symptoms than non-Hispanic women. Additionally, elderly Hispanics who were less acculturated were at greater risk than those who were more acculturated. Female gender, chronic diseases, dissatisfaction with available social support, living alone, and lower income and education enhance risk for more severe depressive symptoms.

There are relatively few studies on psychological distress and depression in elderly Asians and Asian Americans. The most frequently cited of these studies is the Chinese American Psychiatric Epidemiological Study, which found that Chinese Americans between the ages of 50 and 65 were at the greatest risk for becoming depressed (Takeuchi et al., 1998). Those who immigrated at a later stage in their lives were especially vulnerable to the deleterious risks of immigrating to a new country (Hwang et al., in press).

Most of the major epidemiological studies of depression on Asians in Asia also exclude persons over age 65. However, there is some evidence for high prevalence of affective disorders among Asian elderly. For example, Lee et al. (1990) found a high prevalence of major depression among Koreans in Korea ages 18 to 24 (3.8 percent), a decreased prevalence in 25- to 44-year-olds (3 percent), and an increase in those 45 to 65 years old (3.5 percent). In addition, rates of dysthymia increased with age. Rates of major depression in Korean-American elderly in Los Angeles were similar to American elderly in the ECA sample in St. Louis, but lower than elderly Koreans in Korea (Yamamoto, Rhee, and Chang, 1994). However, the rate of alcohol abuse/dependence in Korean Americans was more than twice that of other elderly Americans. Cooper and Sartorius (1996) also found a gradual increase with age in the prevalence of neurotic disorders among Chinese in 12 areas of China. However, Chen et al. (1993) found that the prevalence of major depression was lower among Chinese ages 45 to 64, but that rates of dysthymia were higher compared to younger Chinese. Depression among Chinese elderly has been found to be associated with poor physical health, financial strains, lack of social support and resources, and stressful family environments (Chou and Chi, 2000; Krause and Liang, 1993; Kua, 1990; Woo, Ho, Lau, and Yuen, 1994). Furthermore, depression among elderly immigrants is often associated with social alienation and isolation, disempowerment, loss of support, and increased risk for suicide. In fact, elderly Chinese Americans, especially women, have been found to have higher rates of suicide than elders from other ethnic groups (Yamamoto et al., 1997; Yu, 1986).

Depression in Native American elders is also a common problem. Manson (1992) found significant depressive symptoms in more than 30 percent of elderly Native American adults visiting an urban outpatient medical facility. In addition, nearly 20 percent of Native American elders seeking treatment in primary care settings reported significant psychiatric difficulties (Goldwasser and Badger, 1989; Wilson, Civic, and Glass, 1995), and more than 18 percent of Great Lakes Native Americans endorsed clinically significant levels of depression as measured by the Center for Epidemiologic Study-Depression (Curyto, Chapleski, and Lichtenberg, 1999; Curyto et al., 1998). High prevalence rates of suicide, homelessness, alcohol and drug abuse, poverty, domestic violence, trauma exposure, and comorbidity of health and mental health problems also reflect the significant need for mental health services in this population.

In summary, few studies have examined mental health issues among ethnic minorities, especially ethnic elders. The available evidence is mixed, revealing a higher prevalence of affective disorders among Hispanic Americans and Native Americans across the life course. On the other hand, African Americans and Asian Americans seem to have lower rates of diagnosable disorders, but higher rates of depressive symptomatology overall. Differences in the samples studied (i.e., community versus clinical samples), in the assessment measures used (i.e., symptom measures versus diagnostic interviews), as well as possible differences in expression of distress may partially account for these discrepancies. It is also possible that age-related effects and differences in risk for mental health problems in ethnic elderly may be attributable to a disproportionate burden of accumulated stress, physical health problems, functional and cognitive disability, chronic illness, low social support, and financial difficulties (Blazer et al., 1991; Roberts et al., 1997a). In any event, more systematic research examining the prevalence of psychiatric disorders among ethnic elderly is an important priority.

CONCEPTUAL MODEL OF CUMULATIVE BIOPSYCHOSOCIAL VULNERABILITY AND RESILIENCE IN LATE LIFE

The previous review indicates that the available research on the different ethnic groups is uneven, with limited information on Native Americans and on many racial/ethnic subgroups. Furthermore, few studies of depression and psychological well-being take a developmental life-course perspective in investigating possible ethnic group differences and factors that contribute to such differences. Finally, there is little synergy among the biological, psychosocial, and behavioral explanations that have been offered in accounting for ethnic differences in distress and depression in the elderly. To advance our understanding of the role psychosocial factors might play in ethnic differences in depression and well-being in late life, we offer an integrative biopsychosocial model as a heuristic for organizing our review and discussion of how psychosocial stress and related factors might account for ethnic differences in functional health outcomes. We use depression as an illustrative disorder, but acknowledge that there is substantial evidence that the biopsychosocial factors included in this conceptual model may also apply to many other health outcomes, including but not limited to hypertension, cancer, chronic pain and disability, cognitive decline, and immune-mediated disorders. It is also important to acknowledge that depression is often co-morbid with chronic illnesses (e.g., advanced heart disease, diabetes, cancer), and is often a consequence of the anxiety, pain, and disability associated with these chronic conditions. Therefore, this conceptual framework may have broader applicability to both psychiatric and medical illnesses. We also acknowledge that the evidence supporting many of the hypothesized pathways varies in quality and relevance to explaining ethnic group differences in the health of the elderly. Nevertheless, we believe this model can be helpful in guiding future research efforts.

The proposed model, depicted in Figure 13-1, makes explicit that **(1) sociostructural factors**, such as race/ethnicity, social class, environmental factors (e.g., community, family), and **(2) biological factors** such as genetic vulnerabilities and family medical and psychiatric histories, interact over time to increase **(3) burden of psychosocial adversities**, which is hypothesized to be the primary predictor of risk. Primary among these adversities are a cluster of life stresses that include chronic life stresses, major life events, ethnicity-related stresses, and age-related stresses. Over the life course, we hypothesize that these stresses will accumulate and contribute to vulnerability to disease and dysfunction. The impact of this stress burden is further exacerbated by personality characteristics, such as anger/hostility, neuroticism, and pessimism, and by the clustering of health-endangering behaviors, such as smoking, alcohol and drug abuse, sedentary lifestyle, and obesity (Contrada et al., 2000; Krieger, Rowley, Herman, Avery, and Phillips, 1993; Myers, Kagawa-Singer, Kumanyika, Lex, and Markides, 1995; Williams, Yu, Jackson, and Anderson, 1997).

Our conceptual model builds on the work of several stress and life-course theorists, including McEwen and colleagues' (McEwen, 1998; McEwen and Seeman, 1999) work on "allostatic load," the work by Elder and colleagues (Elder, 1998; Elder and Crosnoe, 2002; Wickrama, Conger, Wallace, and Elder, 1999) on "life course and intergenerational transmission of risk," Singer and Ryff's (1999) work on "life history methodology," and Geronimus's (1992) work on the "weathering hypothesis." These earlier models identify factors that serve as **(4) biobehavioral mediators and moderators** of risk for adverse psychological and health outcomes. Furthermore, lifetime burden of adversities is hypothesized as contributing to disease through biological and behavioral pathways that include the chronic triggering of physiological response mechanisms (i.e., allostasis), constitutional predispositions or vulnerabilities, and allostatic load (i.e., wear and tear on the system). In turn, **allostatic load** is hypothesized to contribute

502

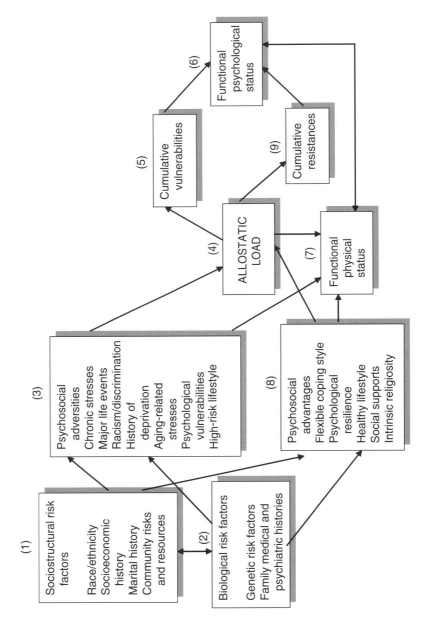

FIGURE 13-1 Biopsychosocial model of cumulative psychological vulnerability and resistance in late life.

over time to (5) **cumulative vulnerability**, and ultimately to (6) **functional outcomes** such as physical and psychological distress and dysfunction (Blanchard, 1996; Geronimus, 1992; Lestra et al., 1998; McEwen, 1998; McEwen and Stellar, 1993; Seeman, Singer, Rowe, Horwitz, and McEwen, 1997). In addition, this burden of biological hyperreactivity is compromised by the clustering of health-endangering behaviors that further enhance risk for adverse health outcomes (Myers et al., 1995; Wickrama et al., 1999).

Furthermore, and consistent with evidence of reciprocal effects between current illness and future stress exposure (McLean and Link, 1994; Harkness, Monroe, Simons, and Thase, 1999), (7) **poor health and functional limitations** are likely to exacerbate the burden of adversities over time by generating new stresses, increasing the demands on coping resources, and increasing the likelihood of greater distress, depression, and functional impairment.

However, the model also acknowledges that the stress-biological processes-disease pathways are influenced by a number of psychosocial and behavioral factors that serve as (8) **psychosocial assets or advantages** that have been shown to moderate risk. These include psychological characteristics, such as dispositional optimism and perceived control (Eizenman, Nesselroade, Featherman, and Rowe, 1997; Holahan and Holahan, 1987; Seeman, Unger, McAvay, and Mendez de Leon, 1999), healthy lifestyles (McEwen, 1998; Myers et al., 1995; Shiono, Rauh, Park, Lederman, and Suskar, 1997), flexible stress appraisal and coping strategies (Stern, Dhanda, and Hazuda, 2001; Wong and Reker, 1985), and the availability and use of adequate social support resources (Kelley, Whitley, Sipe, and Yorke, 2000; Seeman, Lusignolo, Albert, and Berkman, 2001; Walen and Lachman, 2000).

Consistent with the evidence reported by Singer and Ryff (1999) and Elder and Crosnoe (2002), the model therefore hypothesizes that it is the balance between (5) **cumulative adversities or vulnerabilities** and (9) **cumulative advantages or assets** over the life-course and the life transitions experienced that ultimately contributes to differences in functional status and health trajectories in the elderly, both overall and as a function of ethnicity, gender, and social class. Limitations in the available evidence for all pathways as well as space constraints preclude a detailed discussion of all aspects of this conceptual model. Therefore, we give special attention to discussing (1) the role of chronic stress, especially age- and ethnicity-related stressors, as adversities that can enhance risk for depression and other adverse health outcomes, (2) allostatic load and "weathering" or premature aging as hypothesized mediators of disease and dysfunction, and (3) stress coping, perceived control and self-efficacy, social supports, and religiosity as psychosocial advantages that have been shown to moderate the stress-depression relationship.

LIFETIME BURDEN OF ADVERSITIES

A primary hypothesis in our model is that the differential burden of lifetime stresses is responsible for ethnic disparities in health. The additional stress burden that ethnic groups face has yet to be studied thoroughly, but includes racism-related stresses, acculturative stress, and stresses that are particularly salient to ethnic elderly. Although there is a substantial body of evidence linking exposure to many sources of stress to depression, relatively few studies have specifically addressed the particular hypothesized associations between several of these sources of stress and ethnic differences in risk for depression. We suggest that future studies aim toward testing pathways in the proposed model.

Chronic Stress Burden

There is a large and rich interdisciplinary body of research on the complex relationships between stress, generally defined as "environmental demands that tax or exceed the adaptive capacity of an organism, resulting in biological and psychological changes that may be detrimental and place the organism at risk for disease" (Cohen, Kessler, and Gordon, 1995), and functional health outcomes. Most models of stress and disease distinguish among stress exposure, the context of stress exposure, stress appraisal, and stress response (Lobel, Dunkel-Schetter, and Scrimshaw, 1992). Meaningful distinctions are also made among types of stressors, including discrete life changes or events, chronic unresolved stresses and daily hassles, as well as the role that personal predisposition (e.g., anger/hostility, cognitive schemas) (Monroe and Simons, 1991) and situational diatheses (e.g., socioeconomic deprivation, limited social supports) (Dohrenwend et al., 1992) play in increasing vulnerability to physical and psychiatric disorders.

There is also a growing body of evidence that has specifically tested the hypothesis that ethnic differences in physical health may be due, at least in part, to differential exposure to chronic and acute life stressors (Geronimus, 1992; Williams et al., 1997). Ethnic minorities, especially those from lower social classes, often report a greater number of negative life events, greater and more frequent exposure to "generic life stressors" (i.e., stressors that are a usual part of modern life, including those that are financial, occupational, relationship oriented, or parental), and greater psychological distress from these stressful life experiences than their white counterparts (Myers, Lewis, and Parker-Dominguez, 2002b). Therefore, they are likely to be particularly vulnerable to the long-term effects of high chronic stress burden and presumably higher allostatic load. Chronic stressors due to financial strain, inadequate housing, crowding, and violence may also contribute to more frequent activation of stress-response systems and prolonged exposure to stress hormones (Anderson, McNeilly, and Myers, 1992; McEwen, 1998).

In a recent review, Myers, Lewis, and Parker-Dominguez (2002b) discuss the evidence linking psychosocial stress and other factors in accounting for ethnic disparities in a variety of chronic illnesses and adverse health outcomes. For example, studies by Orr et al. (1996) found that exposure to high psychosocial stressors was related to low birthweight for African Americans. Shiono et al. (1997) reported in their study of ethnic differences in birthweight that living in public housing and believing that one's health was largely determined by chance were negatively related to birthweight, and that having a stable residence was associated with higher birthweight. Furthermore, Zambrana and colleagues (1999) found that prenatal stress, drug use and smoking, and attitudes toward the pregnancy accounted for ethnic differences in birthweight between African Americans and Hispanics.

Such differences in exposure to generic life stressors probably account for some of the ethnic disparities in health. However, we argue that such a simple explanation of differential stress burden underestimates the true complexity of the minority stress-health relationships. For example, it has been argued that race conditions social class such that exposure to life stressors are not only greater among the poor, but also that racial/ethnic minorities experience greater stress burden and poorer health outcome at all equivalent levels of SES (Krieger et al., 1993; Williams, 1999). This race-SES relationship can have direct effects on health through additional stress burden and higher allostatic load, as well as indirect effects through structural barriers of access to health care and other social resources (i.e., housing, employment, safety); acceptance of societal stigma of inferiority (i.e., acceptance of minority status); high risk and unhealthy lifestyles (Kumanyika, 1998; Myers et al., 1995; see also Chapter 9, this volume); coercive, restrictive, or neglectful parenting; ineffective coping and negative affective states (e.g., depression, hostility, dispositional pessimism) (Clark, Anderson, Clark, and Williams, 1999; Kreiger et al., 1993; Williams, 1999); and lack of perceived control (Shaw and Krause, 2001).

Minorities, and the elderly in particular, also face a number of neighborhood stresses that add to their stress burdens. These include greater vulnerability to violence, especially from neighborhood youth, inadequate transportation, poor housing, limited access to recreation and other social services geared to the needs of the elderly (e.g., senior centers), as well as increased vulnerability to swindles and other financial schemes. These factors, in addition to their growing burden of health and functional limitations, often contribute to greater sense of lack of control. Some studies suggest there are racial disparities in feelings of perceived control that persist across all age groups (Shaw and Krause, 2001). For a more detailed discussion of these issues, see Chapter 11.

In addition to greater burden of these generic life stresses, persons of color also experience additional stresses related to their race/ethnicity, such as racism-related and acculturative stresses that add to their overall stress burden. Therefore, assessment of stress burden for populations of color will be incomplete without the inclusion of these additional sources of stress.

Racism-Related Stresses

In their recent review of the literature on racism and its effects on African Americans, Clark et al. (1999) discussed the empirical evidence verifying the effects racism has on mental and physical health. They acknowledge that both intergroup and intragroup racism, as well as attitudinal (i.e., prejudice) and behavioral (i.e., overt discrimination) racism, are significant stressors and offer a biopsychosocial model to account for its effects.

Minority elderly may be less likely to experience overt acts of racism and discrimination because they pose less of a threat and are no longer serious competitors for social resources. The one area in which there may be an exception is in access to quality health care (see Smedley, Stith, and Nelson, 2002, for a more detailed discussion of this issue). However, experiences with discrimination over the life course, including exposure to the most blatant forms of discrimination (i.e., discrimination in education, housing, employment, and transportation, and within the legal/judicial system), may have long-term deleterious effects that may become evident in their later years. Elderly African Americans were young adults during the Jim Crow years and the civil rights struggles, many elderly Japanese experienced internment camps, many elderly Mexican Americans experienced the Bracero Movement and the Zoot Suit riots in California, Cuban elders experienced economic losses when forced to leave Cuba followed by racism when they arrived in the United States, and most Native American elders experienced some of the worst treatment by the U.S. government. In addition, many older minority men experienced significant discrimination in the military during World War II and Korea. How they coped with these past and current experiences and how they have resolved these conflicts may have, at least, indirect effects on their current health and functioning. The work by Elder and Crosnoe (2002) on the influence of early behavior patterns on later life illustrates this point. Using data from men born between 1905 and 1914 and tracking their life trajectories in terms of emotional health, career achievement, and civic involvement, Elder and Crosnoe were able to differentiate five behavioral types in terms of overall success and life achievement, and identified factors associated with these life trajectories. Similar longitudinal studies of the life course of racial/ethnic minority men and women would be especially helpful in testing the hypothesized relationship in this conceptual model. For example, it would be especially useful for future research to determine whether there is a measurable difference in health status in minority elderly who experienced more race-related traumas compared to those who were spared such experiences.

One of the methodological challenges facing research on the experience and impact of racism on health is the fact that racism is a "perceived stressor" (i.e., the subjective experience of prejudice or discrimination), and that people of different ethnicities may differ in how they interpret and respond to racist experiences. Clark et al. (1999) argue that traditional models of stress focus primarily on more "objective" stressors such as life events and role strains, and in doing so ignore or underestimate the importance of exposure to more subtle racism because it involves some degree of subjectivity. However, Lazarus and Folkman (1984) note that it is the subjective appraisal of events as stressful that determines the magnitude of a stress response. Therefore, we would expect greater psychological and physiological reactivity and greater allostatic load in those who report greater exposure to both objectively measurable stressors as well as subjectively experienced greater exposure to racism-related stresses (Anderson, McNeilly, and Myers, 1993; Fang and Myers, 2001; Krieger and Sidney, 1996). We might also expect that greater exposure to racism and discrimination will be associated with more health-damaging behaviors and a poorer lifetime health trajectory. Additional studies are needed to investigate these hypotheses and to consider possible ethnic differences in exposure to and impact of racism-related stresses.

Acculturative Stress

Another major source of stress for racial/ethnic minority groups, especially those who are immigrants, is acculturative stress. There is a substantial and growing body of research on acculturation and its effect on psychological and physical health (see Berry, 1998, and Chun, Organista, and Marin, 2002, for a comprehensive review of this literature). Berry (1998) argues that investigations of relationships among acculturation, adjustment, and health need to consider the influences of social and personal variables from the society of origin (i.e., social class, sex roles, opportunity structures for social mobility, and other factors), the society of settlement (i.e., receptivity of cultural differences), and phenomena that exist both prior to (e.g., trauma) and during the process of acculturation. Despite continued debates about how to conceptualize and measure acculturation, the available evidence suggests that acculturation to the majority society has both costs and benefits. For example, research indicates that recent Hispanic and Asian immigrants evidence better mental and physical health than U.S.-born members of the same group (Rogler, Cortes, and Malgady, 1991; Vega et al., 1998), except for those who are refugees, who evidence higher rates of trauma and PTSD (Nicholson, 1997). However, this initial advantage is lost during the early phases of acculturation, primarily through stresses associated with acculturation (e.g., learning a new language, exposure to immigrant-related discrimination, changes in social roles, family disintegration, changes in health behaviors) (Balcazar, Peterson, and Krull, 1997; Nicholson, 1997).

Contrada et al. (2000, p. 138) also note that own-group conformity pressures, defined as "the experience of being pressured or constrained by one's ethnic group's expectations specifying appropriate or inappropriate behavior for the group," are independent of discrimination and are an additional source of stress for those who are upwardly mobile and acculturating, and for children and adults who may be acculturating at different rates. Also, while those who learn to balance their bicultural status (i.e., integrate into majority society yet retain their ethnic identity and cultural roots) seem to reobtain health losses due to acculturation (Cortes, Rogler, and Malgady, 1994; LaFromboise, Coleman, and Gerton, 1995; Moyerman and Forman, 1992; Roysircar-Sodowsky and Maestas, 2000), those who are bicultural but have not learned to negotiate the demands from both worlds may be at increased risk (Hwang et al., 2000).

For minority elderly, acculturation may pose unique challenges. On the one hand, elders are the guardians and conveyors of the culture of origin, and therefore, they are the primary socialization agents and source of knowledge about the cultural values, beliefs, and norms of the group. Thus, they are often at the center of generational conflicts that inevitably emerge as the younger generations embrace the values, beliefs, and norms of the new culture and challenge, adhere less rigidly, or discard those of the culture of origin (e.g., centrality of family loyalty and obligations versus the desire to pursue personal goals). On the other hand, and depending on when minority elders immigrated, they are often the ones who experienced the greatest obstacles and harshest forms of discrimination, and therefore struggle with the competing goals of maintaining cultural integrity versus encouraging the next generation to acculturate (i.e., learn the language and customs of the new society) as quickly as possible in order to improve their odds. This may pose more of a problem for the oldest old, who are either recent immigrants or remain enculturated (e.g., they never learned English or adopted American culture) and are likely to have the greatest difficulty making necessary changes, despite living in the

United States for a significant part of their adult lives. The latter group is more likely to be poorer, to be less educated, to rely entirely on their native community for resources, to have poorer health, and to have less access to health care and other resources of the larger society (Wong and Ujimoto, 1998). Additional studies are needed to explore these issues across different ethnic groups who may differ in their immigration experiences in the United States.

Aging-Related Stresses

In addition to the stresses already described, the elderly face a number of additional stressors related to their life stage. These include adequacy and stability of financial resources, coping with chronic illnesses and the attendant pain and physical limitations, social isolation, assuming caretaking responsibilities for ill spouses or custodial responsibilities for grandchildren, loss of meaningful social roles, decreasing cognitive functioning and dementia, and reductions in their social networks due to death, especially of spouses and friends (Karel, 1997). All of these stresses contribute to enhanced risk for depression and lower life satisfaction in the elderly (Burnette, 1999; Karel, 1997; Kelley et al., 2000; Newsom and Schulz, 1996).

One of the major stressors faced by the elderly is the anxiety over the adequacy and stability of their fixed income. This is especially true for minority elders, who may have experienced lifetime financial obstacles that limited their ability to accumulate savings and who must now rely on Social Security, disability payments, pensions, or veteran's benefits, or on the generosity of family and social services (Gibson, 1993). This is a particularly salient issue for undocumented immigrants as they grow older because they are often not able to capitalize on retirement benefits and may not have been able to accumulate enough savings because many held jobs with low pay and low status.

Ethnic elderly from low socioeconomic backgrounds are also at greater risk for acute and chronic physical illnesses and their sequelae. In Karel's (1997) comprehensive review of the literature on aging and depression, she notes that these functional limitations are more important than life events and psychological factors in contributing to risk for depression and low life satisfaction. She also concludes that these depressogenic effects are greatest in elderly who experience serious illnesses, severe pain, greater functional impairment, and more social isolation, and who must commit more of their limited financial resources to health care. This effect is evident in all ethnic groups, but minority elderly who generally experience greater lifetime socioeconomic deprivation and carry a heavier burden of lifetime medical morbidity are expected to be at higher risk.

Grandparenting Stresses

Minority elderly, especially African-American and Hispanic elderly, are disproportionately burdened by custodial and caretaking responsibilities of grandchildren. The increase in the number of grandparents who are raising grandchildren is one of the unanticipated and underrecognized fallouts of the cocaine/crack abuse, HIV/AIDS, and teen pregnancy epidemics of the 1980s and 1990s (Burnette, 1997; Minkler and Fuller-Thompson, 1999). Data from the U.S. Census reported by Minkler and Fuller-Thompson (1999) indicated that in 1997, approximately 4 million children were living with grandparents, including 4.1 percent of white children, 6.5 percent of Hispanic children, and 13.5 percent of African American children. This is a 44 percent increase from 1980 (Lugaila, 1998), with the greatest increase in skipped-generation families in which the birthparents were not co-resident (Casper and Bryson, 1998). Szinovacz (1998) noted from his analyses of the Wave II data in the National Survey of Families and Households (NSFH) that Census data underestimate the true prevalence of grandchildren living with grandparents. He found custodial grandparenting rates in the NSFH as high as 26 percent in African-American grandmothers and 7.3 percent in white grandmothers.

There is also substantial evidence that caregiving grandparents are especially vulnerable to a host of problems, including depression, social isolation, poverty, and reduced quality of life (Minkler and Fuller-Thompson, 1999; Minkler, Fuller-Thompson, Miller, and Driver, 1997; Rodgers-Farmer, 1999). In their secondary analysis of the NSFH data, Minkler and Fuller-Thompson found that caregiving grandparents were 50 percent more likely to have activities of daily living limitations and lower self-reported satisfaction with health than noncustodial grandparents. Similarly, these grandparents were almost twice as likely as noncaregiving grandparents to report clinically significant levels of depressive symptoms, even after controlling for precaregiving depression and demographic characteristics (Minkler et al., 1997). However, this greater vulnerability to depression cannot be attributed entirely to caregiving per se. Rather, other factors contribute to enhanced risk for depression, such as female gender (Minkler et al., 1997), recency of caregiving, younger age of the dependent child (Strawbridge, Wallhagen, Shema, and Kaplan, 1997), older age and poorer health of the caregiving grandparent (Minkler et al., 1997), having to care for children with special needs (Jendrek, 1994), inadequacy of available social supports (Sands and Goldberg-Glen, 2000), and the reasons for having to assume this responsibility (Minkler and Roe, 1993). Grandparents who had to step in to care for their grandchildren because of parental incarceration due to drug addiction and incapacitation, or death due to AIDS or violent crime, report feeling more anger, shame, and perceptions of entrapment in this "time disordered role" (Minkler et al., 1997). In addition, they may also experience greater feelings of failure in raising their own children, and create more pressure on themselves to do well in raising their grandchildren while trying to adapt to the financial, physical, and mental transitions of growing old.

Several studies have noted, however, that although the additional stress burden associated with assuming caregiving responsibilities for grandchildren increases risk for psychological distress and depression in all groups, there are notable ethnic differences in the relative impact this new source of stress appears to have. In a recent report, Pruchno (1999) compared the experiences of 398 white and 319 African-American caretaking grandmothers and found that the latter reported less distress and less negative impact of their caretaking responsibilities on their mental health and social lives than the former. White grandmothers were more likely to feel trapped in their role; to feel tired, isolated, and alone; and to have less personal time and greater interference with their social lives, and more negative relationships with family members. These differences were evident even though the African-American grandmothers were more likely to be widowed or divorced and to have lower per capita incomes and more children in their households.

The lower impact of childcare burden on African-American grandmothers may be explained by the fact that they traditionally play key roles as support for African-American families during times of crisis. Many African-American grandmothers reported being embedded in large, supportive social networks (e.g., other parenting grandmothers and other sources of support) that provided emotional and other tangible assistance. The same was not true for white grandmothers.

Burnette (1999) reported similar results in her study of Hispanic grandparent caregivers. Using social role theory as a framework, Burnette investigated the effects of caretaking responsibilities on Latina grandmothers. She noted that Hispanic elders tend to have larger families, stronger family bonds, and more interactions with and support from adult children than either African-American or white elders, which may moderate risk for negative outcomes (Lubben and Becerra, 1987; Sabogal, Marin, and Otero-Sabogal, 1987). Older Latinas serve an important central role in kinkeeping, and may identify with this role more than women in other ethnic groups (Kornhaber, 1996; Padgett, 1998). However, while this family status affords them considerable prestige and domestic authority, differences in gender role status also disproportionately burden Latinas with caretaking responsibilities (Hurtado, 1995).

Results from the Burnette (1999) sample of Puerto Rican and Dominican women, most of whom were unmarried, undereducated, and low income, indicated that assuming the responsibility of primary caretaker for grandchildren had significant detrimental effects on their mental health and social lives, such as giving up their jobs, loss of autonomy, and loss of social ties.

In summary, although the evidence clearly indicates that a heavier burden of aging-related stresses is associated with enhanced risk for depression and related dysfunction in both younger and older adults (Bazargan and Hamm-Baugh, 1995; Holahan, Holahan, and Belk, 1984; Karel, 1997; Markides, 1986), stress-depression and well-being relationships are complex and moderated by social class, ethnicity, and a number of psychosocial factors, including social supports, coping, religiosity, and personality traits (Karel, 1997). Most of the available evidence appears to suggest that African-American grandparents who have caretaking responsibilities for their grandchildren may be less vulnerable to the depressogenic effects of this additional source of role strain. The effects for Latina grandmothers, however, appear to be less clear. In any event, simple generalizations to these ethnic groups would be premature. Additional research is still needed to determine to what extent aging-related stresses may contribute to ethnic differences in functional status and health outcomes and for which ethnic groups.

Unfortunately, relatively little research is available on these issues in Asian American or Native American elderly. Therefore, an important priority for future research is to investigate the contributions of chronic stress burden from multiple sources to the health trajectory and functional status of these understudied populations.

ALLOSTATIC LOAD AS A BIOBEHAVIORAL MEDIATOR OF RISK

Modern models of stress, disease, and functional status all acknowledge the importance of identifying the biological pathways through which the burden of life stresses contributes to differences in functional status and health outcomes. The work by McEwen (1998) on allostatic load and by Geronimus (1992) on the weathering hypothesis are especially useful in this regard. In addition, the work by Thayer on heart rate variability (see Chapter 15, this volume, for a review) is a promising alternative mediating mechanism that might be especially useful in future large-scale longitudinal studies.

McEwen and Stellar (1993) coined the term "allostasis" to refer to the normal fluctuations of the autonomic nervous system, the hypothalamic-pituitary-adrenal axis, and the metabolic, cardiovascular, and immune systems that maintain stability and protect the body by responding to stress. However, these normal allostatic responses can become dysregulated, which subsequently overtaxes the system and results in physiologic wear and tear, which they defined as "allostatic load." A good example of this model is essential hypertension, which is conceptualized as a disease that results from the dysregulation of blood pressure control mechanisms due to persistent and pathological autonomic hyperreactivity to stress (Myers, Anderson, and Strickland, 1996).

According to McEwen (1998), allostatic load increases under four conditions: (1) frequent stress exposure, with attendant frequent exposure to stress hormones; (2) exaggerated reactivity and/or inadequate habituation to stressful experiences, which also results in prolonged exposure to stress hormones; (3) inability to recover, where physiological arousal and reactivity continue even after the stressor has been removed or terminated; and (4) an inadequate response to stress because of system fatigue or dysfunction, which triggers pathological compensatory responses in other systems. Recent studies by McEwen and Seeman (1999) and Singer and Ryff (1999) provide compelling empirical support for this argument. In their review, McEwen and Seeman (1999) argue for a more comprehensive model of the effect of stress on disease that includes genetic load, life experiences, individual health habits, and physiological reactivity, all of which interact over time to produce gradients of risk for disease. Specific attention is given to increasing mortality and morbidity rates as one descends the socioeconomic gradient, which reflects the cumulative burden of coping with life demands with inadequate resources for coping. In the case of the elderly, this social class differential, and possible racial/ethnic differential as well, would be expected to be greater given the greater cumulative allostatic load attributable to lifetime accumulation of disadvantage.

Singer and Ryff (1999) tested this hypothesis using data from the predominantly white sample of adults in the Wisconsin Longitudinal Study. Using social relationships (i.e., parental bonding in childhood and relationship intimacy as adults) and household income in childhood and adulthood as their measures of adversity and advantage, and a rating system that characterized distinct life histories based on positive and negative ratings on these two dimensions, they demonstrated that there was a strong direct association between the extent of lifetime adversity relative to advantages in ordering life histories. Those with higher relative disadvantages (i.e., negative economic and social relationships, at each measurement point), especially those with persistent negative social relationships, evidenced higher allostatic loads (i.e., impaired immune function, elevated blood pressure, and later life illness and chronic disease propensity) compared to those with balanced (+, − or −, +) or more advantaged (+, +) histories. Their analyses also confirmed that downward social mobility was more adverse than upward mobility, which provides a more textured glimpse of the substantial variation in the SES-health relationship than is possible using the usual single point in time (i.e., current) measure of SES.

These findings complement the results of the studies by Elder and Crosnoe (2002), who used life-course development methods to track the developmental trajectories of men born in the early 1900s from childhood through later life. They were able to demonstrate that historical events and life transitions exert powerful effects of the life trajectory of these men.

In their more recent work, Elder and colleagues (Wickrama et al., 1999) also demonstrated that health-risk behaviors and health-risk lifestyles are transmitted intergenerationally between parents and teens. These parent health-risk effects were moderated by family social status and by family structure such that parental health-risk lifestyle affected their sons and mothers' health-risk lifestyle affected their daughters. This suggests possible gender-related modeling of health behaviors. Unfortunately, these studies did not specifically address any ethnic differences in these processes, but their findings are somewhat congruent with other studies that indicate a clustering of risk behaviors within minority families, and the role such clustering plays in accounting for the greater burden of illness and disability observed in many racial/ethnic populations (Harris et al., 1997; Moore and Chase-Landsdale, 2001; Myers and Taylor, 1998).

Singer and Ryff (1999) also identified a group of resilient elderly who evidenced lower allostatic loads despite relatively disadvantaged histories, which they attributed to the presence of compensatory social relationship histories. This is an understudied group, especially resilient minority elders, which could yield valuable information for programs designed to foster healthy aging and that might help to close the health disparities gap.

These intriguing ideas and methodologies have not yet been directly applied to investigating ethnic differences in health and well-being in adults and the elderly. However, Geronimus's (1992) "weathering hypothesis," which is hypothesized to account for some of the persistent African-American versus white differences in birth outcomes, demonstrates the utility of investigating health differentials at different developmental stages. Using national infant mortality data comparing African-American and white mothers by age cohorts, Geronimus found that these groups differed in patterns of neonatal mortality rates over the predominant age of having a first child. Her results indicated, as shown in Table 13-2, that compared to white infants, African-American infants of teen mothers experienced a survival advantage relative to infants whose mothers were older and in the prime childbearing years (i.e., 20s and 30s). A similar but weaker trend was also observed for Mexican and Puerto Rican women.

She argued that this evidence indicates that there may be population differences in prime childbearing years, and suggested that African-American (and perhaps also Puerto Rican) women appear to experience an earlier aging or "weathering process." She speculated that this difference was probably a consequence of prolonged, effortful coping with socioeconomic

TABLE 13-2 Neonatal Mortality Rates and Rate Ratios by Maternal Age and Ethnicity: First Births, United States, 1983

Age (years)	Neonatal Mortality Rates*				Rate Ratios		
	White	Black	Mexican	Puerto Rican	Black-white	Mexican-white	Puerto Rican-white
15-19	7.2	9.8	5.3	8.5	1.4	0.7	1.2
20-29	4.6	10.4	4.7	9.2	2.3	1.0	2.0
30-34	5.6	15.0	7.9	11.9	2.7	1.4	2.1
Total	5.4	10.6	5.2	9.0	1.9	0.9	1.7

*Deaths per 1,000 live births.
NOTE: Presented by Geronimus (1992, p. 209).
SOURCE: National Linked Birth/Death Files (1983).

inequality, racial discrimination, and greater risk of exposure to environmental hazards. This burden of risk is likely to be exacerbated as these women get older by the development and untreated progression of chronic illnesses (e.g., hypertension, diabetes), by the development of behavior patterns that are adversarial to health (e.g., obesity, alcohol and drug use), and by increasing stress burden.

It is also important to note that the African-American versus white differentials in adverse birth outcomes, especially low birthweight and infant mortality, are smaller among the less educated and larger among the most educated (Kleinman, Fingerhut, and Prager, 1991; Shiono et al., 1997). This suggests that African-American women may derive less reproductive benefit from upward mobility than white women. Additional research is needed to explore this hypothesis with the other ethnic groups and to determine whether women who experience adverse birth outcomes during their childbearing years evidence early aging in the form of more health difficulties and a heavier burden of medical morbidity in later years.

We believe our understanding of the health disparities would be greatly enhanced by lifespan developmental studies that apply the concepts and methodologies used to test the allostatic load and weathering hypotheses to investigate ethnic differences in health trajectories.

LIFETIME ADVANTAGES AS PSYCHOSOCIAL MODERATORS OF RISK

Substantial empirical evidence shows that a number of psychosocial factors—including psychological resilience, stress appraisal and coping style, the availability of social supports, and religiosity—serve to moderate the stress-health and functional status relationships in adults and the elderly.

Psychological Resilience

In her comprehensive review of depression and aging, Karel (1997) notes that adults appear to become less psychologically vulnerable to depression as they age. This may be because personality characteristics that enhance risk for depression, such as pessimism, self-criticism, interpersonal dependence, and preoccupation with failure (Akiskal, 1991) may be less common among the elderly, despite stereotypes to the contrary (Jones and Meredith, 1996). In fact, Jones and Meredith found patterns of longitudinal changes over 30 to 40 years that indicated stability of personality traits across ages, along with slight increases in self-confidence, extroversion, and dependability as people matured.

Another key moderator of risk for depression is sense of perceived control. Although aging exposes the elderly to more uncontrollable events (i.e., declining physical health and cognitive functioning), this does not appear to result in a decreased sense of overall control. Instead, factors such as an increasing ability to make psychological compensations and accommodations (e.g., adjusting one's goals, making more downward social comparisons to those less well off, seeking assistance from others, and using aids such as wheelchairs and hearing aids to compensate for functional limitations) contribute to protect the elderly from perceived loss of control and corresponding increase in risk for depression (Aldwin, 1992; Heckhausen and Schulz, 1993; Karel, 1997).

Unfortunately, there continues to be inadequate representation of minority elderly in studies investigating factors associated with psychological resilience, especially groups other than African Americans. Therefore, although there is little reason to expect that these factors are likely to operate differently in these populations, current evidence does not allow us to draw any firm conclusions about their effects across ethnic and social class groups.

Stress Appraisal

The impact of exposure to chronic stress on health is moderated by how one interprets or appraises and responds to the stressful experience (Lazarus and Folkman, 1984). Stress appraisal involves the weighing of one's resources against the demands of the stressor in order to determine how large a threat the stressor is to well-being. For ethnic minority elderly, stress appraisal is likely to involve not only the subjective examination of resources versus demands, but also the filtering of stressful experiences through one's unique cultural lens. For example, women of all ethnic groups typically serve as the traditional center of families, and are responsible for the emotional, physical, and spiritual well-being of family members, and in some cases, sharing or carrying the major responsibility for the economic viability of the family, coping with their own burden of life stresses, and moderating the impact stresses have on other family members (Burnette, 1999; Chisholm, 1996; Minkler and Roe, 1993; Reid and Bing, 2000). This is illustrated in the acceptance of the primary responsibility for the care of grandchildren in response to major family crises (Minkler et al., 1997). Accepting this "strong woman" image is an additional burden of stress, and cultural expectations that they should be able to handle life challenges may hinder some minority women (and men) from seeking help with problems from professionals and/or formal assistance programs. On the other hand, fulfilling strong traditional roles may contribute to their resilience, resourcefulness, and flexibility in dealing with stressful situations (Reid and Bing, 2000).

However, and contrary to popular belief, evidence regarding ethnic differences in seeking help is somewhat mixed. Some studies suggest that minorities evidence greater reliance on informal sources of help than whites (Harden, Clark, and Maguire, 1997; Zhang, Snowden, and Sue, 1998), while others indicate that some groups, especially African Americans, tend to rely more on both formal and informal sources of support for mental health needs than whites (Snowden, 1998). More well-designed studies with diverse populations are clearly needed to clarify these apparently contradictory findings, and to identify which factors in which ethnic groups are associated with timely health care seeking versus delayed care seeking.

Coping

As a byproduct of experience and maturity, older adults have been found to use more adaptive coping strategies, including anticipation, sublimation, humor, altruism, and spirituality in coping with life changes (Diehl, Coyle, and Labouvie-Vief, 1996; McCrae, 1982). They may also have a greater ability to accept and reinterpret adverse situations in more positive ways (Diehl et al., 1996), have greater emotional stability and less emotional reactivity (Lawton, Kleban, Rajagopal, and Dean, 1992), and to be more thoughtful and flexible in their response to stress (Diehl et al., 1996).

Again, our ability to investigate the role of coping and psychological distress in minority elderly is severely limited by the dearth of studies that specifically address this issue (Markides, 1986). Nevertheless, useful inferences can be drawn from studies on other populations. For example, in a theoretical discussion of issues surrounding coping in women, Banyard and Graham-Bermann (1993) argued that coping as it is traditionally measured is largely influenced by education and income, such that those with more resources typically cope "better." In this respect, an individual's social position and environment can either constrain or enhance his or her resources and choice of coping strategies (Taylor, Repetti, and Seeman, 1997).

Members of marginalized groups, because of ethnicity, social class, gender, and/or age, may face special challenges to active coping. Limitations in finances, knowledge, access to requisite technical expertise, or other resources and cultural, social, or psychological barriers may discourage active coping. In the case of minority adult men and women, assertiveness is often misperceived as aggressiveness or arrogance, and responded to with fear or punitive action. In the case of the elderly, however, active, assertive coping may not pose the same threat and may not trigger the same adverse outcome. Instead, they may derive greater benefits by being more assertive (e.g., gaining access to needed services). Additional research is needed to investigate this hypothesis and to determine under what conditions and for which ethnic, gender, and age groups does assertive versus emotion-focused coping yield more positive health outcomes.

Ethnic minority status can also influence the efficacy of certain coping strategies, especially when SES is considered. For example, the work by James (1994) on John Henryism illustrates this relationship. John Henryism is defined as active, effortful coping with adversity marked by attitudes that reflect (1) efficacious mental and physical vigor, (2) a strong commitment to hard work, and (3) a single-minded determination to succeed. When compared to higher SES African Americans and whites from all SES groups, John Henryism has been shown to predict higher blood pressure and greater risk for hypertension only in young African-American men with low socioeconomic resources (Dressler, Bindon, and Neggers, 1998; James, 1994). Thus, John Henryism appears to be relatively benign for higher SES African Americans and whites. However, for African-American men with limited resources, the benefits of effortful coping (i.e., economic survival) appear to be tempered by increased health risks.

Given that ethnic minorities are often confronted with chronic stressors that are not easily ameliorated, it is not surprising that effortful, active coping strategies such as John Henryism are likely to yield mixed results. Such coping strategies may not produce the desired changes in status and opportunity and may in fact produce high levels of anger and frustration, which might account for the higher levels of blood pressure seen in these individuals. Unfortunately, we do not know how prevalent this coping strategy is among African-American elderly or what effect long-term use has on their health and well-being. We also do not know whether members of other racial/ethnic minorities use this coping strategy, and whether the effects obtained with low-SES, younger African-American adults will be observed in older and higher SES adults in the other ethnic groups.

Limited attention has been given to identifying coping strategies that are most adaptive for ethnic minority adults and the elderly, especially those with limited resources. It is very likely that healthy functioning in the face of chronic stress exposure from low SES and/or older age requires the development of a different array of active and passive coping strategies than is the case for those who are younger and/or who have more resources.

Religiosity

A substantial literature indicates the salience of religion and religious participation in the lives of the elderly, especially for African Americans, Hispanics, Native Americans, and Asian Americans (Mattis, 1997; McAuley, Pecchioni, and Grant, 2000; Nelson, 1989; Taylor, 1993; Villarosa, 1994; Wade-Gayles, 1995). In addition, both cross-sectional and longitudinal studies indicate that there are aging-related changes in the pattern of predominant religious behaviors, with participation in organized religious activities remaining high until late old age, then dropping off due to increased physical disability. However, religious attitudes and private religious behaviors (i.e., prayer, reading religious materials, watching or listening to religious programs) actually increase with age (Koenig, Smiley, and Gonzalez, 1988).

There is also growing evidence of a positive relationship between religious practices, spirituality, and health. In their recent review of the evidence of the role of spirituality, health, and aging, Musick, Traphagan, Koenig, and Larson (2000) generally conclude that greater religious participation and higher self-rated spirituality have been associated with lower mortality rates (Helm, Hays, Flint, Koenig, and Blazer, 2000; McCullough, Hoyt, Larson, Koenig, and Thoresen, 2000); better self-rated health, both cross-sectionally and over time; and lower risk for hypertension and lower cancer rates, especially in those religions that have strong dietary and other lifestyle restrictions. The evidence for participation and functional status are less clear because of possible reverse causation, but longitudinal studies do suggest that service attendance does influence functional health.

The beneficial effects of religion on health are believed to occur through several mechanisms, including supporting a healthier lifestyle (i.e., proscriptions against smoking, drinking, illicit drug use, more physical activity, and diet) (Idler and Kasl, 1997; Strawbridge et al., 1997), by fostering greater social integration, more social contacts, and the provision of more instrumental and emotional support (Ellison, 1995), greater marital satisfaction and stability, and greater comfort, meaning, and effective coping with major life challenges and transitions (George, Larson, Koenig, and McCullough, 2000; Harrison, Koenig, Hays, Eme-Akwari, and Pargament, 2001; Pargament, Smith, Koenig, and Perez, 1998). (See Musick et al., 2000, for a detailed discussion of this evidence.)

Several authors also note, however, that greater religiosity and religious coping can also have negative health and mental health effects, especially because of ideological rigidity, spiritual discontent, demonic reappraisal, and negative reappraisal of God and his powers (Pargament et al., 1998).

This literature also suggests that there are important ethnic differences in religiosity between ethnic minority versus white elderly. Historically, African Americans and Hispanics have relied on religion and on the church as important sources of spiritual, emotional, and material support in coping with life stresses. In the case of African Americans, the church has also served as a powerful political force for social change and an opportunity for social status (Ellison, 1995). Thus, the prevailing view is that religion is a powerful resource for coping for all groups (George et al., 2000), especially for marginalized minority groups; that ethnic groups may engage in more religious coping with adversity than whites, and that African Americans have a more personal relationship with God (McAuley et al., 2000) and report greater satisfaction with the results of their religious coping efforts (Neighbors, Jackson, Bowman, and Gurin, 1983). For example, in a study of African-American and white elderly women with medical problems, Conway (1985) found that the majority (64 percent) of African-American women employed prayer as a coping strategy, compared to only a third of their white counterparts. Similarly, in a comparative analysis of intrinsic versus extrinsic religious orientation in African-American and white seniors, Nelson (1989) found that although religion was important for both groups, the groups differed in their religious orientation and behaviors. Compared to whites, African-American elders were more intrinsically oriented to religion (i.e., stronger spiritual beliefs and faith and more emphasis on prayer), but there were no differences in extrinsic orientation (i.e., active religious participation). These findings were also confirmed by Ellison (1995) using data from the ECA sample in the southeastern United States, which showed significantly higher rates of church attendance and religious devotion among African Americans compared to their white counterparts.

However, the evidence on the effect of religiosity on well-being, both overall and as a function of ethnicity, is mixed, suggesting the need for better designed studies and more critical analysis (Ellison, 1995; Mickley, Carson, and Soeken, 1995). Many studies suggest that religious beliefs and practices are associated with enhanced health and life satisfaction (Koenig, Siegler, and George, 1989; Levin, Chatters, and Taylor, 1995), greater perceived control (Koenig, Smiley, and Gonzalez, 1989), and greater mobility, less depression, and greater social integration in the elderly (Idler, 1987; Miller, 1998). A number of other studies have suggested, however, that the relationship among religiosity, depression, and well-being is more complex than is generally believed. For example, Nelson (1989) found that African-American elderly who were more active in church attendance and engaged in more private religious practices were more depressed than white elderly. On the other hand, in his sample of adult and elderly southerners, Ellison

(1995) found that religious coping was associated with lower depression in white respondents, but was unrelated to depression in African Americans. He argued that this unexpected finding suggests that other factors might temper the effectiveness of religious experiences and practices in moderating risk for depression in this sample of elderly southern African Americans. Unfortunately, we cannot determine from the data in either the Nelson or Ellison studies whether religious coping was ineffective in preventing depression or whether those who were depressed were simply more likely to engage in more religious coping in an effort to deal with their distress.

Additional evidence in support of the complex relationships between religiosity and health is provided by Strawbridge, Shema, Cohen, Roberts, and Kaplan (1998). They contrasted nonorganizational religiosity (i.e., prayer, importance of religious and spiritual beliefs) versus organizational religiosity (i.e., attendance at services and other religious activities) as moderators on stress and depression in the Alameda County, California Health Survey of adults ages 50 to 102. Their results indicated that although religiosity is protective for mortality and morbidity, it buffers some stressors but appears to exacerbate others. They found that nonorganizational religiosity was unrelated to depression, while organizational religiosity had a weak negative association with depression. However, while both forms of religiosity buffered the effect of nonfamily stressors (i.e., financial, health), nonorganizational religiosity exacerbated the effects of child problems, and organizational religiosity exacerbated the effects of marital problems, child and/or spousal abuse, and caregiving. Thus, religiosity may benefit those facing nonfamilial stressors, but may make coping with family crises worse.

Recent studies of African-American and Hispanic women suffering from chronic illness also found that religious coping was associated with less depression and anxiety, but did not find a similar association with physical health outcomes (Alferi, Culver, Carver, Arena, and Antoni, 1999; Woods, Antoni, Ironson, and Kling, 1999). In this respect, religious coping may be effective in reducing the psychological distress associated with chronic stressors, but may not be effective in ameliorating the negative effects of chronic stressors on health outcomes.

Taken as a whole, the evidence suggests that religion is an important spiritual and social resource for the elderly of all ethnic groups, and that African Americans and other minority elderly evidence greater religious involvement and use of religious coping than white elderly. However, the evidence also indicates that religion does not yield uniformly positive effects, especially as a buffer for depression and feelings of well-being. In fact, several studies indicate higher rates of depression and psychological distress in persons who report high religious participation. It is unclear, however, whether this reflects the ineffectiveness of religious coping or the fact that depressed individuals are more likely to seek more spiritual and social support. Additionally, most of the comparison studies of religiosity and health have been conducted on African Americans and whites, and there are comparatively fewer empirical studies that examined the effects of religiosity on mental health in Native Americans and Asian Americans, which should be an important priority for future research.

Social Support Resources

There is a substantial body of evidence examining the importance of social relationships and availability of adequate instrumental and emotional support on health. The evidence indicates that social supports can serve as both a protector against adverse health outcomes as well as a moderator of stress in reducing its impact on health (Cohen, Underwood, and Gottlieb, 2000; Leppin and Schwarzer, 1990), including improved functional status and quality of life (Seeman, Bruce, and McAvay, 1996; Unger, McAvay, Bruce, Berkman, and Seeman, 1999) and slower cognitive aging in the elderly (Seeman et al., 2001). In addition, social support can also serve as a mediator for depression in the elderly, with lower social support leading to both decreased life satisfaction and increased depressive symptoms (Newsom and Schulz, 1996). Similarly, social isolation, inadequate social support, and problematic interpersonal relationships can have adverse effects on health and well-being, especially for women (Bazargan and Hamm-Baugh, 1995; Burg and Seeman, 1994; Newsom and Schulz, 1996), as well as for those with debilitating physical illnesses, depression, or cognitive decline (Karel, 1997; Musick, Koenig, Hays, and Cohen, 1998; Unger et al., 1999). In fact, there appears to be a reciprocal relationship between physical impairment and social support, such that the availability of social support reduces functional impairment in those with significant chronic illnesses, and in turn, functional impairment is associated with an attenuation of support or reduction in access to supports (e.g., fewer friendship contacts, inability to attend religious services or other social functions, and reduction in perceived self-efficacy) (Holahan and Holahan, 1987; Newsom and Schulz, 1996).

Evidence of the positive effects of social support have been obtained with white and ethnic minority elderly populations, and many studies have reported that ethnic minority adults and elderly tend to rely more on larger family and other informal social networks for support than whites (Antonucci and Jackson, 1987; Delgado and Humm-Delgado, 1982; Lubben and Becerra, 1987; Neighbors et al., 1983; Pruchno, 1999). However, it is unclear whether, after controlling for social class, ethnic differences continue in the number, type, quality, and efficacy of available supports. It is also unclear whether different types of social support and how this variable is conceptualized and measured (e.g., size, type of support received, satisfaction with support received, social network composition, frequency of social contacts) have the same impact on the well-being of elders from diverse ethnic and sociocultural backgrounds. It is also important to note that reliance on informal social networks may exacerbate the stress burden of the elderly by adding to their role demands, by interfering with their autonomy and self-sufficiency, and/or by encouraging greater dependency (Coyne, Wortman, and Lehman, 1988).

Ideally, however, social support serves a positive function across the lifespan and helps maintain an individual's sense of well-being, self-efficacy, and control (Antonucci and Jackson, 1987). In a prospective cohort study of the elderly, instrumental and subjective social support were predictors of longer time to depression remission (Bosworth, McQuoid, George, and Steffens, 2002). Absence of support from a relative or friend also has been found to predict late-life suicide among the elderly (Turvey et al., 2002). Furthermore, being married or unmarried with social support has been found to significantly reduce the impact of functional disabilities on the incidence of depression in the elderly (Schoevers et al., 2000). The role of social support, health, and well-being is addressed in greater detail in Chapter 10.

SUMMARY AND RECOMMENDATIONS FOR FUTURE RESEARCH

In summary, our goal was to offer a multidimensional biopsychosocial framework for understanding the complex relationships among psychosocial, biological, and behavioral adversities and advantages that operate over the lifespan to impact the health and well-being of the elderly. Special attention was paid to identifying some of the primary risks and resources that are likely to be implicated in racial/ethnic differences in health and well-being in late life. The available evidence suggests that adults of color, especially the elderly, carry a disproportionate burden of chronic and life-change stresses compared to white elders, and that lifetime exposure to racism and discrimination (Williams, 1999; Clark et al., 1999), stresses from acculturation (Bastida and Gonzalez, 1995; Contrada et al., 2000; Vega et al., 1998), and the greater likelihood that they will assume caretaking responsibilities for grandchildren and other relatives, should be included in assessments of their stress burdens (Burnette, 1999; Minkler et al., 1997). However, additional caregiving responsibilities do not appear to cause as much distress to minority elders compared to whites, perhaps because of greater cultural congruence of the role, greater access to larger support networks, and exposure to other seniors in their peer group who are also caring for their grandchildren (Pruchno, 1999).

The evidence also suggests that despite overall greater socioeconomic deprivation and stress in this population, there are important differences among ethnic groups in vulnerability to distress and depression, with higher overall rates in whites and Hispanics and lower overall rates in African Americans and Asian Americans (Somervell et al., 1989; Zhang and Snowden, 1999). These ethnic group differences vary by gender, social class, geography, and age of immigration, and there is some evidence that those who immigrate during old age may be at enhanced risk relative to those who immigrated at younger ages. Regardless of ethnicity, greater psychological distress and depression are found in elderly who are older, carrying a heavier burden of medical morbidity and functional impairment, more socially isolated, and who have few family and friend social supports. Higher rates are also found in those who have little perceived control over their circumstances, who fail to use more adaptive and flexible coping strategies, whose autonomy is constrained by their circumstances, who cope with frequent interpersonal conflicts, and who rely heavily on religious coping or have little or no religious or spiritual connections (Diehl et al., 1996; Karel, 1997; Musick et al., 2000; Nelson, 1989).

In addition, the common assumptions that social supports and religiosity have uniformly positive effects for the elderly are not justified. Several studies indicate that although religiosity is protective of mortality and morbidity and appears to buffer nonfamilial stresses, it may exacerbate family conflict stresses (Pargament et al., 1998; Strawbridge et al., 1998), and may yield different results for different ethnic groups depending on what measures of religiosity are used (Ellison, 1995; Nelson, 1989).

Unfortunately, and as in other areas, there is a dearth of information on psychosocial and behavioral issues on racial/ethnic elderly, especially for Native Americans and subgroups of Hispanics and Asian Americans (Markides, 1986). Thus, a major need in the field is for more studies that focus specifically on the psychosocial and behavioral predictors of health and well-being in elderly from these understudied groups. Also, while ethnic comparison studies that investigate group differences in these factors continue to be needed, there is also a substantial need for ethnic-specific studies that can clarify which psychosocial and behavioral factors are most important in increasing and reducing risk for health outcomes in each racial/ethnic group. The latter approach will encourage more focused attention on developing and testing methodologies and measures that are most appropriate for the different ethnic groups.

In this chapter, we also argue for the need for studies that take a lifetime perspective in investigating ethnic disparities in psychological well-being and functioning. To date, most studies are cross-sectional and focus on differences in current or proximal risks and resources in accounting for differences in health and well-being. However, as argued by Geronimus (1992), Elder and Crosnoe (2002), and Singer and Ryff (1999), studies testing such concurrent effects hypotheses are necessarily limited, and substantial additional information can be obtained by investigating the cumulative effects of lifetime advantages and adversities in predicting individual and group differences in health trajectories.

We offer one cumulative advantages and vulnerabilities model as a conceptual tool to guide future studies. This model builds on and expands on the life history approach by Singer and Ryff (1999) and the developmental perspective of Elder and Crosnoe (2002) and Geronimus (1992) by including consideration of lifetime exposure to additional sociostructural and psychosocial adversities and advantages that have specific relevance to ethnic minority elderly. In addition, the model recognizes that these risk and protective factors exert their effects through biological pathways, including genetic predispositions, allostatic load, medical burden, and psychiatric history. Finally, consistent with Singer and Ryff (1999), the model argues that it is the balance between lifetime advantages and adversities that is likely to predict psychological health and well-being over time, with a greater burden of lifetime adversities resulting in greater psychological distress and dysfunction, and an imbalance in favor of assets and advantages resulting in better overall psychological functioning. This approach also should allow for better identification of minority elders who are psychologically resilient despite high lifetime burdens of adversity.

As noted previously, although our review focused specifically on the role these hypothesized risk and protective factors play in accounting for individual and group differences in psychological distress, depression, and well-being, the proposed conceptual perspective should also be useful in investigating health disparities for a variety of other chronic diseases, including but not limited to essential hypertension and other cardiovascular diseases, chronic pain, cognitive decline and dementia, and functional impairment. Future research should consider the following priority issues:

• Ethnic-specific studies are needed that investigate which psychosocial risk and protective factors are the most important contributors to psychological well-being and resilience in each racial/ethnic group. Specific attention is needed to estimate the relative contribution of each risk factor, to include culture-specific variables, and to determine whether there are within-group differences in the relative importance of risk and protective factors. In addition, special focus should be given to problems of particular importance to specific communities (e.g., prevention and intervention research for alcohol and drug abuse, crime and violence, and HIV/AIDS are important for low-SES communities).

• Cross-cultural studies are needed to help us understand the differential roles each risk and protective factor might play in health outcomes for different ethnic groups. Such comparison studies should include representation from as many of the major ethnic groups in the United States as reasonable. Understanding etiological processes across ethnicities may provide additional information and understanding of how early risk exposure predicts differences in health trajectories and what resources are needed to increase resilience in these groups.

• In conducting ethnic-specific and cross-cultural research, measurement issues need to be considered. Basic questions about the validity and generalizability of assessment instruments have yet to be resolved. For example, ethnic differences in the way social support and other coping resources are perceived and utilized have yet to be explicated. Debate also continues regarding differences in the experience, expression, and construct of mental illness, and how such illness should be treated in different ethnic groups. Our ability to understand and treat mental illness will be challenged by our ability to create new assessment measures, verify the reliability and generalizability of existing instruments, and adequately capture the differences and similarities of such constructs.

• Longitudinal studies are also needed that test the hypothesized cumulative effects of lifetime adversities and advantages in predicting functional status in minority elderly. Particular attention should be given to the relationships among lifetime exposure to chronic life stresses, personality dispositions, coping styles, access to and utilization of social supports and formal services, and spirituality and religious participation.

• Additionally, the investigation of ethnic disparities in health also raises a number of important statistical issues. Testing comprehensive, longitudinal models such as the one proposed will require more advanced statistical techniques. One approach that lends itself to this task is multivariate causal modeling that allows the testing of the full model as well as the separate hypothesized pathways within the model. In addition, separate models can be developed and tested for each ethnic group, thus allowing for the possibility that there are ethnic differences in the relative contributions these variables make in predicting health outcomes. For example, exposure to racism and discrimination may have different effects on health in different ethnic groups, perhaps because of differences in appraisal and coping strategies used in coping with this source of stress. This approach also allows other alternative relationships among the variables to be considered. For example, models could test whether race/ethnicity affects SES, and both SES and race/ethnicity in turn affect health.

• Although the evidence is clear that ethnic health disparities are evident at each step in the SES gradient (Williams, 1999), debate continues about what is the best analytic approach to test the interfaces among SES, ethnicity, and health. For example, while conventional practice is to statistically control for SES before testing for ethnic differences on outcomes of interest, many have argued that this may be inappropriate because it assumes that the relationship between SES and health is the same regardless of ethnicity. However, there is ample evidence that race/ethnicity conditions SES such that low SES is associated with greater functional disability and distress in populations of color compared to whites (Kessler and Neighbors, 1986), and persons of color may derive comparatively less health benefit from higher socioeconomic status than whites (Geronimus, 1992). Thus, as suggested by Kessler and Neighbors (1986), it is advisable to test for an SES X ethnicity interaction in order to determine whether the joint effect of SES and ethnicity is most adverse to health.

• Little will be accomplished if most of our attention is focused on studies of group differences that do not inform interventions. A need continues for studies that develop and test interventions that enhance resilience by improving coping, and fostering the development of more effective social support resources, especially among the poorest minority elderly and those who immigrated at older ages. Minority groups who evidence the most difficulty are often underrepresented in research, and their needs are inadequately addressed because interventions used are not specifically tailored to their needs. More studies are needed that investigate psychosocial predictors of risk and resilience in Native American, Asian American, and Hispanic American elderly. Such research needs to recognize the heterogeneity within these larger panethnic or pancultural groups, and test for both within- and between-group differences.

• Finally, studies are also needed to identify factors that predict successful aging and healthy functional status in populations of color. This is perhaps the most understudied issue in the field.

ACKNOWLEDGMENTS

The authors express their appreciation to Carolyn Melton, MSW, for her assistance with the review of the literature on grandparenting stresses, and to the National Research Council Panel on Race, Ethnicity and Health in Later Life and external reviewers for their feedback and recommendations on previous drafts of this manuscript.

REFERENCES

Akiskal, H.S. (1991). An integrative perspective on recurrent mood disorders: The mediating role of personality. In J. Becker and A. Kleinman (Eds.), *Psychosocial aspects of depression* (pp. 215-235). Hillsdale, NJ: Lawrence Erlbaum Associates.

Aldwin, C.M. (1992). Aging, coping, and efficacy: Theoretical framework for examining coping in life-span developmental context. In M.L. Wykle, E. Kahana, and J. Kowal (Eds.), *Stress and health among the elderly* (pp. 96-113). New York: Springer.

Alferi, S.M., Culver, J.L., Carver, C.S., Arena, P.L., and Antoni, M.H. (1999). Religiosity, religious coping, and distress: A prospective study of Catholic and Evangelical Hispanic women in treatment for early-stage breast cancer. *Journal of Health Psychology, 4*(3), 343-356.

Altschuler, L.L., Wang, X.D., Qi, H.Q., Wang, W.Q., and Xia, M.L. (1988). Who seeks mental health care in China? Diagnoses of Chinese outpatients according to DSM-III criteria and the Chinese classification system. *American Journal of Psychiatry, 145*, 872-875.

Anderson, N.B., McNeilly, M., and Myers, H.F. (1992). Autonomic reactivity and hypertension in blacks: Toward a contextual model. In E.H. Johnson, W.D. Johnson, and S. Julius (Eds.), *Personality, elevated blood pressure and essential hypertension* (pp. 197-216). New York: Hemisphere.

Anderson, N.B., McNeilly, M., and Myers, H.F. (1993). A biopsychosocial model of race differences in vascular reactivity. In J.J. Blascovich and E.S. Katkin (Eds.), *Cardiovascular reactivity to psychological stress and disease* (pp. 83-108). Washington, DC: American Psychological Association.

Antonucci, T.C., and Jackson, J.S. (1987). Social support, interpersonal efficacy, and health: A life course perspective. In L.L. Carstensen, B.A. Edelstein, and L. Dornbrand (Eds.), *Handbook of clinical gerontology* (pp. 21-31). New York: Pergamon Press.

Balcazar, H., Peterson, G.W., and Krull, J.L. (1997). Acculturation and family cohesiveness in Mexican American pregnant women: Social and health implications. *Family and Community Health, 20*, 16-31.

Ballenger, J.C., Davidson, J.R., Lecrubier, Y., Nutt, D.J., Kirmayer, L.J., Lepine, J.P., Lin, K.M., Tajima, O., and Ono, Y. (2001). Consensus statement on transcultural issues in depression and anxiety from the International Consensus Group on Depression and Anxiety. *Journal of Clinical Psychiatry, 62*(Suppl. 13), 47-55.

Banyard, V.L., and Graham-Bermann, S.A. (1993). Can women cope? A gender analysis of theories of coping with stress. *Psychology of Women Quarterly, 17*, 303-318.

Bastida, E., and Gonzalez, G. (1995). Mental health status and needs of black and white elderly: Differences in depression. In D.K. Padgett (Ed.), *Handbook on ethnicity, aging, and mental health* (pp. 99-112). Westport, CT: Greenwood Press.

Bazargan, N., and Hamm-Baugh, V.P. (1995). The relationship between chronic illness and depression in a community of urban black elderly persons. *Journals of Gerontology, Series B: Psychological Sciences and Social Sciences, 50*(2), S119-S127.

Beals, J., Manson, S., Shore, J.H., Friedman, M., Ashcraft, M., Fairbanks, J.A., and Schlenger, W.E. (2002). The prevalence of posttraumatic stress disorder among American Indian Vietnam veterans: Disparities and context. *Journal of Traumatic Stress, 15*(2), 89-97.

Berry, J.W. (1998). Acculturation and health: Theory and research. In S. Kazarian and D. Evans (Eds.), *Cultural clinical psychology: Theory, research, and practice* (pp. 39-57). New York: Oxford University Press.

Blanchard, M. (1996). Old age depression—a biological inevitability? *International Review of Psychiatry, 8*(4), 379-385.

Blazer, D., Burchett, B., Service, C., and George, L.K. (1991). The association of age and depression among the elderly: An epidemiologic exploration. *Journal of Gerontology, 46*, 210-215.

Blazer, D.G., Kessler, R.C., McGonagle, K.A., and Swartz, M.S. (1994). The prevalence and distribution of major depression in a national community sample: The National Comorbidity Survey. *American Journal of Psychiatry, 151*, 979-986.

Bosworth, H.B., McQuoid, D.R., George, L.K., and Steffens, D.C. (2002). Time-to-remission from geriatric depression: Psychosocial and clinical factors. *American Journal of Geriatric Psychiatry, 10*(5), 551-559.

Brodaty, H., Luscombe, G., Parker, G., Wilhelm, K., Hickie, I., Austin, M., and Mitchell, P. (2001). Early and late onset depression in old age: Different aetiologies, same phenomenology. *Journal of Affective Disorders, 66,* 225-236.

Brown, D.R., Ahmed, F., Gary, L.E., and Milburn, N.G. (1995). Major depression in a community sample of African Americans. *American Journal of Psychiatry, 152*(3), 373-378.

Burg, M.M., and Seeman, T.E. (1994). Families and health: The negative side of social ties. *The Society of Behavioral Medicine, 16*(2), 109-115.

Burnam, M.A. Hough, R.L., Karno, M., Escobar, J.I., and Telles, C. (1987). Acculturation and lifetime prevalence of psychiatric disorders among Mexican Americans in Los Angeles. *Journal of Health and Social Behavior, 28,* 89-102.

Burnette, D. (1997). Grandparents raising grandchildren in the inner-city. *Families in Society, 78,* 489-499.

Burnette, D. (1999). Social relationships of Hispanic grandparent caregivers: A role theory perspective. *The Gerontologist, 39*(1), 49-58.

Canino, G.J., Bird, H.R., Shrout, P.E., Rubio-Stipec, M., Bravo, M., Martinez, R., Sesman, M., and Guevara, L.M. (1987). The prevalence of specific psychiatric disorders in Puerto Rico. *Archives of General Psychiatry, 44,* 727-735.

Casper, L.M., and Bryson, K.R. (1998). *Coresident grandparents and their grandchildren: Grandparent-maintained families.* Population Division Working Paper No. 26. Washington, DC: U.S. Bureau of the Census.

Centers for Disease Control and Prevention. (2001). *Health, United States: 2001 with urban and rural health chartbook.* Hyattsville, MD: National Center for Health Statistics.

Chen, C.N., Wong, J., Lee, N., Chan-Ho, M.W., Lau, J.T., and Fung, M. (1993). The Shatin community mental health survey in Hong Kong II: Major findings. *Archives of General Psychiatry, 50,* 125-133.

Chisholm, J.F. (1996). Mental health issues in African-American women. *Annals of the New York Academy of Sciences, 789,* 161-179.

Chou, K., and Chi, I. (2000). Stressful events and depressive symptoms among old women and men: A longitudinal study. *International Journal of Aging and Human Development, 51*(4), 275-293.

Chun, K.M., Organista, P.M., and Marin, G. (2002). *Acculturation: Advances in theory, measurement, and applied research.* Washington, DC: American Psychological Association.

Clark, R., Anderson, N.B., Clark, V.R., and Williams, D.R. (1999). Racism as a stressor for African Americans: A biopsychosocial model. *American Psychologist, 54*(10), 805-816.

Cohen, S., Kessler, R.C, and Gordon, L.U. (1995). Strategies for measuring stress in studies of psychiatric and physical disorders. In S. Cohen, R.C. Kessler, and L.U. Gordon (Eds.), *Measuring stress: A guide for health and social scientists* (pp. 3-26). New York: Oxford University Press.

Cohen, S., Underwood, L.G., and Gottlieb, B.H. (2000). *Social support measurement and intervention: A guide for health and social scientists.* New York: Oxford University Press.

Contrada, R.J., Ashmore, R.D., Gary, M.L., Coups, E., Egeth, J.D., Sewell, A., Ewell, K., Goyal, T.M., and Chasse, V. (2000). Ethnicity-related sources of stress and their effects on well-being. *Current Directions in Psychological Science, 9*(4), 136-139.

Conway, K. (1985). Coping with the stress of medical problems among black and white elderly. *International Journal of Aging and Human Development, 21,* 39-48.

Cook, J.M., Pearson, J.L., Thompson, R., Black, B.S., and Rabins, P.V. (2002). Suicidality in older African Americans: Findings from the EPOCH study. *American Journal of Geriatric Psychiatry, 10*(4), 437-446.

Cooper, J.E., and Sartorius, N. (1996). *Mental disorders in China: Results of the national epidemiological survey in 12 areas.* London: Gaskell.

Cortes, D.E., Rogler, L.H., and Malgady, R.G. (1994). Biculturality among Puerto Rican adults in the United States. *American Journal of Community Psychology, 22,* 707-721.

Coyne, J.C., Wortman, C.B., and Lehman, D.R. (1988). The other side of support: Emotional overinvolvement and miscarried helping. In B.H. Gottlieb (Ed.), *Marshalling social support: Format, process, and effects* (pp. 305-330). Thousand Oaks, CA: Sage.

Cross-National Collaborative Group. (1992). The changing rate of major depression: Cross-national comparisons. *Journal of the American Medical Association, 268,* 3098-3105.

Curyto, K.J., Chapleski, E.E., Lichtenberg, P.A., Hodges, E., Kaczynski, R., and Sobeck, J. (1998). Prevalence and prediction of depression in American Indian elderly. *Clinical Gerontologist, 18,* 19-37.

Curyto, K.J., Chapleski, E.E., and Lichtenberg, P.A. (1999). Prediction of the presence and stability of depression in the Great Lakes Native American elderly. *Journal of Mental Health and Aging, 5,* 323-340.

Delgado, M., and Humm-Delgado, D. (1982). Natural support systems: Source of strength in Hispanic communities. *Social Work, 27,* 83-89.

Diehl, M., Coyle, N., and Labouvie-Vief, G. (1996). Age and sex differences in strategies of coping and defense across the life span. *Psychology and Aging, 11,* 127-139.

Dohrenwend, B.P., Levav, I., Shrout, P.E., Schwartz, S., Naveh, G., Link, B.G., Skodol, A.E, and Stueve, A. (1992). Socioeconomic status and psychiatric disorders: The causation-selection issue. *Science, 255*(5047), 946-952.

Dressler, W.W., and Badger, L.W. (1985). Epidemiology of depressive symptoms in black communities: A comparative analysis. *Journal of Nervous and Mental Disorders, 173,* 212-220.

Dressler, W.W., Bindon, J.R., and Neggers, Y.H. (1998). John Henryism, gender, and arterial blood pressure in an African American community. *Psychosomatic Medicine, 60,* 620-624.

Eizenman, D.R., Nesselroade, J.R., Featherman, D.L., and Rowe, J.W. (1997). Intraindividual variability in perceived control in an older sample: The MacArthur successful aging studies. *Psychology and Aging, 12*(3), 489-502.

Elder, G.H. Jr. (1998). The life course as developmental theory. *Child Development, 69*(1), 1-12.

Elder, G.H., Jr., and Crosnoe, R. (2002). The influence of early behavior patterns on later life. In L. Pulkkinen and A. Caspi (Eds.), *Paths to successful development: Personality in the life course* (pp. 157-176). New York: Cambridge University Press.

Ellison, C.G. (1995). Race, religious involvement and depressive symptomatology in a southeastern U.S. community. *Social Science and Medicine, 40*(11), 1561-1572.

Escobar, J.E., Karno, M., Burnam, A., Hough, R.L., and Golding, J. (1988). Distribution of major mental disorders in a U.S. metropolis. *Acta Psychiatrica Scandinavica* (Suppl. 344), 45-53.

Escobar, J.I. (1998). Immigration and mental health: Why are immigrants better off? *Archives of General Psychiatry, 55,* 781-782.

Fabrega, H., Mezzich, J., and Ulrich, R.F. (1988). African American-white differences in psychopathology in an urban psychiatric population. *Comprehensive Psychiatry, 29,* 285-297.

Fang, C.Y., and Myers, H.F. (2001). The effects of racial stressors and hostility on cardiovascular reactivity in African American and white men. *Health Psychology, 20*(1), 64-70.

Flaskerud, J.H., and Hu, L.T. (1994). Participation in and outcome of treatment for major depression among low income Asian Americans. *Psychiatry Research, 53,* 289-300.

George, L.K., Blazer, D., Winfield-Laird, I., Leaf, P.J., and Fischbach, R.I. (1988). Psychiatric disorders and mental health service use in later life: Evidence from the Epidemiologic Catchment Area program. In J. Brody and G. Maddox (Eds.), *Epidemiology and aging* (pp. 189-219). New York: Springer.

George, L.K., Larson, D.B., Koenig, H.G., and McCullough, M.E. (2000). Spirituality and health: What we know, what we need to know. *Journal of Social and Clinical Psychology, 19*(1), 102-116.

Geronimus, A.T. (1992). The weathering hypothesis and the health of African-American women and infants: Evidence and speculations. *Ethnicity and Disease, 2,* 207-221.

Gibson, R.C. (1993). The Black American retirement experience. In J.S. Jackson, L.M. Chatters, and R.J. Taylor (Eds.), *Aging in black America* (pp. 277-297). Thousand Oaks, CA: Sage.

Golding, J.M., Karno, M., and Rutter, C.M. (1990). Symptoms of major depression among Mexican-Americans and non-Hispanic whites. *American Journal of Psychiatry, 147,* 861-866.

Goldwasser, H.D., and Badger, L.W. (1989). Utility of the psychiatric screen among the Navajo of Chinle: A fourth-year clerkship experience. *American Indian Alaska Native Mental Health Research, 3,* 6-15.

Hammen, C.L., Davila, J., Brown, G.P., Gitlin, M.J., and Ellicott, A. (1992). Stress as a mediator of the effects of psychiatric history on severity of unipolar depression. *Journal of Abnormal Psychology, 101,* 45-52.

Harden, A.W., Clark, R., and Maguire, K. (1997). *Informal and formal kinship care.* Report for the Office of the Assistant Secretary for Planning and Evaluation (Task Order HHS-100-95-0021). Washington, DC: U.S. Department of Health and Human Services.

Harkness, K.L., Monroe, S.M., Simons, A.D., and Thase, M. (1999). The generation of life events in recurrent and non-recurrent depression. *Psychological Medicine, 29,* 135-144.

Harris, T.B., Savage, P.J., Tell, G.S., Haan, M., Kumanyika, S., and Lynch, J.C. (1997). Carrying the burden of cardiovascular risk in old age: Associations of weight and weight change with prevalent cardiovascular disease, risk factors, and health status in the Cardiovascular Health Study. *American Journal of Clinical Nutrition, 66*(4), 837-844.

Harrison, M.O., Koenig, H.G., Hays, J.C., Eme-Akwari, A.G., and Pargament, K.I. (2001). The epidemiology of religious coping: A review of recent literature. *International Review of Psychiatry, 13*(2), 86-93.

Heckhausen, J., and Schulz, R. (1993). Optimization by selection and compensation: Balancing primary and secondary control in life span development. *International Journal of Behavioral Development, 16,* 287-303.

Helm, H.M., Hays, J.C., Flint, E.P., Koenig, H.G., and Blazer, D.G. (2000). Does private religious activity prolong survival? A six-year follow-up study of 3,851 older adults. *Journals of Gerontology, Series A: Biological Sciences and Medical Sciences, 55*(7), M400-M405.

Holahan, C.K., and Holahan, C.J. (1987). Life stresses, hassles, and self-efficacy in aging: A replication and extension. *Journal of Applied Social Psychology, 17*(6), 574-592.

Holahan, C.K., Holahan, C.J., and Belk, S.S. (1984). Adjustment in aging: The roles of life stresses, hassles, and self-efficacy. *Health Psychology, 3*(4), 315-328.

Hurtado, A. (1995). Variations, combinations, and evolutions: Hispanic families in the United States. In R.E. Zanbrana (Ed.), *Understanding Hispanic families: Scholarship, policy, and practice* (pp. 40-61). Thousand Oaks, CA: Sage.

Husaini, B.A., Moore, S.T., Castor, R.S., Neser, W., Whitten-Stovall, R., Linn, J.G., and Griffin, D. (1991). Social density, stressors, and depression: Gender differences among the black elderly. *Journal of Gerontology: Psychological Sciences, 46*(5), 236-242.

Hwang, W., Myers, H., and Takeuchi, D. (2000). Psychosocial predictors of first-onset depression in Chinese Americans. *Social Psychiatry and Psychiatric Epidemiology, 35*, 133-145.

Hwang, W., Chun, C., Takeuchi, D.T., Myers, H.F., and Prabha, S. (in press). Age at first-onset depression among Chinese Americans. *Journal of Consulting and Clinical Psychology*.

Hwu, H., Yeh, E., and Chang, L. (1989). Prevalence of psychiatric disorders in Taiwan defined by the Chinese Diagnostic Interview Schedule. *Acta Psychiatrica Scandinavica, 79*, 136-147.

Idler, E.L. (1987). Religious involvement and the health of the elderly: Some hypotheses and an initial test. *Social Forces, 66*(1), 226-238.

Idler, E.L., and Kasl, S.V. (1997). Religion among disabled and nondisabled persons II: Attendance at religious services as a predictor of the course of disability. *Journal of Gerontology, Series B: Psychology and Social Science, 52*(6), S306-S316.

James, S.A. (1994). John Henryism and the health of African-Americans. *Culture, Medicine and Psychiatry, 18*(2), 163-182.

Jendrek, M.P. (1994). Grandparents who parent their grandchildren: Circumstances and decisions. *Gerontologist, 34*, 206-216.

Jones, C.J., and Meredith, W. (1996). Patterns of personality change across the life span. *Psychology and Aging, 11*, 57-65.

Kales, H.C., Blow, F.C., Bingham, C.R., Copeland, L.A., and Mellow, A.M. (2000). Race and inpatient psychiatric diagnoses among elderly veterans. *Psychiatric Services, 51*(6), 795-800.

Karel, M.J. (1997). Aging and depression: Vulnerability and stress across adulthood. *Clinical Psychology Review, 17*(8), 847-879.

Kasch, K.L., and Klein, D.N. (1996). The relationship between age of onset and comorbidity in psychiatric disorders. *Journal of Nervous and Mental Disease, 184*(11), 703-707.

Kelley, S.J., Whitley, D., Sipe, J., and Yorke, B.C. (2000). Psychological distress in grandmother kinship care providers: The role of resources, social support, and physical health. *Child Abuse and Neglect, 24*(3), 311-321.

Kessler, R.C., and Neighbors, H.W. (1986). A new perspective on the relationships among race, social class and psychological distress. *Journal of Health and Social Behavior, 27*, 107-115.

Kinzie, J.D., Leung, P.K., Boehnlein, J., Matsunaga, D., Johnson, R., Manson, S., Shore, J.H., Heinz, J., and Williams, M. (1992). Psychiatric epidemiology of an Indian village: A 19-year replication study. *Journal of Nervous and Mental Disease, 180*(1), 33-39.

Kirmayer, L.J., and Young, A. (1998). Culture and somatization: Clinical, epidemiological, and ethnographic perspectives. *Psychosomatic Medicine, 60*, 420-430.

Klein, D.N., Taylor, E.B., Harding, K., and Dickstein, S. (1988). Double depression and episodic major depression: Demographic, clinical, familial, personality, and socioenvironmental characteristics and short-term outcome. *American Journal of Psychiatry, 145*, 1226-1231.

Klein, D.N., Schatzberg, A.F., McCullough, J.P., Dowling, F., Goodman, D., Howland, R.H., Markowitz, J.C., Smith, C., Thase, M.E., Rush, A.J., LaVange, L., Harrison, W.M., and Keller, M.B. (1999). Age of onset in chronic major depression: Relation to demographic and clinical variables, family history, and treatment response. *Journal of Affective Disorders, 55*, 149-158.

Kleinman, J.C., Fingerhut, L.A., and Prager, K. (1991). Differences in infant mortality by race, nativity status, and other maternal characteristics. *American Journal of Diseases of Childhood, 145*, 194-195.

Koenig, H., Smiley, M., and Gonzalez, J.A.P. (1988). *Religion, health, and aging*. Westport, CT: Greenwood Press.

Koenig, H.G., Siegler, I.C., and George, L.K. (1989). Religious and non-religious coping: Impact on adaptation in later life. *Journal of Religion and Aging, 5,* 73-94.

Kornhaber, A. (1996). *Contemporary grandparenting*. Thousand Oaks, CA: Sage.

Krause, N., and Liang, J. (1993). Stress, social support, and psychological distress among the Chinese elderly. *Journal of Gerontology, 48*(6), 282-291.

Krieger, N., and Sidney, S. (1996). Racial discrimination and blood pressure: The CARDIA study of young black and white adults. *American Journal of Public Health, 86,* 1370-1378.

Krieger, N., Rowley, D.L., Herman, A.A., Avery, B., and Phillips, M.T. (1993). Racism, sexism, and social class: Implications for studies of health, disease, and well-being. *American Journal of Preventive Medicine, 9*(Suppl. 6), 82-122.

Kua, E.H. (1990). Depressive disorder in elderly Chinese people. *Acta Psychiatrica Scandinavica, 81*(4), 386-388.

Kumanyika, S.K. (1998). Obesity in African Americans: Biobehavioral consequences of culture. *Ethnicity and Disease, 8*(1), 93-96.

Kuo, W. (1984). Prevalence of depression among Asian-Americans. *Journal of Nervous and Mental Disease, 172,* 449-457.

LaFromboise, T., Coleman, H.L.K., and Gerton, J. (1995). Psychological impact of biculturalism: Evidence and theory. In N.R. Goldberger, J.B. Veroff et al. (Eds.), *The culture and psychology reader* (pp. 489-535). New York: New York University Press.

Lawton, M.P., Kleban, M.H., Rajagopal, D., and Dean, J. (1992). Dimensions of affective experience in three age groups. *Psychology and Aging, 7,* 171-184.

Lazarus, R.S., and Folkman, S. (1984). *Stress, appraisal and coping*. New York: Springer.

Lee, C.K., Kwak, Y.S., Yamamoto, J., Rhee, H., Kim, Y.S., Han, J.H., Choi, J.O., and Lee, Y.H. (1990). Psychiatric epidemiology in Korea, Part I: Gender and age differences in Seoul. *Journal of Nervous and Mental Disease, 175*(4), 242-246.

Leppin, A., and Schwarzer, R. (1990). Social support and physical health: An updated meta-analysis. In L.R. Schmidt, P. Schwenkmezzger, P.J. Weinman, and S. Maes (Eds.), *Theoretical and applied aspects of health psychology* (pp. 185-202). Chur, Switzerland: Harwood Academic Press.

Lestra, C., D'Amato, T., Ghaemmaghami, C., Perret-Liaudet, A., Broyer, M., Renaud, B., Dalery, J., and Chamba, G. (1998). Biological parameters in major depression: Effects of paroxetine, viloxazine, moclobemide, and electroconvulsive therapy: Relation to early clinical outcome. *Biological Psychiatry, 44*(4), 274-280.

Levin, J.S., Chatters, L.M., and Taylor, R.J. (1995). Religious effects on health status and life satisfaction among black Americans. *Journals of Gerontology, Series B: Psychological Sciences and Social Sciences, 50*(3), S154-S163.

Lewinsohn, P.M., Fenn, S., Stanton, A.K., and Franklin, J. (1986). Relation of age at onset to duration of episode in unipolar depression. *Journal of Psychology and Aging, 1*(1), 63-68.

Lewinsohn, P.M., Rohde, P., Seeley, J.R., and Fischer, S.A. (1991). Age and depression: Unique and shared effects. *Psychology and Aging, 6*(2), 247-260.

Lobel, M., Dunkel-Schetter, C., and Scrimshaw, S. (1992). Prenatal maternal stress and prematurity: A prospective study of socioeconomically disadvantaged women. *Health Psychology, 11*(1), 32-40.

Lubben, J.E., and Becerra, R.M. (1987). Social support among black, Mexican, and Chinese elderly. In D.E. Gelfand and C.M. Barresi (Eds.), *Ethnic dimensions in aging* (pp. 18-34). New York: Springer.

Lugaila, T. (1998). *Marital status and living arrangements: March, 1997*. Current Population Reports Series. Washington, DC: U.S. Bureau of the Census.

Lyons, M.J., Eisen, S.A., Goldberg, J., True, W., Lin, N., Meyer, J.M., Toomey, R., Faraone, S.V., Merla-Ramos, M., and Tsuang, M.T. (1998). A registry-based twin study of depression in men. *Archives of General Psychiatry, 55*(5), 468-472.

Manson, S.M. (1992). Long-term care of older American Indians: Challenges in the development of institutional services. In C. Barresi and D.E. Stull (Eds.), *Ethnicity and long-term care* (pp. 130-143). New York: Springer.

Manson, S.M. (1995). Mental health status and needs of the American Indian and Alaska Native elderly. In D.K. Padgett (Ed.), *Handbook on ethnicity, aging, and mental health* (pp. 132-141). Westport, CT: Greenwood Press.

Markides, K.S. (1986). Minority status, aging, and mental health. *International Journal of Aging and Human Development, 23*(4), 285-300.

Mattis, J. (1997). Spirituality and religiosity in the lives of black women. *African American Research Perspectives, 3,* 56-60.

McAuley, W.J., Pecchioni, L., and Grant, J.A. (2000). Personal accounts of the role of God in health and illness among older rural African American and white residents. *Journal of Cross-Cultural Gerontology, 15*(1), 13-35.

McCrae, R.R. (1982). Age differences in the use of coping mechanisms. *Journal of Gerontology, 37,* 454-460.

McCullough, M.E., Hoyt, W.T., Larson, D.B., Koenig, H.G., and Thoresen, C. (2000). Religious involvement and mortality: A meta-analytic review. *Health Psychology, 19*(3), 211-222.

McEwen, B.S. (1998). Stress, adaptation, and disease: Allostasis and allostatic load. In S.M. McCann, J.M. Lipton et al. (Eds.), *Annals of the New York Academy of Sciences. Vol. 840. Neuroimmunomodulation: Molecular aspects, integrative systems, and clinical advances* (pp. 33-44). New York: New York Academy of Sciences.

McEwen, B.S., and Seeman, T. (1999). Protective and damaging effects of mediators of stress: Elaborating and testing the concepts of allostasis and allostatic load. In N.E. Adler, M. Marmot, B.S. McEwen, and J. Stewart (Eds.), *Socioeconomic status and health in industrial nations: Social, psychological, and biological pathways* (pp. 30-47). New York: New York Academy of Sciences.

McEwen, B.S., and Stellar, E. (1993). Stress and the individual mechanisms leading to disease. *Archives of Internal Medicine, 153,* 2093-2101.

McLean, D.E., and Link, B.G. (1994). Unraveling complexity: Strategies to refine concepts, measures, and research designs in the study of life events and mental health. In W.R. Avison and I.H. Gotlib (Eds.), *Stress and mental health: Contemporary issues and prospects for the future* (pp. 15-42). New York: Plenum Press.

Mickley, J.R., Carson, V., and Soeken, K.L. (1995). Religion and mental health: State of the science in nursing. *Issues in Mental Health Nursing, 16*(4), 345-366.

Miller, K.J. (1998). Life satisfaction in older adults: The impact of social support and religious maturity. *Dissertation Abstracts International: Section B: The Sciences and Engineering, 59*(6-B), 3067.

Minkler, M., and Fuller-Thompson, E. (1999). The health of grandparents raising grandchildren: Results of a national study. *American Journal of Public Health, 89*(9), 1384-1389.

Minkler, M., and Roe, K.M. (1993). Grandparents as surrogate parents. *Generation, 20,* 304-338.

Minkler, M., Fuller-Thompson, E., Miller, D., and Driver, D. (1997). Depression in grandparents raising grandchildren: Results of a national longitudinal study. *Archives of Family Medicine, 6,* 445-452.

Monroe, S.M., and Simons, A.D. (1991). Diathesis-stress theories in the context of life stress research: Implications for the depressive disorders. *Psychology Bulletin, 110*(3), 406-425.

Moore, M.R., and Chase-Landsdale, P.L. (2001). Sexual intercourse and pregnancy among African American girls in high-poverty neighborhoods: The role of family and perceived community environment. *Journal of Marriage and the Family, 63*(4), 1146-1157.

Moyerman, D.R., and Forman, B.D. (1992). Acculturation and adjustment: A meta-analytic study. *Hispanic Journal of Behavioral Sciences, 14,* 163-200.

Musick, M.A, Koenig, H.G., Hays, J.C, and Cohen, H.J. (1998). Religious activity and depression among community-dwelling elderly persons with cancer: The moderating effect of race. *Journal of Gerontology, Series B: Psychology and Social Science, 53*(4), S218-227.

Musick, M.A., Traphagan, J.W., Koenig, H.G., and Larson, D.B. (2000). Spirituality in physical health and aging. *Journal of Adult Development, 7*(2), 73-86.

Myers, H.F., and Taylor, S. (1998). Family contributions to risk and resilience in African American children. *Journal of Comparative Family Studies, 29*(1), 215-229.

Myers, H.F., Kagawa-Singer, M., Kumanyika, S.K., Lex, B.W., and Markides, K.S. (1995). Panel III: Behavioral risk factors related to chronic diseases in ethnic populations. *Health Psychology, 14*(7), 613-621.

Myers, H.F., Anderson, N.B., and Strickland, R. (1996). Biobehavioral perspective for research on stress and hypertension in black adults. Theoretical and empirical issues. In R. Jones (Ed.), *African American mental health* (pp. 1-36). Hampton, VA: Cobb and Henry.

Myers, H.F., Lesser, I., Rodrigues, N., Mira, C.B., Hwang, W., Camp, C., Anderson, D., Erickson, L., and Wohl, M. (2002a). Ethnic differences in clinical presentation of depression in adult women. *Cultural Diversity and Ethnic Minority Psychology, 8*(2), 138-156.

Myers, H.F., Lewis, T.T., and Parker-Dominguez, T. (2002b). Stress, coping and minority health: Biopsychosocial perspective on ethnic health disparities. In G. Bernal, J. Trimble, K. Burlew, and F. Leong (Eds.), *Handbook of racial and ethnic minority psychology.* Thousand Oaks, CA: Sage.

Nakane, Y., Ohta, Y., Radford, M., Yan, H., et al. (1991). Comparative study of affective disorders in three Asian countries: II. Differences in prevalence rates and symptom presentation. *Acta Psychiatrica Scandinavica, 84,* 313-319.

National Center for Post-Traumatic Stress Disorder and National Center for American Indian and Alaska Native Mental Health Research Center. (1996). *Matsunaga Vietnam Veterans Project.* White River Junction, VT.

Neighbors, H.W., Jackson, J.S., Bowman, P.J., and Gurin, G. (1983). Stress, coping, and black mental health: Preliminary findings from a national study. *Prevention and Human Services, 2,* 5.

Nelson, P.B. (1989). Ethnic differences in intrinsic/extrinsic religious orientation and depression in the elderly. *Archives of Psychiatric Nursing, 3*(4), 199-204.

Newsom, J.T., and Schulz, R. (1996). Social support as a mediator in the relation between functional status and quality of life in older adults. *Psychology of Aging, 11*(1), 34-44.

Nicassio, P.M. (1985). The psychosocial adjustment of the Southeast Asian refugee: An overview of empirical findings and theoretical models. *Journal of Cross-Cultural Psychology, 16*(2), 153-173.

Nicholson, B.L. (1997). The influence of pre-emigration and postemigration stressors on mental health: A study of Southeast Asian refugees. *Social Work Research, 21*(1), 19-31.

Orr, S.T., James, S.A., Miller, C A., Barakt, B., Daikoku, N., Pupkin, M., Engstrom, K., and Huggins, G. (1996). Psychosocial stressors and low birthweight in an urban population. *American Journal of Preventive Medicine, 12*(6), 457-466.

Padgett, D. (1998). Aging minority women: Issues in research and health policy. *Women and Health, 14,* 213-225.

Pargament, K.I., Smith, B.W., Koenig, H.G., and Perez, L. (1998). Patterns of positive and negative religious coping with major life stressors. *Journal of the Scientific Study of Religion, 37*(4), 710-724.

Pruchno, R. (1999). Raising grandchildren: The experiences of black and white grandmothers. *The Gerontologist, 39*(2), 209-221.

Raskin, A., Crook, T.H., and Herman, K.D. (1975). Psychiatric history and symptom differences in black and white depressed patients. *Journal of Consulting and Clinical Psychology, 43*, 73-80.

Regier, D.A., Boyd, J.H., Burke, J.D., Rae, D.S., Myers, J.K., Kramer, M., Robins, L.N., George, L.K., Karno, M., and Locke, B.Z. (1988). One-month prevalence of mental disorders in the United States. Based on five epidemiologic area sites. *Archives of General Psychiatry, 45*, 977-986.

Regier, D.A., Farmer, M.E., Rae, D.S., Myers, J.K., Kramer, M., Robins, L.N., George, L.K., Karno, M., and Locke, B.Z. (1993). One-month prevalence of mental disorders in the United States and sociodemographic characteristics: The Epidemiologic Catchment Area Study. *Acta Psychiatrica Scandinavica, 88*, 35-47.

Reid, P.T., and Bing, V.M. (2000). Sexual role of girls and women: An ethnocultural lifespan perspective. In C.B. Travis, J.W. White, et al. (Eds.), *Sexuality, society, and feminism* (pp. 141-166). Washington, DC: American Psychological Association.

Roberts, R.E., Kaplan, G.A., Shema, S.J., and Strawbridge, W.J. (1997a). Does growing old increase the risk for depression? *American Journal of Psychiatry, 154*(10), 1384-1390.

Roberts, R.E., Roberts, C.R., and Chen, Y.R. (1997b). Ethnocultural differences in prevalence of adolescent depression. *American Journal of Community Psychology, 25*, 95-109.

Rodgers-Farmer, A.Y. (1999). Parenting stress, depression, and parenting in grandmothers raising their grandchildren. *Children and Youth Services Review, 21*(5), 377-388.

Rogler, L., Cortes, D.E., and Malgady, R.G. (1991). Acculturation and mental health status among Hispanics: Convergence and new directions of research. *American Psychologist, 6*, 585-597.

Roysircar-Sodowsky, G., and Maestas, M.V. (2000). Acculturation, ethnic identity, and acculturative stress: Evidence and measurement. In R.H. Dana et al. (Eds.), *Handbook of cross-cultural and multicultural personality assessment* (pp. 131-172). Hillsdale, NJ: Lawrence Erlbaum Associates.

Ruiz, D.S. (1995). A demographic and epidemiologic profile of the ethnic elderly. In D. Padget (Ed.), *Handbook on ethnicity, aging, and mental health* (pp. 3-21). Westport, CT: Greenwood Press.

Sabogal, F., Marin, G., and Otero-Sabogal, R. (1987). Hispanic familism and acculturation: What changes and what doesn't? *Hispanic Journal of Behavioral Sciences, 9*, 397-412.

Sands, R.G., and Goldberg-Glen, R.S. (2000). Factors associated with stress among grandparents raising their grandchildren. *Family Relations, 49*, 97-105.

Schoevers, R.A., Beekman, A.T.F., Deeg, D.J.H., Geerlings, M.I., Jonker, C., and Van Tilburg, W. (2000). Risk factors for depression in later life: Results of a prospective community based study (AMSTEL). *Journal of Affective Disorders, 59*(2), 127-137.

Seeman, T.E., Bruce, M.L., and McAvay, G.J. (1996). Social network characteristics and onset of ADL disability: MacArthur studies of successful aging. *Journals of Gerontology, Series B: Psychological Sciences and Social Sciences, 51*(4), S191-S200.

Seeman, T.E., Singer, B.H., Rowe, J.W., Horwitz, R.I., and McEwen, B.S. (1997). Price of adaptation—allostatic load and its health consequences: MacArthur studies of successful aging. *Archives of Internal Medicine, 157*, 2259-2268.

Seeman, T.E, Unger, J.B, McAvay, G., and Mendes de Leon, C.F. (1999). Self-efficacy beliefs and perceived declines in functional ability: MacArthur studies of successful aging. *Journals of Gerontology, Series B: Psychological Sciences and Social Sciences, 54*(4), P214-222.

Seeman, T.E., Lusignolo, T.M., Albert, M., and Berkman, L. (2001). Social relationships, social support, and patterns of cognitive aging in healthy, high functioning older adults: MacArthur studies of successful aging. *Health Psychology, 20*(4), 243-255.

Shaw, B.A., and Krause, N. (2001). Exploring race variations in aging and personal control. *Journals of Gerontology, Series B: Psychological Sciences and Social Sciences, 6*(2), S119-S124.

Shiono, P.H., Rauh, V.A., Park, M., Lederman, S.A., and Suskar, D. (1997). Ethnic differences in birthweight: Lifestyle and other factors. *American Journal of Public Health, 87*(5), 787-793.

Siegel, J.M., Aneshensel, C.S., Taub, B., Cantwell, D.P., and Driscoll, A.K. (1998). Adolescent depressed mood in a multiethnic sample. *Journal of Youth and Adolescence, 27*(4), 413-427.

Singer, B., and Ryff, C.D. (1999). Hierarchies of life histories and associated health risks. In N.E. Adler, M. Marmot, B.S. McEwen, and J. Stewart (Eds.), *Socioeconomic status and health in industrial nations: Social, psychological, and biological pathways* (pp. 96-115). New York: New York Academy of Sciences.

Smedley, B.D., Stith, A.Y., and Nelson, A.R. (Eds.). (2002). *Unequal treatment: Confronting racial and ethnic disparities in health care.* Washington, DC: National Academy Press.

Snowden, L.R. (1998). Racial differences in informal help-seeking for mental health problems. *Journal of Community Psychology, 26*(5), 429-438.

Snowden, L.R., and Cheung, F.K. (1990). Use of inpatient mental health services by members of ethnic minority groups. *American Psychologist, 45*, 347-355.

Somervell, P.D., Leaf, P.J., Weissman, M.M., Blazer, D.G., and Bruce, M.L. (1989). The prevalence of major depression in black and white adults in five United States communities. *American Journal of Epidemiology, 130*(4), 725-735.

Sorenson, S.B., Rutter, C.M., and Aneshensel, C.S. (1991). Depression in the community: An investigation into age of onset. *Journal of Consulting and Clinical Psychology, 59*, 541-546.

Strawbridge, W.J., Wallhagen, M.I., Shema, S.J., and Kaplan, G.A. (1997). New burdens or more of the same? Comparing grandparent, spouse, and adult child caregivers. *The Gerontologist, 37*(4), 505-510.

Strawbridge, W.J., Shema, S.J., Cohen, R.D., Roberts, R.E., and Kaplan, G.A. (1998). Religiosity buffers effects of some stressors on depression but exacerbates others. *Journals of Gerontology, Series B: Psychological Sciences and Social Sciences, 53*(3), S118-S126.

Stern, S.L., Dhanda, R., and Hazuda, H.P. (2001). Hopelessness predicts mortality in older Mexican and European Americans. *Psychosomatic Medicine, 63*(3), 344-351.

Sue, D., and Sue, S. (1987). Cultural factors in the clinical assessment of Asian Americans. *Journal of Consulting and Clinical Psychology, 55*(4), 479-487.

Sue, S., Fujino, D., Hu, L., Takeuchi, D., and Zane, N. (1991). Community mental services for ethnic minority groups: A test of the cultural responsiveness hypothesis. *Journal of Consulting and Clinical Psychology, 59*, 533-540.

Swenson, C.J., Baxter, J., Shetterly, S.M., Scarbro, S.L., and Hamman, R.F. (2000). Depressive symptoms in Hispanic and non-Hispanic white rural elderly: The San Luis Valley Health and Aging Study. *American Journal of Epidemiology, 152*(11), 1048-1055.

Szinovacz, M.E. (1998). Grandparents today: A demographic profile. *The Gerontologist, 38*, 37-52.

Takeuchi, D.T., Leaf, P.J., and Kuo, H.S. (1988). Ethnic differences in the perception of barriers to help-seeking. *Social Psychiatry and Psychiatric Epidemiology, 23*(4), 273-280.

Takeuchi, D.T., Chung, R.C., Lin, K.M., Shen, H., Kurasaki, K., Chun, C., and Sue, S. (1998). Lifetime and twelve-month prevalence rates of major depressive episodes and dysthymia among Chinese Americans in Los Angeles. *American Journal of Psychiatry, 155,* 1407-1414.

Taylor, R.J. (1993). Religion and religious observances. In J.S. Jackson, L.M. Chatters, and R.J. Taylor (Eds.), *Aging in black America* (pp. 101-123). Thousand Oaks, CA: Sage.

Taylor, S.E., Repetti, R.L., and Seeman, T.E. (1997). Health psychology: What is an unhealthy environment and how does it get under the skin? *Annual Review of Psychology, 48,* 411-447.

Turnbull, J.E., and Mui, A.C. (1995). Mental health status and needs of black and white elderly: Differences in depression. In D.K. Padgett (Ed.), *Handbook on ethnicity, aging, and mental health* (pp. 73-98). Westport, CT: Greenwood Press.

Turvey, C.L., Conwell, Y., Jones, M.P., Phillips, C., Simonsick, E., Pearson, J.L., and Wallace, R. (2002). Risk factors for late-life suicide: A prospective community-based study. *American Journal of Geriatric Psychiatry, 10*(4), 398-406.

Unger, J.G., McAvay, G., Bruce, M.L., Berkman, L., and Seeman, T. (1999). Variation in the impact of social network characteristics on physical functioning in elderly persons: MacArthur studies of successful aging. *Journals of Gerontology, Series B: Psychological Sciences and Social Sciences, 54*(5), S245-S251.

U.S. Census Bureau. (2001). United States Census 2000. Available: http://www.census.gov [accessed March 2003].

Van den Berg, M.D., Oldehinkel, A.J., Bouhuys, A.L., Brilman, E.I., Beekman, A.T.F., and Ormel, J. (2001). Depression in later life: Three etiologically different subgroups. *Journal of Affective Disorders, 65,* 19-26.

Vega, W.A., Kolody, B., Aguilar-Gaxiola, S., Alderete, E., Catalano, R., and Caraveo-Anduaga, J. (1998). Lifetime prevalence of DSM-III-R psychiatric disorders among urban and rural Mexican Americans in California. *Archives of General Psychiatry, 55,* 771-782.

Villarosa, L. (Ed.). (1994). *Body and soul: The black women's guide to physical health and emotional well-being.* A National Black Women's Health Project Book. New York: HarperCollins.

Wade-Gayles, G. (Ed.). (1995). *My soul is a witness: African-American women's spirituality.* Boston: Beacon Press.

Walen, H.R., and Lachman, M.E. (2000). Social support and strain from partner, family, and friends: Costs and benefits for men and women in adulthood. *Journal of Social and Personal Relationships, 17*(1), 5-30.

Weissman, M.M., Bruce, M.L., Leaf, P.J., Florio, L.P., and Holzer, C., III. (1991). Affective disorders. In L.N. Robins and D.A. Regier (Eds.), *Psychiatric disorders in America: The epidemiologic catchment area study* (pp. 53-80). New York: The Free Press.

Weissman, M.M., Bland, R.C., Canino, G.J., Faravelli, C., Greenwald, S., Hwu, H., Joyce, P.R., Karam, E.G., Lee, C., Lellouch, J., Lepine, J., Newman, S.C., Rubio-Stipec, M., Wells, J.E., Wickramaratne, P.J., Wittchen, H., and Yeh, E. (1996). Cross-national epidemiology of major depression and bipolar disorder. *Journal of the American Medical Association, 276*(4), 293-299.

Wickrama, K.A.S., Conger, R.D., Wallace, L.E., and Elder, G.J., Jr. (1999). The intergenerational transmission of health-risk behaviors: Adolescent lifestyles and gender moderating effects. *Journal of Health and Social Behavior, 40*(3), 258-272.

Williams, D.R. (1999). Race, socioeconomic status, and health: The added effects of racism and discrimination. In N.E. Adler, M. Marmot, B.S. McEwen, and J. Stewart (Eds.), *Socioeconomic status and health in industrial nations: Social, psychological, and biological pathways* (pp. 173-188). New York: New York Academy of Sciences.

Williams, D.R., Takeuchi, D.T., and Adair, R. (1992). Socioeconomic status and psychiatric disorder among blacks and whites. *Social Forum, 71*, 179-194.

Williams, D.R., Yu, Y., Jackson, J.S., and Anderson, N.B. (1997). Racial differences in physical and mental health: Socio-economic status, stress and discrimination. *Journal of Health Psychology, 2*(3), 335-351.

Wilson, C., Civic, D., and Glass, D. (1995). Prevalence and correlates of depressive syndromes among adults visiting an Indian Health Service primary care clinic. *American Indian Alaska Native Mental Health Research, 6*(2), 1-12.

Wong, P.T., and Reker, G.T. (1985). Stress, coping and well-being in Anglo and Chinese elderly. *Canadian Journal on Aging, 4*(1), 29-37.

Wong, P.T.P., and Ujimoto, V K. (1998). The elderly: The stress, coping, and mental health. In L.C. Lee and N.W.S. Zane (Eds.), *Handbook of Asian American psychology* (pp. 165-209). Thousand Oaks, CA: Sage.

Woo, J., Ho, S.C., Lau, J., and Yuen, Y.K. (1994). The prevalence of depressive symptoms and predisposing factors in an elderly Chinese population. *Acta Psychiatrica Scandinavica, 89*(1), 8-13.

Woods, T.E., Antoni, M.H., Ironson, G.H., and Kling, D.W. (1999). Religiosity is associated with affective status in symptomatic HIV-infected African-American women. *Journal of Health Psychology, 4*(3), 317-326.

Yamamoto, J., Rhee, S., and Chang, D. (1994). Psychiatric disorders among elderly Koreans in the United States. *Community Mental Health Journal, 30*(1), 17-27.

Yamamoto, J., Chung, C., Nukariya, K., Ushijima, S., Kim, J., Dai, Y., Zhang, S., Ao, M., Cheung, F., Chang, D., and Winn, T. (1997). Depression prevention, suicide prevention in elderly Asian Americans. *American Journal of Forensic Psychiatry, 18*, 75-83.

Yu, E.S. (1986). Health of the Chinese elderly in America. *Research on Aging, 8*, 84-109.

Zambrana, R.E., Dunkle-Schetter, C., Collins, N.L., and Scrimshaw, S.C. (1999). Mediators of ethnic-associated differences in infant birth weight. *Journal of Urban Health, 76*(1), 102-116.

Zane, N., Enomoto, K., and Chun, C.-A. (1994). Treatment outcomes of Asian and white American clients in outpatient therapy. *Journal of Community Psychology, 22*, 177-191.

Zhang, A.Y., and Snowden, L.R. (1999). Ethnic characteristics of mental disorders in five U.S. communities. *Cultural Diversity and Ethnic Minority Psychology, 5*(2), 134-146.

Zhang, A.Y., Snowden, L.R., and Sue, S. (1998). Differences between Asian and white Americans' help seeking and utilization patterns in the Los Angeles area. *Journal of Community Psychology, 26*(4), 317-326.

Zheng, Y.P., Lin, K.M., Takeuchi, D.T., Kurasaki, K.S., and Cheung, F. (1997). An epidemiological study of neurasthenia in Chinese-Americans in Los Angeles. *Comprehensive Psychiatry, 38*(5), 249-259.

14

Significance of Perceived Racism: Toward Understanding Ethnic Group Disparities in Health, the Later Years

Rodney Clark

Numerous indices could be used to characterize health status in the later years. These indices include mortality (e.g., all causes, life expectancy, heart diseases, malignant neoplasms, and cerebrovascular diseases), chronic conditions (e.g., hypertension and cancer), and subjective health status. Many of the major racial (Asian, black, Native American, Pacific Islander, and white) and ethnic (Hispanic) groups in the United States, heretofore referred to as ethnic groups, differ with respect to these health indices. For example, research indicates that relative to their peers in other ethnic groups, more seasoned blacks (65 to 84 years of age) have shorter life expectancies, poorer subjective health, higher rates of hypertension, and higher death rates from all causes, heart diseases, malignant neoplasms, cerebrovascular diseases, and diabetes (National Center for Health Statistics [NCHS], 1998; Pamuk, Makuc, Heck, Reuben, and Lochner, 1998; Pappas, Queen, Hadden, and Fisher, 1993). With one rather consistent exception of non-Hispanic white males having higher mortality rates than black males in the oldest age group (85 years and older), the observation of poorer health profiles for black males and females tended to persist, even after stratifying by socioeconomic status. Among the other ethnic groups, non-Hispanic whites generally had the second poorest profiles, with Hispanics having the most favorable profiles and Asians or Pacific Islanders and Native Americans having intermediary profiles. Notable exceptions to this trend include age-adjusted death rates for chronic liver disease/cirrhosis and diabetes mellitus, where Native Americans have the highest and second highest mortality rates.

If these ethnic group disparities in health are not secondary to genetic or biological differences between the ethnic groups (American Anthropological Association, 1998; Barnett et al., 2001; Casper et al., 2000; Lewontin, 1995; Lieberman and Jackson, 1995; Williams, 1997), to what could the ethnic group disparities in health be attributed? Recent research suggests that behavioral risk profiles (NCHS, 1998) as well as direct and indirect effects of environmental and sociopolitical conditions are among the factors that contribute to these health disparities (Smith, Shipley, and Rose, 1990; Tennstedt and Chang, 1998). Racism is one environmental and sociopolitical condition that might help to explain the persisting disparities (Barnett et al., 2001; Casper et al., 2000; Krieger, 1999). The primary purpose of this chapter is to examine probable associations between racism and interethnic group health differences in the later years. Toward this end, the first section explores the ways in which racism has been conceptualized. In the context of a proposed conceptual model, the second section reviews research investigating the relationship of racism to different indices of health, and the final section highlights several directions for future research.

CONCEPTUALIZATIONS OF RACISM

Throughout this chapter, racism is used to refer to "beliefs, attitudes, institutional arrangements, and acts that tend to denigrate individuals or groups because of phenotypic characteristics [e.g., skin color, hair texture, width of nose, size of lips] or ethnic group affiliation" (Clark, Anderson, Clark, and Williams, 1999, p. 805). Defined in this way, racism can exist at both the individual and institutional levels and include subjective and more objective experiences of racism. Consistent with Clark et al. (1999), perceived racism involves perceptions of prejudiced attitudes and discriminatory behaviors, and is not limited to more overt expressions of behaviors (e.g., being called a "nigger"). That is, perceived racism may also include perceptions of subtler forms of racism (e.g., symbolic beliefs and behaviors) (McConahay and Hough, 1976; Sears, 1991; Yetman, 1985). Although perceived racism will be the focus of this chapter, institutional racism (discussed in detail elsewhere in this volume), which may not be perceived, is also included, given its complex and often overlooked relationship to perceived racism and health status.

Although several terms have been used in the scientific literature to describe perceived racism, it is important to note that using the definition of racism forwarded by Clark et al. (1999), perceived racism is not necessarily characterized by feelings of racial superiority, an ethnic group's control over valued resources, or the power of an ethnic group to impose its beliefs and values on others. Any member of a given ethnic group has the capacity to be racist against members of other ethnic groups (interethnic group racism) or against members of their own ethnic group (intraethnic group racism; also referred to as "colorism" by Hall [1992]). Because perceived racism is conceptualized herein as an umbrella term that includes prejudice and discrimination, it differs from other conceptualizations that describe racism as an ideologically based set of beliefs that direct relationships between oppressed and nonoppressed groups (Jones, 1997). Additionally, because relationships between ethnic groups are emphasized, racism perpetuated by members within an ethnic minority group is nonexistent.

Although a large body of research has examined the prevalence of interethnic group racism (both institutional and individual), relatively few have explored the existence of intraethnic group racism—a likely byproduct of how racism has been conceptualized to date in the scientific literature (Clark, in press). Among the limited number of studies exploring the existence of intraethnic group racism, research suggests that U.S. blacks once endorsed the idea of lighter skinned superiority (Gatewood, 1988; Okazawa-Rey, Robinson, and Ward, 1986) and routinely blocked darker skinned blacks from valued resources (e.g., matriculation at select historically black colleges and universities, as well as membership in some predominantly black fraternities and sororities, churches, and social/business organizations) (Neal and Wilson, 1989; Okazawa-Rey et al., 1986). Published research investigating the independent effects of intraethnic group racism, as well as the interactive or additive effects of intraethnic group racism and interethnic group racism, on health has yet to be published.

Jones (1972, p. 131) described institutional racism as "established laws, customs, and practices, which systematically reflect and produce racial inequities in American society." The institutionalization of these laws, customs, and practices are significant because their "effects are widespread and because they can result either from overt racism by an individual, or from a negative race-based policy, or as a systematic racial effect of a bias-free practice or policy" (Jones, 1997, p. 437). Institutional racism, whether overt/covert or intentional/unintentional, refers to social conditions such as residential segregation, occupational steering, and racial profiling. These social conditions in turn are posited to contribute to (1) socioeconomic disparities, (2) greater exposure to hazards (e.g., dangerous jobs and toxic environments), (3) coping responses, and (4) perceptions of unfair treatment and injustices—all of which may influence health (Bird and Bogart, 2001; Charatz-Litt, 1992; Cooper, 2001; Ferguson et al., 1998; Fernando, 1984; Jackson, Anderson, Johnson, and Sorlie, 2000; Kennedy, Kawachi, Lochner, Jones, and Prothrow-Stith, 1997; Klassen, Hall, Saksvig, Curbow, and Klassen, 2002; Landrine and Klonoff, 2000; Polednak, 1996; Utsey, Payne, Jackson, and Jones, 2002; Williams and Collins, 1995).

PERCEIVED RACISM AND HEALTH DISPARITIES:
A PROPOSED MODEL

Racism as a Source of Stress

An emerging body of research indicates that racism (whether or not it is perceived) is a potential source of acute and chronic stress for many ethnic group members (Clark, in press; Harrell, 2000; Kessler, Mickelson, and Williams, 1999; Krieger, 1999; Noh, Beiser, Kaspar, Hou, and Rummens, 1999; Utsey and Ponterotto, 1996; Williams and Neighbors, 2001), including Caucasians (Williams, 1997b). As an additional source of stress, individual and institutional racism may contribute to interethnic group and intraethnic group disparities in health via distal and proximal pathways (Figure 14-1). Distal pathways include internal and external factors that are hypothesized to mediate the relationship between environmental events and perceptions of these events as involving racism and involving harm, a threat, or a challenge. Importantly, the subjective component of perceived racism precludes an *a priori* determination of stressfulness (i.e., perception of harm, a threat, or a challenge). Proximal pathways, on the other hand, are postulated to influence psychological (e.g., anger) and physiological (e.g., sympa-

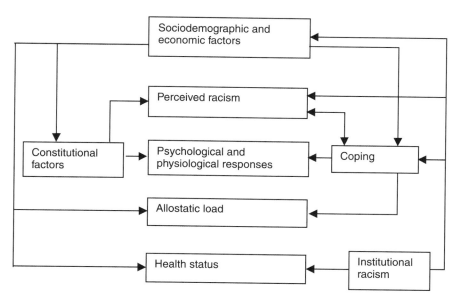

FIGURE 14-1 Conceptual model to examine the contribution of racism to health disparities.

thetic nervous system and immune activity) stress responses or tertiary outcomes (e.g., cardiovascular disease, depression, low birthweight, and cancer) more directly.

Building on existing conceptualizations proposed by Lazarus and Folkman (1984), McEwen (1998), and Clark et al. (1999), the underlying premise of this proposed model is that perceptions of an environmental stimulus as involving racism and involving harm, a threat, or a challenge are mitigated by sociodemographic factors, constitutional factors, and coping resources. Once the stimulus is perceived as involving racism and involving harm, a threat, or a challenge, psychological and physiological stress responses will result, followed by coping responses. *Over time,* the repeated activation and adaptation of these psychological and physiological systems are posited to lead to an allostatic burden, which, in turn, increases the risk of negative health outcomes (McEwen and Seeman, 1999). To the extent that (1) perceived racism evokes psychological and physiological responses with which people cope, and (2) the differential allostatic burden associated with perceived racism is observed along ethnic-gender lines, this model may provide a more context-specific framework for understanding the relationship between perceived racism and health disparities in the later years. Although it is probable that perceptions of discrimination associated with other "isms" (e.g., ageism, classism, and sexism), as well as perceptions of other stressors (e.g., acculturative stress), are related in similar ways to psychological and physiological functioning, this chapter will be relegated to a discussion of ethnically based injustices and inequities.

Sociodemographic and Economic Factors

Ethnicity

Research conducted in various countries indicates that ethnically based injustices and inequities are evident across different ethnic groups (Collier and Burke, 1986; Gilvarry et al., 1999; Karlsen and Nazroo, 2002; Lowell, Teachman, and Jing, 1995; McKeigue, Richards, and Richards, 1990; Sakamoto, Wu, and Tzeng, 2000; Villarruel, Canales, and Torres, 2001), which may have implications for health among Southeast Asian refugees in Canada (Noh et al., 1999), Asian-American Vietnam veterans in the United States (Loo et al., 2001), Southeast Asian refugees and Pacific Islander immigrants in New Zealand (Pernice and Brook, 1996), former Soviet immigrants in the United States (Aroian, Norris, Patsdaughter, and Tran, 1998), Chinese Canadians in Canada (Pak, Dion, and Dion, 1991; Tang and Trovato, 1998), Chinese Americans in the United States (Gee, 2002), Native Americans in the United States (Whitbeck, Hoyt, McMorris, Chen, and Stubben, 2001), Latin Americans in Australia (McDonald, Vechi, Bowman, and Sanson-Fisher, 1996), Aboriginals in Australia (Lowe, Kerridge, and Mitchell, 1995), and Mexican Americans in the United States (Finch, Kolody, and Vega, 2000).

In the United States, blacks are disproportionately exposed to environmental stimuli that might be perceived as involving racism (Collier and Burke, 1986; James, 1993; Jones, 1997; Krieger, 1999; Krieger, Sidney, and Coakley, 1998; Outlaw, 1993; Sears, 1991; Sigelman and Welch, 1991; Utsey, 1998). Although members of other ethnic groups report experiences of racism in the United States (Aroian et al., 1998; Finch et al., 2000; Krieger, 1990; Krieger and Sidney, 1996; Whitbeck et al., 2001; Williams, Yu, Jackson, and Anderson, 1997b), the sociopolitical history of racism in the United States as it relates to blacks (e.g., statement regarding slaves in the U.S. Constitution) has been more pervasive (James, 1993; Jones, 1997) and has contributed to acute and chronic perceptions that may be especially toxic for blacks (Cooper, 1993). In a multistage probability sample of 1,139 black and white adults (18 years and over) in three counties in southeastern Michigan, Williams et al. (1997a) found that blacks were nearly 10 times more likely to attribute perceptions of unfair treatment to ethnicity. Additionally, blacks were four times more likely to report ever being treated unfairly because of their ethnicity compared to whites. These attributions were positively related to chronic health conditions, and lifetime experiences of racism were positively associated with bed days and chronic health conditions in black but not white adults. Were these findings to be replicated among persons in the later years, and were the cumulative psychological and physiological effects of perceived racism associated with coping resources and allostatic burden, a more informed understanding of probable contributors to the health divide in the later years might be evinced.

Socioeconomic Status

Research indicates that socioeconomic status (SES) is one of the strongest predictors of health status (Krieger, Rowley, Herman, Avery, and Phillips, 1993; Marmot, Kogevinas, and Elston, 1987; Williams and Collins, 1995). Although space limitations preclude a detailed discussion of the direct and indirect effects of SES and health status, several reports have discussed these relationships and are suggested for further reading (Anderson and Armstead, 1995; Kaufman, Long, Liao, Cooper, and McGee, 1998; Krieger, 1999; Krieger et al., 1993; Marmot et al., 1987; NCHS, 1998; West, 1997; Whitfield, Weidner, Clark, and Anderson, 2002; Williams and Collins, 1995). Per the proposed model, SES differences could influence health disparities directly or indirectly. As an example of the former, secondary to sociopolitical conditions such as institutional racism, black elders are disproportionately represented in lower SES groups (Pamuk et al., 1998). Accordingly, they would be more likely to experience financial barriers to health care (beyond that provided by Medicare, e.g., out-of-pocket expenses for deductibles and co-payments) (McBean and Gornick, 1994) and reside in areas with limited access to quality health services and personnel, leading to elevated morbidity and mortality rates.

If the SES associated with institutional racism is related to elevated morbidity and mortality in some black elders, what accounts for their ability not to succumb to these ailments in young and middle adulthood? Cross-sectional data suggest that many chronic health conditions observed in young and middle adulthood persist into late adulthood, thereby contributing to higher rates of major activity limitations and higher percentages of respondent-assessed fair and poor health observed among blacks (65 years of age and older) compared to their white counterparts (NCHS, 1998). Regarding mortality, the cumulative effects of perceived racism probably do not lead to physiological exhaustion until the associated allostatic burden has taken its toll in late adulthood.

SES might also affect ethnic group health disparities indirectly via its relationship to the quantity and type of racist stimuli to which individuals are exposed, constitutional factors, and coping resources. For example, the equivocal findings with regard to the relationship between SES and the prevalence of racism (Gary, 1995; Landrine and Klonoff, 1996; Sigelman and Welch, 1991) probably are secondary to the dimension of racism assessed, with higher and lower SES blacks having greater exposures to subtle and overt forms of racism, respectively (Clark et al., 1999). To the extent that the magnitude of psychological and physiological stress responses are similar for overt and more subtle forms of perceived racism, contributing to comparable allostatic burdens, the deleterious effects of perceived racism would be observed across SES groups among those disproportionately exposed to environmental stimuli perceived as involving racism and involving harm, a threat, or a challenge. This interpretation is consistent with the observation that many ethnic disparities in health persist after adjusting for SES.

Age

Age is another sociodemographic factor that is rather consistently related to health status, with more seasoned persons being at greater risk for negative health outcomes (NCHS, 1998). In addition to its relationship to health status, age is also related to the frequency with which blacks and whites (Bledsoe, Combs, Sigelman, and Welch, 1996), as well as Southeast Asian refugees (Noh et al., 1999), perceive racism. For example, Forman, Williams, and Jackson (1997) found that perceptions of lifetime discrimination (e.g., "Do you think that you have ever been unfairly stopped, searched, questioned, physically threatened or abused by the police?"), recent discrimination (same as lifetime discrimination questions, except exposure is limited to the past 12 months), and everyday discrimination (e.g., "In your day-to-day life how often have any of the following things happened to you: You receive poorer service than other people at restaurants or stores?") decreased with advancing age in blacks and whites. Relative to the older age cohort (65+ years of age), for instance, blacks and whites in the youngest age cohort (18 to 34 years) had scores on the measure of everyday discrimination that were 44 percent and 53 percent higher (blacks and whites, respectively) (Figure 14-2). Despite decreases in reports of discrimination across the two ethnic groups, black-white differences in these reports remained consistent across the four age groups. However, the direction of these relationships has varied. Although some studies have found positive relationships between age and perceived racism/discrimination (Sigelman and Welch, 1991), the association in other studies has been negative (Adams and Dressler, 1988; Forman et al., 1997; Gary, 1995), and the relationship in still other investigations has been curvilinear (with the

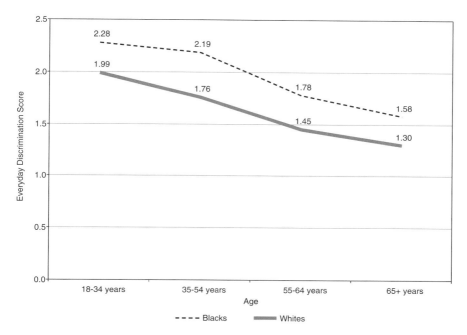

FIGURE 14-2 Reports of everyday discrimination as a function of ethnicity and age. SOURCE: Forman et al. (1997).

apex occurring during middle adulthood) (Forman et al., 1997; Schuman and Hatchett, 1974). The observed black-white differences with respect to perceived discrimination should be interpreted cautiously in the Forman et al. (1997) study, given that participants were not instructed to limit their reports to ethnic group discrimination. Therefore, it is possible that whites were reporting on experiences of discrimination that they perceived as being secondary to their gender, sexual orientation, SES, or weight. Although the discrimination scores for blacks probably were also inflated with respect to perceived ethnic discrimination—as opposed to discrimination from all causes—research indicates that blacks overwhelmingly attribute such unfair treatment to racism, whereas whites do not (Williams et al., 1997b).

To address the curvilinear relationship they observed between age and subjective experiences of racism, Schuman and Hatchett (1974) reasoned that higher reports of racism during middle adulthood, relative to early and late adulthood, might reflect their greater exposure to workplace discrimination. Studies that have found an inverse association between age and perceptions of racism should not necessarily be interpreted as meaning that black elders habituate (psychologically or physiologically) to perceptions of racism. In addition to habituation, several explanations are plausible. First, in the later years, blacks may come to accept racism as a way of life and not attribute the unfair treatment to racism (Adams and Dressler, 1988). Second, because of their disproportionate exposure to racist stimuli, more seasoned blacks may have come to use racism-specific coping strategies (e.g., anticipatory coping) that mitigate the negative psychological effects associated with these stimuli (Essed, 1991). As a result, they may not perceive the stimulus as being stressful or involving as much stress (e.g., possibly secondary to habituation) as their white counterparts. Third, given that blacks who are 65 and older were teenagers and young adults before and just after the Civil Rights Movement, it is also probable that by comparison, black elders do not consider many of the subtler forms of racism prevalent in the United States today as involving the same type of racism to which many of them may have been exposed. Thus, they may not perceive these more subtle forms of racism as really involving racism. Finally, if blacks in the later years use denial (i.e., not reporting perceptions of racism) as a way of coping with the untoward effects associated with their higher perceptions of racism (Forman et al., 1997), and if this method of coping is used repeatedly to deal with perceived racism or is associated with prolonged psychological or physiological reactivity, a greater allostatic burden would be expected to develop in this group (Krieger, 1999; McEwen and Seeman, 1999). Although speculative, this increased allostatic burden may contribute to more negative health profiles among blacks in the later years.

Gender

With the exception of health outcomes that occur in an inordinately higher frequency in one gender group (e.g., breast and prostate cancer), females generally have more favorable health profiles than males across ethnic and socioeconomic groups (Barnett et al., 2001; Casper et al., 2000; NCHS, 1998; Pamuk et al., 1998). Exceptions to this general trend include higher cerebrovascular mortality rates for black and white females (relative to males) who are 85 years and over, and higher hypertension prevalence rates for females (relative to males) who are 55 years and over. Similar to the observed relationships between age and perceived racism, the findings with respect to gender and perceived racism have been mixed, with some research showing that black males and females perceive equal amounts of racism (Landrine and Klonoff, 1996) and other investigations indicating that black men perceive more racism than black women (Sigelman and Welch, 1991; Utsey et al., 2002). In one study of black and white adults, Forman et al. (1997) used two indices to measure major perceptions of discrimination: lifetime discrimination and recent (past 12 months) discrimination. They found that black males and white males perceived more discrimination than black females and white females, respectively, although the gender effect was stronger in blacks. In another study using a more seasoned sample of blacks (mean age = 71.62 years), Utsey et al. (2002) assessed perceptions of cultural, institutional, individual, and collective racism. Their findings indicated that the stress associated with perceptions of institutional and collective racism was significantly higher for black males relative to black females. These findings, coupled with the previously mentioned observations that blacks perceive more racism than whites, suggest that black males may be the most vulnerable to the allostatic burden associated with perceived racism—a pattern that mirrors the health risk profiles of black males (highest risk).

Constitutional

The constitutional factors are qualities with which people are born, and include genes, skin tone, and family history of disease (e.g., hypertension, cancer, heart disease, and psychological disorders). These factors are not only related to perceived racism, but may interact with other components of the model to influence health status (Clark, 2003a; Dressler, Baleiro, and Dos Santos, 1999; Klag, Whelton, Coresh, Grim, and Kuller, 1991; Knapp et al., 1995). For example, although nil findings have been reported (Krieger et al., 1998), research indicates that darker skin blacks perceive more racism (Keith and Herring, 1991; Klonoff and Landrine, 2000; Udry, Bauman, and Chase, 1971), have lower incomes (Keith and Herring, 1991), are employed in less prestigious positions (Hughes and Hertel, 1990; Keith and Herring, 1991), and have higher diastolic blood pressure (Gleiberman, Harburg, Frone, Russell, and Cooper, 1995) than lighter skin blacks. Whereas the posited mechanisms underlying the relationship of skin tone to socioeconomic and health factors in blacks (e.g., the associations explicated in Figure 14-1) may be different than those in other ethnic groups, it is noteworthy that with some exceptions (Mosley et al., 2000), similar patterns have also been observed in other ethnic groups. In one study of Brazilians, for instance, Telles and Lim (1998) showed that after controlling for human capital and labor market factors, whites earned 26 percent more than "browns" (a racial classification in Brazil), and browns earned 13 percent more than blacks. In another study of 763 white Hispanics and non-Hispanic whites, Gleiberman, Harburg, Frone, Russell, and Cooper (1993) found that darker skin tone was associated with higher systolic blood pressure.

Psychological and Physiological Responses

Several responses from different systems are posited to follow perceptions of racism (e.g., psychological and physiological). The psychological responses include anger, helplessness, hopelessness, anxiety, resentment, and fear (Armstead, Lawler, Gorden, Cross, and Gibbons, 1989; Bullock and Houston, 1987; Clark, 2000; Fernando, 1984), and the physiological responses involve the cardiovascular, immune, and neuroendocrine systems (Clark et al., 1999). Whereas cardiac contraction, vasodilation, venoconstriction, vasoconstriction, and decreased excretion of sodium are among the cardiovascular responses, immune response to chronic stress most notably involve cellular and humoral reactions and include lower natural-killer cell activity and suppression of B- and T-lymphocytes, which increase susceptibility to disease (Cohen and Herbert, 1996). Lastly, activation of the pituitary-adrenocortical and hypothalamic-sympathetic-adrenal medullary systems is the primary response of the neuroendocrine system (Burchfield, 1979; Herd, 1991).

Although published research in this area is lacking (in general) and is nonexistent among the elderly, a limited number of studies using young- and middle-adulthood samples have examined the relationship of perceived racism to resting blood pressure and cardiovascular responses. These studies have shown that perceptions of racism are positively related to stress-induced changes in diastolic blood pressure in blacks (Fang and Myers, 2001; Guyll, Matthews, and Bromberger, 2001). In one study of black females that measured blood pressure responses during a standardized laboratory-speaking task, Clark (2000) found that perceptions of racism (during past year) were related to more exaggerated diastolic blood pressure responses. Even though participants who scored in the upper and lower quartile on perceived racism had similar baseline diastolic blood pressure levels, participants in the upper quartile had higher diastolic blood pressure levels during the prespeech and speech periods, and poorer posttask recovery (Figure 14-3).

Coping Responses

Coping responses and behaviors (coping responses) involve efforts used by or resources available to persons to manage intrinsic and extrinsic stimuli that are perceived as stressful. Although numerous conceptualizations of coping exist (e.g., approach, avoidance, emotion focused, problem focused, and cognitive), these strategies can be characterized as active or passive. Responses that are more active involve efforts to change the nature of the person-environment interaction (e.g., problem solving), whereas more passive responses include efforts to manage "distress" resulting from the perceived stressor (e.g., self-medication) (Lazarus and Folkman, 1984). It remains to be determined if individuals use similar coping responses to

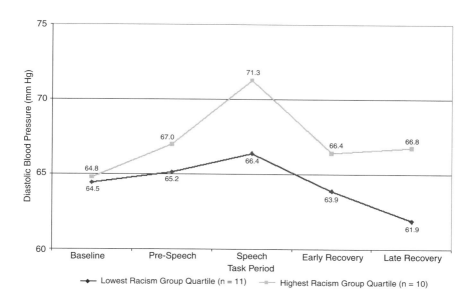

FIGURE 14-3 Absolute diastolic blood pressure levels for participants scoring in the upper and lower quartiles on perceived racism measure.
SOURCE: Clark (2000).

negotiate stressors (Carver, Scheier, and Weintraub, 1989) or if coping responses are context dependent (Lazarus and Folkman, 1984).

To the extent that individual differences in psychological and physiological responses to perceived racism are mitigated in part by coping responses (Clark, 2003b; Clark and Adams, in press), these responses are expected to influence allostatic loads in late adulthood. Ethnic minority group members who advance to late adulthood in light of life histories riddled with chronic exposures to racism probably have done so because of the mitigating effects associated with their coping responses and attribution styles. For example, in one probability sample of black adults, LaVeist, Sellars, and Neighbors (2001) found that individuals who are exposed to racism and who attribute these negative experiences to institutional and societal practices—as opposed to personal deficiencies—were more likely to survive the 13-year follow-up period.

Relatively few studies have examined the relationships among perceived racism, coping, and health status. Among the studies that have been conducted, the directions of the relationships have been outcome dependent. For example, in a sample of black college females, Clark and Anderson (2001) found that although some passive and active coping responses were positively related to blood pressure and heart rate responses, both strategies were also inversely related to cardiovascular responses. In a probability sample of black and white adults, Williams et al. (1997a) also found that passive and active coping responses to unfair treatment (including ethnic group discrimination) were positively associated with psychological distress, poorer well-being, and chronic conditions in blacks and whites. In another study exploring the effects of coping with unfair treatment and resting blood pressure, Krieger and Sidney (1996) found that more passive strategies were related to higher resting blood pressure levels in working-class blacks. In yet another study, Noh et al. (1999) found that depression symptoms were higher in Asian refugees who were high in perceived discrimination and high in the use of passive coping strategies, relative to those who were high in perceived discrimination and low in the use of passive coping strategies.

Consistent with Sterling and Eyer (1988) and McEwen (1998), allostasis involves achieving or maintaining physiological systems through change. Although not originally discussed in this way, allostasis could be thought of as the physiological equivalent of coping. For example, if Mr. Leach, a lower SES black male with a dark skin tone in his middle 60s, has come to respond to relatively chronic perceptions of interethnic group and intraethnic racism by briefly removing himself from the environment to "collect himself and regroup," a coping response that leads to the blunting and elimination of hostile feelings and to a marked reduction in heart rate, he would be said to have coped successfully and to have achieved allostasis. Although possibly adaptive in the short term (e.g., observable decrease in psychological and physiological responses), repeated attempts to maintain psychological and physiological systems in response to chronic perceptions of racism may have associated "costs." All things equal (e.g., age, socioeconomic resources, occupational status, and education attainment), compare Mr. Leach's psychological and physiological health risk profile to that of a white male peer who has not perceived racism or whose perceptions of racism have been more discrete, or to that of a black male peer who has perceived approximately the same amount of interethnic group racism but has not perceived intraethnic group racism because his skin tone is slightly lighter than a brown paper bag.

Institutional Racism

Even when racism is not perceived, institutional forms of racism may also influence health directly by restricted access to health care or high-quality health care (King, 1996; Kuno and Rothbard, 2002; Sheifer, Escarce, and Schulman, 2000; Whaley, 1998; Williams, 1997). For example, amid some nil findings (Farley et al., 2001; Taylor, Meyer, Morse, and Pearson, 1997), research suggests that ethnic minorities (usually blacks) are less likely than whites to receive select cardiovascular procedures (Gregory, Rhoads, Wilson, O'Dowd, and Kostis, 1999; Johnson, Lee, Cook, Rouan, and Goldman, 1993; Peterson et al., 1997; Schulman et al., 1999; Whittle, Conigliaro, Good, and Lofgren, 1993) and renal procedures (Alexander and Sehgal, 1998; Epstein et al., 2000; Kasiske, London, and Ellison, 1998; McCauley et al., 1997; Soucie, Neylan, and McClellan, 1992). MacLean, Siew, Fowler, and Graham (1987) also found that relative to their elderly French-Canadian, English-Canadian, and Portuguese counterparts, institutional racism contributed to limited or blocked social and health services for Chinese elders in Montreal. Similarly, the contribution of institutional practices to health access problems has been observed among older Mexican Americans (Parra and Espino, 1992). Research indicates that these ethnic group biases (1) begin in medical school (Rathore et al., 2000), (2) are observed among black and white physicians (Chen, Rathore, Radford, Wang, and Krumholz, 2001), and (3) are present in the treatment of patient populations before adulthood (Cuffe, Waller, Cuccaro, Pumariega, and Garrison, 1995).

Allostatic Load and Health Outcomes

The cumulative negative effects associated with the maintenance of psychological and physiological systems are referred to as allostatic load (McEwen and Seeman, 1999). The systems that are involved in the stress response (e.g., psychological, immune, cardiovascular, and neuroendocrine) are the same as those posited to contribute to allostatic load. This load is postulated to increase risk of negative health outcomes. Importantly, these systems do not act in isolation. Rather, they are often related in complex ways (Burchfield, 1985; Cacioppo, 1994; Herd, 1991).

Psychological sequelae include cognitive declines and persisting mood state alterations (Fernando, 1984; McEwen and Seeman, 1999; Seligman, 1975). To the extent that acute perceptions of racism are associated with increased neuroendocrine responses and excitatory amino acid neurotransmitter activity, resulting in reduced hippocampal volume, chronic perceptions of racism might be related to cognitive deficits in the later years among those who are disproportionately exposed (McEwen, 2000; Seeman, Singer, Rowe, Horwitz, and McEwen, 1997). Although the literature is mixed with regard to mental health disparities, research does suggest that perceptions of racism are positively related to mood deficits (Rumbaut, 1994). Ethnic differences in the prevalence of depression in later years could develop secondary to the untoward effects of perceived racism via chronic feelings of uncontrollability, helplessness, and threats to self-esteem (Fernando, 1984).

Cardiovascular and cerebrovascular outcomes include hypertension, stroke, and heart disease (Burchfield, 1979; Cacioppo, 1994; Clark et al., 1999; Herd, 1991; McEwen and Seeman, 1999). If perceptions of racism are related to acute elevations in vascular reactivity, which over time lead to hyper-reactivity, structural changes in the vasculature, and baroreceptor alterations, it is plausible that over the lifespan, chronic perceptions of racism might contribute to the eventual development of hypertension in the later years (Anderson, McNeilly, and Myers, 1991). This cascade of physiological events (namely hyperactivity and exaggerated catecholamine secretions) has also been associated with the progression of arterial plaque formation (Manuck, Kaplan, Adams, and Clarkson, 1995; Manuck, Kaplan, Muldoon, Adams, and Clarkson, 1991), which may place people who are disproportionately exposed to racism at increased risk of developing coronary heart disease.

Although no published studies could be found that have explicitly examined the relationship between perceived racism and immune outcomes, there is no reason to believe that as a stressor, chronic perceptions of racism are associated with different humoral and cellular reactions. The one caveat is that unlike other chronic stressors to which individuals may habituate, it is not known to what extent persons habituate to perceptions of racism. This notwithstanding, the possible cumulative toxic effects from immuno-suppression (e.g., lower natural-killer cell cytotoxic activity, B- and T-lymphocyte suppression, and suppression of the delayed-type hypersensitivity response) include prolonged respiratory infections and increased susceptibility to a myriad of health outcomes (Cohen and Herbert, 1996; Kiecolt-Glaser, Dura, Speicher, Trask, and Glaser, 1991).

DIRECTIONS FOR FUTURE RESEARCH

Theory and Assessment

Recent reviews suggest that research investigating the untoward effects of racism is on the rise (Brondolo, Rieppi, Kelly, and Gerin, 2003; Harrell, Hall, and Taliaferro, 2003; Meyer, 2003; Williams, Neighbors, and Jackson, 2003). As the empirical literature exploring associations between racism and health continues to emerge, the development of an equally strong theoretical literature is also needed that explicates the multiple biological, psychological, and social pathways through which perceived racism and institutional racism are posited to influence health outcomes. Concomitantly, special attention should be given to theoretically based assessments of racism that are reliable and valid (Utsey, 1998). Suggestions for future research examining theoretical and assessment issues are delineated below.

- Because perceptions of racism are among the psychosocial stressors that are posited to contribute to health disparities in the later years, assessments of perceived racism should be conducted in the context of a comprehensive evaluation of psychosocial stressors (e.g., those that might be culture specific). Although perceptions of interethnic group racism and intraethnic group racism are important considerations, the extent to which racism interacts with acculturation to influence the psychological and physiological risk profiles of black elders would probably lead to a more informed understanding of the complex interplay between racism and cultural factors. For example, consistent with the research of Landrine and Klonoff (1996), black elders may report fewer perceptions compared to their less seasoned counterparts because they are more acculturated. To assess racism in isolation of the other powerful psychosocial predictors of physiological activity would likely limit the potential to more fully explain ethnic group health disparities in the later years. Also, conceptual differences notwithstanding (e.g., researchers who assert that blacks lack the social and economic "power" to be racist but can discriminate against members of the in-group versus researchers who contend that intraethnic group racism involves the perpetuation of racism among in-group members), further research is needed that explores the additive and interactive relationships of interethnic group and intraethnic group racism to psychological and physiological functioning, which might further elucidate the mechanisms that contribute to within-group and between-group disparities in health during the later years.
- Although research suggests that perceptions of events as stressful are more predictive of psychological and physiological functioning than objective demands, comparative research exploring the relationship between a

person's perceptions and objective demands might provide additional concurrent validity. Further research is also needed to be able to more clearly interpret observed findings with respect to perceived racism. For example, some persons who perceive stimuli as involving racism probably do so because it is less anxiety provoking than attributing the failure of being promoted at work to personal deficits. Furthermore, some persons who do not report perceiving racism probably fail to do so because of denial or as an attempt to avoid the expected psychological distress that would be associated with negotiating an uncontrollable stressor. Accordingly, in addition to assessing perceptions of racism, the simultaneous measurement of other contributory factors such as attribution style, impression management, self-deception, and affective state would help to delineate the possible mitigating effects of these variables.

• According to Krieger (1999), of the 20 published studies that have assessed the effects of unfair treatment (including racism), more than half used measures with questionable or unreported psychometric properties. When psychometric data were presented, little to no attention was devoted to the generalizability of these data for the gender and/or ethnic groups being studied. Additionally, almost without exception, each author used different measures or response formats to assess racism. As a result of these methodological caveats, comparisons of findings across studies remain somewhat limited. Measures used to assess racism should (1) be reliable and valid for the target groups and subgroups (e.g., native-born Hispanics and immigrant Hispanics) as well as ethnic-gender groups and subgroups (e.g., Filipino males and Filipino females) being studied, (2) be specific enough to capture the reported multidimensional nature of racism, and (3) be developed with equivalent shorter and longer versions to facilitate use with different study designs.

• Systematic efforts by national agencies to "unpack" the broad ethnic groupings are needed. In addition to unpacking such broad ethnic grouping as Asians, Hispanics, and Pacific Islanders, ethnic groups who are presumed to be more or less homogeneous (e.g., blacks and whites) should also be unpacked to provide a more informed understanding of the cumulative perceptions of racism by ethnic subgroups. For example, although viewing whites as a homogeneous group probably has been convenient, the health profiles of white ethnic groups (e.g., Irish, Turks, and Cypriots) probably are influenced by differences in the amount of discrimination to which these ethnic groups are exposed and perceived (Aspinall, 1998).

Research Design

Given the dearth of data exploring the relationship between perceived racism and other components of the model proposed herein, studies using different research designs are warranted. These research designs should take the multidimensional nature of racism into consideration (Harrell, 2000), as well as the different levels (e.g., individual, cultural, and institutional) at which racism is perpetuated (Jones, 1997). In the section that follows, suggestions for future research using different designs are presented.

- National and large-scale studies exploring perceptions of interethnic group and intraethnic group racism within and between ethnic groups across the lifespan would provide the necessary baseline information, as well as identify groups who may be at increased risk. If allostatic load results from the cumulative effects of efforts to maintain psychological and physiological systems, the assessment of perceived racism in these studies (e.g., longitudinal) should begin prior to the later years and include cross-sectional and longitudinal designs. Because of the often cited monetary limitations of funding numerous longitudinal studies and the time involved in the collection of longitudinal data, cross-sectional and shorter term prospective studies are essential and may provide the necessary data for more targeted longitudinal research. For example, if cross-sectional research indicates that the perceptual base rates of racism (peak in middle adulthood and presumably the allostatic burden associated with these perceptions), targeted longitudinal research could be initiated during this period to explore concomitant changes in psychological and physiological systems.

- Studies exploring the relationship of perceived racism to the cascade of shorter term (e.g., psychological and physiological stress responses) and longer term (e.g., hippocampal volume, depression, cognitive declines, arterial elasticity) processes posited to contribute to allostatic load are needed, as well as integrated/multilevel research that examines how perceived racism interacts with psychological factors (e.g., coping efficacy), behavioral risk factors (e.g., smoking and alcohol consumption), and constitutional factors (e.g., genetic predisposition) to influence allostatic burden and health status. For example, among persons high in perceived racism, are different types of coping (e.g., problem focused and emotion focused) related to arterial elasticity and blood pressure reactivity, and, if so, are racism-specific coping strategies reflective of styles used to deal with other stressors (consistent with a trait approach)? Does the efficacy of a given racism coping strategy depend on the context in which it is perceived (e.g., work versus public realm), the ethnicity of the perpetrator (i.e., interethnic group or intraethnic group), or the position of the perpetrator (e.g., supervisor or subordinate)? These types of inquiries are essential to understanding how perceived racism "gets under the skin" and concomitantly contributes to psychological and physiological vulnerabilities in more seasoned adults.

• Given the history of *de jure* and *de facto* racism in the United States, more systematic studies exploring the extent to which these forms of racism continue to influence health status directly (e.g., access to services) and indirectly (e.g., nonequivalent returns on education, residential segregation, median household income, and educational attainment) are needed. For example, the observation that black males and white males differ with respect to returns on education is often cited as an example of interethnic group racism. Given the rather crude and descriptive nature of these data, however, a number of alternate hypotheses could be forwarded to explain these differences and should be explored to examine the robustness of these findings. For example, given a larger proportion of bachelor's degrees earned by blacks are in the liberal arts relative to the proportion of those earned by whites in the liberal arts, it is conceivable that the observed income differences are secondary to career-specific income differences. A stronger argument for the persistence of racism could be made if, for example, black males and white males with doctorates in psychology from Wayne State University, who currently work in the private sector of Detroit as consultants, earn different incomes.

The exploration of alternate hypotheses would also be important when interpreting data on ethnic group disparities in receiving medical treatments. For example, to the extent that atypical symptom presentations are associated with lower intervention rates (Summers, Cooper, Woodward, and Finerty, 2001), it could be argued that secondary to culturally sanctioned differences in symptom presentations, older members of ethnic minority groups do not present in ways that would lead to standard medical treatments. A cautionary note is in order, however, if in fact typical symptom presentations or standard assessment procedures are based or normed primarily on nonethnic minority group members and used to determine treatment options for ethnic minority elders. For example, Miles (2001) advised against the use of standard screening tools to assess cognitive functioning in elderly blacks. She reasoned that because cognitive functioning determines the course of various treatments for older adults, and black elders more than any other age cohort have been systematically deprived of access to quality education, the continued use of standard cognitive batteries, which are more likely to incorrectly label those whose education level does not exceed the seventh grade as being mildly demented, would perpetuate the untoward effects of institutional racism.

• In addition to studies examining interethnic group differences, coordinated federal efforts are needed to advocate for the importance of intraethnic group investigations. These efforts would help to serve at least two purposes. First, they might help to dismantle the erroneous belief, but widely accepted practice of many federal grant reviewers and journal editors, that "acceptable" research designs must include a white comparison group. Second, although it is important to decrease interethnic group disparities in the later years, it seems as if it would be equally important to decrease the prevalence of (dis)ease—regardless of interethnic group disparities.

ACKNOWLEDGMENTS

Preparation of this manuscript was supported by grants (1R03 MH56868 and 1 K01 MH01867) to the author from the National Institute of Mental Health.

REFERENCES

Adams, J.P., and Dressler, W.W. (1988). Perceptions of injustice in a black community: Dimensions and variations. *Human Relations, 41,* 753-767.

Alexander, G.C., and Sehgal, A.R. (1998). Barriers to cadaveric renal transplantation among blacks, women, and the poor. *Journal of the American Medical Association, 280,* 1148-1152.

American Anthropological Association. (1998). Statement on race. *American Anthropologist, 100,* 712-713.

Anderson, N.B., and Armstead, C.A. (1995). Toward understanding the association of socioeconomic status and health: A new challenge for the biopsychosocial approach. *Psychosomatic Medicine, 57,* 213-225.

Anderson, N.B., McNeilly, M., and Myers, H. (1991). Autonomic reactivity and hypertension in blacks: A review and proposed model. *Ethnicity and Disease, 1,* 154-170.

Armstead, C.A., Lawler, K.A., Gorden, G., Cross, J., and Gibbons, J. (1989). Relationship of racial stressors to blood pressure responses and anger expression in black college students. *Health Psychology, 8,* 541-556.

Aroian, K.J., Norris, A.E., Patsdaughter, C.A., and Tran, T.V. (1998). Predicting psychological distress among former Soviet immigrants. *International Journal of Social Psychiatry, 44,* 284-294.

Aspinall, P.J. (1998). Describing the "white" ethnic group and its composition in medical research. *Social Science and Medicine, 47,* 1797-1808.

Barnett, E., Casper, M.L., Halverson, J.A., Elmes, G.A., Braham, V.E., Majeed, Z.A., Bloom, A.S., and Stanley, S. (2001). *Men and heart disease: An atlas of racial and ethnic disparities in mortality* (1st ed.). Office for Social Environment and Health Research. Morgantown: West Virginia University.

Bird, S.T., and Bogart, L.M. (2001). Perceived race-based and socioeconomic status (SES)-based discrimination in interactions with health care providers. *Ethnicity and Disease, 11,* 554-563.

Bledsoe, T., Combs, M., Sigelman, L., and Welch, S. (1996). Trends in racial attitudes in Detroit, 1968-1992. *Urban Affairs Review, 31,* 508-528.

Brondolo, E., Rieppi, R., Kelly, K.P., and Gerin, W. (2003). Perceived racism and blood pressure: A review of the literature and conceptual and methodological critique. *Annals of Behavioral Medicine, 25,* 55-65.

Bullock, S.C., and Houston, E. (1987). Perceptions of racism by black medical students attending white medical schools. *Journal of the National Medical Association, 79,* 601-608.

Burchfield, S.R. (1979). The stress response: A new perspective. *Psychosomatic Medicine, 41,* 661-672.

Burchfield, S.R. (1985). Stress: An integrative framework. In S.R. Burchfield (Ed.), *Stress: Psychological and physiological interactions* (pp. 381-394). New York: Hemisphere.

Cacioppo, J. (1994). Social neuroscience. Autonomic, neuroendocrine, and immune responses to stress. *Psychophysiology, 31,* 113-128.

Carver, D.P., Scheier, M.F., and Weintraub, J.K. (1989). Assessing coping strategies: A theoretically based approach. *Journal of Personality and Social Psychology, 56,* 267-283.

Casper, M.L., Barnett, E., Halverson, J.A., Elmes, G.A., Braham, V.E., Majeed, Z.A., Bloom, A.S., and Stanley, S. (2000). *Women and heart disease: An atlas of racial and ethnic disparities in* mortality (2nd ed.). Office for Social Environment and Health Research. Morgantown: West Virginia University.

Charatz-Litt, C. (1992). A chronicle of racism: The effects of the white medical community on black health. *Journal of the National Medical Association, 84,* 717-725.

Chen, J., Rathore, S.S., Radford, M.J., Wang, Y., and Krumholz, H.M. (2001). Racial differences in the use of cardiac catheterization after acute myocardial infarction. *New England Journal of Medicine, 344,* 1443-1449.

Clark, R. (2000). Perceptions of interethnic group racism predict increased blood pressure responses to a laboratory challenge in college women. *Annals of Behavioral Medicine, 22,* 214-222.

Clark, R. (2003a). Parental history of hypertension and coping responses predict blood pressure changes to a perceived racism speaking task in black college volunteers. *Psychosomatic Medicine, 65,* 1012-1019.

Clark, R. (2003b). Self-reported racism and social support predict blood pressure reactivity in blacks. *Annals of Behavioral Medicine, 25,* 127-136.

Clark, R. (in press). Inter-ethnic group and intra-ethnic racism: Perceptions and coping in Black university students. *Journal of Black Psychology.*

Clark, R., and Adams, J.H. (in press). Moderating effects of perceived racism on John Henryism and blood pressure reactivity in Black college females. *Annals of Behavioral Medicine.*

Clark, R., and Anderson, N.B. (2001). Efficacy of racism-specific coping styles as predictors of cardiovascular functioning. *Ethnicity and Disease, 11,* 286-295.

Clark, R., Anderson, N.B., Clark, V.R., and Williams, D.R. (1999). Racism as a stressor for African Americans: A biopsychosocial model. *American Psychologist, 54,* 805-816.

Cohen, S., and Herbert, T.B. (1996). Health psychology: Psychological factors and physical disease from the perspective of human psychoneuroimmunology. *Annual Review of Psychology, 47,* 113-142.

Collier, J., and Burke, A. (1986). Racial and sexual discrimination in the selection of students for London medical schools. *Medical Education, 20,* 86-90.

Cooper, R.S. (1993). Health and the social status of blacks in the United States. *Annals of Epidemiology, 3,* 137-144.

Cooper, R.S. (2001). Social inequality, ethnicity and cardiovascular disease. *International Journal of Epidemiology, 30,* S48-S52.

Cuffe, S.P., Waller, J.L., Cuccaro, M.L., Pumariega, A.J., and Garrison, C.Z. (1995). Race and gender differences in the treatment of psychiatric disorders in young adolescents. *Journal of the American Academy of Child and Adolescent Psychiatry, 34,* 1536-1543.

Dressler, W.W., Baleiro, M.C., and Dos Santos, J.E. (1999). Culture, skin color, and arterial blood pressure in Brazil. *American Journal of Human Biology, 11,* 49-59.

Epstein, A.M., Ayanian, J.Z., Keogh, J.H., Noonan, S.J., Armistead, N., Cleary, P.D., Weissman, J.S., David-Kasdan, J.A., Carlson, D., Fuller, J., Marsh, D., and Conti, R.M. (2000). Racial disparities in access to renal transplantation—clinically appropriate or due to underuse or overuse? *New England Journal of Medicine, 343,* 1537-1544.

Essed, P. (1991). *Everyday racism.* Claremont, CA: Hunter House.

Fang, C.Y., and Myers, H.F. (2001). The effects of racial stressors and hostility on cardiovascular reactivity in African American and Caucasian men. *Health Psychology, 20,* 64-70.

Farley, J.H., Hines, J.F., Taylor, R.R., Carlson, J.W., Parker, M.F., Kost, E.R., Rogers, S.J., Harrison, T.A., Macri, C.I., and Parham, G.P. (2001). Equal care ensures equal survival for African-American women with cervical carcinoma. *Cancer, 91,* 869-873.

Ferguson, J.A., Weinberger, M., Westmoreland, G.R., Mamlin, L.A., Segar, D.S., Greene, J.Y., Martin, D.K., and Tierney, W.M. (1998). Racial disparity in cardiac decision making: Results from patient focus groups. *Archives of Internal Medicine, 158,* 1450-1453.

Fernando, S. (1984). Racism as a cause of depression. *International Journal of Social Psychiatry, 30,* 41-49.

Finch, B.K., Kolody, B., and Vega, WA. (2000). Perceived discrimination and depression among Mexican-origin adults in California. *Journal of Health and Social Behavior, 41,* 295-313.

Forman, T.A., Williams, D.R., and Jackson, J.S. (1997). Race, place, and discrimination. *Social Problems, 9,* 231-261.

Gary, L. (1995). African American men's perceptions of racial discrimination: A sociocultural analysis. *Social Work Research, 19,* 207-217.

Gatewood, W.B., Jr. (1988). Aristocrats of color: South and North, the black elite, 1880-1920. *Journal of Southern History, 54,* 3-20.

Gee, G.C. (2002). A multilevel analysis of the relationship between institutional and individual racial discrimination and health status. *American Journal of Public Health, 92,* 615-623.

Gilvarry, C.M., Walsh, E., Samele, C., Hutchinson, G., Mallet, R., Rabe-Hesketh, S., Fahy, T., van Os, J., and Murray, R.M. (1999). Life events, ethnicity and perceptions of discrimination in patients with severe mental illness. *Social Psychiatry and Psychiatric Epidemiology, 34,* 600-608.

Gleiberman, L., Harburg, E., Frone, M.R., Russell, M., and Cooper, M.L. (1993). Skin color, ancestry, and blood pressure among whites in Erie County, New York. *Ethnicity and Disease, 3,* 378-386.

Gleiberman, L., Harburg, E., Frone, M.R., Russell, M., and Cooper, M.L. (1995). Skin colour, measures of socioeconomic status, and blood pressure among blacks in Erie County, NY. *Annals of Human Biology, 22,* 69-73.

Gregory, P.M., Rhoads, G.C., Wilson, A.C., O'Dowd, K.J., and Kostis, J.B. (1999). Impact of availability of hospital-based invasive cardiac services on racial differences in the use of these services. *American Heart Journal, 138,* 507-517.

Guyll, M., Matthews, K.A., and Bromberger, J.T. (2001). Discrimination and unfair treatment: Relationship to cardiovascular reactivity among African American and European American women. *Health Psychology, 20,* 315-325.

Hall, D.E. (1992). Bias among African-Americans regarding skin color: Implications for social work practice. *Research on Social Work Practice, 2,* 479-486.

Harrell, J.P., Hall, S., and Taliaferro, J. (2003). Physiological responses to racism and discrimination: An assessment of the evidence. *American Journal of Public Health, 93,* 243-248.

Harrell, S.P. (2000). A multidimensional conceptualization of racism-related stress: Implications for the well-being of people of color. *American Journal of Orthopsychiatry, 70,* 42-57.

Herd, J.A. (1991). Cardiovascular responses to stress. *Physiological Reviews, 71,* 305-330.

Hughes, M., and Hertel, B.R. (1990). The significance of color remains: A study of life chances, mate selection, and ethnic consciousness among black Americans. *Social Forces, 68,* 1105-1120.

Jackson, S.A., Anderson, R.T., Johnson, N.J., and Sorlie, P.D. (2000). The relation of residential segregation to all cause mortality: A study in black and white. *American Journal of Public Health, 90,* 615-617.

James, S.A. (1993). Racial and ethnic differences in infant mortality and low birthweight: A psychosocial critique. *Annals of Epidemiology, 3,* 130-136.

Johnson, P.A., Lee, T.H., Cook, E.F., Rouan, G.W., and Goldman, L. (1993). Effect of race on the presentation and management of patients with acute chest pain. *Annals of Internal Medicine, 118,* 593-601.

Jones, J.M. (1972). *Prejudice and racism.* Reading, MA: Addison-Wesley.

Jones, J.M. (1997). *Prejudice and racism* (2nd ed.). New York: McGraw-Hill.

Karlsen, S., and Nazroo, J.Y. (2002). Relation between racial discrimination, social class, and health among ethnic minority groups. *American Journal of Public Health, 92,* 624-631.

Kasiske, B.L., London, W., and Ellison, M.D. (1998). Race and socioeconomic factors influencing early placement on the kidney transplant waiting list. *Journal of the American Society of Nephrology, 9,* 2142-2147.

Kaufman, J.S., Long, A.E., Liao, Y., Cooper, R.S., and McGee, D.L. (1998). The relationship between income and mortality in U.S. blacks and whites. *Epidemiology, 9,* 147-155.

Keith, V.M., and Herring, C. (1991). Skin tone and stratification in the black community. *American Journal of Sociology, 97,* 760-778.

Kennedy, B.P., Kawachi, I., Lochner, K., Jones, C., and Prothrow-Stith, D. (1997). (Dis)respect and black mortality. *Ethnicity and Disease, 7,* 207-214.

Kessler, R.C., Mickelson, K.D., and Williams, D.R. (1999). The prevalence, distribution, and mental health correlates of perceived discrimination in the United States. *Journal of Health and Social Behavior, 40,* 208-230.

Kiecolt-Glaser, J.K., Dura, J.R., Speicher, C.E., Trask, O.J., and Glaser, R. (1991). Spousal caregivers of dementia victims: Longitudinal changes in immunity and health. *Psychosomatic Medicine, 53,* 345-362.

King, G. (1996). Institutional racism and the medical/health complex: A conceptual analysis. *Ethnicity and Disease, 6,* 30-46.

Klag, M.J., Whelton, P.K., Coresh, J., Grim, C.E., and Kuller, L.H. (1991). The association of skin color with blood pressure in U.S. blacks with low socioeconomic status. *Journal of the American Medical Association, 265,* 599-602.

Klassen, A.C., Hall, A.G., Saksvig, B., Curbow, B., and Klassen, D.K. (2002). Relationship between patients' perceptions of disadvantage and discrimination and listing for kidney transplantation. *American Journal of Public Health, 92,* 811-817.

Klonoff, E.A., and Landrine, H. (2000). Is skin color a marker for racial discrimination? Explaining the skin color-hypertension relationship. *Journal of Behavioral Medicine, 23,* 329-338.

Knapp, R.G., Keil, J.E., Sutherland, S.E., Rust, P.F., Hames, C., and Tyroler, H.A. (1995). Skin color and cancer mortality among black men in the Charleston Heart Study. *Clinical Genetics, 47,* 200-206.

Krieger, N. (1990). Racial and gender discrimination: Risk factors for high blood pressure? *Social Science Medicine, 12,* 1273-1281.

Krieger, N. (1999). Embodying inequality: A review of concepts, measures, and methods for studying health consequences of discrimination. *International Journal of Health Services, 29,* 295-352.

Krieger, N., and Sidney, S. (1996). Racial discrimination and blood pressure: The CARDIA Study of young black and white adults. *American Journal of Public Health, 86,* 1370-1378.

Krieger, N., Rowley, D.L., Herman, A.A., Avery, B., and Phillips, M.T. (1993). Racism, sexism, and social class: Implications for studies of health, disease, and well-being. *American Journal of Preventive Medicine, 9,* 82-122.

Krieger, N., Sidney, S., and Coakley, E. (1998). Racial discrimination and skin color in the CARDIA study: Implications for public health research. *American Journal of Public Health, 88,* 1308-1313.

Kuno, E., and Rothbard, A.B. (2002). Racial disparities in antipsychotic prescription patterns for patients with schizophrenia. *American Journal of Psychiatry, 159,* 567-572.

Landrine, H., and Klonoff, E.A. (1996). The schedule of racist events: A measure of racial discrimination and a study of its negative physical and mental health consequences. *Journal of Black Psychology, 22,* 144-168.

Landrine, H., and Klonoff, E.A. (2000). Racial discrimination and cigarette smoking among blacks: Findings from two studies. *Ethnicity and Disease, 10,* 195-202.

LaVeist, T.A., Sellars, R., and Neighbors, H.W. (2001). Perceived racism and self and system blame attribution: Consequences for longevity. *Ethnicity and Disease, 11,* 711-721.

Lazarus, R.S., and Folkman, S. (1984). *Stress, appraisal, and coping.* New York: Springer.

Lewontin, R. (1995). *Human diversity.* New York: Scientific American Books.

Lieberman, L., and Jackson, F.L. (1995). Race and three models of human origin. *American Anthropologist, 97,* 231-242.

Loo, C.M., Fairbank, J.A., Scurfield, R.M., Ruch, L.O., King, D.W., Adams, L.J., and Chemtob, C.M. (2001). Measuring exposure to racism: Development and validation of a Race-Related Stress Scale (RRSS) for Asian American Vietnam veterans. *Psychological Assessment, 13,* 503-520.

Lowe, M., Kerridge, I.H., and Mitchell, K.R. (1995). "These sorts of people don't do very well": Race and allocation of health care resources. *Journal of Medical Ethics, 21,* 356-360.

Lowell, B.L., Teachman, J., and Jing, Z. (1995). Unintended consequences of immigration reform: Discrimination and Hispanic employment. *Demography, 32,* 617-628.

MacLean, M.J., Siew, N., Fowler, D., and Graham, I. (1987). Institutional racism in old age: Theoretical perspectives and a case study about access to social services [Special issue]. *Canadian Journal on Aging, 6,* 128-140.

Manuck, S.B., Kaplan, J.R., Muldoon, M.F., Adams, M.R., and Clarkson, T.B. (1991). The behavioral exacerbation of atherosclerosis and its inhibition by propranolol. In P.M. McCabe, N. Schneiderman, T.M. Field, and J.S. Skyler (Eds.), *Stress, coping and disease* (pp. 51-72). Hillsdale, NJ: Lawrence Erlbaum.

Manuck, S.B., Kaplan, J.R., Adams, M.R., and Clarkson, T.B. (1995). Studies of psychosocial influences on coronary artery atherosclerosis in cynomolgus monkeys. *Health Psychology, 7,* 113-124.

Marmot, M.G., Kogevinas, M., and Elston, M.A. (1987). Social/economic status and disease. *Annual Review of Public Health, 8,* 111-135.

McBean, A.M., and Gornick, M. (1994). Differences by race in the rates of procedures performed in hospitals for Medicare beneficiaries. *Health Care Financing Review, 15,* 77-90.

McCauley, J., Irish, W., Thompson, L., Stevenson, J., Lockett, R., Bussard, R., and Washington, M. (1997). Factors determining the rate of referral, transplantation, and survival on dialysis in women with ESRD. *American Journal of Kidney Diseases, 30,* 739-748.

McConahay, J.B., and Hough, J.C. (1976). Symbolic racism. *Journal of Social Issues, 32,* 23-45.

McDonald, R., Vechi, C., Bowman, J., and Sanson-Fisher, R. (1996). Mental health status of a Latin American community in New South Wales. *Australian and New Zealand Journal of Psychiatry, 30,* 457-462.

McEwen, B.S. (1998). Protective and damaging effects of stress mediators. *New England Journal of Medicine, 338,* 171-179.

McEwen, B.S. (2000). The neurobiology of stress: From serendipity to clinical relevance. *Brain Research, 886,* 172-189.

McEwen, B.S., and Seeman, T. (1999). Protective and damaging effects of mediators of stress: Elaborating and testing the concepts of allostasis and allostatic load. *Annals of the New York Academy of Sciences, 896,* 30-47.

McKeigue, P.M., Richards, J.D., and Richards, P. (1990). Effects of discrimination by sex and race on the early careers of British medical graduates during 1981-1987. *British Medical Journal, 301,* 961-964.

Meyer, I.H. (2003). Prejudice as stress: Conceptual and measurement problems. *American Journal of Public Health, 93,* 262-265.

Miles, T.P. (2001). Dementia, race, and education: A cautionary note for clinicians and researchers. *Journal of the American Geriatrics Society, 49,* 490.

Mosley, J.D., Appel, L.J., Ashour, Z., Coresh, J., Whelton, P.K., and Ibrahim, M.M. (2000). Relationship between skin color and blood pressure in Egyptian adults: Results from the National Hypertension Project. *Hypertension, 36,* 296-302.

National Center for Health Statistics. (1998). *Health, United States, 1998 with socioeconomic status and health chartbook.* Hyattsville, MD: Author.

Neal, A.M., and Wilson, M.L. (1989). The role of skin color and features in the black community: Implications for black women and therapy. *Clinical Psychology Review, 9,* 323-333.

Noh, S., Beiser, M., Kaspar, V., Hou, F., and Rummens, J. (1999). Discrimination and emotional well-being. *Journal of Health and Social Behavior, 40,* 193-207.

Okazawa-Rey, M., Robinson, T., and Ward, J.V. (1986). Black women and the politics of skin color and hair. *Women's Studies Quarterly, 14,* 13-14.

Outlaw, F.H. (1993). Stress and coping: The influence of racism on the cognitive appraisal processing of African Americans. *Issues in Mental Health Nursing, 14,* 399-409.

Pak, A.W., Dion, K.L., and Dion, K.K. (1991). Social-psychological correlates of experienced discrimination: Test of the double jeopardy hypothesis. *International Journal of Intercultural Relations, 15,* 243-254.

Pamuk, E., Makuc, D., Heck, K., Reuben, C., and Lochner, K. (1998). *Socioeconomic status and health chartbook: Health, United States, 1998.* Hyattsville, MD: National Center for Health Statistics.

Pappas, G., Queen, S., Hadden, W., and Fisher, G. (1993). The increasing disparity and mortality between socioeconomic groups in the United States, 1960 and 1986. *New England Journal of Medicine, 329,* 103-109.

Parra, E.O., and Espino, D.V. (1992). Barriers to health care access faced by elderly Mexican Americans [Special issue]. *Clinical Gerontologist, 11,* 171-177.

Pernice, R., and Brook, J. (1996). Refugees and immigrants' mental health: Association of demographic and post-migration factors. *Journal of Social Psychology, 136,* 511-519.

Peterson, E.D., Shaw, L.K., DeLong, E.R., Pryor, D.B., Califf, R.M., and Mark, D.B. (1997). Racial variation in the use of coronary-revascularization procedures. Are the differences real? Do they matter? *New England Journal of Medicine, 336,* 480-486.

Polednak, A.P. (1996). Segregation, discrimination and mortality in U.S. blacks. *Ethnicity and Disease, 6,* 99-108.

Rathore, S.S., Lenert, L.A., Weinfurt, K.P., Tinoco, A., Taleghani, C.K., Harless, W., and Schulman, K.A. (2000). The effects of patient sex and race on medical students' ratings of quality of life. *American Journal of Medicine, 108,* 561-566.

Rumbaut, R.G. (1994). The crucible within: Ethnic identity, self-esteem, and segmented assimilation among children of immigrants. *International Migration Review, 28,* 748-794.

Sakamoto, A., Wu, H.H., and Tzeng, J.M. (2000). The declining significance of race among American men during the latter half of the twentieth century. *Demography, 37,* 41-51.

Schulman, K.A., Berlin, J.A., Harless, W., Kerner, J.F., Sistrunk, S., Gersh, B.J., Dube, R., Taleghani, C.K., Burke, J.E., Williams, S., Eisenberg, J.M., and Escarce, J.J. (1999). The effect of race and sex on physicians' recommendations for cardiac catheterization. *New England Journal of Medicine, 340,* 618-626.

Schuman, H., and Hatchett, S. (1974). *Black racial attitudes.* Ann Arbor, MI: Institute for Social Research.

Sears, D.O. (1991). Symbolic racism. In P.A. Katz and D.A. Taylor (Eds.), *Eliminating racism: Profiles in controversy* (pp. 53-84). New York: Plenum Press.

Seeman, T.E., Singer, B.H., Rowe, J.W., Horwitz, R.I., and McEwen, B.S. (1997). Price of adaptation-allostatic load and its health consequences: MacArthur studies of successful aging. *Archives of Internal Medicine, 157,* 2259-2268.

Seligman, M.E.P. (1975). *Helplessness: On depression, development and death.* San Francisco: W. H. Freeman.

Sheifer, S.E., Escarce, J.J., and Schulman, K.A. (2000). Race and sex differences in the management of coronary artery disease. *American Heart Journal, 139,* 848-857.

Sigelman, L., and Welch, S. (1991). *Black Americans' views of racial inequality: The dream deferred.* New York: Cambridge University Press.

Smith, D.G., Shipley, R., and Rose, G. (1990). Magnitude and causes of socioeconomic differentials in mortality: Further evidence from the Whitehall Study. *Journal of Epidemiology and Community Health, 44,* 265-270.

Soucie, J.M., Neylan, J.F., and McClellan, W. (1992). Race and sex differences in the identification of candidates for renal transplantation. *American Journal of Kidney Diseases, 19,* 414-419.

Sterling, P., and Eyer, J. (1988). Allostasis: A new paradigm to explain arousal pathology. In S. Fisher and J. Reason (Eds.), *Handbook of life stress, cognition and health* (pp. 629-649). New York: John Wiley and Sons.

Summers, R.L., Cooper, G.J., Woodward, L.H., and Finerty, L. (2001). Association of atypical chest pain presentations by African Americans and the lack of utilization of reperfusion therapy. *Ethnicity and Disease, 11,* 463-468.

Tang, Z., and Trovato, R. (1998). Discrimination and Chinese fertility in Canada. *Social Biology, 45,* 172-193.

Taylor, A.J., Meyer, G.S., Morse, R., and Pearson, C.S. (1997). Can characteristics of a health care system mitigate ethnic bias in access to cardiovascular procedures? Experience from the Military Health Services System. *Journal of the American College of Cardiology, 30,* 901-907.

Telles, E.E., and Lim, N. (1998). Does it matter who answers the race question? Racial classification and income inequality in Brazil. *Demography, 35,* 465-474.

Tennstedt, S., and Chang, B.H. (1998). The relative contribution of ethnicity versus socioeconomic status in explaining differences in disability and receipt of informal care. *Journals of Gerontology. Series B, Psychological Sciences and Social Sciences, 53,* 61-70.

Udry, J.R., Bauman, K.E., and Chase, C. (1971). Skin color, status, and mate selection. *American Journal of Sociology, 76,* 722-733.

Utsey, S.O. (1998). Assessing the stressful effects of racism: A review of instrumentation. *Journal of Black Psychology, 24,* 269-288.

Utsey, S.O., and Ponterotto, J.G. (1996). Development and validation of the Index of Race-Related Stress (IRRS). *Journal of Counseling Psychology, 43,* 490-501.

Utsey, S.O., Payne, Y.A., Jackson, E.S., and Jones, A.M. (2002). Race-related stress, quality of life indicators, and life satisfaction among elderly African Americans. *Cultural Diversity and Ethnic Minority Psychology, 8,* 224-233.

Villarruel, A.M., Canales, M., and Torres, S. (2001). Bridges and barriers: Educational mobility of Hispanic nurses. *Journal of Nursing Education, 40,* 245-251.

West, P. (1997). Health inequalities in the early years: Is there equalisation in youth? *Social Science and Medicine, 44,* 833-858.

Whaley, A.L. (1998). Racism in the provision of mental health services: A social-cognitive analysis. *American Journal of Orthopsychiatry, 68,* 47-57.

Whitbeck, L.B., Hoyt, D.R., McMorris, B.J., Chen, X., and Stubben, J.D. (2001). Perceived discrimination and early substance abuse among American Indian children. *Journal of Health and Social Behavior, 42,* 405-424.

Whitfield, K., Weidner, G., Clark, R., and Anderson, N.B. (2002). Sociodemographic diversity in behavioral medicine. *Journal of Consulting and Clinical Psychology, 70,* 463-481.

Whittle, J., Conigliaro, J., Good, C.B., and Lofgren, R.P. (1993). Racial differences in the use of invasive cardiovascular procedures in the Department of Veterans Affairs medical system. *New England Journal of Medicine, 329,* 621-627.

Williams, D.R. (1997). Race and health: Basic questions, emerging directions. *Annals of Epidemiology, 7,* 322-333.

Williams, D.R., and Collins, C. (1995). Socioeconomic and racial differences in health. *Annual Review of Sociology, 21,* 349-386.

Williams, D.R., and Neighbors, H. (2001). Racism, discrimination and hypertension: Evidence and needed research. *Ethnicity and Disease, 11,* 800-816.

Williams, D.R., Yu, Y., and Jackson, J. (1997a, July). *The costs of racism: Discrimination, race, and health.* Paper presented at the joint meeting of the Public Health Conference on Records and Statistics and Data User's Conference, Washington, DC.

Williams, D.R., Yu, Y., Jackson, J., and Anderson, N. (1997b). Racial differences in physical and mental health: Socioeconomic status, stress and discrimination. *Journal of Health Psychology, 2,* 335-351.

Williams, D.R., Neighbors, H.W., and Jackson, J.S. (2003). Racial/ethnic discrimination and health: Findings from community studies. *American Journal of Public Health, 93,* 200-208.

Yetman, N. (1985). Introduction: Definitions and perspectives. In N. Yetman (Ed.), *Majority and minority: The dynamics of race and ethnicity in American life* (4th ed., pp. 1-20). Boston: Allyn and Bacon.

15

A Neurovisceral Integration Model of Health Disparities in Aging

Julian F. Thayer and Bruce H. Friedman

Significant ethnic disparities exist in the health of elderly Americans that cover a broad range of disorders, from the psychological to the physiological, and that are manifested in both morbidity and mortality differences. The life expectancies of minority groups in the United States and other industrialized countries are often dramatically reduced (see Chapter 2, this volume; Williams, 1997). Moreover, morbidity is often greater in ethnic minorities. For example, hypertension rates in African Americans are among the highest in the world, with the age-adjusted rate being more than 50 percent higher than for white Americans. African Americans also develop hypertension earlier and have much higher average blood pressures and higher rates of stage 3 hypertension than whites. These factors combine to produce higher rates of stroke mortality (80 percent higher), heart disease mortality (50 percent higher), and hypertension-related end-stage renal disease (320 percent higher) than whites (National High Blood Pressure Education Program, 1997). The prevalence of diabetes also varies greatly by ethnic group. The prevalence of known diabetes in African Americans is more than 1.7 times the rate of whites, whereas for some Native American tribes, the rate is more than 5.2 times that of whites (Black, 2002).

A number of potential pathways, both institutional and individual, to these health disparities have been identified, and include differential access to care, differential treatment, differential exposure to environmental pathogens, and differential exposure to chronic stress (Krieger, 2000). In this latter category, discrimination and racism have been implicated. This stressor is believed to be able to elicit the perception of threat from the environment, which in turn leads to a plethora of negative affective states, such as fear, anxiety, anger and hostility, and depression. Both acutely and chronically, these affective states may lead to negative health outcomes (Kiecolt-Glaser, McGuire, Robles, and Glaser, 2002; Krantz and McCeney, 2002). That ethnic minorities might be differentially exposed to racism-related stress and negative affect has been proposed as a possible causal factor in the observed health disparities (Clark, Anderson, Clark, and Williams, 1999; Williams and Neighbors, 2001). However, any comprehensive model of emotions and health must account for the complex mix of cognitive, affective, behavioral, and physiological concomitants of normal and pathological affective states and dispositions, and how these might impact health. In addition, the concept of stress is often invoked to explain the impact of psychosocial factors on physiological processes and health. However, this concept is plagued by a lack of a precise and widely accepted definition, and by a lack of specificity in the organismic mechanisms by which stress produces its effects (Eriksen and Ursin, 2002). Despite recent attempts to reconceptualize stress effects in terms of allostatic load (McEwen, 1998), the situation has not substantially improved (Eriksen and Ursin, 2002; Kiecolt-Glaser et al., 2002).

The impact of multiple pathways on ethnic health disparities must be acknowledged, but this chapter focuses on psychosocial factors. Broadly defined in terms of stress, negative emotion, and perceived racism, the core question is how these psychosocial factors are instantiated in physiological processes that can lead to disease and death. With the added premise that ethnic minorities are differentially and excessively exposed to discrimination and racism, the underlying causes of the health disparities begin to be revealed.

Due to the scope of the issues involved, coverage of the literature will be more illustrative than comprehensive. However, wherever possible, references to more comprehensive reviews and key primary sources are provided. We begin in a broad context within which to view the observed health disparities in the elderly by presenting evidence for the role of autonomic imbalance in disease and negative affective states and dispositions. The notion of appropriate energy regulation as a factor in health and disease is emphasized. Next, a brief description of a neurovisceral model of emotion regulation and dysregulation is offered, in which heart rate variability (HRV) is used to index important aspects of autonomic, affective, and cognitive system regulation. This model may help to explicate the complex interrelationships that exist in the connection between psychosocial factors on the one hand and health and disease on the other. This model utilizes a dynamical systems approach, and stresses the role of inhibitory processes via parasympathetic mechanisms in maintaining optimal energy regulation. A discussion follows in which perseverative thinking is viewed as the core cognitive toxic factor. Evidence is presented on the relationship among perseverative thinking, HRV, and poor health outcomes. The central concomitants of perseverative behavior and their links to hypervigilance also will be considered. Next, the relevance of this model to health disparities is shown. Relevant experimental and correlational data in support of elements of the model are supplied, including how they might relate to health disparities. Finally, we offer recommendations for future research that might flesh out the model and further guide the understanding of health disparities in the elderly.

AUTONOMIC IMBALANCE IN DISEASE AND NEGATIVE EMOTIONS

There is growing evidence for the role of the autonomic nervous system (ANS) in a wide range of diseases. The ANS is generally conceived to have two major branches—the sympathetic system, associated with energy mobilization, and the parasympathetic system, associated with vegetative and restorative functions. Normally, the activity of these branches is in dynamic balance. For example, there is a well-documented circadian rhythm such that sympathetic activity is higher during daytime hours and parasympathetic activity increases at night. Other periodicities are present, and the activity of the two branches can be rapidly modulated in response to changing environmental demands. More modern conceptions of organism function based on complexity theory hold that organism stability, adaptability, and health are maintained through variability in the dynamic relationship among system elements (Friedman and Thayer, 1998a, 1998b; Thayer and Friedman, 1997; Thayer and Lane, 2000). Thus, patterns of organized variability, rather than static levels, are preserved in the face of constantly changing environmental demands. This conception, in contrast to homeostasis, posits that the system has multiple points of stability, which necessitate a dynamic organization of resources to match specific situational demands. These demands can be conceived in terms of energy regulation such that the points of relative stability represent local energy minima required by the situation. For example, in healthy individuals, average heart rate (HR) is greater during the day, when energy demands are higher, than at night, when energy demands are lower. Thus, the system has a local energy minimum or attractor for daytime and another for nighttime. Because the system operates "far from equilibrium," the system is always searching for local energy minima to minimize the energy requirements of the organism. Consequentially, optimal system functioning is achieved via lability and variability in its component processes, and rigid regularity is associated with mortality, morbidity, and ill health (Lipsitz and Goldberger, 1992; Peng et al., 1994).

Another corollary of this view is that autonomic imbalance, in which one branch of the ANS dominates over the other, is associated with a lack of dynamic flexibility and health. Empirically, there is a large body of evidence to suggest that autonomic imbalance, in which typically the sympathetic system is hyperactive and the parasympathetic system is hypoactive, is associated with various pathological conditions (Malliani, Pagani, and Lombardi, 1994). In particular, when the sympathetic branch dominates for long periods of time, the energy demands on the system become excessive and ultimately cannot be met, eventuating in death. The prolonged state of alarm associated with negative emotions likewise places an excessive energy demand on the system. On the way to death, however, premature aging and disease characterize a system dominated by negative affect and autonomic imbalance.

Like many organs in the body, the heart is dually innervated. Although a wide range of physiologic factors determines HR, the ANS is the most prominent. Importantly, when both cardiac vagal (the primary parasympathetic nerve) and sympathetic inputs are blocked pharmacologically (for example, with atropine plus propranolol, the so-called double blockade), intrinsic HR is higher than the normal resting HR (Jose and Collison, 1970). This fact supports the idea that the heart is under tonic inhibitory control by parasympathetic influences. Thus, resting cardiac autonomic balance favors energy conservation by way of parasympathetic dominance over sympathetic influences. In addition, the HR time series is characterized by beat-to-beat variability over a wide range, which also implicates vagal dominance. Lowered HRV is associated with increased risk of mortality, and HRV has been proposed as a marker for disease (Task Force of the European Society of Cardiology and the North American Society of Pacing Electrophysiology, 1996).

Resting HR can be used as a rough indicator of autonomic balance, and several large studies have shown a largely linear, positive dose-response relationship between resting HR and all-cause mortality (see Habib, 1999, for review). This association was independent of gender and ethnicity, and showed a threefold increase in mortality in persons with HR over 90 beats per minute (bpm) compared to those with HRs of less than 60 bpm. It was suggested that this relationship is due to the role of HR as a major determinant of myocardial oxygen demand and the direct link of HR to the rate of myocardial energy use.

Brook and Julius (2000) have recently detailed how autonomic imbalance in the sympathetic direction is associated with a range of metabolic, hemodynamic, trophic, and rheologic abnormalities that contribute to elevated cardiac morbidity and mortality. Although the relationship between HR and cardiovascular morbidity and mortality may be assumed, the fact that autonomic imbalance and HR are related to other diseases may not be as obvious. However, links do exist. For example, HRV has been shown to be associated with diabetes mellitus, and decreased HRV has been shown to precede evidence of disease provided by standard clinical tests (Ziegler, Laude, Akila, and Elgwhozi, 2001). In addition, immune dysfunction and inflammation have been implicated in a wide range of conditions associated with aging including cardiovascular disease, diabetes, osteoporosis, arthritis, Alzheimer's disease, periodontal disease, and certain types of cancers as well as declines in muscle strength and increased frailty and disability (Ershler and Keller, 2000; Kiecolt-Glaser et al., 2002). The common mechanism seems to involve excess proinflammatory cytokines such as interleuken 1 and 6 and tumor necrosis factor. Importantly, increased parasympathetic tone and acetylcholine (the primary parasympathetic neurotransmitter) have been shown to attenuate release of these proinflammatory cytokines, and sympathetic hyperactivity is associated with their increased production (Das, 2000; Maier and Watkins, 1998; Tracey, 2002). Thus, autonomic imbalance may be a final common pathway to increased morbidity and mortality from a host of conditions and diseases.

Although the idea is not new (Sternberg, 1997), several recent reviews have provided strong evidence linking negative affective states and dispositions to disease and ill health (Friedman and Thayer, 1998b; Kiecolt-Glaser et al., 2002; Krantz and McCeney, 2002; Musselman, Evans, and Nemeroff, 1998; Rozanski, Blumenthal, and Kaplan, 1999; Verrier and Mittleman, 2000). All of these reviews implicate altered ANS function and decreased parasympathetic activity as a possible mediator in this link.

An additional pathway between psychosocial stressors and ill health is an indirect one, in which psychosocial factors lead to poor lifestyle choices, including a lack of physical activity and the abuse of tobacco, alcohol, and drugs. Both sedentary lifestyle and substance abuse are associated with autonomic imbalance and decreased parasympathetic tone (Ingjaldsson, Laberg, and Thayer, 2003c; Nabors-Oberg, Sollers, Niaura, and Thayer, 2002; Reed, Porges, and Newlin, 1999; Rossy and Thayer, 1998; Weise, Krell, and Brinkhoff, 1986). In fact, the therapeutic effectiveness of smoking cessation, reduced alcohol consumption, and increased physical activity rest in part on their ability to restore autonomic balance and increase parasympathetic tone.

In sum, autonomic imbalance and decreased parasympathetic tone in particular may be the final common pathway linking negative affective states and dispositions, including the indirect effects via poor lifestyle, to numerous diseases and conditions associated with aging as well as increased morbidity and mortality.

THE MODEL IN A NUTSHELL

A comprehensive model of emotions and health must account for the complex mix of cognitive, affective, behavioral, and physiological

concomitants of normal and pathological affective states and dispositions, and how these might impact health. In this chapter, a model is
outlined that integrates some of these components into a functional and
structural network that may help to guide the understanding of emotion
and health. Functionally, this network involves autonomic, affective,
and cognitive regulation, and structurally it entails reciprocal inhibitory
circuits between prefrontal cortex and subcortical evolutionarily primitive motivational structures, that can be indexed by rhythmic activity of
the cardiovascular system. Research that relates functional aspects of
this circuitry to psychophysiological regulation will be briefly reviewed.
We emphasize the relationships among autonomic, affective, and cognitive regulation in organism health, and propose a group of underlying
physiological systems that integrate these functions in the service of self-
regulation and adaptability. This network is placed in the context of a
dynamical systems model that involves feedback and feedforward circuits, with special attention to negative feedback mechanisms and inhibitory processes. It will be shown that the negative behavioral states
and dispositions associated with a relative autonomic sympathetic imbalance reflect a disinhibition of positive feedback circuits that are normally under tonic inhibitory control.

Other models have also been proposed to account for the effects of
emotions and stress on health and disease. The allostatic load model has
garnered much recent attention, particularly in medical circles (McEwen,
1998). The recently proposed psychoneuroimmunology model highlights
the increasing role that inflammation has been shown to play in a wide
variety of diseases, including cardiovascular disease (Kiecolt-Glaser et al.,
2002). The reactivity model has been the stalwart in psychophysiology
and behavioral medicine (see Krantz and McCeney, 2002). The
neurovisceral integration model (NIM) builds on these prior models, but
has important differences from them as well. First, the NIM is a true
multilevel model incorporating factors from the sociopolitical to the molecular. Second, the NIM specifies in detail the core cognitive toxic factor,
that of perseverative thinking, and explicates its neural and physiological
concomitants. Third, the NIM proposes the autonomic nervous system,
with an emphasis on the parasympathetic nervous system, as the final
common pathway linking psychological and physiological states and dispositions. Fourth, the NIM is based on a nonlinear dynamical systems
perspective and highlights the role of feedback and feedforward networks
and their interplay in the maintenance of the dynamic flexibility of the
organism. Finally, the NIM emphasizes inhibitory, negative feedback processes and explicates their physiological substrates at both the central and
peripheral levels. Thus the NIM incorporates many aspects of the prior
models and is not contradictory to them, but expands on them in ways

that are needed to account for the extant data and to generate testable hypotheses for future research.

The Central Autonomic Network

Investigators have identified functional units within the central nervous system (CNS) that support goal-directed behavior and adaptability. One such entity is the central autonomic network (CAN) (Benarroch, 1993, 1997). Functionally, this network is an integrated component of an internal regulation system through which the brain controls visceromotor, neuroendocrine, and behavioral responses that are critical for goal-directed behavior, adaptability, and health. Structurally, the CAN includes the anterior cingulate, insular, orbitofrontal, and ventromedial prefrontal cortices, the central nucleus of the amygdala, the paraventricular and related nuclei of the hypothalamus, the periaquaductal gray matter, the parabrachial nucleus, the nucleus of the solitary tract (NTS), the nucleus ambiguous, the ventrolateral medulla, the ventromedial medulla, and the medullary tegmental field (see Figure 15-1). These components are reciprocally interconnected such that information flows bidirectionally between lower and higher levels of the CNS. The primary output of the CAN is mediated through preganglionic sympathetic and parasympathetic neurons that innervate the heart via the stellate ganglia and vagus nerve, respectively. The interplay of these inputs to the cardiac sino-atrial node produces the complex variability that characterizes the HR time series (Saul, 1990). Thus, the output of the CAN is directly linked to HRV. Notably, vagal influences dominate cardiac chronotropic control (Levy, 1990). In addition, sensory information from peripheral end organs such as the heart and the immune system are fed back to the CAN. Thus, HRV is an indicator of central-peripheral neural feedback and CNS-ANS integration.

Moreover, the CAN has many features of a dynamical system. First, the components of the CAN are reciprocally interconnected, allowing for unbroken positive and negative feedback interactions and integration of autonomic responses. Second, the CAN consists of numerous parallel, distributed pathways, which permit multiple avenues to a given response. For example, a HR change of 72 to 90 bpm can be attained by various permutations of sympathetic and vagal input, including increased sympathetic or decreased vagal activity or some combination of the two, or by other processes such as circulating hormones. Moreover, within the CAN, direct and indirect paths can regulate output to preganglionic sympathetic and parasympathetic neurons. Third, CAN activity is state dependent and thus sensitive to initial conditions (see Glass and Mackey, 1988).

The CAN receives and integrates visceral, humoral, and environmental information; organizes autonomic, endocrine, and behavioral responses to

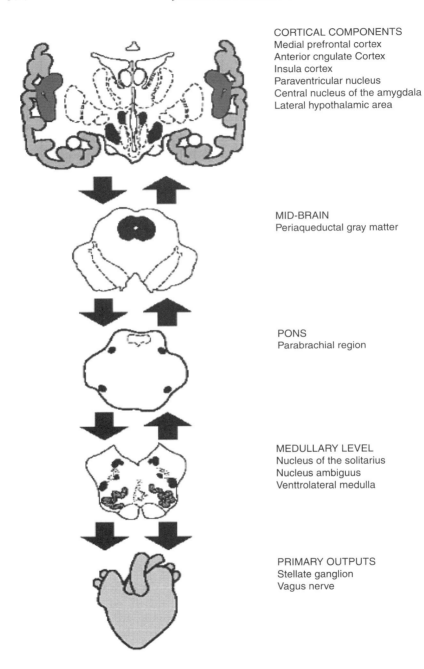

CORTICAL COMPONENTS
Medial prefrontal cortex
Anterior cngulate Cortex
Insula cortex
Paraventricular nucleus
Central nucleus of the amygdala
Lateral hypothalamic area

MID-BRAIN
Periaqueductal gray matter

PONS
Parabrachial region

MEDULLARY LEVEL
Nucleus of the solitarius
Nucleus ambiguus
Venttrolateral medulla

PRIMARY OUTPUTS
Stellate ganglion
Vagus nerve

FIGURE 15-1 Central nervous system structures involved in neurovisceral integration.

environmental challenges; and is under tonic inhibitory control. This inhibition is achieved by γ-aminobutyric acid (GABA), the main inhibitory CNS neurotransmitter, emanating from interneurons within the NTS. Disruption of this pathway may lead to hypertension and sinus tachycardia, and represents a disinhibition of sympathoexcitatory circuits in the CAN (Benarroch, 1993, 1997; Masterman and Cummings, 1997; Spyer, 1989).

Other functional units within the CNS serving executive, social, affective, attentional, and motivated behavior in humans and animals have been identified (Damasio, 1998; Devinsky, Morrell, and Vogt, 1995; Masterman and Cummings, 1997; Spyer, 1989). One such network has been termed the anterior executive region (AER; Devinsky et al., 1995). The AER and its projections regulate behavior by monitoring the motivational quality of internal and external stimuli. The AER network has been called the "rostral limbic system" and includes the anterior, insular, and orbitofrontal cortices, amygdala, periaquaductal gray, ventral striatum, and autonomic brainstem motor nuclei. Damasio (1998) has recognized a similar neural "emotion circuit" for which there is considerable structural overlap with the CAN and the AER (Thayer and Lane, 2000).

We propose that the CAN, the AER network, Damasio's (1998) "emotion circuit," and related systems (Masterman and Cummings, 1997; Spyer, 1989) represent a common central functional network recognized by different researchers from diverse approaches. This CNS network is associated with the processes of response organization and selection, and serves to control psychophysiological resources in attention and emotion (Friedman and Thayer, 1998a, 1998b; Thayer and Friedman, 1997). Additional structures are flexibly recruited to manage specific behavioral adaptations. This sparsely interconnected neural complex allows for maximal organism flexibility in accommodating rapidly changing environmental demands. When this network is either rigidly coupled or completely uncoupled, the ability to recruit and utilize appropriate neural support to meet a particular demand is hampered, and the organism is thus less adaptive.

Autonomic Regulation

Autonomically mediated HRV is useful as an index of neurovisceral integration and organismic self-regulation. The interaction of sympathetic and parasympathetic outputs of the CAN at the sino-atrial node produces the complex beat-to-beat variability that marks a healthy, adaptive organism. Vagal activity dominates HR control, and thus HR is under tonic inhibitory vagal control (Levy, 1990; Uijtdehaage and Thayer, 2000). HRV is also associated with prefrontal cortex activity (Lane, Reiman, Ahern, and Thayer, 2001), and the prefrontal cortex has been inversely related to subcortical activity in structures such as the amygdala that have been implicated in primitive motivation systems (Davidson, 2000).

Several lines of research point to the significance of HRV in emotions and health. Decreased HRV is linked with a number of disease states, including cardiovascular disease, diabetes, obesity, and lack of physical exercise (Stein and Kleiger, 1999). Reduced vagally mediated HRV is also associated with a number of psychological disease states, such as anxiety, depression, and hostility. For example, low HRV is consistent with the cardiac symptoms of panic anxiety as well as with its psychological expressions in poor attentional control and emotion regulation, and behavioral inflexibility (Friedman and Thayer, 1998a, 1998b). Similar reductions in HRV have been found in depression (Thayer, Smith, Rossy, Sollers, and Friedman, 1998), generalized anxiety disorder (Thayer, Friedman, and Borkovec, 1996), and posttraumatic stress disorder (Cohen, Matar, Kaplan, and Kotler, 1999). Low levels of vagal cardiovascular influence serve to disinhibit sympathoexcitatory influences. Due to differences in the temporal kinetics of the autonomic neuroeffectors, sympathetic effects on cardiac control are relatively slow (order of magnitude seconds) compared to vagal effects (order of magnitude milliseconds; see Saul, 1990). Thus, when this rapid vagal cardiac control is low, HR cannot change as quickly in response to environmental changes. In this view, the prefrontal cortex modulates subcortical motivational circuits to serve goal-directed behavior. When the prefrontal cortex is taken "offline" for whatever reason, a relative sympathetic dominance associated with disinhibited defensive circuits is released.

Human evidence for the inhibitory role of the frontal cortex comes from a recent study of HR and HRV before and after right- and left-side intracarotid sodium amobarbital (ISA) injection (Ahern et al., 1994). HR changes were similar during each hemisphere's pharmacological inactivation. During the 10-minute inactivations of either hemisphere, HR increased, peaked around the third minute, and gradually declined toward baseline values. These data indicate that the frontal cortex exerts tonic inhibition on brainstem sympathoexcitatory circuits. There were lateralized effects: larger and faster HR increases occurred during right-hemisphere inactivation. Moreover, vagally mediated HRV decreases were also greater in the right-hemisphere inactivations, mirroring the hemispheric effects on HR. These results support anatomical and physiological findings that right-hemispheric autonomic cardiac inputs are associated with greater chronotropic (rate) control.

The effects of the ISA test are largely restricted to anterior neural structures, which include the orbital and medial prefrontal cortices (Ahern et al., 1994; Hong et al., 2000). These areas are linked broadly with biopsychological functions such as affective, cognitive, and autonomic regulation (Thayer and Lane, 2000). Additionally, these structures are related to inhibitory control of behavior in general (Roberts and Wallis, 2000) and cardiac behavior in particular (Verberne and Owens, 1998). It is noteworthy that direct and indirect pathways connect these areas with vagal motor output regions (Ter Horst, 1999). Many researchers have proposed inhibitory cortical-subcortical circuits (Benarroch, 1993, 1997; Masterman and Cummings, 1997; Mayberg et al., 1999; Spyer, 1989), but our group is the first to tie these circuits to HRV (Thayer and Friedman, 2002; Thayer and Lane, 2000). The ISA test results provide compelling evidence that cortical structures tonically inhibit sympathoexcitatory circuits by way of vagal mechanisms.

It has been proposed that the prefrontal cortex is taken "offline" during emotional stress to let automatic, prepotent processes regulate behavior (Arnsten and Goldman-Rakic, 1998). This selective prefrontal inactivation may be adaptive by facilitating predominantly nonvolitional behaviors associated with subcortical neural structures such as the amygdala to organize responses without delay from the more deliberative and consciously guided prefrontal cortex. In modern society, however, inhibition, delayed response, and cognitive flexibility are vital for successful adjustment and self-regulation, and prolonged prefrontal inactivity can lead to hypervigilance, defensiveness, and perseveration.

A common reciprocal inhibitory cortical-subcortical neural circuit may structurally link psychological processes such as emotion with health-related physiology, and this circuit can be indexed with HRV. This neural network permits the prefrontal cortex to inhibit subcortical structures associated with defensive behaviors, and thus promote flexible responsiveness to environmental changes. For example, when faced with threat, tonic inhibitory subcortical control can be withdrawn quickly, leading to sympathoexcitatory survival ("fight or flight") responses. However, when this network is disrupted, a rigid, defensive pattern emerges with associated perseverations in cognitive, affective, and autonomic behavior. This protracted state of action readiness and associated sympathetic activity may be the pathogenic state underlying the increased morbidity and mortality found in chronic negative psychological states and dispositions.

Affective Regulation

Affect regulation is a valuable skill that has clear implications for health. Emotions represent a distillation of an individual's perception of personally relevant environmental interactions, including not only challenges and threats but also the ability to respond to them (Frijda, 1988). Viewed as such, emotions reflect the integrity of one's ongoing adjustment to constantly changing environmental demands. Emotions have also been characterized as an organism's response to the environment that allows for rapid mobilization of multiple action subsystems (Levenson, 1988). In this context, emotions are the uninterrupted output of continuous sequential behavior. These lawful behavioral sequences are organized around biologically important functions and have been termed "behavioral systems" (Timberlake, 1994). Put another way, emotions act to coordinate efficient responses for goal-directed behavior. For example, when faced with danger, a defensive behavioral system might be activated. The first stage of this sequence might involve the experience of anxiety, increased HR and a general shift toward sympathetic autonomic activity, and vigilant scanning of the environment for signs of danger. If a threat is identified, the next stage might involve fear and mobilization for "fight or flight." However, in contemporary life, fully aggressive or escape responses are rarely appropriate. As Frijda (1988) noted, specific emotions imply specific eliciting stimuli, specific action tendencies including selective attention to relevant stimuli, and specific reinforcers. When this system works properly, it promotes flexible adaptation to shifting environmental demands. In another sense, an emotional response represents a selection of an optimal response and the inhibition of less functional ones from a broad behavioral repertoire, with the goal of matching energy use to fit situational requirements.

Several psychophysiological measures have proven to be useful indices of affect regulation. One is the reflexive startle blink, the magnitude of which can be affected by emotional state. The emotion-modulated startle is a robust phenomenon that has been demonstrated in a wide range of experimental situations, and has been broadly linked to affective and motivational phenomena (Lang, 1995). Similarly, HRV has been associated with a diverse range of processes, including affective and attentional regulation (Porges, 1992; Porges, Doussard-Roosevelt, and Maita, 1994). The relationship between these two important measures of affective regulation was recently investigated (Ruiz-Padial, Sollers, Vila, and Thayer, 2003). Ninety female participants viewed pleasant, neutral, and unpleasant pictures while exposed to acoustic startle stimuli. Eyeblink strength to startle probes was recorded both during affective foregrounds and intertrial intervals, and the relationship between resting HRV and startle magnitudes was examined. Resting HRV was found to be inversely related to both intertrial interval and emotion-modulated startle magnitude. In addition, subjects with the highest HRV showed the most differentiated emotion-modulated startle effects, whereas those with the lowest HRV showed significant augmentation of startle to neutral foregrounds and marginally potentiated startle to pleasant foregrounds. Thus, individuals with low HRV reacted to neutral, harmless stimuli as if they were aversive and threatening, and also had a tendency to react similarly to positive stimuli. In addition, individuals with high HRV were able to best match their response to situational demands and thus respond most appropriately to the energy requirements of the situation. The findings are consistent with our model that posits that pre-frontal cortical activity modulates subcortical motivation circuits in the service of goal-directed behavior and appropriate energy regulation. More-over, persons with low HRV showed evidence of hypervigilance and the activation of a defensive behavioral system in response to nonthreatening stimuli.

Numerous studies in both animals and humans suggest that an intact amygdala is associated with larger startle magnitude and emotion-potenti-ated startle during an unpleasant foreground (Aggleton and Young, 2000; Angrilli et al., 1996). A related structure, the bed nucleus of the stria terminalis, has been implicated in the general startle sensitivity associated with anxiety in rats and negative affect in humans (Bradley and Lang, 2000). Evidence for a role of medial prefrontal activity in startle response regulation can be found in its inverse association with amygdaloid activity (Davidson, 2000). The reported relationship between startle modulation and HRV provides further support for the notion that prefrontal activity is inversely related to structural functions associated with defensiveness, and thereby moderates interactions with the environment (Thayer and Lane, 2000). These results also further suggest that HRV can be used to index activity in this network of neural structures associated with emotional regu-lation.

Attentional Regulation and Executive Function

Attentional regulation and the ability to inhibit prepotent but inappro-priate responses are also important for health in a complex environment. Many tasks important for survival in today's world involve cognitive func-tions such as working memory, sustained attention, behavioral inhibition, and general mental flexibility. These tasks are all associated with prefrontal cortical activity (Arnsten and Goldman-Rakic, 1998). Deficits in these cog-nitive functions tend to accompany aging, and are also present in negative affective states and dispositions such as depression and anxiety. Stress can also impair cognitive function and may contribute to the cognitive deficits observed in various mental disorders. It is also possible that autonomic dysregulation contributes to decline in attention and cognitive performance. A series of experiments in our lab have been conducted to examine this issue, and will be described.

In a recent experiment, Johnsen et al. (2003) examined inhibitory re-sponses in an emotional Stroop paradigm. Dental phobics were first ex-posed to recorded scenes of dental procedures and then administered the emotional Stroop test. In addition to the traditional color-congruent and color-incongruent words, phobic subjects also were asked to respond to neutral words and dental-related words (e.g., "drill" and "cavity") that were threatening to them. All subjects exhibited longer reaction times to the color-incongruent words and the dental-related threat words, and thus displayed a difficulty in inhibiting prepotent responses. However, greater HRV was associated with faster reaction times to these words, consistent with the link among vagally mediated HRV, inhibitory ability, and frontal lobe function. These results support the idea that vagally mediated HRV is associated with efficient attentional regulation and greater ability to inhibit prepotent but inappropriate responses.

Subsequent studies further examined executive function and working memory in healthy individuals. In the first experiment, subjects performed a number of tasks involving continuous performance, including a simple reaction time task, a choice reaction time task, and three tasks that involved delayed responding and working memory (Hansen, Johnsen, and Thayer, 2003; Johnsen, Hansen, Murison, and Thayer, 2001). These latter tasks involved the presentation of a sequence of digits that required a response when a digit was identical to one that appeared either one or two back in the series, and have been shown to be associated with prefrontal activity (Goldman-Rakic, 1998). HRV and cortisol responses were recorded, and subjects were grouped into low and high HRV groups. Performance on tasks involving simple and choice reaction times did not differ between these groups. However, on tasks associated with prefrontal activity, subjects in the low HRV group performed more poorly in terms of reaction time, number of errors, and number of correct responses than those in the high HRV group. In addition, the groups did not differ in baseline, morning, or evening cortisol, but the low HRV group showed larger cortisol responses to cognitive tasks that lasted into the posttask recovery period. Stress is associated with an increased cortisol release, and cortisol plays a major role in immune function through its association with proinflammatory cytokines (Kiecolt-Glaser et al., 2002). Cortisol is also known to impair function on cognitive tasks associated with prefrontal cortex (Lupien, Gillin, and Hauger, 1999). Thus, the low HRV group was less stress tolerant as indexed by cortisol responses and more impaired cognitively than the high HRV group.

In another study in the series, subjects performed the same tasks as described earlier, but half did so under threat of electric shock (Hansen, Johnsen, Sollers, and Thayer, 2002). Again, subjects were divided into two groups based on resting HRV levels. In the shock threat condition, task performance involving delayed responding and prefrontal activity was significantly impaired in the low HRV group. Thus, persons with high HRV were more stress tolerant and less affected by the threat compared to those with low HRV. In yet another study, HRV was manipulated by having half of the subjects in a physically active group undergo mild detraining for 4 weeks. Aerobic capacity and HRV were significantly reduced in this group compared to those who maintained their fitness and HRV levels. All subjects again performed the above cognitive tasks: once before the 4-week detraining period, and once after. The detrained, lower HRV group failed to show the expected learning effect associated with repeated performance of the cognitive tasks, and thus did not reap the typical benefit of previous task exposure.

Taken together, these results support the usage of HRV to index efficient allocation of attentional and cognitive resources needed for efficient functioning in a challenging environment in which delayed responding and behavioral inhibition are key. In addition, these data show that low HRV marks increased risk to stress exposure. Significantly, these results provide a connection among stress-related cognitive deficits, high negative affect, and negative health consequences via the common mechanism of autonomic imbalance and low parasympathetic activity.

Summary of the Model

Autonomic, cognitive, and affective regulation assist an organism in facing the challenge of an environment in constant flux. However, the importance of inhibitory processes in self-regulatory behavior has not yet made its way into the dominant thinking in this area. From a systems perspective, inhibitory processes can be viewed as negative feedback circuits that permit the interruption of ongoing behavior and redeployment of resources to other tasks. When these negative feedback mechanisms are compromised, positive feedback loops may develop as a result of disinhibition. These positive circuits can have disastrous consequences by promoting hypervigilance, perseveration, and continued system activation, thereby limiting resource availability for other processes. This state of affairs can provide a chronic pathogenic substrate for psychological processes and emotions to negatively impact health. For example, at the synaptic level, ". . . substances which interfere with inhibitory synaptic action would cause unfettered excitatory action of neuron onto neuron and so lead to convulsions" (McGeer, Eccles, and McGeer, 1978, p. 134).

Healthy systems involve both positive and negative feedback circuits (Glass and Mackey, 1988; Goldberger, 1992). That inhibitory circuits may be indexed by vagally mediated HRV has several implications. First, vagal influences on the cardiovascular system represent negative chronotropic and dromotropic (conduction) mechanisms that are associated with system flexibility, responsivity, and stability (Levy, 1990; Porges, 1992). Second, as an index of central-peripheral neural feedback mechanisms, vagally mediated HRV represents a psychophysiological resource that the organism can bring to bear on environmental challenges (Friedman and Thayer, 1998b). Third, framing the diverse self-regulatory functions and dysfunctions observed in terms of vagal as opposed to sympathetic processes may be a more parsimonious representation of the data (Friedman and Thayer, 1998b; Thayer and Friedman, 1997). From this perspective, the relative sympathetic activation and autonomic imbalance seen in psychological and physiological disorders may represent disinhibition due to faulty inhibitory mechanisms. One key additional factor makes this conceptualization in terms of autonomic imbalance particularly relevant to the health disparities in aging. Whereas the traditional risk factors such as smoking, total cholesterol, obesity, and even hypertension, many of which are used to index allostatic load (Seeman, Singer, Rowe, Horwitz, and McEwen, 1997), lose their predictive value in old age, autonomic imbalance continues to be predictive of morbidity and mortality (Kiecolt-Glaser et al., 2002; Palatini and Julius, 1999).

Perseverative Thinking as the Core Cognitive Toxic Factor

Perseverative thinking, common to a number of negative affective states and dispositions, including depression, anxiety disorders, posttraumatic stress disorder, and perhaps many medically unexplained syndromes, is repetitive, abstract, and involuntary and represents a failure of inhibitory neural processes (Thayer and Lane, 2000). This cognitive mode is thought to serve several different functions. The most straightforward function attributed to worry and perseverative thinking is an attempt, albeit thwarted, at constructive mental problem solving (Davey, 1994). In support of this role, Davey (1994) and coworkers found positive correlations between worry and problem-focused coping, but only after partialing out the effect of trait anxiety. Thus, worry appeared to be associated with a habitual tendency for active problem solving combined with low confidence in succeeding in it. This is similar to the concept of "John Henryism" that has been related to exaggerated stress responses and poor health (James, 1994). Tallis and Eysenck (1994) proposed a tripartite function of worry. First, worry serves an alarm function, acting to interrupt ongoing behavior and directing awareness toward an issue demanding immediate solution. Second, worry has a prompt function, continuously representing unresolved threatening situations to awareness. Third, worry is proposed to have a preparation function, anticipating threat and readying the organism for a situation in which intense motor activation is needed. Obviously, such a situation is rare relative to typical levels of worry and perseverative thinking. Thus, perseverative thinking theoretically engenders a protracted state of psychophysiological "action preparation" without resolution.

Thus, perseverative thought reflects a disinhibition of a potentially adaptive frontal lobe mechanism in higher organisms. The frontal lobes have reciprocal neural connections with more evolutionarily primitive subcortical structures that are partially responsible for basic approach and avoidance behavior. When these structures are disinhibited, a number of processes associated with threat response are unleashed, including hypervigilance and fear, as well as changes such as increased HR and blood pressure associated with autonomic imbalance. These processes could be viewed as sensitization-like as well as disinhibitory, and their behavioral "hallmarks" of hypervigilance and fear might pertain to any threat, including that associated with discrimination and racism.

The classical finding of a large orienting response followed by habituation is an example of sensitization (Ursin, 1998). Similarly, the phenomenon of long-term potentiation, so important for memory, can be viewed as a type of sensitization (Thayer and Friedman, 2002). The tuning of the organism to novel stimuli followed by habituation to innocuous stimuli is characteristic of healthy and adaptive functioning. In contrast, failure to habituate to innocuous stimuli leads to vigilance and defensiveness that is the hallmark of pathologies such as anxiety disorders. This maladaptive mode exemplifies perseverative behavior that can be seen as a positive feedback loop. Interruption of this ongoing state is associated with inhibition and negative feedback. In the context of our model of neurovisceral integration, vagal control of cardiovascular function (as well as activity of the prefrontal cortex) is associated with these inhibitory processes.

This phenomenon was examined in a study that compared generalized anxiety disorder (GAD) patients to a matched control group who were exposed to threat and nonthreat words in an S1—S2 paradigm (Thayer, Friedman, Borkovec, Johnsen, and Molina, 2000). Briefly, the S1—S2 paradigm involves the presentation of a series of paired stimuli in which an initial cue stimulus (S1) is followed after a fixed interstimulus interval (ISI) by a second stimulus (S2). A robust triphasic HR response has been described during the ISI (Bohlin and Kjellberg, 1979). An initial HR deceleration following S1 is followed by HR acceleration over the next several cardiac beats. Finally, just prior to S2, a second HR deceleration occurs. The initial deceleration has been interpreted as an orienting response to novelty (Sokolov, 1963). Phasic cardiac changes found in the S1—S2 paradigm have been shown to be vagally mediated (Porges, 1992). It was reasoned that GAD entails excess vigilance to environmental threat and low disengagement from unimportant events. This attentional style would produce a failure to habituate to novel innocuous stimuli in the GAD group, whereas nonanxious controls would show habituation. Because HR response magnitude is positively related to vagally mediated HRV (Porges, 1992), it was predicted that relative to persons with GAD, nonanxious controls initially would show larger orienting responses that would habituate rapidly.

These predictions were supported by data that showed the GAD group to have smaller cardiac orienting responses and impaired habituation to neutral words, relative to the nonanxious controls. Diminished orienting is consistent with findings of low HRV in GAD, and the impaired habituation suggests excess vigilance to a perceived perpetually threatening environment. The inability to inhibit attention to harmless stimuli leads to a positive feedback loop that spirals out of control. Thus, worry becomes the preferred response to an ever-widening range of situations, maintaining anxiety in the face of disconfirming data. However, the chronic perception of threat may lead to a restriction of behavior such that the individual is paradoxically exposed to less novel, disconfirming information. Particularly in the elderly, this limitation can lead to social isolation and physical inactivity. Again, positive feedback perpetuates the existing dysfunctional state.

These mechanisms could operate outside of conscious awareness at a precognitive or preconscious level. One of us recently found similar phenomena in alcoholics exposed to briefly presented (Ingjaldsson, Thayer, and Laberg, 2003a) and nonconsciously presented alcohol stimuli (Ingjaldsson, Thayer, and Laberg, 2003b). These findings are consistent with classic work on perceptual defense (see Mackinnon and Dukes, 1962, for review) and the psychophysiology of attention (e.g., Graham and Clifton, 1966; Sokolov, 1963), as well as more contemporary notions of preattentive discrimination and selective processing of threat in anxiety (Mathews, 1990). Furthermore, the rapid mobilization of resources for action fits the dynamical systems view of emotion as an emergent response or attractor driven by motivational factors (see Globus and Arpaia, 1994; Thayer and Lane, 2000).

Several recent studies further highlight the fact that perseverative thinking can have effects outside of conscious awareness. In one study, healthy individuals were brought into a sleep laboratory and randomly divided into two groups (Hall et al., 2004). One group was told that in the morning they would be asked to give a speech that would be evaluated (stress group). The other participants were told that they would be allowed to read popular magazines upon awakening (control group). The results indicated that relative to the control group, the stress group had decreased HRV during both rapid eye movement (REM) and non-REM sleep. They also had poorer sleep maintenance and lower automated delta counts assessed via electroencephalography. Another recent study found that daytime worry and daily hassles were associated with decreased HRV and increased HR on the succeeding night (Brosschot, van Dijk, and Thayer, 2003). Taken together, these studies suggest that the effects of perseverative cognition are not restricted to periods when such activity is consciously perceived, but can have effects that extend to periods in which perseverative cognition is not accessible to conscious awareness.

Perseverative Thinking and Poor Health

Perseverative thinking is a central feature of many psychological disorders that also have been associated with poor physical health outcomes. For example, chronic and transient episodes of anxiety, depression, and anger all have been associated with cardiovascular disease (Musselman et al., 1998; Rozanski et al., 1999; Verrier and Mittleman, 2000). A core characteristic of these perseverative states is the perception that control over a stressor is threatened. Only when a threat to control is perceived is the stressor's full potential for activating the organism manifested, because there is no apparent way to cope with the stressor. Perceived uncontrollability of stress (or related concepts like hopelessness) has been documented as a chief characteristic of both stressors and individuals that accounts for potentially pathogenic physiological states and health problems (Brosschot et al., 1998; Everson et al., 1996; Frankenhäuser, 1980; Lundberg and Frankenhäuser, 1978; Steptoe and Appels, 1989; Ursin, 1987; Ursin and Hytten, 1992).

From this perspective, perseverative thinking might be viewed as the cognitive manifestation and source of nourishment of the deeper underlying experience of perceived uncontrollability. The concept of perseverative thinking thus may help to explain the health effects of perceived uncontrollability by accounting for the prolongation of its physiological effects. Specifically, perseverative thinking sustains the physiological response to a stressor by prolonging uncertainty over stressor control in the coping process. A theoretical implication of this concept is an emphasis on the time dimension in stress research. Associations between perseverative thinking on the one hand and physiological and health consequences on the other are implicit in view of the crucial role of uncertainty and uncontrollability in the stress-disease link.

Indeed, preliminary evidence for a positive association between dispositional worry and general health exists (Brosschot et al., unpublished data). In this exploratory study of more than 250 first-year psychology students, the disposition to worry (Borkovec, 1985) was found to be correlated with subjective health complaints ($r = 0.64$, $p < 0.001$). The association was lower when the effect of trait anxiety was controlled (partial $r = 0.18$, $p < 0.05$), which suggests that the association was at least partly due to "pure" worry tendencies and not entirely to the disposition to express negative affect. In a related study from the same lab in older, part-time students, further evidence accrued for a causal role for worry. Seven students were instructed to limit worry every day to a 30-minute designated "worry period" late in the day, for one week. Compared to 3 days prior to initiating this procedure, the worry "postponement" group had fewer health complaints during the last 3 days of the intervention week, as opposed to 10 control students who only registered their worry periods ($p < 0.05$). Effects were stronger for common cold or flu-like complaints and coughing than for more conventional psychosomatic complaints like headache or dizziness. Although sample sizes were too small for strong conclusions, these results collectively imply that time spent worrying and health complaints are positively related. A psychoneuroimmunological path from perseverative thinking to infectious and perhaps other immune-related diseases may be inferred. As noted earlier, autonomic imbalance and decreased parasympathetic activity have been shown to be associated with immune function via excess proinflammatory cytokines (Das, 2000; Tracey, 2002).

Another way in which perseverative thinking may be causally related to autonomic imbalance and disease is by decreased vagally mediated HRV. Diminished tonic HRV and the associated reduction of vagally mediated cardiovascular control has been associated with a variety of pathological states and dispositions, including diabetes, myocardial infarction, congestive heart failure, and hypertension (for review see Friedman and Thayer, 1998b; Malliani et al., 1994; Stein, Bosner, Kleiger, and Conger, 1994; Stein and Kleiger, 1999). As an index of vagally mediated cardiovascular activity, HRV reflects a negative feedback mechanism that is crucial for the self-regulation of behavior. Vagal activity has negative cardiac chronotropic and dromotropic effects that promote efficient cardiovascular function by restraining cardiac rate and electrical conduction speed, which is vital to attain cardiac stability, responsiveness, and flexibility (Levy, 1990; Verrier, 1987).

Chronic worry was recently shown to be related to increased risk of coronary heart disease (Kubzansky et al., 1997). Thus, the perseverative thinking characteristic of worry not only can lead to increased anxiety, but is also associated with an increased cardiovascular disease risk. Transition worry is associated with decreased vagal activity (Thayer et al., 1996). Thus, one mechanism that might link worry to elevated disease risk is low vagal activity. Similar models of decreased vagal activity have been proposed to describe the relationship between other psychological factors and physiological health. For example, Brosschot and Thayer (1998) relate diminished vagal activity to hostility and cardiovascular disease risk, and vagal depression has been suggested as the link between psychological factors and myocardial ischemia (Kop et al., 2001; Sroka, Peimann, and Seevers, 1997).

A possible key role in this process is played by decreased medial prefrontal cortex activity. The frontal cortex may tonically inhibit limbic (amygdala) activity (Skinner, 1985), and this limbic activity has been associated with autonomically mediated defensive behavior, including increased HR and blood pressure. More recently, direct and indirect pathways by which the frontal cortex modulates limbic activity, especially via parasympathetic activity, have been identified (Ter Horst, 1999; Ter Horst and Postema, 1997). Ter Horst relates these connections to increased risk of reinfarction and death in postmyocardial infarction depression. The thrust of this line of thought is that when faced with threat, tonic inhibitory limbic control can be rapidly decreased, leading to sympathoexcitatory fight or flight survival responses. Disruption of this inhibitory control allows a rigid, defensive behavioral pattern to emerge with associated hypervigilance and perseverative behavior, manifested in cognitive, affective, and autonomic inflexibility.

Perseverative thinking and low HRV may, in fact, reflect the breakdown of a common reciprocal inhibitory cortical-subcortical neural circuit. This network of reciprocally interconnected structures allows the prefrontal cortex to inhibit subcortical activity associated with defensive behavior, and thus foster flexible control of behavior in response to changing environmental demands. As noted earlier, disruption of this network might lead to disinhibition of defensive perseverative behaviors, including hypervigilance.

Perseverative Thinking and HRV

In a study of the autonomic characteristics of GAD and its cardinal feature, worry, spectral analysis of HRV was used to investigate the effects of a 10-minute relaxation period and a 10-minute worry period in persons with GAD and nonanxious controls (Thayer et al., 1996). Results highlighted two main effects. First, persons with GAD had lower vagally mediated HRV compared to controls across all experimental conditions, including baseline. The second main effect indicated that worry in both GAD and nonanxious control groups was associated with reduced HRV. A similar effect was observed in an HRV study in which an analogue sample of GADs and a nonanxious control group engaged in periods of imagery and worry (Lyonfields, Borkovec, and Thayer, 1995). Resting HRV was recorded both at the beginning and at the end of the experimental session. GAD subjects showed reduced HRV across all recording periods, with little change from one period to the next. Although the nonanxious controls did show differences among experimental conditions, the worry condition was associated with the greatest reduction in HRV. This reduction during worry was greater than the reduction during imagery of the same topic.

Tonic low HRV in GAD, as well as the phasic HRV reduction during worry in nonanxious subjects, represents a breakdown of inhibitory processes that assist efficient self-regulation, including the interruption of ongoing behavior. Thus, an excitatory positive feedback loop emerges, leading to, or perhaps reflected in, perseverative thinking. Thus, the normally fine-tuned ability to adjust to change becomes a rigid, inflexible response disposition. In behavioral terms, the defensive attentional style that characterizes GAD is ultimately detrimental to functioning because it impairs adaptive, versatile responding. Such defensiveness constrains one's behavioral repertoire by limiting the range of appropriate responses through the compromised ability to inhibit inappropriate responses. In other words, behavioral options become restricted to the more automatic and prepotent anxious cognitive and behavioral tendencies. More extreme examples of this perseverative behavior have been associated with frontal lobe dysfunction.

Central Concomitants of Perseverative Behavior

Perseverative behavior is associated with depression, anxiety, and hostility among other negative affective states and dispositions. The current discussion will be restricted to anxiety and hostility, based on a recent review of the physiological concomitants of rumination and depression (Siegle and Thayer, 2003). As mentioned earlier, the main inhibitory CNS neurotransmitter is GABA. Animal and human work often converge to suggest that anxiety and its associated perseverative activity are related to decreased GABA receptor binding in the medial prefrontal and orbital frontal cortices. For example, in a murine model of anxiety, decreased $GABA_A$-receptor clustering was associated with harm avoidance behavior and an explicit memory bias for threat cues (Crestani et al., 1999). Mice with reduced $GABA_A$-receptor clustering showed enhanced reactivity to threat stimuli (an effect that was reversed by diazepam), a facilitation of trace conditioning in a fear conditioning paradigm, and a deficit in ambiguous cue discrimination. These findings are remarkably similar to the HR acceleration to and explicit memory bias for threat words, and failure to habituate to neutral words, found in generalized anxiety disorder patients in a conditioning paradigm (Friedman, Thayer, and Borkovec, 2000; Thayer et al., 2000).

Positron emission tomography (PET) has been used to examine benzodiazepine $GABA_A$-receptor kinetics in humans with and without panic disorder (Malizia et al., 1998). Compared to nonanxious controls, panic disorder patients showed a global decrease in benzodiazepine site binding, with the largest decreases in the orbitofrontal and insular cortices. Decreased blood flow in the right medial frontal cortex also has been reported in self-induced anxiety (Kimbrell et al., 1999). These cortical areas have been implicated in anxiety and are also associated with HRV (Lane et al., 2001). Similar altered orbitofrontal chemistry has been found in anxious humans (Grachev and Apkarian, 2000). Relative to low anxious subjects, high anxious subjects showed reduced levels of a number of orbitofrontal neurochemicals, including GABA.

Recent neuroimaging studies have also examined patterns of cerebral blood flow associated with anger and aggressive behavior. Using single photon emission computed tomography, decreased prefrontal activity was found in 40 psychiatric patients who exhibited aggressive behavior within the 6-month period prior to scanning compared to psychiatric patients without a history of aggression (Amen, Stubblefield, Carmichael, and Thisted, 1996). In nonaggressive individuals, it is clear that anger inhibition is the most common response to provocation, mainly due to social norms

(Brosschot and Thayer, 1998). Consistent with this notion, PET data showed lateral orbitofrontal cortex (LOFC) activation during imagery-driven anger in men (Dougherty et al., 1999). These researchers noted that the LOFC and the associated "prefrontal" circuit are considered pivotal to response inhibition and the mediation of social behavior. Therefore, the reported LOFC activation was hypothesized to represent inhibition of an aggressive response during the anger provocation. Similar right prefrontal activation during self-induced anger, as compared to self-induced anxiety, has been reported (Kimbrell et al., 1999). However, in this study both self-induced anxiety and self-induced anger were associated with decreased frontal activity relative to a neutral condition, suggesting that inhibition pertains in general to emotional behavior.

The amygdala is often held to be the key limbic structure in emotional behavior. For example, electrical stimulation of the amygdala has been associated with a range of defensive behaviors, including increased cortisol, heart rate, and blood pressure (see Davis and Whalen, 2001, for review). Brain imaging data show that both depression severity and dispositional negative affect are correlated with amygdala activity (Davidson, 2002; Drevets, 1999). Although there is evidence that the amygdala responds to both appetitive and aversive stimuli, recent conceptualizations suggest that vigilance regulation and the detection of biologically relevant stimuli is the basic function of the amygdala (Davis and Whalen, 2001). Prolonged amygdaloid activation can lead to excess threat awareness and may form the foundation of psychiatric disorders such as anxiety and depression. This overalert state also has been linked to decreased cardiac output and increased peripheral vascular resistance (Winters, McCabe, Green, and Schneiderman, 2000). Interestingly, this cardiovascular pattern is relatively more prevalent in African Americans and may be a factor in the increased levels of hypertension and related morbidity and mortality in this group (Anderson, McNeilly, and Myers, 1991; Brosschot and Thayer, 1998, 1999). Furthermore, variation in alpha-adrenergically mediated vascular tone may be associated with insulin resistance and thus provide a link to the increased diabetes risk found in African Americans (Brook and Julius, 2000).

In sum, decreased prefrontal activity as well as increased amygdala activity have been associated with anxiety, depression, and related pathological states and dispositions. These structures are both part of the CAN and form the core of an emotion regulation system that may become dysfunctional as reflected in perseverative behavior.

Perseverative Thinking as a Balance Between Inhibition and Excitation

In a normal, relaxed, and safe environment, the prefrontal cortex tonically inhibits limbic activity while it is responsively monitoring internal and external stimuli and guiding goal-directed behavior. The prefrontal cortex is receptive to a broad range of information, but is not specifically directed to potential concerns (e.g., fears such as racism and discrimination) of the organism. Such is the case in situations in which the organism does not expect threat or immediate danger. However, when the situation becomes ambiguous or threat becomes more imminent, or is ever present as it might be for minorities under the constant threat of potential discrimination, prefrontal inhibition of the limbic brain is partially released, potentially generating hypervigilance and perseverative thinking. This partial disinhibition is associated with a hyperalert state of action readiness. In this situation, the organism is obviously not switched completely into a defensive, fight-flight excitatory state. Instead, under limbic influence, the nature of prefrontal function is converted from flexible and open to experience into a state of anticipatory rehearsal of feared scenarios, and vigilant scanning of available information. Under immediate threat, however, the prefrontal cortex is disengaged nearly completely, albeit temporarily, in normal or healthy subjects, resulting in the full and sometimes explosive manifestation of the emotion (anger attack, actual flight, shouting, panicking).

Thus, perseverative thinking can be viewed as a demonstration of the reciprocal nature of prefrontal-amygdala communication. The amygdala sends signals of threat warning to the prefrontal cortex, leading to hypervigilance and rehearsal of feared scenarios, but it is able to do this because of prefrontal disinhibition itself. The disinhibition is in turn due to the rapid and rough perception of immediate threat, which emerges from the integration of ongoing environmental perception with memory associations (conditioned responses), the storage and activation of which is, again, largely under amygdala influence (LeDoux, 2000). In other words, in a bottom-up manner, lower brain centers, in cooperation with memory, demand the prefrontal cortex to occupy itself with rehearsing feared scenarios and stimulate vigilant and biased scanning of internal and external information. At the same time, in a top-down mode, the prefrontal inhibition of lower brain centers is maintained. Perseverative thinking may in fact lead to solutions to the threat, resulting in diminished activation and restoration of the relaxed state dominated by prefrontal inhibition of subcortical sympathoexcitatory circuits.

Finally, it is clear from these findings and theoretical considerations that hypervigilance and perseveration have physiological consequences, that is, signs of stress and limbic-induced autonomic imbalance such as low HRV, elevated HR and cortisol, and particularly elevated blood pressure and peripheral resistance (the so-called "vigilance reaction"; see Winters et al., 2000). Due to partially maintained limbic inhibition by the prefrontal cortex, this activation is often moderate and may appear blunted (cf. Young, Nesse, Weder, and Julius, 1998). But prolonged vagal withdrawal renders the ANS inflexible and unresponsive to changing environmental demands. Therefore autonomic activation is still high enough (but sustained) to cause damage (e.g., hypertension and cardiovascular disease) (Brosschot and Thayer, 1998), but also low enough, for example, for anxious subjects to learn to worry to prevent full manifestation of fear responses (Borkovec and Hu, 1999). Thus, the autonomic imbalance associated with anticipatory coping and delayed physiological recovery from discrete stressors may be associated with hypervigilance and perseveration due to partial release of prefrontal inhibition of the amygdala. That these anticipatory and recovery responses have been associated with increased blood pressure and peripheral resistance (Gregg, James, Matyas, and Thorsteinsson, 1999) has special importance because this pattern has been linked to increased hypertension and related morbidity and mortality in African Americans.

We have written extensively about perseverative thinking and its physiological and psychological concomitants (Brosschot and Thayer, in press; Brosschot et al., 2003; Friedman and Thayer, 1998a; Ingjaldsson et al., 2003c; Siegle and Thayer, 2003; Thayer and Friedman, 2002; Thayer and Lane, 2002; Thayer and Ruiz-Padial, 2002; Thayer et al., 1996). Physiological concomitants include autonomic imbalance as indexed by decreased HRV, decreased prefrontal cortex activity, increased amygdala activity, excess and prolonged cortisol responsivity, altered immune function, increased blood pressure and peripheral resistance responses in anticipatory coping, increased blood pressure and peripheral resistance during recovery from stress, sustained and prolonged pupil dilation, and poor tolerance to and delayed recovery from stress in general. All of these physiological responses are associated with poor health outcomes.

In addition, a psychological profile associated with perseverative thinking has emerged. This profile is marked by hypervigilance to threat and failure to habituate to innocuous stimuli, impaired cognitive function on tasks demanding delayed responding and executive functions, a lack of inhibitory behavior, denial and an avoidant coping style, increased neuroticism, decreased conscientiousness and impulse control, thought intrusions, lack of perceived control, and greater levels of depression, anxiety, and hostility. Again, all of these psychological responses are linked to poor health outcomes.

RELEVANCE TO HEALTH DISPARITIES

Discrimination and racism have been strongly implicated in the health disparities between ethnic minorities and majority group members (Clark et al., 1999; Gee, 2002; Karlsen and Nazroo, 2002; Krieger, 2000; Williams and Neighbors, 2001). Among the various institutional and individual paths by which discrimination and racism may to lead health disparities, one at the individual level posits that minority group members are exposed to chronic excess stress. The NIM model details how such stress might "get under one's skin," as it were, and lead to both pathophysiology and psychopathology. The final common path of these conditions may be autonomic imbalance, but the question remains as to whether minority group members show evidence of chronic and excessive levels of stress exposure that might lead to an autonomic imbalance that favors poor health outcomes.

The answer to this question appears to be an unqualified yes. Supportive evidence has been provided in the cases of African Americans (Clark et al., 1999), Chinese Americans (Gee, 2002), and of minority groups in England and Wales (Karlsen and Nazroo, 2002). In the United States, for example, perceived interpersonal discrimination has been associated with a number of factors associated with autonomic imbalance, such as depression and psychological stress, high blood pressure, low birthweight, poor self-rated health, smoking, and physical inactivity (Karlsen and Nazroo, 2002).

The literature paints a vivid picture of persons exposed to discrimination and racism. These people tend to show signs of anger, frustration, anxiety, depression, helplessness, hopelessness, resentment, fear, and paranoia (Clark et al., 1999). In addition, such individuals tend to be hypervigilant, distrustful, and wary; often find themselves in ambiguous situations with respect to unfair treatment; interpret ambiguous and harmless situations as threatening; are prone to rumination about the causes and consequences of perceived unfair treatment; engage in anticipatory coping in response to the potential discrimination; and engage in denial and avoidant coping with respect to discrimination (Williams and Neighbors, 2001). It is important to note the similarity between the psychological profiles associated with perseverative thinking and that of persons exposed to discrimination. Moreover, minority status is associated with numerous diseases and increased morbidity and mortality, as discussed at the beginning of this chapter.

Several recent investigations further support this psychological profile of minority group members as distrustful, engaging in anticipatory coping in response to potential discrimination, and hypervigilant. For example, Hunt (2000) recently reported that African Americans in Southern California, when compared to whites and Latinos, have the weakest "belief in a just world." This concept measures the perceived fairness of a person's interactions with the world and suggests that African Americans have greater mistrust. That this mistrust may be adaptive and appropriate in a society characterized by discrimination does not lessen its potential deleterious effects via hypervigilance. Similarly, Blascovich, Spencer, Quinn, and Steele (2001) have shown that African Americans exposed to stereotype threat have elevated mean arterial pressure (MAP) responses during a mild cognitive challenge. Stereotype threat occurs when members of stereotyped groups find themselves in situations in which others may view them stereotypically such that the pressure to perform well is increased. Importantly, they also found that MAP was elevated during an intervening rest period when performance was not expected, but rumination or perseverative thinking may have occurred. Finally, Chen and Matthews (2001) have recently reported that low socioeconomic status (SES) and African-American children interpret ambiguous scenarios as conveying more hostile intent and inducing greater feelings of anger. In addition, these appraisals were associated with increased vascular responses as measured by impedance cardiography. Importantly, for low-SES African-American children, these appraisals and feelings were associated with vascular responses 3 years later. Thus these appraisal biases grew stronger over time in the African-American children and appeared to sensitize them to interpret ambiguous situations as more and more threatening over time. The authors suggest that this may be the result of the greater exposure of the African American children to discrimination and racism. Similar results have been reported in adult African Americans. Merritt, Bennett, and Williams (2002) found that in response to a story about a negative social interaction in which the actors were ambiguous with respect to ethnicity, the African-American males showed elevated MAP and diastolic blood pressure responses when they reported greater perceptions of racism evident in the story. Again, these elevated responses persisted into recovery periods when the actual stressor was no longer present, but when rumination and perseverative thinking were likely to occur. Taken together, these studies provide empirical support for the psychological profile described earlier and its deleterious effects in African Americns.

Due to the excess energy demand that autonomic imbalance places on the organism, individuals exposed to discrimination and racism may have a kind of premature aging that speeds their way to death and disability. The fact that autonomic imbalance continues to predict morbidity and mortality into old age when other risk factors have lost their predictive power adds further to the utility of the neurovisceral integration model in the understanding of health disparities in the elderly.

Preliminary Data in Support of the Model

We recently completed a pilot study that sought to examine in an elderly African-American sample some of the aspects of the model we have outlined. The total sample included 445 African Americans residing in east Baltimore. Psychophysiological assessment was completed on a subsample of 106 participants (50 males, 56 females) as part of the Healthy Aging in Nationally Diverse Samples (HANDLS) study that has been initiated at the

Intramural Research Program of the National Institute on Aging. This study was designed to examine the nature of health disparities using a multilevel approach ranging from the molecular to the social. Briefly, blood pressure and HR were continuously monitored during administration of two subtasks of the Perception of Affect Test (PAT) in this African-American sample. The PAT involved asking subjects to evaluate emotional expressions (and their intensity) in faces and sentences. Those who were able to correctly identify emotions in these stimuli showed lower blood pressure and total peripheral resistance responses as well as decreased depression scores. Older persons (age 52 and higher) performed more poorly than younger ones at correctly identifying emotions, and older men specifically had more difficulty in correctly identifying disgust and fear than their female counterparts. Older African-American males, therefore, showed the greatest deficits in emotional processing and the largest total peripheral resistance responses to the tasks.

A more thorough examination of the physiological responses indicated that HR and blood pressure increased from baseline in response to completion of the PAT tasks. Notably, blood pressure remained elevated during the subsequent recovery period. Indices of blood pressure, cardiac output, and total peripheral resistance revealed signs of elevated peripheral resistance during recovery. In addition, sympathetic (vascular) measures of HRV (reduced high-frequency and increased low-frequency power) and blood pressure variability (reduced high-frequency power) increased during recovery. Previous research showing vascular hyperreactivity among African Americans supports the present results (Brosschot and Thayer, 1999; Jones, Andrawis, and Abernethy, 1999).

The present data further suggest that high vascular reactivity may be associated with psychosocial factors. In this sample, higher levels of depressive symptoms were related to larger total peripheral resistance during task and recovery. In older women, self-reported loneliness was positively correlated with total peripheral resistance at baseline and recovery. These results underscore the multiple levels of system function that may contribute to health disparities in cardiovascular disease, especially hypertension.

A series of carefully selected genetic polymorphisms implicated in cardiovascular disease will be studied in future work to assess genetic contributions to autonomic balance. These are (1) angiotensin-converting enzyme (ACE) insertion/deletion mutation, (2) endothelial nitric oxide synthase (eNOS) G894T mutation, (3) eNOS T786C mutation, (4), angiotensinogen M235T mutation, (5) apolipoprotein E polymorphisms, and (6) serotonin transporter 5-HTTLPR polymorphism. Common features of these mutations are allelic frequency in populations studied greater than 0.2, association with cardiovascular disease (congestive heart failure, hypertension, myocardial infarction) and/or specific personality traits, and relation to a measurable physiological difference among genotypes (e.g., decreased nitric oxide production, impaired angiotensin II formation, altered lipoprotein pattern, decreased serotonin transporter transcription efficiency). The study population will be genotyped for this array, and genotype patterns of the six genes as well as single polymorphisms will be linked to variability subgroups in ANS function using quartile analyses.

Preliminary observations indicate that high-frequency HRV is decreased in the basal state in the DD genotype of the ACE insertion/deletion polymorphism (Thayer et al., 2003), and that the allelic frequency of the eNOS G894T allele is markedly decreased in the HANDLS study population as compared to a white control group. This finding is intriguing because the T allele has been associated with increased likelihood of cardiovascular disease in other populations. If confirmed, this observation would exclude this source of cardiovascular risk in this African-American population. The DD phenotype of the ACE insertion/deletion gene has been associated with increased levels of circulating ACE and increased risk of sudden cardiac death in some populations. Our finding of decreased HRV and decreased baroreflex sensitivity in the DD phenotype is consistent with the literature linking this phenotype with increased cardiovascular disease risk. These preliminary findings attest to the promise of the candidate gene approach to better understand sources of variability in ANS function.

These preliminary data also suggest that psychosocial factors are related to physiological processes that have major implications for the health disparities observed in the United States. For example, depression, which has been suggested as a primary factor in the greater rates of hypertension in African Americans, was associated with both poor affective regulation and increased peripheral resistance. As detailed earlier, increased peripheral resistance is associated with autonomic imbalance via sustained activity in the amygdala and with hypervigilance and perseverative thinking. Increased peripheral resistance is also related to established hypertension and insulin resistance, and thus plays a role in both cardiovascular disease and diabetes (Brook and Julius, 2000).

Genetic factors also have been implicated in the health disparities, but our data suggest that at least one genetic polymorphism associated with increased risk in whites may not be a factor in African Americans (see Chapter 8, this volume). Another polymorphism, however, was found to have a relationship with HRV, and thus may interact with psychosocial factors to produce individual differences in disease risk. It is notable in this context that merely having a particular polymorphism is not sufficient to produce risk—the polymorphism must be expressed. Gene expression is a result of a complex process that includes exposure to environmental factors that can determine the expression of a cascade of genetic influences, the outcome of which is difficult to predict.

FUTURE DIRECTIONS AND RECOMMENDATIONS
FOR RESEARCH

There are a number of important directions for future research. First and foremost, this research must take into account the requisite multiple levels of analysis to explicate the complex factors that contribute to the health disparities (Anderson, 1999; Brosschot and Thayer, 1998). The interaction of factors across these levels will be the source of many insights. This type of multidisciplinary research must face the current grant review system that often establishes narrowly focused study sections, which may miss the value of multilevel initiatives.

In addition, longitudinal, prospective studies will be necessary to untangle the causal factors that lead to the observed health disparities. These studies will require a major commitment on the part of funding agencies. It will also be necessary to examine factors across generations, and this will also tax the current review and funding structure.

More specific recommendations for research are also justified, such as the need to examine within-ethnic group variability. That is, individual differences exist within each ethnic group. For example, preliminary results of the ACE insertion/deletion polymorphism reported earlier suggest an intraethnic group source of variability that may modify the impact of other genetic as well as psychosocial influences. Such factors need to be identified and explored. Related to this need is the call for examination of intraindividual variability as distinct from interindividual variability. Relationships found among variables between individuals may not generalize to the relationships found among the same variables within individuals (Thayer and Lane, 2000). Thus, the repeated measurement of individuals over time is necessary to explicate those relationships at the individual level (Friedman, 2003).

Finally, studies must address the interplay of physiological, behavioral, affective, cognitive, and social processes and their impact on health, health behaviors, and disease. The neurovisceral integration model offers a framework to integrate such work across levels of analysis. It is key that the central nervous system be included, which entails neuroimaging and neuropsychological research to tap brain processes that support and accompany the many complex factors involved in health and disease in aging.

REFERENCES

Aggleton, J.P., and Young, A. (2000). The enigma of the amygdala: On its contribution to human emotion. In R.D. Lane and L. Nadel (Eds.), *Cognitive neuroscience of emotion* (pp. 106-128). New York: Oxford University Press.

Ahern, G.L., Labiner, D.M., Hutzler, R., Osburn, C., Talwar, D., Herring, A.M., et al. (1994). Quantitative analysis of the EEG in the intracarotid amobarbital test: I. Amplitude analysis. *Electroencephalography and Clinical Neurophysiology, 91,* 21-32.

Amen, D.G., Stubblefield, M., Carmichael, B., and Thisted, R. (1996). Brain SPECT findings and aggressiveness. *Annals of Clinical Psychiatry, 8,* 129-137.

Anderson, N.B. (1999). Solving the puzzle of socioeconomic status and health: The need for integrated, multilevel, interdisciplinary research. *Annals of the New York Academy of Sciences, 896,* 302-312.

Anderson, N.B., McNeilly, M., and Myers, H. (1991). Autonomic reactivity and hypertension in blacks: A review and proposed model. *Ethnicity and Disease, 1,* 154-170.

Angrilli, A., Mauri, A., Palomba, D., Flor, H., Birbaumer, N., Sartori, G., and di Paola, F. (1996). Startle reflex and emotion modulation impairment after a right amygdala lesion. *Brain, 119,* 1991-2000.

Arnsten, A.F.T., and Goldman-Rakic, P.S. (1998). Noise stress impairs prefrontal cortical cognitive function in monkeys: Evidence for a hyperdopaminergic mechanism. *Archives of General Psychiatry, 55,* 362-368.

Benarroch, E.E. (1993). The central autonomic network: Functional organization, dysfunction, and perspective. *Mayo Clinic Proceedings, 68,* 988-1001.

Benarroch, E.E. (1997). The central autonomic network. In P.A. Low (Ed.), *Clinical autonomic disorders* (2nd ed., pp. 17-23). Philadelphia: Lippincott-Raven.

Black, S.A. (2002). Diabetes, diversity, and disparity: What do we do with the evidence? *American Journal of Public Health, 92,* 543-548.

Blascovich, J., Spencer, S.J., Quinn, D., and Steele, C. (2001). African Americans and high blood pressure: The role of stereotype threat. *Psychological Science, 12,* 225-229.

Bohlin, G., and Kjellberg, A. (1979). Orienting activity in two-stimulus paradigms as reflected in heart rate. In H.D. Kimmel, E.H. van Olst, and J.F. Orlebeke (Eds.), *The orienting reflex in humans* (pp. 169-197). Hillsdale, NJ: Lawrence Erlbaum Associates.

Borkovec, T.D. (1985) Worry: A potentially valuable concept. *Behaviour Research and Therapy, 23*(4), 481-482.

Borkovec, T.D., and Hu, S. (1999). The effect of worry on cardiovascular response to phobic imagery. *Behavioral Research Therapy, 28*(1), 69-73.

Bradley, M.M., and Lang, P.J. (2000). Measuring emotion: Behavior, feeling, and psysiology. In R.D. Lane and L. Nadel (Eds.), *Cognitive neuroscience of emotion* (pp. 106-128). New York: Oxford University Press.

Brook, R.D., and Julius, S. (2000). Autonomic imbalance, hypertension, and cardiovascular risk. *American Journal of Hypertension, 13,* 112S-122S.

Brosschot, J.F., and Thayer, J.F. (1998). Anger inhibition, cardiovascular recovery, and vagal function: A model of the link between hostility and cardiovascular disease. *Annals of Behavioral Medicine, 20*(4), 1-8.

Brosschot, J.F., and Thayer, J.F. (1999). Cardiovascular recovery after harassment with anger expression or inhibition. *Gedrag & Gezondheid, 27*(1/2), 8-14.

Brosschot, J.F., and Thayer, J.F. (in press). Worry, perseverative thinking and health. In L. Temoshok (Ed.), *The expression and non-expression of emotion in health and disease.* Hillsdale, NJ: Lawrence Erlbaum Associates.

Brosschot, J.F., Godaert, G.L.R., Benschop, R.J., Olff, M., Ballieux, R.E., and Heijnen, C.J. (1998). Experimental stress and immunological reactivity: A closer look at perceived uncontrollability. *Psychosomatic Medicine, 60*(3), 359-361.

Brosschot, J.F., van Dijk, E., and Thayer, J.F. (2003). Daily worrying and stressors increase daytime-and night-time cardiac activity. *Psychosomatic Medicine, 65,* A-4.

Chen, E., and Matthews, K.A. (2001). Cognitive appraisal biases: An approach to under-standing the relation between socioeconomic status and cardiovascular reactivity in children. *Annals of Behavioral Medicine, 23,* 101-111.

Clark, R., Anderson, N.B., Clark, V.R., and Williams, D.R. (1999). Racism as a stressor for African Americans: A biopsychosocial model. *American Psychologist, 54,* 805-816.

Cohen, H., Matar, M.A., Kaplan, Z., and Kotler, M. (1999). Power spectral analysis of heart rate variability in psychiatry. *Psychotherapy and Psychosomatics, 68,* 59-66.

Crestani, F., et al. (1999). Decreased $GABA_A$-receptor clustering results in enhanced anxiety and a bias for threat cues. *Nature Neuroscience, 2,* 833-839.

Damasio, A.R. (1998). Emotion in the perspective of an integrated nervous system. *Brain Research Reviews, 26,* 83-86.

Das, U.N. (2000). Beneficial effect(s) of n-3 fatty acids in cardiovascular disease: But, why and how? *Prostaglandins, Leukotrienes, and Essential Fatty Acids, 63,* 351-362.

Davey, G.C.L. (1994). Pathological worrying as exacerbated problem-solving. In G.C.L. Davey and F. Tallis (Eds.), *Worrying: Perspectives on theory, assessment and treatment* (pp. 35-60). New York: Wiley.

Davidson, R.J. (2000). The functional neuroanatomy of affective style. In R.D. Lane and L. Nadel (Eds.), *Cognitive neuroscience of emotion* (pp. 106-128). New York: Oxford University Press.

Davidson, R.J. (2002). Anxiety and affective style: Role of prefrontal cortex and amygdala. *Biological Psychiatry, 51,* 68-80.

Davis, M., and Whalen, P.J. (2001). The amygdala: Vigilance and emotion. *Molecular Psychiatry, 6,* 13-34.

Devinsky, O., Morrell, M.J., and Vogt, B.A. (1995). Contributions of anterior cingulate cortex to behavior. *Brain, 118,* 279-306.

Dougherty, D.D., Shin, L.M., Alpert, N.M., Pitman, R.K., Orr, S.P., Lasko, M., Macklin, M.L., Fischman, A.J., and Rauch, S.L. (1999). Anger in healthy men: A PET study using script-driven imagery. *Biological Psychiatry, 46,* 466-472.

Drevets, W.C. (1999) . Prefrontal cortical-amygdalar metabolism in major depression. *Annals of the New York Academy of Sciences, 877,* 614-637.

Eriksen, H.R., and Ursin, H. (2002). Sensitization and subjective health complaints. *Scandinavian Journal of Psychology, 4*(2), 189-196.

Ershler, W., and Keller, E. (2000). Age-associated increased interleukin-6 gene expression, late life diseases, and frailty. *Annual Review of Medicine, 51,* 245-270.

Everson, S.A., Goldberg, D.E., Kaplan, G.A., Cohen, R.D., et al. (1996). Hopelessness and risk of mortality and incidence of myocardial infarction and cancer. *Psychosomatic Medicine, 58*(2), 113-121.

Frankenhäuser, M. (1980). Psychobiologic aspects of life stress. In S. Levine and H. Ursin (Eds.), *Coping and health* (Series III, Vol. 12). NATO Conference Series. New York: Plenum.

Friedman, B.H. (2003). Idiodynamics vis-a-vis psychophysiology: An idiodynamic portrayal of cardiovascular activity. *Journal of Applied Psychoanalytic Studies, 5,* 425-441.

Friedman, B.H., and Thayer, J.F. (1998a). Anxiety and autonomic flexibility: A cardiovascular approach. *Biological Psychology, 49,* 303-323.

Friedman, B.H., and Thayer, J.F. (1998b). Autonomic balance revisited: Panic anxiety and heart rate variability. *Journal of Psychosomatic Research, 44,* 133-151.

Friedman, B.H., Thayer, J.T., and Borkovec, T.D. (2000). Explicit memory bias for threat words in generalized anxiety disorder. *Behavior Therapy, 31,* 745-756.

Frijda, N.H. (1988). The laws of emotion. *American Psychologist, 43,* 349-358.

Gee, G.C. (2002). Multilevel analysis of the relationship between institutional and individual racial discrimination and health status. *American Journal of Public Health, 92,* 615-623.

Glass, L., and Mackey, M.C. (1988). *From clocks to chaos*. Princeton, NJ: Princeton University Press.

Globus, G.G., and Arpaia, J.P. (1994). Psychiatry and the new dynamics. *Biological Psychiatry, 35*, 352-364.

Goldberger, A.L. (1992). Applications of chaos to physiology and medicine. In J.H. Kim and J. Stringer (Eds.), *Applied chaos* (pp. 321-331). New York: Wiley.

Goldman-Rakic, P.S. (1998). The prefrontal landscape: Implications of the functional architecture for understanding human mentation and the central executive. In A.C. Roberts, T.W. Robbins, and L. Weiskrantz (Eds.), *The prefrontal cortex: Executive and cognitive functions* (pp. 87-102). Oxford, England: Oxford University Press.

Grachev, I.D., and Apkarian, A.V. (2000). Anxiety in healthy humans is associated with orbital frontal chemistry. *Molecular Psychiatry, 5*, 482-488.

Graham, F.K., and Clifton, R.K. (1966). Heart-rate change as a component of the orienting response. *Psychological Bulletin, 65*, 305-320.

Gregg, M.E., James, J.E., Matyas, T.A., and Thorsteinsson, E.B. (1999). Hemodynamic profile of stress-induced anticipation and recovery. *International Journal of Psychophysiology, 34*, 147-162.

Habib, G.B. (1999). Reappraisal of heart rate as a risk factor in the general population. *European Heart Journal Supplements, 1*(H), H2-H10.

Hall, M., Vasko, R., Buysse, D., Thayer, J.F., Ombao, H., Chen, Q., Cashmere, J.D., and Kupfer, D. (2004). Acute stress affects autonomic tone during sleep. *Psychosomatic Medicine, 66*, 56-62.

Hansen, A.L., Johnsen, B.H., Sollers, J.J., and Thayer, J.F. (2002). Neural control of the heart modulates cognitive processing during stress. *Clinical Autonomic Research, 12*, 167 (abstract).

Hansen, A.L., Johnsen, B.H., and Thayer, J.F. (2003). Vagal influence in the regulation of attention and working memory. *International Journal of Psychophysiology, 48*, 263-274.

Hong, S.B., Kim, K.W., Seo, D.W., Kim, S.E., Na, D.G., and Byun, Y.S. (2000). Contralateral EEG slowing and amobarbital distribution in Wada test: An intracarotid SPECT study. *Epilepsia, 41*, 207-212.

Hunt, M.O. (2000). Status, religion, and the "belief in a just world": Comparing African Americans, Latinos, and whites. *Social Science Quarterly, 81*, 325-343.

Ingjaldsson, J.T., Thayer, J.F., and Laberg, J.C. (2003a). Preattentive processing of alcohol stimuli. *Scandinavian Journal of Psychology, 44*, 161-165.

Ingjaldsson, J.T., Thayer, J.F., and Laberg, J.C. (2003b). Craving for alcohol and preattentive processing of alcohol stimuli. *International Journal of Psychophysiology, 49*, 29-39.

Ingjaldsson, J.T., Laberg, J.C., and Thayer, J.F. (2003c). Reduced heart rate variability in chronic alcohol abuse: Relationship with negative mood, chronic thought suppression, and compulsive drinking. *Biological Psychiatry, 54*, 1427-1436.

James, S.A. (1994). John Henryism and the health of African-Americans. *Culture Medicine and Psychiatry, 18*(2), 163-182.

Johnsen, B.H., Hansen, A.L., Sollers, J.J., Murison, R., and Thayer, J.F. (2001). Heart rate variability is inversely related to cortisol reactivity during cognitive stress. *Psychosomatic Medicine, 64*, 148 (abstract).

Johnsen, B.H., Thayer, J.F., Laberg, J.C., Wormnes, B., Raadal, M., Skaret, E., Kvale, G., and Berg, E. (2003). Attentional and physiological characteristics of patients with dental anxiety. *Journal of Anxiety Disorders, 17*, 75-87.

Jones, D.S., Andrawis, N.S., and Abernethy, D.R. (1999). Impaired endothelial-dependent forearm vascular relaxation in black Americans. *Clinical Pharmacology Therapy, 65*(4), 408-412.

Jose, A.D., and Collison, D. (1970). The normal range and determinants of the intrinsic heart rate in man. *Cardiovascular Research, 4,* 160-167.

Karlsen, S., and Nazroo, J.Y. (2002). Relation between discrimination, social class, and health among ethnic minority groups. *American Journal of Public Health, 92,* 624-631.

Kiecolt-Glaser, J.K., McGuire, L., Robles, T.F., and Glaser, R. (2002). Emotions, morbidity, and mortality: New perspectives from psychoneuroimmunology. *Annual Review of Psychology, 53,* 83-107.

Kimbrell, T.S., George, M.S., Parekh, P.I., Ketter, T.A., Podell, D.M., Danielson, A.L., Repella, J.D., Benson, B.E., Willis, M.W., Herscovitch, P., and Post, R.M. (1999). Regional brain activity during transient self-induced anxiety and anger in healthy adults. *Biological Psychiatry, 46*(4), 454-465.

Kop, W.J., Verdino, R.J., Gottdiener, J.S., O'Leary, S.T., Merz, C.N.B., and Krantz, D.S. (2001). Changes in heart rate and heart rate variability before ambulatory ischemic events. *Journal of the American College of Cardiology, 38,* 742-749.

Krantz, D.S., and McCeney, M.K. (2002). Effects of psychological and social factors on organic disease: A critical assessment of research on coronary heart disease. *Annual Review of Psychology, 53,* 341-369.

Krieger, N. (2000). Discrimination and health. In L. Berkman and I. Kawachi (Eds.), *Social epidemiology* (pp. 36-75). New York: Oxford University Press.

Kubzansky, L.D., Kawachi, I., Spiro, A., Weiss, S.T., Vokonas, P.S., and Sparrow, D. (1997). Is worrying bad for your heart? A prospective study of worry and coronary heart disease in the Normative Aging Study. *Circulation, 95,* 818-824.

Lane, R.D., Reiman, E.M., Ahern, G.L., and Thayer, J.F. (2001). Activity in medial prefrontal cortex correlates with vagal component of heart rate variability during emotion. *Brain and Cognition, 47,* 97-100.

Lang, P.J. (1995). The emotion probe—studies of motivation and attention. *American Psychologist, 50,* 372-385.

LeDoux, J.E. (2000). Emotion circuits in the brain. *Annual Review of Neuroscience, 23,* 155-184.

Levenson, R.W. (1988). Emotion and the autonomic nervous system: A prospectus for research on autonomic specificity. In H.L. Wagner (Ed.), *Social psychophysiology and emotion: Theory and clinical applications* (pp. 17-42). Chichester, England: Wiley.

Levy, M.N. (1990). Autonomic interactions in cardiac control. *Annals of the New York Academy of Sciences, 601,* 209-221.

Lipsitz, L.A., and Goldberger, A.L. (1992). Loss of complexity and aging: Potential applications of fractals and chaos theory to senescence. *Journal of the American Medical Association, 267*(13), 1806-1809.

Lundberg, U., and Frankenhäuser, M. (1978). Psychophysiological reactions to noise as modified by personal control over noise intensity. *Biological Psychology, 6,* 51-59.

Lupien, S.J., Gillin, C.J., and Hauger, R.L. (1999). Working memory is more sensitive than declarative memory to the acute effects of corticosteroids: A dose-response study in humans. *Behavioral Neuroscience, 113*(3), 420-430.

Lyonfields, J.D., Borkovec, T.D., and Thayer, J.F. (1995). Vagal tone in generalized anxiety disorder and the effects of aversive imagery and worrisome thinking. *Behavioral Therapy, 26,* 457-466.

Mackinnon, D.W., and Dukes, W. (1962). Repression. In L. Postman (Ed.), *Psychology in the making: Histories of selected research problems* (pp. 662-744). New York: Alfred A. Knopf.

Maier, S.F., and Watkins, L.R. (1998). Cytokines for psychologists: Implications of bi-directional immune-to-brain communication for understanding behavior, mood, and cognition. *Psychological Review, 105,* 83-107.

Malizia, A.L., Cunningham, V.J., Bell, C.J., Liddle, P.F., Jones, T., and Nutt, D.J. (1998). Decreased brain GABA$_A$-benzodiazepine receptor binding in panic disorder. *Archives of General Psychiatry, 55*, 715-720.

Malliani, A., Pagani, M., and Lombardi, F. (1994). Methods for assessment of sympatho-vagal balance: Power spectral analysis. In M.N. Levy and P.J. Schwartz (Eds.), *Vagal control of the heart: Experimental basis and clinical implications* (pp. 433-454). Armonk, NY: Futura.

Masterman, D.L., and Cummings, J.L. (1997). Frontal-subcortical circuits: The anatomical basis of executive, social and motivated behaviors. *Journal of Psychopharmacology, 11*, 107-114.

Mathews, A. (1990). Why worry? The cognitive function of anxiety. *Behaviour Research and Therapy, 28*, 455-468.

Mayberg, H.S., et al. (1999). Reciprocal limbic-cortical function and negative mood: Converging PET findings in depression and normal sadness. *American Journal of Psychiatry, 156*, 675-682.

McEwen, B.S. (1998). Protective and damaging effects of stress mediators. *New England Journal of Medicine, 338*, 171-179.

McGeer, P.L., Eccles, J.C., and McGeer, E.G. (1978). *Molecular neurobiology of the mammalian brain*. New York: Plenum.

Merritt, M.M., Bennett, G.G., and Williams, R.B. (2002). Subtle racism and elevated cardiovascular reactivity among black males. *Annals of Behavioral Medicine, 24*, S18 (abstract).

Musselman, D.L., Evans, D.L., and Nemeroff, C.B. (1998). The relationship of depression to cardiovascular disease. *Archives of General Psychiatry, 55*, 580-592.

Nabors-Oberg, R., Sollers, J.J., Niaura, R., and Thayer, J.F. (2002). The effects of controlled smoking on heart period variability. *IEEE Engineering in Medicine and Biology Magazine, 21*, 65-70.

National High Blood Pressure Education Program. (1997). *The sixth report of the Joint National Committee on Prevention, Detection, Evaluation, and Treatment of High Blood Pressure*. NIH Publication no. 98-4080. Bethesda, MD: U.S. Department of Health and Human Services, National Heart, Lung, and Blood Institute.

Palatini, P., and Julius, S. (1999). The physiological determinants and risk correlations of elevated heart rate. *American Journal of Hypertension, 12*, 3S-8S.

Peng, C.K., Buldyrev, S.V., Hausdorff, J.M., Havlin, S., Mietus, J.E., Simons, M., Stanley, H.E., and Goldberger, A.L. (1994). Non-equilibrium dynamics as an indispensable characteristic of a healthy biological system. *Integrated Physiologic Behavioral Science, 3*, 283-293.

Porges, S.W. (1992). Autonomic regulation and attention. In B.A. Campbell, H. Hayne, and R. Richardson (Eds.), *Attention and information processing in infants and adults* (pp. 201-223). Hillsdale, NJ: Lawrence Erlbaum Associates.

Porges, S.W., Doussard-Roosevelt, J.A., and Maita, A.K. (1994). Vagal tone and the physiological regulation of emotion. *Monographs of the Society for Research in Child Development, 59*(2-3), 167-186, 250-283.

Reed, S.W., Porges, S.W., and Newlin, D.B. (1999). Effect of alcohol on vagal regulation of cardiovascular function: Contributions of the polyvagal theory to the psychophysiology of alcohol. *Experimental and Clinical Psychopharmacology, 7*(4), 484-492.

Roberts, A.C., and Wallis, J.D. (2000). Inhibitory control and affective processing in the prefrontal cortex: Neuropsychological studies in the common marmoset. *Cerebral Cortex, 10*, 252-262.

Rossy, L.A., and Thayer, J.F. (1998). Fitness and gender-related differences in heart period variability. *Psychosomatic Medicine, 60*, 773-781.

Rozanski, A., Blumenthal, J.A., and Kaplan, J. (1999). Impact of psychological factors on the pathogenesis of cardiovascular disease and implications for therapy. *Circulation, 99*, 2192-2217.

Ruiz-Padial, E., Sollers, J.J., III, Vila, J., and Thayer, J.F. (2003). The rhythm of the heart in the blink of an eye: Emotion-modulated startle magnitude covaries with heart rate variability. *Psychophysiology, 40*, 306-313.

Saul, J.P. (1990). Beat-to-beat variations of heart rate reflect modulation of cardiac autonomic outflow. *News in Physiological Science, 5*, 32-37.

Seeman, T.E., Singer, B.H., Rowe, J.W., Horwitz, R.I., and McEwen, B.S. (1997). Price of adaptation—allostatic load and its health consequences: McArthur studies of successful aging. *Archives of Internal Medicine, 157*, 2259-2268.

Siegle, G.J., and Thayer, J.F. (2003). Physiological aspects of depressive rumination (pp. 79-104). In C. Papageorgiou and A. Wells (Eds.), *Depressive rumination: Nature, theory, and treatment.* New York: Wiley.

Skinner, J.E. (1985). Regulation of cardiac vulnerability by the cerebral defense system. *Journal of the American College of Cardiology, 5*, 88B-94B.

Sokolov, E.N. (1963). *Perception and the orienting response.* New York: MacMillan.

Spyer, K.M. (1989). Neural mechanisms involved in cardiovascular control during affective behavior. *Trends in Neuroscience, 12*, 506-513.

Sroka, K., Peimann, C.J., and Seevers, H. (1997). Heart rate variability in myocardial ischemia during daily life. *Journal of Electrocardiology, 30*, 45-56.

Stein, P.K., and Kleiger, R.E. (1999). Insights from the study of heart rate variability. *Annual Review of Medicine, 50*, 249-261.

Stein, P.K., Bosner, M.S., Kleiger, R.E., and Conger, B.M. (1994). Heart rate variability: A measure of cardiac autonomic tone. *American Heart Journal, 127*, 1376-1381.

Steptoe, A., and Appels, A. (1989). *Stress, personal control and health.* Chicester, England: Wiley.

Sternberg, E.M. (1997). Emotions and disease: From balance of humors to balance of molecules. *Nature Medicine, 3*, 264-267.

Tallis, F., and Eysenck, M.W. (1994). Worry: Mechanisms and modulating influences. *Behavioural and Cognitive Psychotherapy, 22*(1), 37-56.

Task Force of the European Society of Cardiology and the North American Society of Pacing Electrophysiology. (1996). Heart rate variability: Standards of measurement, physiological interpretation, and clinical use. *Circulation, 93*, 1043-1065.

Ter Horst, G.J. (1999). Central autonomic control of the heart, angina, and pathogenic mechanisms of post-myocardial infarction depression. *European Journal of Morphology, 37*, 257-266.

Ter Horst, G.J., and Postema, F. (1997). Forebrain parasympathetic control of heart activity: Retrograde transneuronal viral labeling in rats. *American Journal of Physiology, 273*, H2926-H2930.

Thayer, J.F., and Friedman, B.H. (1997). The heart of anxiety: A dynamical systems approach. In A. Vingerhoets (Ed.), *The (non) expression of emotions in health and disease.* Amsterdam: Springer Verlag.

Thayer, J.F., and Friedman, B.H. (2002). Stop that! Inhibition, sensitization, and their neurovisceral concomitants. *Scandinavian Journal of Psychology, 43*, 123-130.

Thayer, J.F., and Lane, R.D. (2000). A model of neurovisceral integration in emotion regulation and dysregulation. *Journal of Affective Disorders, 61*, 201-216.

Thayer, J.F., and Lane, R.D. (2002). Perseverative thinking and health: Neurovisceral concomitants. *Psychology and Health, 17*, 685-695.

Thayer, J.F., and Ruiz-Padial, E. (2002). Neurovisceral integration in emotion and health. *International Congress Series: Proceedings of the 16th World Congress on Psychosomatic Medicine, 1241,* 321-327.

Thayer, J.F., Friedman, B.H., and Borkovec, T.D. (1996). Autonomic characteristics of generalized anxiety disorder and worry. *Biological Psychiatry, 39,* 255-266.

Thayer, J.F., Smith, M., Rossy, L.A., Sollers, J.J., and Friedman, B.H. (1998). Heart period variability and depressive symptoms: Gender differences. *Biological Psychiatry, 44,* 304-306.

Thayer, J.F., Friedman, B.H., Borkovec, T.D., Johnsen, B.H., and Molina, S. (2000). Phasic heart period to cued threat and non-threat stimuli in generalized anxiety disorder. *Psychophysiology, 37,* 361-368.

Thayer, J.F., Merritt, M.M., Sollers, J.J., III, Zonderman, A.B., Evans, M.K., Yie, S., and Abernethy, D.R. (2003). Effect of angiotensin-converting enzyme insertion/deletion polymorphophism DD genotype on high-frequency heart rate variability in African Americans. *American Journal of Cardiology, 92,* 1487-1490.

Timberlake, W. (1994). Behavior systems, associationism, and Pavlovian conditioning. *Psychonomic Bulletin and Review, 1,* 405-420.

Tracey, K.J. (2002). The inflammatory reflex. *Nature, 420,* 853-859.

Uijtdehaage, S.B.H., and Thayer, J.F. (2000). Accentuated antagonism in the control of human heart rate. *Clinical Autonomic Research, 10,* 107-110.

Ursin, H. (1987). Personality, activation, and psychosomatic disease. In D. Magnusson, A. Oehman et al. (Eds.), *Psychopathology: An interactional perspective. Personality, psychopathology, and psychotherapy* (pp. 273-287). Orlando, FL: Academic Press.

Ursin, H. (1998). The psychology in psychoneuroendocrinology. *Psychoneuroendocrinology, 23,* 555-570.

Ursin, H., and Hytten, K. (1992). Outcome expectancies and psychosomatic consequences. In B.N. Carpenter et al. (Eds.), *Personal coping: Theory, research, and application* (pp. 171-184). Westport, CT: Praeger/Greenwood.

Verberne, A.J.M., and Owens, N.C. (1998). Cortical modulation of the cardiovascular system. *Progress in Neurobiology, 54,* 149-168.

Verrier, R.L. (1987). Mechanisms of behaviorally induced arrhythmias. *Circulation,* 76(Suppl. I), I48-I56.

Verrier, R.L., and Mittleman, M.A. (2000). The impact of emotions on the heart. *Progress in Brain Research, 122,* 369-380.

Weise, F., Krell, D., and Brinkhoff, N. (1986). Acute alcohol ingestion reduces heart rate variability. *Drug and Alcohol Dependence, 17,* 89-91.

Williams, D.R. (1997). Race and health: Basic questions, emerging directions. *Annals of Epidemiology, 7,* 322-333.

Williams, D.R., and Neighbors, H. (2001). Racism, discrimination and hypertension: Evidence and needed research. *Ethnicity and Disease, 11,* 800-816.

Winters, R.W., McCabe, P.M., Green, E.J., and Schneiderman, N. (2000). Stress responses, coping, and cardiovascular neurobiology: Central nervous system circuitry underlying learned and unlearned affective responses to stressful stimuli. In P.M. McCabe, N. Schneiderman, T. Field, and A.R. Wellens (Eds.), *Stress, coping, and cardiovascular disease.* Hillsdale, NJ: Lawrence Erlbaum Associates.

Young, E.A., Neese, R.M., Weder, A., and Julius, S. (1998). Anxiety and cardiovascular reactivity in the Tecumseh population. *Journal of Hypertension,* 16(12), 1727-1733.

Ziegler, D., Laude, D., Akila, F., and Elghozi, J.L. (2001). Time and frequency domain estimation of early diabetic cardiovascular autonomic neuropathy. *Clinical Autonomic Research,* 11(6), 369-376.

16

Geography and Racial Health Disparities

Amitabh Chandra and Jonathan S. Skinner

During the past several decades, many studies have documented racial, ethnic, gender, and socioeconomic disparities in both medical care treatments and health outcomes.[1] There are no easy economic explanations for such differences: African Americans seem less likely to receive invasive treatments even in the Veteran's Affairs (VA) system, where doctors' economic incentives are likely to be blunted (Peterson, Wright, Daley, and Thibault, 1994; Whittle, Conigliaro, Good, and Lofgren, 1993). Nor do differences in insurance coverage seem to eliminate racial or ethnic gaps (Carlisle, Leake, and Shapiro, 1997); indeed Ross and Mirowsky (2000) believe public insurance such as Medicare and Medicaid lead to worse health. More recently, racial differences in cardiac surgery were hypothesized to depend on the race of the physician; however, no significant differences were found (Chen et al., 2001). The Institute of Medicine's (IOM's) landmark study (Smedley, Stith, and Nelson, 2002) has conducted a comprehensive survey of the evidence and concluded that racial disparities in medical care treatments and outcomes are pervasive; this topic also has been an integral part of the National Research Council's research agenda (National Research Council, 1997).

Collectively these papers clearly document important racial differences in treatments, intensity of care, and outcomes. In this chapter, we consider a complicating factor that has implications for both statistical inference and policy recommendations regarding racial disparities: the *geography* of health care and health outcomes, and its relationship to the measurement of racial health disparities. This is a broad topic (see for example, Chapter 11, this volume), and so we will organize our contribution along five basic points.

(1) There is considerable variation in the utilization of health care, and in outcomes, by region.

The phenomenon of "small area variation" in utilization rates has been studied for a number of decades. Most recently the *Dartmouth Atlas of Health Care* has used nearly 100 percent samples of Medicare enrollees to measure such differences across 306 Hospital Referral Regions (HRRs) in the United States (Wennberg and Cooper, 1999). Even after controlling for differences in underlying health status across regions, there is clear evidence of persistent and large differences in treatment patterns, even in contiguous areas. Much of the current debate is how to interpret such differences—are they "demand" driven by patient preferences, or "supply" driven by physician beliefs and historical patterns of hospital location? In addition to disparities in treatment patterns, there are also substantial variations in health outcomes by region. Recent research has documented race-specific and gender-specific variations at the county or state level in overall mortality rates as well as disease-specific mortality rates (Barnett et al., 2001; Casper et al., 2001).[2]

(2) People who are African American or Hispanic or belong to other minority groups tend to seek care from different hospitals and from different physicians compared to non-Hispanic whites.

It is not surprising that African-American and Hispanic patients tend to see different physicians and are admitted to different hospitals compared to non-Hispanic whites. This is largely the consequence of where people live: there are far fewer African Americans seeking care in eastern Tennessee hospitals than in Mississippi hospitals, and many more Hispanic patients seeking care in hospitals in Florida, Texas, and California than in Maine and New Hampshire. Furthermore, patients of color who live in the same neighborhood as whites may go to different hospitals or (more clearly) see different physicians and in different settings for a variety of reasons, including financial barriers, as well as racial barriers to care (Lillie-Blanton, Martinez, and Salganicoff, 2001). Patients also tend to be seen by physicians of the same race, although one study (Harrison and Thurston, 2001) suggested this matching is in part the consequence of minority physicians being more likely to live near minority neighborhoods.

(3) Racial disparities are pronounced in some areas, but are less so (or may not be present) in other areas.

In most regions of the United States, there are pronounced racial differences in utilization and outcomes. But in other areas, there are no significant racial differences. In some sense, this is welcome news, in that the medical profession is not some monolithic and uniform "system" that treats patients identically regardless of where they live. Such differences, however, are not easily explained, and may rely on one or two surgeons who account for the majority of procedures in their region. In other cases, the differences in racial disparities may arise from spatial "mismatches" of patients and physicians, for example, because of segregation in residential areas or the location of hospital facilities.

(4) These three facts create strong statistical interactions between geography and racial identity: one may falsely diagnose geographical variation as racial disparities, and conversely.

On average, Hispanic Medicare enrollees account for the same level of expenditures as their non-Hispanic elderly counterparts (Centers for Medicare and Medicaid Services, 2000, Table 4.8). Although this might reassure observers that there are no obvious utilization disparities between Hispanic and non-Hispanic Medicare enrollees, there is one complicating factor: geography. Medicare expenditures on average are substantially higher in Florida, Texas, and California (Wennberg and Cooper, 1999). Because a large fraction of Hispanic Medicare patients live in these three states, the researcher might find that within each state, Hispanic patients experience lower utilization rates than their non-Hispanic counterparts.

More generally, in typical regression analysis when minority patients live in regions with systematically different rates of utilization (e.g., African Americans in the south), and the region of residence is not controlled for, one can estimate larger or smaller racial "disparities" that are in fact the consequence of where people live, and not how they are treated or their outcomes within their community. Nor are typical regional measures, such as Metropolitan Statistical Area (MSA), necessarily accurate mirrors of "local" effects.

It is important to note here that we do *not* argue against the existence of racial disparities, nor do we argue that they are necessarily mitigated by geographical variation. If African Americans live in regions with poor hospital quality, then that in itself represents a valid source of racial disparities. Instead, our central thesis is that ignoring geography (or misspecifying it) will cause the analyst to "cry wolf" when true differences are nonexistent, or to falsely conclude that there are no differences when in fact there are substantial differences in the outcomes of interest. Furthermore, as we argue next, the policy prescriptions may differ, depending on whether the racial disparities are caused by regional variations instead of by differences in treatment within hospitals or communities.

(5) A potentially large part of overall health disparities in the United States may be the consequence of regional differences in treatment and outcomes. Reducing geographic disparities in quality of care will benefit all Americans, but is likely to yield greater benefits to minority patients.

The policy implications of racial disparities are different depending on their proximate causes. Racial differences arising within a hospital or even within a physician's practice may reasonably be ascribed to differences in underlying health status, patient preferences, financial barriers, provider biases, or some combination of these four factors. Here, however, the insights of the regional variation literature is relevant; it is not the case that the rate of therapeutic interventions for whites should be necessarily viewed as the "correct" or "desired" rate (Tu et al., 1997; Wennberg, 1986). This is because the white rate might reflect inappropriate care—whites get too much done to them, as discussed by Schneider et al. (2001). Alternatively, preferences for care may differ by race or gender.

When aggregate racial differences in outcomes are the consequence of minority patients being more likely to live in regions where everyone in the region experiences poorer outcomes, then the policy focus should be on disparities in *geography*—that specific regions be targeted to improve quality of care or reduce "flat of the curve" health care spending.[3] Such policies would ensure that disadvantaged racial groups would be the major beneficiaries of quality improvements.

THE GEOGRAPHY OF HEALTH CARE

The measurement of regional variation in health care utilization is difficult for a variety of reasons. First, a great deal of statistical power is necessary to measure utilization at the local level; even a sample of 50,000 observations quickly loses power when the data are partitioned into separate regions, and used to focus on specific diseases. Small sample sizes and inadequate statistical power can generate spurious "area variation" just because of random noise in measured average rates.[4] Second, the problem of migration to hospitals must be considered; Boston hospitals accept referrals from all over New England, and if these patients were counted, it might appear falsely that Boston residents are at elevated risk of hospitalization. Third, one needs a sample that is not subject to selectivity bias. For example, the sample of Medicaid patients, or of managed care patients, is not likely to be representative of the general population; Medicaid patients can become eligible because of serious illness, and managed care patients tend to be healthier than the general population. Finally, the regions should correspond to actual migration patterns of patients rather than artifacts of historical compromises such as state or county boundaries.

In this section, we use data from the *Dartmouth Atlas of Health Care* that go far to avoid these four shortfalls (Wennberg and Cooper, 1996, 1999). The data comprise a nearly 100 percent sample of Medicare enrollees over age 65, often for 2 years, so the sample sizes are as much as 60 million person-years in a given map or graph; this provides considerable power for regional analysis. Second, the *Atlas* defines one's location by the zip code of residence, rather than where one actually gets care. So if a patient from the Burlington, Vermont, region is admitted to a Boston hospital, that hospital stay (and any procedures done there) is assigned to Burlington, not Boston.

Third, the Medicare data provide nearly 100 percent coverage of the population over age 65 and is the nearest thing to a national database of utilization in the United States. There have been increases in the population of risk-bearing Health Maintenance Organizations (HMOs) in the Medicare population (now referred to as Medicare+Choice), but that ratio never exceeded 12 percent and has fallen as many insurance carriers have dropped the Medicare+Choice option. In some urban regions the ratio of HMO patients in the Medicare population has been higher than the national average, and this has engendered more concern about selection bias.[5]

The *Dartmouth Atlas* has divided the United States into 306 Hospital Referral Regions (HRRs). An HRR is the unit of analysis at which health care for the elderly is delivered. Its geographic boundaries are computed by examining the complex pattern of commuting patterns to major referral hospitals.[6] HRRs are named for the hospital service area containing the referral hospital or hospitals most often used by residents of the region. The regions sometimes cross state boundaries—an attribute that is by its very nature ruled out by cross-state analysis. Intuitively, one may think of HRRs as representing the geographic level at which "tertiary" services such as cardiac surgery are received.

To demonstrate the construction of the HRRs, in Figure 16-1 we detail the construction of the Evansville, Indiana, HRR. This region includes three states: Illinois, Indiana, and Kentucky. In this region, three hospitals provide cardiovascular surgery services: two in Evansville and one in Vincennes, Indiana. The Evansville HRR also demonstrates that the inclusion of simple MSA fixed effects does not account adequately for geography: the U.S. Census' Evansville-Henderson MSA is actually comprised of three HRRs. This is not a problem in itself. However, if different HRRs have different practice styles, then it blurs the measure of true regional differences in utilization by aggregating up to the state or MSA level. To demonstrate the

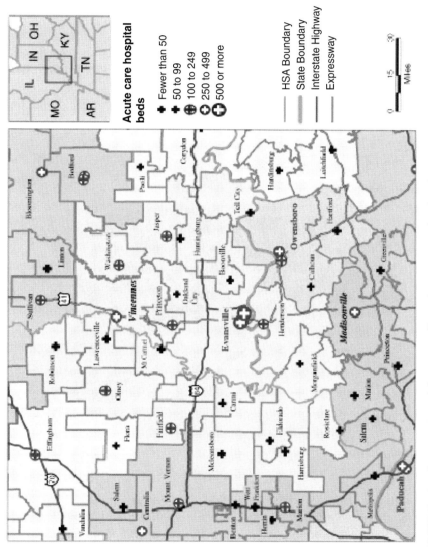

FIGURE 16-1 Construction of the Evansville, Indiana, Hospital Referral Region.

overwhelming degree to which even adjacent HRRs practice different "styles" of medicine, we now draw on the findings of the *Dartmouth Atlas of Health Care*.

Figure 16-2 demonstrates that there is substantial variation in Medicare payments for services reimbursed on a fee-for-service basis (including non-risk-bearing health maintenance organizations). Even after controlling for age, sex, race, illness patterns, and differences in regional prices, reimbursements per enrollee varied greatly: as noted in the *Atlas*, even though the average payment was $4,993 per beneficiary, payments ranged from

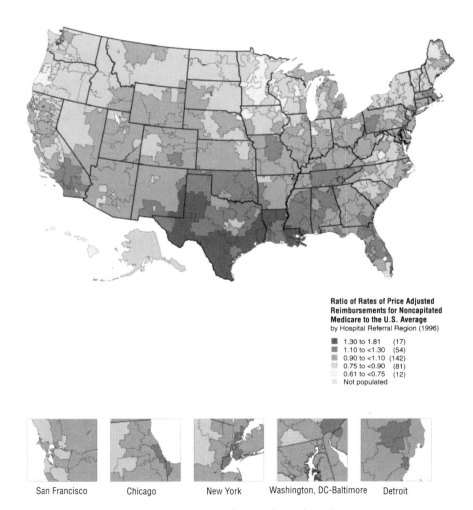

FIGURE 16-2 Geographic variation in illness-adjusted Medicare payments.

$9,033 in the McAllen, Texas, hospital referral region to $3,074 in Lynchburg, Virginia.[7]

In Figure 16-3 the *Atlas* illustrates the enormous geographic variation in a relatively standard procedure—Percutaneous Coronary Intervention (PCI), which includes the use of angioplasty and the placement of stents. PCI is an invasive procedure in which a catheter is inserted into the thigh and guided to the narrowed artery, where a balloon is expanded to clear the blockage and improve blood flow. Percutaneous Transluminal Coronary Angioplasty (PTCA) is often used immediately following a heart attack, or shortly thereafter, or to relieve pain for patients with ischemic heart disease. In 1996 more than 200,000 of these procedures were conducted with an average rate of 7.5 per 1,000 Medicare enrollees. As in previous figures, the data have been standardized for demographic characteristics, and the unit of reporting is a HRR. Note how in Texas, Pennsylvania, and California, the ratio of rates (to the U.S. average) can vary drastically even across adjacent HRRs.

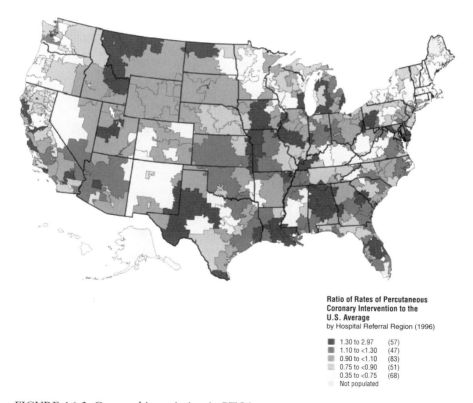

Ratio of Rates of Percutaneous Coronary Intervention to the U.S. Average
by Hospital Referral Region (1996)

■ 1.30 to 2.97 (57)
■ 1.10 to <1.30 (47)
▨ 0.90 to <1.10 (83)
▧ 0.75 to <0.90 (51)
  0.35 to <0.75 (68)
  Not populated

FIGURE 16-3 Geographic variation in PTCA rates.

The same pattern exists for other surgical procedures. Figure 16-4 summarizes the variation in rates (on a log scale) at which 10 common surgical procedures are used relative to the U.S. average (in 1996). Similar results have been documented for the variation in rates at which different diagnostic tests are utilized. Together the ten procedures listed in Figure 16-4 made up 42 percent of Medicare inpatient surgery and accounted for 44 percent of reimbursements for surgical care in 1995-1996. For many of these procedures, regional variation occurs because of fundamental uncertainty about the effectiveness of the procedure and ambiguity about the efficacy of alternatives. For example, variation in rates of radical prostatectomy might be partly attributable to the lack of controlled clinical trials comparing the risks and benefits of surgery, radiation therapy, and watchful waiting. For other procedures, even the best clinical trials are often not sufficient to eliminate variation in procedure rates: physicians vary in how they interpret findings from the carefully controlled settings of clinical trials to decision making for individual patients in other settings. The variation for hip fractures is small because the fracture can be diagnosed easily and virtually all physicians agree on the appropriate treatment therapy. For this procedure, the observed variation more accurately reflects variation in the

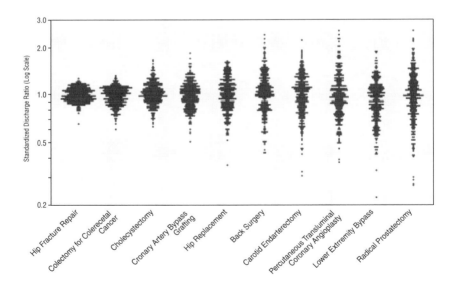

FIGURE 16-4 Surgical variation for ten common procedures. Each data point represents an observation for a Hospital Referral Region relative to the U.S. average standardized for age-gender-race and illness.
SOURCE: Wennberg and Cooper (1996).

actual rate of the hip fractures. Similarly, hospitalizations for colectomy reflect variations in the incidence of colorectal cancer, rather than differences in treatment strategies.

One might suspect these variations may be in part the consequence of differences in underlying patterns of cardiovascular disease. Certainly one might expect that HRR-level rates of PTCA should be associated with HRR-level rates of heart attacks (acute myocardial infarctions, or AMIs). This is because nearly one-third of heart attack patients are treated with PTCA and community rates of AMI should be correlated with true (diagnosed and undiagnosed) levels of ischemic heart disease. However, the correlation coefficient (weighted by the Medicare population) between PTCA rates and AMI rates is essentially zero (correlation = 0.05, p = 0.35) and not significant, meaning that these variations are unlikely to be explained by differences in cardiovascular health status.

The provocative nature of these results has not gone unnoticed, and several hypotheses have been put forward to explain these variations. These include the role of sampling variation, differences in underlying severity, patient preferences, the role of capacity, and the nature of physician learning. Wennberg et al. (2002) demonstrate that higher Medicare spending does not result in more high-quality care, such as flu vaccines, use of beta blockers when appropriate, or better health outcomes. Instead, higher spending is typically associated with more "supply-sensitive services" such as physician visits, specialist consultations, and days in the intensive care unit. Supply-sensitive services are those that are provided in the absence of specific clinical guidelines on frequency of use, and where medical texts provide little guidance. Utilization rates for such services appear to be highly correlated with the supply of resources—the number of physicians, specialists, labs, and beds. As such, there appears to be little support for the notion that costs or inadequate training drive practice variation.

Another class of rationalizations is developed by Phelps and Mooney (1993) and Bikhchandani et al. (2002), who suggest that explanations based on the nature of physician learning are most likely to account for much of the empirically observed locality of treatment. In the Phelps-Mooney model, physicians are Bayesian learners who attempt to reach an optimal rate for the application of a particular treatment. Eventually, as physicians sample both their own and their colleagues' experiences, the two will converge toward an optimal rate. This hypothesis suggests a number of implications: a physician's propensity to treat converges toward the community norm, and faster if the community is more informed and the doctor is less informed (e.g., younger). Among the implications of this theory is the hypothesis that the provision of more precise medical information in medical studies can enhance the learning of physicians, and thus offer dramatic social efficiency gains. Bikhchandani and colleagues (2002) consider a modification of this model and demonstrate that it is possible for physicians to fall into a localized "cascade" because of the difficulty in experimenting with alternative treatment choices.

The message of Figures 16-2, 16-3, and 16-4 is that the practice or "intensity" of medicine varies tremendously across space. But there are also large differences within states and even within cities. Fisher, Wennberg, Stukel, and Sharp (1994) construct cohorts of Medicare beneficiaries on the basis of initial hospitalization for AMI, stroke, gastro-intestinal bleeding, hip fracture, or surgery for breast, colon, or lung cancer. They find substantial differences in the intensity with which beneficiaries were treated (as measured by readmission rates) even across similar teaching hospitals in the Boston area. Specifically, there is substantial variation across readmission rates for Massachusetts General Hospital, Brigham and Women's Hospital, Beth Israel, and Boston University Medical Center. Most interestingly, there is no relationship between mortality (both 30 day and over the entire study period) and the intensity of hospitalization. Clearly, racial differences in migration patterns to hospitals of patients within Boston could have first-order effects on utilization rates, although in this case, probably not with respect to outcomes.

RACIAL DIFFERENCES IN WHERE (AND FROM WHOM) HEALTH CARE IS PROVIDED

A variety of studies have documented the large differences in insurance status and presence of regular providers (versus emergency room visits) among African Americans, Hispanics, and non-Hispanic whites (e.g., Lillie-Blanton, Martinez, and Salganicoff, 2001). In addition, simple differences in where people live will lead to minority patients being seen at different hospitals, and by different providers, from whites. This is not terribly surprising; clearly, hospitals in Washington, DC, will be more likely utilized by African Americans and Hispanics than those in Minot, South Dakota.

To capture this difference, we use a nearly 100 percent sample of Medicare fee-for-service patients who were admitted for a heart attack, or AMI, in 1998-1999; these data come from the National Bureau of Economic Research Medicare claims panel developed by McClellan and Staiger (1999). There were a total of 468,663 admissions in those two years to 4,737 hospitals. Nonblack admissions totaled 439,350, while black admissions were 29,313. We use a Lorenz curve approach to characterize the extent to which black and nonblack AMI patients tend to be admitted to different hospitals, as shown in Figure 16-5. The 4,737 hospitals were sorted according to the total number of black AMI Medicare patients admitted during 1998-1999, starting with the lowest number (to the left) and ranging to the right of the graph showing hospitals with the largest number

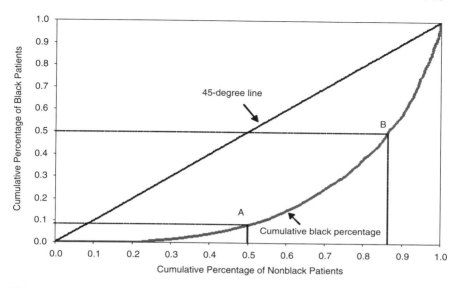

FIGURE 16-5 Lorenz curve showing distribution of black and nonblack AMI patients by hospital of admission.

of black patients. The scale on the horizontal axis is the percentage of total nonblack patients in the sample. The scale on the vertical axis is the percentage of black patients in the sample. Given that we have sorted hospitals in this way, we then plot the cumulative percentage of black admissions on the vertical axis, and the cumulative number of nonblack admissions on the horizontal axis.

The 45-degree line in Figure 16-5 is the hypothetical line one would get if perfect equality held in the distribution of black and nonblack patients by hospital. That is, if every hospital admitted 6.25 black patients per 100 nonblack patients (i.e., 0.0625 = 29,313/468,663), then the hospitals accounting for 50 percent of nonblack patients would also account for the cumulative total of 50 percent of black patients. (The analogy in the economics literature is that the 45-degree line in the Lorenz curve characterizes perfect equality of income.)

As is clear from the graph, however, there is little equality with regard to hospital admissions. Slightly more than one-fifth of nonblack AMI patients are admitted to hospitals with *no* black AMI patients. Point A shows that 50 percent of nonblack Medicare patients are admitted to hospitals that account for just 9 percent of black patients. Point B shows the converse statistic, that 50 percent of black AMI patients are admitted to hospitals that combined account for just 14 percent of nonblack AMI patients. The Gini coefficient (or the ratio of the area between the 45-degree line and the curved line, divided by the total area underneath the 45-degree line) is 0.61. Thus, the results of Figure 16-5 suggest that even 35 years after the passage of Title VI and VII of the Civil Rights Act that forbade de jure segregation and discrimination, considerable de facto segregation by race still occurs in the hospitals where whites and blacks seek care.

These patterns are not unique to hospital admissions, and it is likely that differences in where whites and minorities seek care may ultimately reflect differences in where they live. The important work of Massey (2001) on residential segregation confirms our intuition on this fact. Using data on 30 major U.S. cities, Massey finds that *dissimilarity indices* (the relative number of minorities who would have to migrate in order to establish a uniform distribution of race across neighborhoods) range from 67 in southern cities to 78 in northern ones;[8] larger cities such as Chicago, Cleveland, Detroit, and New York had *isolation indices* of over 80 (implying that in these cities the average African American inhabits a neighborhood that is more than 80 percent black).[9]

A story similar to racial differences in the hospitals where minorities seek care holds for physicians. In a recent study, Harrison and Thurston (2001) first demonstrated considerable "matching" between minority physicians and minority patients. The degree to which racial matching occurs is striking—in 1991, 47 percent of patients seen by black physicians were black (versus 17 percent for white non-Hispanic physicians), and 30 percent of patients seen by Hispanic physicians were Hispanic (versus 9 percent for white non-Hispanic physicians). However, the differences between white and minority physicians are reduced substantially when the analysis controls for location according to the zip code of the physician's practice. As the authors suggest, improving health care services for minority populations can be addressed both by increasing the number of physicians (of any race) who live in the area, as well as by increasing the numbers of minority physicians. (See also Cooper-Patrick et al., 1999; however, this study finds greater patient satisfaction and treatment adherence when there is concordance in racial identity between provider and patient.)

These results are useful reminders that when health care more generally exhibits such wide variations across areas, these area differences could be reflected as racial differences at the aggregate level. What is not as well known is how much of the actual differences in where one lives (i.e., the zip code of residence) and selective migration to different hospitals are *conditional on* where one lives (i.e., whether blacks and whites in a given zip code go to different hospitals).

Furthermore, it is important to put these differences in health care providers in the context of the many other effects of neighborhood on health status more generally. Morenoff and Lynch (see Chapter 11, this volume) have documented the multiple and dynamic causal pathways by which neighborhood-specific factors can influence long-term health outcomes independent of the type or nature of health care. Thus, access to health care and quality of health care are only two of a variety of factors affecting health that are likely to vary by neighborhood of residence. The work of Oliver and Shapiro (1995) and, more quantitatively, Smith and Kington (1997) provides additional perspective on understanding these facts. Smith and Kingston emphasize noting the difference between income (a relatively transitory measure of socioeconomic status, or SES) and wealth (a more permanent index of SES). Smith and Kington document that wealth disparities across race are substantially larger than income disparities. What is not well understood is the extent to which wealth as well as income can explain racial variations in health care utilization and health care outcomes.

GEOGRAPHIC VARIATIONS IN THE EXTENT OF RACIAL DISPARITIES: AN EXAMPLE

Few studies of racial disparities treat such differences at a regional level. In part, this is the consequence of power considerations; there are not enough observations in most data sets to distinguish racial differences in utilization across regions. In recent work Baicker (2002) utilizes data on heart attack treatments assembled by researchers at Dartmouth College and Stanford University to examine state-level differences in treatment patterns. Figure 16-6 uses these data to provide measures of angioplasty use for several selected states during 1990-1995 using a sample of fee-for-service Medicare patients admitted to hospital for AMI.[10] In addition, the U.S. national rates are presented based on a sample size of more than 1 million Medicare patients. These estimates are adjusted for two broad age categories (ages 65 to 80 or greater than 80), gender, and income (whether in the bottom quintile of zip codes as sorted by race-specific income). Generally, sample sizes were very large, and the 95 percent confidence intervals for black PTCA rates were (at most) ±0.025 in the smallest state, Massachusetts, and generally an order of magnitude smaller among nonblacks and in larger states (e.g., ±0.0063 for blacks in New York).

Figure 16-6 shows the remarkable heterogeneity in PTCA rates across selected states and across race in these states. On average, there was a large gap in PTCA rates in the United States, with rates for blacks just 69 percent of those for nonblacks; this result has been established in many other studies. However, a state-by-state analysis suggests some variability in the magnitude of the disparities. In Massachusetts, rates are slightly higher among black Medicare patients, although the results are by no means statistically significant. By contrast, black PTCA rates in Arkansas are just 23 percent of the nonblack rates (p < 0.001). Most states are closer to the national mean difference, such as New York (black rates are 62 percent of

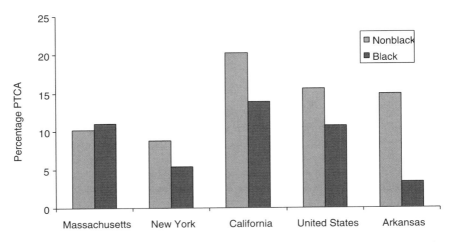

FIGURE 16-6 Ninety-day PTCA rates per AMI patient in the Medicare population, by selected states, 1990-1995.

nonblack rates) and California (69 percent of nonblack rates). Note also the considerable degree of variation *across* states, so that the PTCA rates for black Medicare patients in California (13.9 percent) are higher than nonblack rates in New York (8.8 percent).

These results are obviously quite preliminary and have not been fully risk adjusted, so they should be interpreted cautiously. Nonetheless, they suggest that racial disparities in utilization are not entirely uniform across regions.

THE INTERACTION BETWEEN GEOGRAPHY AND RACIAL DISPARITIES: STATISTICAL ISSUES

The standard approach to measuring racial disparities in health data makes careful efforts to control for a variety of risk adjusters, including health status, co-morbidities, possibly clinical data on admission, demographic information, and, where possible, income. Often, in quantitative studies, region is not included, either because region is suppressed because of concerns about confidentiality or because of difficulty in how to interpret regional differences.

To see how region can interact with measures of health disparities in a statistical sense, it is useful to begin with a simple example. Table 16-1 shows cardiovascular deaths by race for men in two states, Massachusetts and Mississippi; these statistics were developed by a team of researchers and published by the Centers for Disease Control and Prevention (for details see Barnett et al., 2001). (Results are similar but not as pronounced for

TABLE 16-1 Cardiovascular Deaths per 100,000 Population for Men: Mississippi and Massachusetts

	Black Mortality Rate	White Mortality Rate	Ratio: Black/White
Both states combined	900	668	1.35
Mississippi	1,028	835	1.23
Massachusetts	580	616	0.94

SOURCES: Cardiovascular data from Barnett et al. (2001), black and white state population numbers (total, not by sex) and for 1998.

women.) Were we to combine the data and consider the difference in age-adjusted mortality rates for cardiovascular disease for both states, we would find black mortality rates of 900 per 100,000, and for whites, a corresponding rate of 668.[11] In other words, cardiovascular disease is 35 percent higher for blacks than for whites.

However, note that rates of cardiovascular deaths in Mississippi are higher for both blacks and whites. Within Mississippi, rates are 24 percent higher for men, and within Massachusetts, black cardiovascular rates are actually 6 percent below those for white men. Indeed, the overall weighted elevated risk for cardiovascular disease is 15 percent once state-level differences are taken into account. Furthermore, all of the additional mortality is occurring not in Massachusetts, but in Mississippi.

There are many scenarios in which the 35 percent elevated rate would be relevant; for example, how much at risk are African Americans overall to cardiovascular disease? From a policy viewpoint it is useful to decompose that 35 percent difference into two parts: that part attributable to within-state differences (15 percent) and the remaining 20 percent that is caused by African Americans being more likely to live in a state where *everyone* experiences higher cardiovascular mortality rates. The latter 20 percent (which comprises nearly 60 percent of the total 35 percent disparity) is perhaps best addressed by improving health behaviors and health care for all citizens of Mississippi.

The point of this exercise is not to argue that the 35 percent elevated rate observed in these two states is not the consequence of deep-rooted discrimination, nor does it rule out the presence of disparities in health among blacks even in Massachusetts. Instead, we are trying to suggest that it is useful to decompose overall black-white differences in health outcomes (or health care utilization) into two parts. First, there could be discrimination by providers and hospitals (or the health care system), and second, there could be economic and social discrimination (or a historical legacy) that affects the location decisions of minorities. This chapter focuses on the role of the first source of disparities, not on the second. It is critical to note that ruling out the first does not rule out the second (or for that matter, vice versa).

A similar issue can be seen in evaluating quality of care for blacks and whites as measured by specific treatment regimes for AMI patients. For example, beta blockers are effective in extending survival because they lower blood pressure and reduce the demands placed on a weakened heart following AMI. Most clinicians would agree that the rate of beta blockers among patients who are not contraindicated for such therapy should be near 100 percent. Yet as one important study demonstrated using data from the Cooperative Cardiovascular Project (CCP) during 1993-1994, actual rates of compliance were considerably below 100 percent, and in some states were below 50 percent (Jencks et al., 2000). Figure 16-7 graphs on the vertical axis the percentage of AMI patients for whom chart review indicated that beta blockers were appropriate, while the horizontal axis graphs the percentage of people living in that state who were African American; the lowest rate of compliance was in Mississippi (47 percent). (For the moment, we exclude Washington, DC.) There is a distinct and significant negative correlation between the percentage of the state that is African American and the quality of care as measured by the use of beta blockers.[12] A state-level regression implies that black rates of beta-blocker compliance are 32 percentage points lower than for nonblacks.

However, another study that used the same CCP data found little overall difference in the use of beta blockers at discharge by race (Rathore et al., 2000). Unadjusted odds ratios were 0.90, but after adjusting for differences in clinical presentation, the odds ratio was just 0.96, which, although significant, implied just a 1 percentage point lower rate in the use of beta blockers for African Americans.

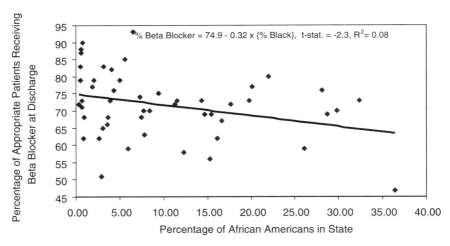

FIGURE 16-7 Percentage of appropriate AMI patients treated with beta blockers at discharge and percentage African American, by state.

Why the difference? One reason may be that the model also adjusts for differences in poverty rates, which do exert a significant influence on beta-blocker use (odds ratio = 0.93). More importantly, however, the regression controlled for Census region and for hospital volume, and while Census regions are crude measures of regional variation, they effectively limit differences in utilization of beta blockers to within-region comparisons. In other words, it is not simply the large African-American population in Mississippi that leads to such low compliance with the use of beta blockers where appropriate; it would appear that white AMI patients in Mississippi are not getting beta blockers either.[13] Nonetheless, this example illustrates the risks of making inferences about individual behavior based on aggregated data.

This problem is generally referred to as "ecological fallacy" and is well known in both the public health literature and in the political science literature (King, 1997; Susser, 1994a, 1994b). In theory, one can "solve" the ecological fallacy problem with the use of microlevel data with both race and location identifiers, but in practice that is often difficult. Often one must aggregate data at some level to identify community or region-specific effects that may themselves reflect a variety of unmeasured confounding variables.[14]

The results shown in Figure 16-8 illustrate state-level performance of general measures of health care quality by Jencks et al. (2000) and are taken from Fisher and Skinner (2001).[15] They show a southward progression from the Northeast (New Hampshire and Vermont, ranked numbers 1 and 2 in state-level quality) to the Deep South (Louisiana and Mississippi ranked 49 and 50, respectively; Washington, DC, dropped to 34 in the ranking). The first point is that conventional t-statistics in state-level regressions are overstated; these are not independent draws of 50 states.

Figures 16-8 also displays Medicare spending by state in 1996. The estimated spending values are adjusted for the fact that some states have more elderly people in the population or a sicker population. (The elderly in states such as Louisiana and West Virginia are indeed sicker—and we allow for their greater health needs in calculating per-capita Medicare spending.) The spending data, from the Dartmouth Atlas of Health Care Working Group (http://www.dartmouthatlas.org), do show remarkable differences in per-capita Medicare spending across states, ranging from $2,763 in Oregon to $5,668 in Texas and $6,307 in Alaska. The pattern of the dots, each of which represents a state, shows that more spending per capita does not appear to be related to better quality; if anything, it appears to be associated with worse care (Fisher and Skinner, 2001). We do not believe that increasing spending will reduce the quality of care. Connecticut and Massachusetts are both high-cost states, but ranked in the top 10 in terms of quality. Instead, we think that spending on Medicare is largely indepen-

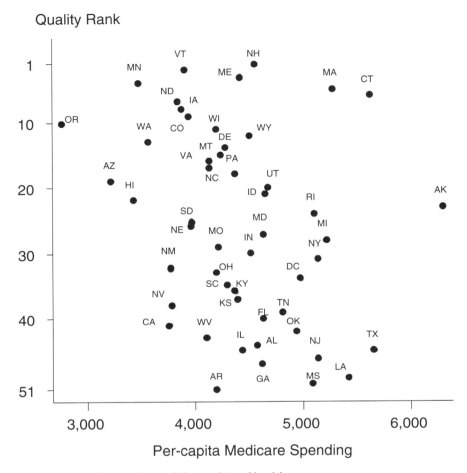

FIGURE 16-8 Geography and the quality of health care.

dent of how well physicians follow clinical guidelines for appropriate care, such as prescribing the right set of drugs for heart attack patients or screening for common and treatable diseases. High-quality care is not necessarily expensive care (Wennberg et al., 2002).

The second point is that this pattern is replicated in other studies showing a correlation between outcomes and percentage African American (Deaton and Lubotsky, 2001), rather than a correlation, as earlier hypothesized, between income inequality and mortality (Kennedy, Kawachi, and Prothrow-Stith, 1996).[16] Because there are many factors that seem to align themselves along this geographical dimension from New England to the

South (percentage black, income inequality, quality of health care), the ecological fallacy problem is particularly relevant here. The point to note from Figure 16-8 is that the states where many blacks live—Mississippi, Louisiana, Georgia, and Alabama—are all "low-quality" providers. The Northeast tends to comprise the "high-quality" providers, but as is well known, with the exception of the New York City area, these states have a small African-American population.

Even when researchers do specify regional covariates, they are often not specific to actual geographical patterns of health care use and outcomes; while incorporating state or MSA fixed effects is an improvement over ignoring them, they are still a highly simplistic characterization of the data, because patient migration patterns are not necessarily constrained by state or MSA boundaries. For example, blacks who live in Covington, Kentucky, will find it much easier to seek care in Cincinnati, Ohio (1 mile away across the Ohio river) versus driving to Louisville, Kentucky, or Lexington, Kentucky. The same story can be told for any large urban population center that encompasses several states (consider, e.g., large east coast cities such as Boston, Providence, Philadelphia, New York, Washington, DC).[17] Although the *Dartmouth Atlas'* use of HRR attempts to circumvent these problems by using zip code location and migration data to assign individuals to hospitals, even these measures likely understate true differences across HRRs in utilization variability.[18]

We next consider the statistical issues at a more general level: how specification of risk adjusters and geography can dramatically affect the bias in estimated regression coefficients. To illustrate the importance of geography and focus the discussion, we simplify the analysis and assume that high-quality data have been obtained which avoids problems with unmeasured confounding variables; any errors in measuring the "true" relationship arises because of model specification. For the purpose of these pictures, geography may be thought to be a variable such as hospital quality; this link is especially persuasive if we recall the previous discussion on hospital quality and residential segregation.

Figures 16-9a-9c simulate the estimation of simple regressions, where the parameter of interest is the coefficient on race (in our simple example, the coefficient on an indicator variable for "black"). In Figure 16-9a, we illustrate two data "clouds" for blacks and whites. Mortality is plotted on the y-axis and the x-axis measures the quality of health care provided at the relevant regional level. Ideally, this would be at the level of individual HRRs. Blacks are shown to have higher mortality than whites. However, this is entirely shown to be driven by geography—blacks live in regions or seek care at hospitals that provide low-quality care. Blacks and whites who live in the same region have the same outcomes. As we showed earlier, omitting quality or the correct measure of geography from the regression

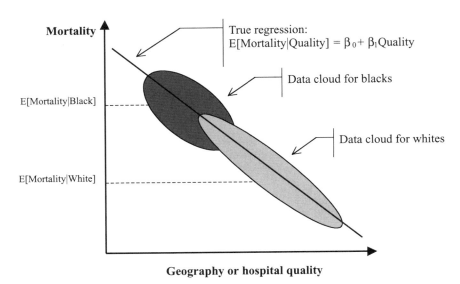

FIGURE 16-9a Geography and the measurement of racial disparities. Omitting quality or the correct measure of geography from the regression and comparing the racial difference in mortality (risk adjusted or otherwise) will yield an estimate of $\Delta = E[Mortality|Black] - E[Mortality|White]$. However, if whites are more likely to be seen at high-quality hospitals than blacks, Δ is overstated. In the true regression, there is no effect of race on mortality within hospitals or geographic area.

and comparing the racial difference in mortality (risk adjusted or otherwise) will yield an estimate of

$$\Delta = E[Mortality|Black] - E[Mortality|White].$$

However, if whites are more likely to be seen at high-quality hospitals than blacks, Δ is overstated. In the true regression, there is no effect of race on mortality within hospitals or geographic area.

In Figure 16-9b we assume that within-area blacks receive worse care than whites, but that this differential is constant over areas. Here, African Americans have worse outcomes even within the same hospitals. This correct race difference is β_2 (the distance between the lines for blacks and whites at the same level of quality, or within the same geographical unit). Omitting quality or the correct measure of geography from the regression and comparing the racial difference in mortality (risk adjusted or otherwise) will yield an estimate of $\Delta = E[Mortality|Black] - E[Mortality|White]$. It can be seen that Δ considerably overstates β_2.

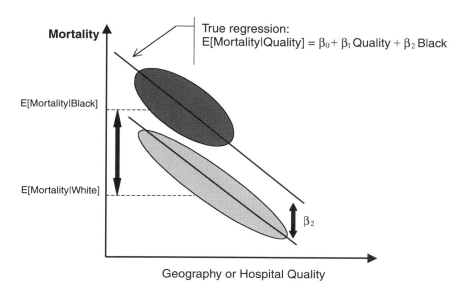

FIGURE 16-9b   Geography and the measurement of racial disparities. Here, African Americans have worse outcomes even within the same hospitals. This correct race difference is β_2 (the distance between the lines for blacks and whites at the same level of quality, or within the same geographical unit). Omitting quality or the correct measure of geography from the regression and comparing the racial difference in mortality (risk adjusted or otherwise) will yield an estimate of $\Delta =$ *E[Mortality|Black] – E[Mortality|White]*. It can be seen that Δ considerably overstates β_2.

An indirect example of estimating this model may be seen in the careful work of Morrison, Wallerstein, Natale, Senzel, and Huang (2000), who study the relationship between the racial composition of neighborhoods in New York and the degree to which pharmacies in these neighborhoods carried opioid supplies.[19] After controlling for the fraction of the local population that is elderly at the Census block level, the authors find that only 25 percent of the pharmacies in the largely nonwhite neighborhoods (those with nonwhite populations of 60 percent or larger) carried opioids. In contrast, in predominately white neighborhoods (those where more than 80 percent of the residents are white), over 72 percent of pharmacies carried the requisite supplies. The Morrison studies provide an intuitive description of Figures 16-9a and 16-9b: If the researcher does not control for geography and simply asks whether minorities are less likely to be near a well-stocked pharmacy (relative to whites), the conclusion would be yes. However, the point of Figure 16-9b is to note that whites who live in predominately nonwhite neighborhoods are also not near an adequately stocked pharmacy.

In Figure 16-9c, we illustrate the problems of ignoring differential quality effects. Here, African Americans have worse outcomes even within the same hospitals, and the race difference grows in worse hospitals. This correct race differential is β_1 *Quality* + β_2. Graphically, this is the height of the larger arrow. Omitting the Quality × Race interaction leads to severely understating the gap (the regression line will be weighted heavily by the white data), and the height of the smaller arrow is incorrectly estimated to be the race difference.

In practice, of course, the problem of unmeasured confounding variables is quite serious, even for very good data sets such as the CCP. Suppose the researcher estimates a model of the form:

$$Mortality_i = \beta_0 + Z\Gamma + \beta_1\ Black_i + u_i$$

Mortality (say 30-day mortality after AMI) for the ith individual is regressed on a vector of risk-adjustment controls (the Z matrix), and an indicator variable for whether the individual was African American. Here, the coefficient on race (here, an indicator variable for whether the respon-

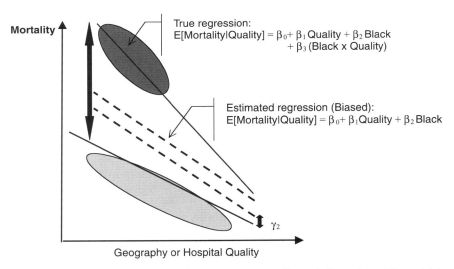

FIGURE 16-9c Geography and the measurement of racial disparities. Here, African Americans have worse outcomes even within the same hospitals and the race difference grows in worse hospitals. This correct race differential is β_1 *Quality* + β_2. Graphically, this is the height of the larger arrow. Omitting the quality × race interaction leads to severely understating the gap (the regression line will be weighted heavily by the white data), and the height of the smaller arrow is incorrectly estimated to be the race difference.

dent is an African American) is the parameter of interest. If the risk adjusters Z are complete, then it is possible to interpret the estimated coefficient β_1 as the effect of being black on mortality. However, the assumptions necessary to justify such a conclusion are very strong. First, as noted earlier, the presumption is that racial differences are the same across regions (as in Figure 16-9b), a finding that does not appear to be true in practice. (One might still interpret the coefficient as a weighted average, of course.)

Second, it presumes that the researcher has controlled for all biological or genetic differences that persist even once measurable risk adjustment has been made. If controls for co-morbidities are not complete and blacks are unobservably sicker than whites, we will overstate the coefficient estimate for β_1; otherwise the categorical variable on race will "pick up" all the unmeasured variables that differ by race. For example, in evaluating the use of thrombolytics (medications that dissolve blot clots) for the treatment of coronary disease, it is of first-order importance to know that such interventions are contraindicated for those patients who have had a recent hemorrhagic stroke. If blacks are more likely to have suffered from a stroke, documenting lower thrombolytic prescription rates alone, without appropriate covariates, is not meaningful.

Third, the model as estimated presumes that the influence of either co-morbidities or treatments are the same for both whites and blacks. Barbara McNeil, in her Shattuck Lecture, emphasized the importance of noting clinically relevant drug and race interactions (McNeil, 2001). For example, biological differences between races in receptor polymorphisms will cause different responses to the same drugs. A series of papers in the *New England Journal of Medicine* reflects these concerns. Among patients with congestive heart failure and left ventricular dysfunction, the use of Enalaprin or Bucindolol (angiotensin-converting enzyme inhibitors) reduced hospitalizations for whites and nonwhites respectively, but not for blacks (Exner et al., 2001). Similarly, Chen et al. (2001) note that African-American patients who have had an AMI are more likely to have negative or oftentimes unclear cardiograms at the moment of presentation, thereby complicating the ensuing diagnoses.

One approach to avoiding such statistical pitfalls is to use the insights of the Oaxaca-Blinder decomposition approach, used previously in the economics literature to evaluate racial wage disparities (Blinder, 1973; Oaxaca, 1973, 1975); more recently this approach has been used to measure racial disparities in health care (Balsa and McGuire, 2002). This approach counsels against pooling patient data across race or ethnic identity, but instead prescribes estimating the type of model above for just (say) whites. One can then ask: What would be the implied results (whether utilization or health outcome) for blacks or Hispanics given their own levels of covariates Z and the set of coefficients estimated for whites, Γ_w?

Skinner, Staiger, Chandra, Lee, and McClellan (2002), for example, used this approach to measure differences in average hospital quality for African-American AMI patients. They did not attempt to directly measure differences in outcomes between blacks and nonblacks within a given hospital. Instead, they used only nonblack AMI adjusted mortality rates to measure hospital "quality" for both blacks and nonblacks. Thus if blacks tended to be admitted to hospitals with higher *nonblack* mortality rates, hospital quality was deemed to be lower for blacks than for nonblacks. (The critical assumption in using nonblack mortality rates as a measure of quality is that the authors can adjust for differences in underlying health status for nonblacks living in largely black areas compared to nonblacks living in largely white areas.) This focus on identifying the degree to which the observed racial disparities are explained by hospital quality alone has the strength of not being contaminated by other potentially important factors, such as provider-patient interactions and patient preferences.

In equation form, average 30-day mortality rates for whites at the national level, M_w, can be written as the weighted average of mortality rates for each of the $i = 1,\ldots, N$ hospitals in the United States:

$$M_w = \Sigma_i f_w(i)\ Q2_w(i)$$

where $f_w(i)$ is the transformed mean of Z_w, and is equal to the fraction of nonblack Medicare AMI patients who are admitted to hospital i (so that $S_i f(i) = 1$) and $Q_{2w}(i)$ is the quality measure, in terms of differential 30-day mortality, for hospital i among nonblack patients. The alternative counterfactual measure of mortality M_w^* is predicted mortality under the assumption that nonblack AMI Medicare patients are admitted to the same distribution of hospitals as are black AMI Medicare patients:

$$M_w^* = \Sigma i\ f_b(i)\ Q_{2w}(i)$$

where $f_b(i)$ is again the transformed value of Z_b, the distribution of hospitals to which black AMI patients are admitted. The difference, $M_w - M_w^*$, is defined to be the component of mortality rates for black AMI patients that is the consequence of differential admission (by race) to high- or low-quality hospitals (see Figure 16-10). Preliminary results by Skinner et al. (2002) suggested lower quality levels among hospitals to which African Americans were admitted, but little difference in mortality within hospitals.

At first glance, this study may appear to contradict many of the findings reviewed in the recent IOM study (Smedley et al., 2002). It seeks to explain the observed racial disparity that has been noted in the countless other studies (reviewed in the IOM report) as a function of differences in where care is sought. It does not rule out the role of provider discrimination

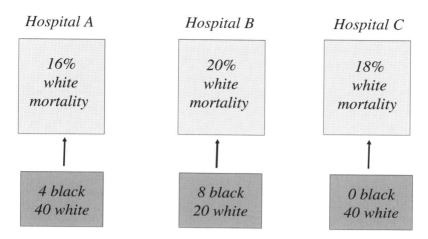

FIGURE 16-10 Differential migration of AMI patients: An example with 100 whites, 12 African Americans.

NOTE: In this example, the "true" mortality rate for whites is determined by the share of white patients going to each hospital times the 30-day mortality rate for whites within each hospital, or M = (16 × 40 + 20 × 20 + 18 × 40)/100 = 17.6 percent. The counterfactual mortality rate is determined by imposing the migration patterns for blacks, who largely are admitted to Hospital B, to whites, leading to an alternative mortality measure M* = (16 × 4 + 20 × 8 + 18 × 0)/12 = 18.7 percent. If whites were to be admitted to the same hospitals as African Americans in this simple example, mortality rates would be predicted to rise by 1.1 percent, or the difference between 18.7 percent and 17.6 percent.

in explaining outcomes, but notes the striking degree to which whites and blacks who are seen at similar hospitals tend to have similar outcomes. In fact, many of the studies reviewed in the IOM report are consistent with the findings of this chapter. Consider, for example, the IOM discussion of the 13 high-quality studies on racial and ethnic disparities in cardiovascular care. Out of the hundreds of studies that IOM reviewed, these 13 are highlighted because they use clinical (chart) data to adjust for co-morbidities, which is superior to the use of administrative data. Furthermore, they accounted for the use of cardiovascular services by including measures of the appropriateness of care. Of these studies, only two, Carlisle et al. (1997) and Leape et al. (1999), and found no racial and ethnic disparities in care after controlling for insurance status, co-morbidities, and severity.

What separates these studies from the others? We note that the Leape study uses data from 13 New York hospitals and tests for racial differences in revascularization. On the basis of the RAND appropriateness criteria, all patients in the study were classified as being proper candidates for the requisite intervention. However, it is important to note that the analysis also controls for the hospital that the patient was treated at (through the inclusion of a hospital fixed effect). As noted earlier, regions vary substantially with regard to the degree of racial differences in utilization; controlling for hospital effects could have further attenuated such differences.

These studies taken together suggest an additional focus for improving quality of care among the black elderly population. If African Americans are more likely to be seen at low-quality hospitals, public policies that attempt to improve hospital quality would disproportionately benefit African Americans. This conclusion remains consistent with one of the salient conclusions of the IOM report:

> Significantly, minority access to better quality facilities is often limited by the geographic distribution of care facilities and patterns of residential segregation, which results in higher quality facilities being less accessible (Smedley et al., 2002, Chapter 3, p. 114).

GEOGRAPHY AND RACIAL DISPARITIES: POLICY IMPLICATIONS AND CONCLUSIONS

Most studies in the literature on health disparities find dramatic differences in utilization by race, but are generally vague on the question of whether differences are driven by demand (e.g., blacks do not want the more intensive care) or supply (e.g., physicians treat blacks with otherwise identical characteristics differently) or perhaps that blacks and whites differ by unmeasured health characteristics (e.g., Johnson, Lee, Cook, Rouan, and Goldman, 1993) or respond to different nonmedical incentives such as insurance coverage. Hence most studies do not provide strong policy prescriptions on how one goes about fixing the problem. It is often useful to characterize such differences into three general categories:

1. Preferences, or the underlying demand "function" by patients.
2. "Supply" or physician, health professional, and hospital behavior.
3. Implicit and explicit "prices," or differences in insurance coverage, travel time, and other factors without explicit prices such as location of residence that are likely to affect behavior.

A massive body of literature in social science and medicine may be classified under the first two categories. Indeed, the recent IOM report provides a detailed literature review of these two categories. The report concludes that while a small number of studies demonstrate that minority patients are more likely to refuse care, these differences in refusal rates are insufficiently large to explain a significant share of the observed disparities. A smaller subset of studies has also considered the impact of insurance coverage and travel time on utilization. We group location in this third categorization; in theory, an individual could travel 300 miles to a different hospital, but the costs of travel broadly defined (including the potential for adverse outcomes during the travel) are too high to make it feasible. Most health care is local, and we believe that this third category is critical in evaluating evidence for racial disparities and developing policies to reduce such disparities.

We would suggest that, if possible, racial disparities be decomposed into their proximate causes, for example, with respect to "across hospital" variation (i.e., patients are more likely to be admitted to hospitals with perhaps less aggressive treatment protocol) and "within hospital" variation (i.e., black, Hispanic, and non-Hispanic white patients are treated differently within a hospital). Both variations can lead to lower utilization rates for minority populations; the difference, however, lies in the policy implications. The latter type of variation clearly involves the internal workings of specific hospitals or provider groups, and further inquiry into causes of such differences (financial barriers, preferences of patients, or provider behavior) is clearly warranted. The former type of variation, however, relates less to race per se and more to geographical variations in treatment patterns of all patients.

The research on regional variations, health outcomes, and shared decision making provides illuminating lessons particularly with theses types of variations. For example, a cursory examination of the medical and social science literature on racial disparities in outcomes reveals that for nearly every study, the white treatment rate is seen as the "gold standard" against which to evaluate black outcomes. This may or may not be the right approach: For economists interested in the study of the racial wage gap, for example, it makes sense to view white wages or white test scores as the standard against which black outcomes should be measured (Chandra, 2000, 2002). Increases in incomes, wealth, or test scores are viewed as being desirable, and decreases in these measures are viewed unanimously as being adverse events. However, with medical outcomes there are at least two reasons why the above logic may not translate over.

First, a number of recent studies suggest that "more is not necessarily better." Simply put, the fact that whites have higher rates of PCI or bypass surgery following AMI does not necessarily mean that blacks should have the same rate (Schwartz et al., 1999).[20] This is because it is entirely possible that the white rate of PTCA is a consequence of aggressive medicine and is therefore not the desired benchmark. In the technical jargon of economics, if physicians are operating in a region of negative marginal product on the production function, then scaling back on intensity could actually improve outcomes. Similar issues are considered in asking whether some regions that practice more intensive health care are in fact practicing "flat of the curve" medicine with no observable benefit in terms of better health outcomes (Skinner, Fisher, and Weinberg, 2001).

For example, in a widely publicized study, actors of different races and gender described identical symptoms in videos that were then shown to physicians, who were then asked whether they would prescribe cardiac catheterization (Schulman et al., 1999).[21] The results of the study indicated that for the actors who were white males, black males, and white females, prescribed catheterization rates of about 91 percent were identical. For the two actresses who were African American, prescribed catheterization rates were 79 percent. (These findings were reported to the media in a quite different way; see Schwartz et al., 1999.) The researchers suggested such differences were evidence of provider discrimination, but what is not known is whether the 91 percent rate is too high or the 79 percent rate is too low (or both) (Schwartz et al., 1999). This question also has been confronted in studies of geographical variation; we don't know which rate is correct (Tu et al., 1997; Wennberg, 1986).

This point also constitutes the central thesis of a recent paper by Schneider et al. (2001). In this important paper, the authors use RAND criteria to classify Coronary Artery Bypass Grafting (CABG) and PTCA procedures on a sample of Medicare beneficiaries who had undergone coronary angiography. The sample was drawn from more than 170 hospitals, and each beneficiary's treatment was classified as being appropriate, uncertain, or inappropriate.[22] The authors found that there was substantial cross-state variation in the inappropriate use of both bypass surgery (CABG) and PTCA; for PTCA inappropriate rates were 24 percent in California, 14 percent in Pennsylvania, 8 percent in Georgia, and 12 percent in Alabama. These regional differences clearly have implications for the percentage of Hispanics and African Americans receiving inappropriate care. Furthermore, they find almost all of the measured racial gap in PTCA revascularization is explained by the higher rate of inappropriate care for whites as well as higher rate of PTCA that is viewed as being of "uncertain" legitimacy. By contrast, they found lower rates of CABG use where appropriate among African-American patients.

The null hypothesis in the racial disparities literature always appears to be that there should be no differences in utilization. This is reasonable for procedures where nearly 100 percent of patients should be in favor of such treatments (immunization, eye exams for diabetics) or where 100 percent of patients should be against treatment (inappropriate PTCA as mentioned earlier). It is not unreasonable, however, that preferences for certain types of care may differ across patients, even for demonstrably effective elective surgical procedures (where appropriate) such as hip replacements. It is highly unlikely that observed differences in utilization can be attributed solely to preferences, however. Preferences for a kidney transplant were slightly lower among African-American men and women, but these differences in preferences could explain only a fraction of overall racial differences in transplant rates (Ayanian, Cleary, Weissman, and Epstein, 1999). When seriously ill patients were asked about preferences for life-sustaining technology, preferences among African Americans were stronger for more intensive care (Hopp and Duffy, 2000). Still, it should be kept in mind that the null hypothesis is not exact equality across racial or ethnic groups, but instead that rates of procedures (by race) match with informed preferences for that procedure.

In summary, this chapter has argued that local area variations need to be taken seriously in considering racial disparities in health care. This is true for two reasons: First, statistical pitfalls can trip up otherwise careful and valid empirical research documenting the existence and prevalence of disparities. Second, the policy solutions to racial disparities that occur because African Americans and Hispanics tend to live in different places from non-Hispanic whites are quite different from the more obvious sources of racial differences in treatment within a hospital or provider group. A potentially important, but not well understood, source of racial disparities cannot be solved by equal access to health care at the local level, or by universal health insurance for everyone. Instead, the disparities that occur when hospital or provider quality is worse in regions with a larger percentage of African Americans can be solved only by addressing the problem of *geographic* disparities in health care. Furthermore, reducing geographic disparities is likely to have a first-order impact on improving racial disparities in health care and health outcomes.

ACKNOWLEDGMENTS

We have benefited from conversations with Elliott Fisher, Douglas Staiger, Kate Baicker, and Jack Wennberg, and this chapter draws on our work with these individuals. We are grateful to the National Institute of Aging for generous support and to Angus Deaton, Christopher Jencks, Jim Smith, Richard Suzman, two anonymous reviewers, and other participants at the National Research Council Workshop on Ethnic Disparities for useful comments. Chandra also acknowledges support from the Nelson A. Rockefeller Center through the Rockefeller Faculty Fellowship program. All errors are our own.

Annex to Chapter 16
DEFINITIONS USED IN THE
DARTMOUTH ATLAS OF HEALTH CARE[23]

Hospital Service Areas

Hospital Service Areas (HSAs) represent local health care markets for community-based inpatient care. The definitions of HSAs used in the 1996 edition of the *Atlas* were retained in the 1999 edition. HSAs were originally defined in three steps using 1993 provider files and 1992-1993 utilization data. First, all acute care hospitals in the 50 states and the District of Columbia were identified from the American Hospital Association Annual Survey of Hospitals and the Medicare Provider of Services files and assigned to a location within a town or city. The list of towns or cities with at least one acute care hospital (N = 3,953) defined the maximum number of possible HSAs. Second, all 1992 and 1993 acute care hospitalizations of the Medicare population were analyzed according to zip code to determine the proportion of residents' hospital stays that occurred in each of the 3,953 candidate HSAs. Zip codes were initially assigned to the HSA where the greatest proportion (plurality) of residents were hospitalized. Approximately 500 of the candidate HSAs did not qualify as independent HSAs because the plurality of patients resident in those HSAs were hospitalized in other HSAs. The third step required visual examination of the zip codes used to define each HSA. Maps of zip code boundaries were made using files obtained from Geographic Data Technologies, and each HAS's component zip codes were examined. To achieve contiguity of the component zip codes for each HSA, "island" zip codes were reassigned to the enclosing HSA, and/or HSAs were grouped into larger HSAs. This process resulted in the identification of 3,436 HSAs, ranging in total 1996 population from 604 (Turtle Lake, North Dakota) to 3,067,356 (Houston) in the 1999 edition of the *Atlas*. Intuitively, one may think of HSAs as representing the geographic level at which "front end" services such as diagnoses are received.

Hospital Referral Region

Hospital Service Areas make clear the patterns of use of local hospitals. A significant proportion of care, however, is provided by referral hospitals that serve a larger region. Hospital Referral Regions were defined in the *Atlas* by documenting where patients were referred for major cardiovascular surgical procedures and for neurosurgery. Each Hospital Service Area was examined to determine where most of its residents went for these services. The result was the aggregation of the 3,436 HSAs into 306 HRRs. Each HRR had at least one city where both major cardiovascular surgical procedures and neurosurgery were performed. Maps were used to make sure that the small number of "orphan" hospital service areas—those surrounded by HSAs allocated to a different HRR—were reassigned, in almost all cases, to ensure geographic contiguity. HRRs were pooled with neighbors if their populations were less than 120,000 or if less than 65 percent of their residents' hospitalizations occurred within the region. HRR were named for the HSA containing the referral hospital or hospitals used most often by residents of the region. The regions sometimes cross state boundaries. Intuitively, one may think of HRRs as representing the geographic level at which "back end" services such as invasive surgery are received.

ENDNOTES

1. For a partial list of references, see Alter et al. (1999); Blustein and Weitzman (1995); Chen et al. (2001); Gornick et al. (1996); Peterson et al. (1997); Rathore et al. (2000); and references therein.

2. Also see Skinner et al. (2001) for measures of morbidity (i.e., heart attacks, stroke, gastrointestinal bleeding, colon cancer, lung cancer) across HRRs as developed in the *Dartmouth Atlas of Health Care* (Wennberg and Cooper, 1999).

3. The "flat of the curve" refers to a region where the marginal health intervention has zero impact on outcomes. For economists, this corresponds to the region of zero marginal product. This notion is formalized by Skinner and colleagues (2001); and Wennberg et al. (2002).

4. It is possible that much of the observed variation reflects random deviations from identical practice patterns across communities (Diehr, Cain, Kreuter, and Rosenkranz, 1992). While this possibility must be considered for smaller samples, the very large samples in the Medicare claims data preclude this explanation; also see McPherson, Strong, Epstein, and Jones (1981).

5. In statistical analysis, controlling implicitly for selection using the percentage of HMO enrollees in the area has not affected empirical estimates. Beginning in 2000, HMOs were expected to report hospital procedures to the Centers for Medicare and Medicaid Services, suggesting better data on managed care enrollees in the future.

6. For further details on the construction methods, see http://www.dartmouthatlas.org/99US/toc8.php.

7. Illness has been controlled for by using age-sex-race-specific mortality and hospitalization rates for five conditions: hip fracture, cancer of the colon or lung treated surgically, gastrointestinal hemorrhage, acute myocardial infarction, or stroke. These conditions were chosen because hospitalization for them is a proxy for the incidence of disease. The cost of living indices were computed by using nonmedical regional price measures. Doing so avoids contaminating the analysis with physician workforce or hospital market conditions.

8. Values of the index over 60 are considered high. It means that 60 percent of the members of one group would need to move to a different neighborhood in order for the two groups to be equally distributed.

9. The isolation index measures the extent to which minority members are exposed only to each other, and is calculated as the minority-weighted average of the minority proportion in each area.

10. States are used instead of HRRs to increase statistical power.

11. Population weights are for the state-specific African-American and non-African American population for both men and women, not just men alone.

12. We are grateful to Melinda Pitts for pointing out this correlation to us.

13. Furthermore, the means for beta-blocker use differ substantially between the two studies—56 percent versus 72 percent, suggesting different criteria may have been used to determine appropriateness.

14. When Washington, DC, is included in the sample, the observed (unweighted) negative correlation disappears. This is because DC is an "outlier"—the population is 61 percent African American, but exhibits 93 percent beta-blocker use.

15. Jenks et al. (2000) rank states on the basis of whether interventions that are known to be correct were administered for conditions such as AMI, heart failure, stroke, pneumonia, screening for breast cancer for women aged over 53, and eye exams and lipid profiles for diabetics.

16. Thus, percentage African American may be a better proxy for SES than income or other indirect measures of economic well-being. This interpretation is one that will be consistent with the results presented in this chapter. However, it would not be a proxy for income or social inequality, as is demonstrated conclusively by Deaton and Lubotsky (2001).

17. More technically, one might think of this error as being identical to measurement error in a covariate (geography, in our example). For a subset of observations, the wrong state has been included (Kentucky instead of Ohio). In general, measurement error biases the coefficient toward zero, implying that the researcher is prone to incorrectly concluding that geography does not matter.

18. For example, if 15 percent of the residents in HRR A seek care in the more aggressive HRR B, then because HRR measures of utilization are based on residence, the measured level of utilization for HRR A would be higher than is the true level of utilization in its local hospitals.

19. Opioids refer to codeine, morphine, and other drugs whose effects are mediated by specific receptors in the central and peripheral nervous systems. They are used for severe pain management in cancer patients.

20. CABG is surgery in which a vein is harvested from the leg, or an artery is harvested from the internal mammary artery, to bypass the coronary artery that has narrowed because of the buildup of atherosclerotic plaque.

21. Cardiac catheterization (or an angiogram) is a nonsurgical procedure performed under X-ray guidance in a cardiac catheterization lab to aid in the diagnosis of coronary artery disease.

22. The RAND appropriateness criteria for CABG and PTCA are discussed by Leape et al. (1999). These criteria are not based on the cost of the procedure, and classify a procedure as being appropriate or inappropriate based on the expected health benefit (quality of life or longevity) versus the expected health costs (probability of death or disability). The criteria are constructed for nearly 3,000 clinical scenarios or indications.

23. We have duplicated the definitions used by Wennberg and Cooper (1998, 1999). For further details on the construction methods, see http://www.dartmouthatlas.org/99US/toc8.php.

REFERENCES

Alter, D.A., et al. (1999). Effects of socioeconomic status on access to invasive cardiac procedures and on mortality after acute myocardial infarction. *New England Journal of Medicine, 341*(19), 1359-1368.

Ayanian, J.Z., Cleary, P.D., Weissman, J.S., and Epstein, A.M. (1999). The effect of patients' preferences on racial differences in access to renal transplantation. *New England Journal of Medicine, 341*(22), 1359-1368.

Baicker, K. (2002). *The government subsidization of hospital care and health care outcomes.* Unpublished, Dartmouth College.

Balsa, A.I., and McGuire, T.G. (2002). *Testing for statistical discrimination: An application to health care disparities.* Unpublished, Department of Health Care Policy, Harvard Medical School.

Barnett, E., Casper, M., Halverson, J., et al. (2001). *Men and heart disease: An atlas of racial and ethnic disparities in mortality.* Atlanta: Centers for Disease Control and Prevention.

Bikhchandani, S., Chandra, A., Goldman, D., and Welch, I. (2002). *The economics of Iatroepidemics and Quakeries: Physician learning, informational cascades and geographic variation in medical practice.* Department of Economics, Dartmouth College, working paper.

Blinder, A.S. (1973). Wage discrimination: Reduced form and structural estimates. *Journal of Human Resources, 8*(4), 436-455.

Blustein, J., and Weitzman, B.C. (1995). Access to hospitals with high-technology cardiac services: How is race important? *American Journal of Public Health, 85,* 345-351.

Carlisle, D.M., Leake, B.D., and Shapiro, M.R. (1997). Racial and ethnic disparities in the use of cardiovascular procedures: Associations with type of health insurance. *American Journal of Public Health, 87,* 263-267.

Casper, M., Barnett, E., Halverson, J., et al. (2001). *Women and heart disease: An atlas of racial and ethnic disparities in mortality.* Atlanta: Centers for Disease Control and Prevention.

Centers for Medicare and Medicaid Services. (2000). *Health and health care of the elderly population: Data from the 1996 Current Beneficiary Survey.* Washington, DC: U.S. Department of Health and Human Services.

Chandra, A. (2000). Labor market dropouts and the racial wage gap. *American Economic Review, 90*(2), 333-338.

Chandra, A. (2002). *Is the convergence in the racial wage gap illusory?* Unpublished, Department of Economics, Dartmouth College.

Chen, J., Rathore, S.S., Radford, M.J., Wang, Y., and Krumholz, H.M. (2001). Racial differences in the use of cardiac catheterization after acute myocardial infarction. *New England Journal of Medicine, 344*(19), 1443-1449.

Cooper-Patrick, L., Gallo, J.J., Gonzales, J.J., Vu, H.T., Powe, N.R., Nelson, C., and Ford, D.E. (1999). Race, gender and partnership in the patient-physician relationship. *Journal of the American Medical Association, 282*(6), 583-589.

Deaton, A., and Lubotsky, D. (2001). *Mortality, inequality and race in American cities and states.* (NBER Working Paper No. 8370). Cambridge, MA: National Bureau of Economic Research.

Diehr, P., Cain, K.C., Kreuter, W., and Rosenkranz, S. (1992). Can small area analysis detect variation in surgery rates? The power of small area variations analysis. *Medical Care, 30*(6), 484-502.

Exner, D.V., Dries, D.L., Domanski, M.J., and Cohn, J.N. (2001). Lesser response to angiotensin-converting-enzyme inhibitor therapy in black as compared with white patients with left ventricular dysfunction. *New England Journal of Medicine, 344,* 1351-1357.

Fisher, E.S., and Skinner, J. (2001). Geography and the debate over Medicare reform. *Health Affairs, 21*(1).

Fisher, E.S., Wennberg, J.E., Stukel, T.A., and Sharp, S. (1994). Hospital readmission rates for cohorts of Medicare beneficiaries in Boston and New Haven. *New England Journal of Medicine, 331,* 989-995.

Gornick, M.E., Eggers, P.W., Reilly, T.W., et al. (1996). Effects of race and income on mortality and use of services among Medicare beneficiaries. *New England Journal of Medicine, 335,* 791-799.

Harrison, M., and Thurston, N.K. (2001). Racial matching among African-American and Hispanic physicians and patients: Causes and consequences. *Journal of Human Resources, 37*(2), 410-428.

Hopp, F.P., and Duffy, S.A. (2000). Racial variations in end-of-life care. *Journal of the American Geriatrics Society, 48*(6), 658-663.

Jencks, S.F., Cuerdon, T., Burwen, D.R., Fleming, B., Houck, P.M., et al. (2000). Quality of medical care delivered to Medicare beneficiaries: A profile at state and national levels. *Journal of the American Medical Association, 284*(13), 1670-1676.

Johnson, P.A., Lee, T.H., Cook, E.F., Rouan, G.W., and Goldman, L. (1993). Effect of race on the presentation and management of patients with acute chest pain. *Annals of Internal Medicine, 118,* 593-601.

Kennedy, B.P., Kawachi, K.I., and Prothrow-Stith, D. (1996). Income distribution and mortality: Cross-sectional ecological study of the Robin Hood Index in the United States. *British Medical Journal, 312*, 1004-1007.

King, G. (1997). *A solution to the ecological inference problem.* Princeton, NJ: Princeton University Press.

Leape, L.L., Hilborne, L.H., Bell, R., Kamberg, C., and Brook, R.H. (1999). Underuse of cardiac procedures: Do women, ethnic minorities, and the uninsured fail to receive needed revascularization? *Annals of International Medicine, 130*(3), 183-192.

Lillie-Blanton, M., Martinez, R.M., and Salganicoff, A. (2001). Site of medical care: Do racial and ethnic differences persist? *Yale Journal of Health Policy, Law, and Ethics, 1*(1), 1-17.

Massey, D.G. (2001). Residential segregation and neighborhood conditions in US metropolitan areas. In N.J. Smelser, W.J. Wilson, and F. Mitchell (Eds.), *America becoming: Racial trends and their consequences* (Vol. I). Washington, DC: National Academy Press.

McClellan, M., and Staiger, D. (1999, revised 2000). *The quality of health care providers.* (NBER Working Paper #7327). Cambridge, MA: National Bureau of Economic Research.

McNeil, B.J. (2001, November). Shattuck Lecture: Hidden barriers to improvement in the quality of care. *New England Journal of Medicine, 345*(22).

McPherson K, Strong, P.M., Epstein, A, and Jones, L. (1981). Regional variations in the use of common surgical procedures: Within and between England and Wales, Canada and the United States of America. *Social Science and Medicine, 15A*, 273-288.

Morrison, R.S., Wallerstein, S., Natale, D.K., Senzel, R.S., and Huang, L. (2000). We don't carry that—failure of pharmacies in predominately non-white neighborhoods to stock opioid analgesics. *New England Journal of Medicine, 342*(14), 1023-1026.

National Research Council. (1997). *Racial and ethnic differences in the health of older Americans.* L.G. Martin and B.J. Soldo (Eds.), Committee on Population, Commission on Behavioral and Social Sciences and Education. Washington, DC: National Academy Press.

Oaxaca, R. (1973). Male-female wage differentials in urban labor markets. *International Economic Review, 14*(3), 693-709.

Oaxaca, R. (1975). Estimation of union/nonunion wage differentials within occupational/regional subgroups. *Journal of Human Resources, 10*(4), 529-537.

Oliver, M.L., and Shapiro, T.M. (1995). *Black wealth/white wealth: A new perspective on racial inequality.* New York: Routledge.

Peterson, E.D., Wright, S.M., Daley, J., and Thibault, G.E. (1994). Racial variation in cardiac procedure use and survival following AMI in the Department of Veterans Affairs. *Journal of the American Medical Association, 271*, 1175-1180.

Peterson, E.D., Shaw, L.K., DeLong, E.R., Pryor, D.B., Califf, R.M., and Mark, D.B. (1997). Racial variation in the use of coronary-revascularization procedures: Are the differences real? Do they matter? *New England Journal of Medicine, 336*, 480-486.

Phelps, C.E., and Mooney, C. (1993). Variations in medical practice use: Causes and consequences. In R.J. Arnauld, R.F. Rich, and W. White (Eds.), *Competitive approaches to health care reform.* Washington, DC: The Urban Institute Press.

Rathore, S.S., Berger, A.K., Weinfurth, K.P., et al. (2000). Race, sex, poverty, and the medical treatment of acute myocardial infarction in the elderly. *Circulation, 102*(6), 642-648.

Ross, C.E., and Mirowsky, J. (2000). Does medical insurance contribute to socioeconomic differentials in health? *The Millbank Quarterly, 72*(2), 291-321.

Schneider, E.C., Leape, L.L., Weissman, J.S., Piana, R.N., Gatsonis, C., and Epstein, A.M. (2001). Racial differences in cardiac revascularization rates: Does "overuse" explain higher rates among white patients? *Annals of Internal Medicine, 135*(5), 328-337.

Schulman, K.A., et al. (1999). The effect of race and sex on physicians' recommendations for cardiac catheterization. *New England Journal of Medicine, 340*(8), 618-626.

Schwartz, L.M., et al. (1999). Misunderstandings about the effects of race and sex on physicians' referrals for cardiac catheterization. *New England Journal of Medicine, 341*(4), 279-283.

Skinner, J., Fisher, E., and Wennberg, J.E. (2001). *The efficiency of Medicare.* (NBER Working Paper 8395). Cambridge, MA: National Bureau of Economic Research.

Skinner, J., Staiger, D., Chandra, A., Lee, J., and McClellan, M. (2002). *Racial differences in hospital quality for the treatment of acute myocardial infarction: Evidence from the Medicare population* (Unpublished). Dartmouth Medical School.

Smedley, B.D., Stith, A.Y., and Nelson, A.R. (2002). *Unequal treatment: Confronting racial and ethnic disparities in health care.* Washington, DC: National Academies Press.

Smith, J.P., and Kington, R.S. (1997). Race, socioeconomic status, and health in late life. In L.G. Martin and B.J. Soldo (Eds.), *Racial and ethnic differences in the health of older Americans.* Committee on Population, Commission on Behavioral and Social Sciences and Education, National Research Council. Washington, DC: National Academy Press.

Susser, M. (1994a). The logic in ecological. The logic of analysis. *American Journal of Public Health, 84*(5), 825-829.

Susser, M. (1994b). The logic in ecological. The logic of design. *American Journal of Public Health, 84*(5), 830-835.

Tu, J.V., Naylor, C.D., Kumar, D., DeBuono, B.A., McNeil, B.J., and Hannan, E.L. (1997). Coronary artery bypass graft surgery in Ontario and New York State: Which rate is right? *Annals of Internal Medicine, 126*(1), 13-19.

Wennberg, J. (1986). Which rate is right? *New England Journal of Medicine, 314*(5), 310-311.

Wennberg, J.E., and Cooper, M. (Eds.). (1996). *Dartmouth atlas of health care.* Chicago: Dartmouth Medical School and American Hospital Association.

Wennberg, J.E., and Cooper, M. (Eds.). (1999). *Dartmouth atlas of health care 1999.* Chicago: Dartmouth Medical School and American Hospital Association.

Wennberg, J.E., Fisher, E., and Skinner, J. (2002). Geography and the debate over Medicare reform. *Health Affairs,* February, 1-19.

Whittle, J., Conigliaro, J., Good, C.B., and Lofgren, R.P. (1993). Racial differences in the use of invasive cardiovascular procedures in the Department of Veterans Affairs medical system. *New England Journal of Medicine, 329,* 621-627.

SECTION IV

THE CHALLENGE OF IDENTIFYING
EFFECTIVE INTERVENTIONS

17

Behavioral Health Interventions: What Works and Why?

David M. Cutler

Behavioral interventions are interventions designed to affect the actions that individuals take with regard to their health. The typical medical intervention is a clinical trial of a particular drug, surgery, or device. In the trial, doctors provide different services to different people, and then evaluate the outcomes. Variation in patient behavior is generally shunned; a strong emphasis is placed on making sure that patients do exactly what is expected from them. With behavioral interventions, in contrast, patient behavior is the key and the goal is to change it. In considering issues such as the high rate of preventable illness (McGinness and Foege, 1993) or racial disparities in health, behavioral interventions are key. This chapter reviews what is known about the success and failure of behavioral interventions and speculates about why some interventions are more successful than others.

Behavioral interventions can be implemented at three levels.[1] The first is the individual level. These interventions encourage people who are at high risk for a particular disease to do something about it. Examples are programs to encourage smokers to quit, hypertensives to take medications, or diabetics to exercise. These steps involve lifestyle changes (eating well and exercising) and medical changes (regular testing of blood pressure and cholesterol). In both cases, though, the actions taken are controlled by the individual.

The most important individual intervention trial is the Multiple Risk Factor Intervention Trial (MRFIT) conducted in the 1970s. MRFIT enrolled more than 12,000 men at high risk for heart disease in a program to lower their blood pressure and cholesterol and to stop smoking. The men received counseling and help with behavior modification. But the trial was only partly successful. Risk factors changed more in the treatment group than in the control group, but the impact was less than was hypothesized. Furthermore, mortality outcomes for the treatment group improved only slightly more than did outcomes for the control group.

The relative failure of individual interventions was interpreted by many as evidence of the importance of environmental factors in health. Individuals are products of their environment, the theory went, and thus one cannot change the individual without changing the community in which he or she lives. This led to a second type of intervention—the community intervention, designed to change behaviors by modifying the environment that supports them. Several community-level interventions were implemented in the 1980s, again focusing on cardiovascular disease. These interventions used mass media, population screening, and community organizations to convey messages encouraging healthy behavior. The results of these trials were disappointing. Risk factors and health outcomes did not improve any more rapidly in the intervention sites than in the control sites.

In contrast to the failure of community-level encouragement, public policies have been shown to have large effects on health behaviors. When governments tax cigarettes, smoking rates drop. Restrictions on where people are allowed to smoke also lower cigarette consumption. People respond to prices and regulations, even if they do not respond to reinforcing messages.

The third level of health intervention is at the national level. The federal government or private groups often convey health information to people, with the goal of encouraging behavioral change. In at least some cases, these national interventions have a much more successful record than do community interventions. This chapter presents evidence that the campaign launched by the Surgeon General in 1964 to warn people of the harms of tobacco had a role in the reduction in smoking in the past four decades. Similarly, the movement against drunk driving pushed by Mothers Against Drunk Driving and the designated driver campaign have reduced the share of traffic fatalities involving drunk drivers. National information campaigns about the danger of high cholesterol have led to sustained reductions in consumption of red meat, eggs, and high-fat dairy products. Each of these behaviors is quite responsive to interventions.

Determining why the national interventions had salient effects while individual- and community-level interventions had smaller effects is difficult. This chapter does not present a definitive answer, but several theories are discussed. The first is intensity. People would prefer not to change their behavior. Inertia is strong, and changing behaviors requires major changes in thinking and action. Health messages are easier to ignore when the intervention is small; there is no pressing need to respond to each such impulse. But when information permeates widely, it is difficult to continue on the old path without contemplation. Doing nothing becomes a choice in itself that individuals must make. At such moments, people may be more willing to undertake large changes in behavior.

The second theory is one of externalities. Many of the national interventions justified individual action by noting that people conducting the activities were hurting others in addition to themselves. Examples of these externalities include the movement against drunk driving (drunk driving kills children) and the argument against smoking (passive smoking has adverse health consequences). Highlighting these external consequences may induce more behavioral change than simply stressing the benefits of behavioral change to one's self.

The third theory is of peer effects. People may judge appropriate behavior on the basis of what others are doing, in addition to their own utility from the activity under question. Thus, changes in the share of people who engage in a certain behavior, for example smoking, may affect the decision of other people to quit.

This chapter presents these theories, but does not offer direct evidence for or against them. Such evidence will need to be part of further research.

Several other theories are highlighted that have been proposed but do not seem supported by the data. Some speculate that individual and community interventions do not have major effects because they are not implemented for a long enough period of time. But this chapter shows that many national interventions achieve large behavioral changes within a shorter period of time than typical individual- and community-level interventions. Similarly, the nature of the information provided does not seem to be so important. National intervention campaigns have succeeded when their message is positive (you should help yourself by quitting smoking) or negative (you are evil if you drive while drunk). Something more than the framing of the message is at issue.

This chapter is structured as follows: The next section briefly outlines the nature of behavioral interventions. The following three sections consider evidence on the effectiveness of interventions at the individual, community, and national levels. The final section concludes by discussing the theories that are consistent and inconsistent with successful change.

THE NATURE OF BEHAVIORAL INTERVENTIONS

Health behavior encompasses many facets, and so behavioral interventions are broad as well. To introduce the subject, it is helpful to consider a particular example. Many of the interventions that have been attempted have focused on cardiovascular disease, and this chapter does the same.

To set the stage, information on cardiovascular disease health is presented. Figure 17-1 shows cardiovascular disease mortality over time for different racial and gender groups. Since 1950, cardiovascular disease mortality has declined across the board. Among white males, for example, mortality fell by 52 percent. For both men and women, the racial gradient in cardiovascular disease mortality has increased. The relative change was largest for men. Compared to the 52 percent decline in cardiovascular disease mortality among whites, mortality for blacks declined by only 36 percent. Among women, there was a 54 percent decline in mortality for whites and a 46 percent decline in mortality for blacks. The increased racial gradient in mortality suggests the importance of understanding how interventions affect particular racial and gender groups.

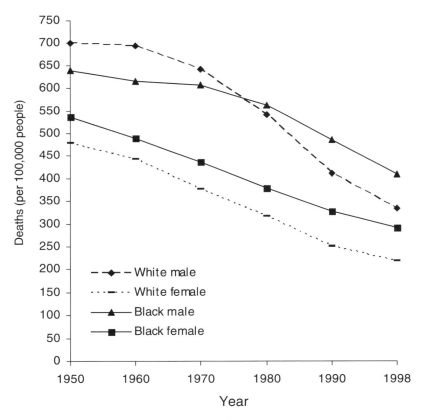

FIGURE 17-1 Cardiovascular disease mortality by race.
SOURCE: U.S. Department of Health and Human Services (2001).

The process of cardiovascular disease begins with risk factors—attributes of individuals that make them more likely to have a serious medical event. Some risk factors are exogenous to the individual, such as a family history of heart disease or genetic abnormalities. Other risk factors are (at least partly) under the control of the person. These factors include hypertension, high cholesterol, smoking, obesity, and diabetes. People with elevated risk factors are more likely to suffer a serious adverse event than people at lower risk, the most common of which are heart attacks and strokes. For those who survive the acute event, risk remains high for a subsequent time period.

The classic medical intervention is in the treatment of people with a heart attack. There are a range of possible therapies, from medications to balloon angioplasty to coronary artery bypass surgery. The relative efficacy of these therapies has been evaluated in clinical trials. Similarly, clinical trials have examined which medications are most effective in managing hypertension, high levels of cholesterol, and diabetes.

Behavioral interventions are targeted to the other factors. A "simple" intervention would be encouraging people to stop smoking (simple in the goals at least; smoking cessation is quite complex to achieve). A more complex intervention would target people with several risk factors and encourage a variety of behavioral changes: eliminating cigarette smoking, lowering consumption of fatty foods, reducing overall caloric intake, exercising more regularly, visiting physicians for hypertension and cholesterol screening, and adhering to medication guidelines. Behavioral changes are not independent of medical care; indeed, appropriate medical care requires behavioral changes. But the idea is to change the actions of people rather than to act on individuals passively.

There are other interventions that bridge medical and behavioral factors. For example, physicians may not order the appropriate tests for measuring cholesterol, or may not prescribe the correct medications for reducing it. Some recent interventions have targeted physician behavior to correct these limitations. In the interest of considering widespread interventions, such programs are not considered in depth in this chapter.

Individual behaviors might be modified in several ways. One possibility is to target particularly high-risk individuals and encourage behavioral changes among this group. This is the right strategy if individuals are autonomous actors and the greatest health damage is from people with very high risk. An alternative strategy, though, is to target the (usually) many more people with moderate risk. This would be more appropriate if many people with a small excess risk produce more adverse health outcomes than a few people with very substantial risk (Rose, 1992), or if there are peer effects that link the behaviors of particularly high-risk people to the average risk in the population. In considering the population strategy, one is naturally led to community or national interventions. All individual, community, and national interventions can rely on changes in information or the environment. In the next sections of the chapter, I evaluate the efficacy of interventions at these three levels.

INDIVIDUAL INTERVENTIONS

The most important individual interventions in health behavior were conducted in the 1970s. Knowledge about cardiovascular disease risk factors solidified in the 1960s. Results from the Framingham Heart Study and other research efforts demonstrated the importance of several risk factors for cardiovascular disease: hypertension (or high blood pressure), high cholesterol, obesity, smoking, and diabetes. The natural policy goal was to intervene to change these risk factors. In the 1970s, experiments were designed to do just this. The most important of these interventions was the Multiple Risk Factor Intervention Trial (Gotto, 1997; Multiple Risk Factor Intervention Trial Research Group, 1982, 1990, 1996).

The MRFIT was initiated in 1972. More than 350,000 men aged 35 to 57 were screened to produce a sample of 12,866 men at high risk for coronary heart disease. The screening focused on blood pressure, cholesterol, and smoking status. Individuals in the top 10 percent of the risk distribution were eligible for the trial and were enrolled if they agreed to the trial and randomization, and had no doubts about their ability to manage the heavily involved intervention.

Eligible individuals were divided into two groups. Members of the control, or usual care, group were examined once a year for medical history, physical examination, and laboratory results. The results of the screening and lab exams were conveyed to their primary care physicians, but no other intervention was undertaken. Members of the treatment, or special intervention, group received several interventions. Smokers were counseled by physicians to quit smoking. All intervention members were invited to attend weekly discussion groups addressing control of risk factors. After an intensive initial phase, participants in the intervention group were seen every 4 months, when they received individual counseling from a team of behavioral scientists, nutritionists, nurses, physicians, and general health counselors. The intervention lasted 6 years, at a total cost of $180 million in 1980 (about $350 million today).

The MRFIT investigators expected significant reductions in all three risk factors. It was hypothesized that cholesterol would decline by 10 percent for men with elevated levels ($\geq$220 mg/dL), diastolic blood pressure would decline by 10 percent for those with high levels ($\geq$95 mm Hg), and smoking would decline by 20 to 40 percent, depending on the initial level smoked (Sherwin, Kaelber, Kezdi, Kjelsberg, and Thomas, 1981). If achieved, these changes would translate into a 27 percent reduced chance of coronary heart disease mortality.

Table 17-1 shows the results the trial actually produced. For each of the three risk factors, there were improvements in risk factors for the intervention group. Blood pressure declined by 12 percent, smoking fell nearly in half, and cholesterol was lower by 5 percent.[2] But there were also favorable changes in the three risk factors in the control group. Aside from smoking, where some reduction was expected in the control group, these risk factor changes in the control group were unexpected. As a result, the net change in risk factor control for the intervention group was below expectations. Cigarette smoking declined by more than the forecast amount, but the decline in blood pressure was only 75 percent of expected levels, and the decline in cholesterol was only half of expected levels. The behavioral intervention worked, but not to the extent forecast.

Before moving on to the mortality outcomes, the racial homogeneity of the MRFIT results must be noted. Figure 17-2 shows the relative change in risk factors for whites and blacks in the intervention group compared to the treatment group (Connett and Stamler, 1984).[3] For each risk factor—blood pressure, cholesterol, and smoking status—changes were similar for blacks and whites; if anything, changes were a bit larger for blacks than whites. Because blacks are more likely to be hypertensive than whites, this part of the intervention reduced racial disparities in health.

TABLE 17-1 Effects of the MRFIT on Risk Factors and Mortality

Measure	Experimental Results			Percentage of Hypothesized Effect
	Intervention Group	Control Group	Difference-in-Difference	
Diastolic blood pressure	−12%	−8%	−4%	75%
Smoking rate	−46	−29	−17	145
Serum cholesterol	−5	−3	−2	50
Coronary heart disease (CHD) mortality*	17.9	19.3	−7	26
Overall mortality*	41.2	40.4	2	—
10-year CHD mortality*	31.4	35.1	−11	—
10-year overall mortality*	77.2	83.4	−8	—
16-year CHD mortality*	57.6	64.7	−11	—
16-year overall mortality*	154.2	163.1	−6	—

*Deaths are per 1,000 people.

NOTE: Difference-in-difference is the percentage change for the intervention group less the percentage change for the control group. In the mortality rate rows, the difference-in-difference is the percentage reduction in mortality rate. Differential changes in blood pressure, cigarette smoking, and cholesterol were statistically significant; changes in mortality rate were not.

SOURCE: Data are from Multiple Risk Factor Intervention Trial Research Group, 1982, 1990, 1996.

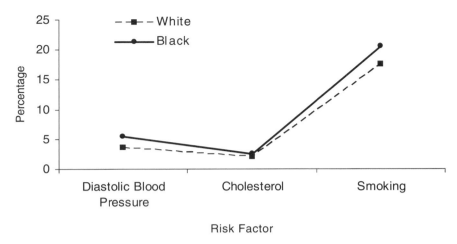

FIGURE 17-2 Decline in risk factors by race, MRFIT.
SOURCE: Multiple Risk Factor Intervention Trial Research Group (1982).

The ultimate end-point for the study was mortality. The mortality effects are also shown in Table 17-1. These effects are even smaller. Coronary heart disease mortality was only 7 percent lower in the treatment group than in the control group, and overall mortality was slightly higher. Neither estimate is statistically significant.

The failure of the MRFIT trial to effect significant behavioral change does not imply that all individual intervention trials have had no impact. There have been a large number of individual intervention trials (many using much smaller samples of people), and some have shown positive behavioral effects (Orleans et al., 1999). But MRFIT is the largest behavioral change trial, and its failure casts a shadow over all of the results. Thus, it is worth considering that experiment in some detail.

There are two disappointments in the MRFIT trial—the lower than expected effect of interventions on risk factors and the small translation between risk factor changes and mortality. The second issue has been investigated more extensively than the first. The leading hypothesis put forward is that risk factor reduction did not translate into large net mortality improvements because one of the antihypertensive medications used was actually harmful to some men. For men with electrocardiogram abnormalities at baseline, use of hydrochlorothiazide (a type of diuretic) was associated with increased mortality. On the basis of this evidence, in the fifth year of the intervention, a decision was made to replace use of hydrochlorothiazide with chlorthalidone (a different diuretic).

In a follow-up several years after the intervention was completed and 10½ years after the trial began, the differences in mortality between the treatment and control groups were larger (11 percent for coronary heart disease mortality, 8 percent for total mortality), but still not statistically significant (one-tailed p = 0.12 and 0.10). This change was consistent with an adverse effect of the antihypertensive medication. The same conclusion was reached at a 16-year evaluation published late in the 1990s. Mortality was lower for the treatment group compared to the control group (11 percent for coronary heart disease mortality, 6 percent for total mortality), although again the results were not statistically significant.

Perhaps more important for this chapter is the fact that the behavioral interventions had mixed effects. Smoking cessation was more successful than expected and hypertension control (largely through medication) was close to expectations, but cholesterol reduction (largely through weight reduction) was further away. The social component of the experiment was not a failure, but it was not a big victory.

There are several possible explanations for this mixed record. A first explanation is that the 6-year trial was not long enough to effect significant behavioral changes. Without continuing the experiment longer, it is impossible to test this theory. The theory may be incorrect, however. If this theory were correct, the change in risk factors between the treatment and control groups should be increasing over time, as more treatment group members adopt healthier lifestyles. In fact, however, the risk factor change is relatively constant from year 1 to year 6 (Multiple Risk Factor Intervention Trial Research Group, 1982).[4]

A second theory is the effect of background changes. In the study design, it was assumed that there would be no major change in risk factors in the control group, other than a modest reduction in smoking. In fact, large changes occurred in all three of the risk factors. It is possible that even the modest intervention for the control group—annual risk factor measurement and referral to a doctor for care—led to changes in behavior for this group. A related possibility is that disappointment at not being in the intervention group led these men to change their behavior. However, a comparison of those in the control group with those at high risk but not in the trial suggests this is not the case (Luepker, Grimm, and Taylor, 1984). Rather, the control group improved because the population as a whole was improving. The treatment had some impact above that, but not an enormous amount.

The reasons for these background changes are not hard to divine. Over this time period, a great deal of public attention was focused on the dangers of hypertension and smoking, and attention was also paid to cholesterol. The issue is not why behaviors in the control group improved, but why the intensive intervention was not even more successful.

One possibility is that the background knowledge dissemination was close to mimicking what the treatment group received. Thus, there might have been little additional information from the intervention. A more refined version of this theory is that only a certain number of people are "ready to change," and that this ready population in both the treatment and control groups was reached through general information. The intervention had little effect because only a small push was needed to get the trial participants to do better. This explanation is not very satisfying, though. One of the premises of the MRFIT trial was that information itself is not enough. Just telling people to quit smoking or exercise more, it was assumed, would not be sufficient to induce smoking cessation or greater physical activity.

A second explanation is that the trial was unsuccessful because the behavioral intervention was poorly designed. There are two possible reasons for this. First, the focus on individual behavior leads to a fear of "blaming the victim." If people are told high-risk factors are their fault, they may resist change to avoid admitting responsibility. In this theory, one needs more positive messages than negative ones. A second issue is that the intervention focused on individual change, but ignored the environment in which the person lived. Eating better is difficult if one's family and friends do not change their eating patterns. Smoking cessation is harder when a person's co-workers and family continue to smoke. In this theory, the focus should be on community-level interventions rather than individual-level interventions.[5]

This latter argument was convincing to many. The failure of the MRFIT to achieve risk reduction on the scale hypothesized led to a series of community-level interventions to reduce cardiovascular disease risk. These community-level interventions are described in the next section. The community-level interventions were not very successful either, however, so this interpretation is probably not right.

From today's perspective, it is not clear why the MRFIT trial failed to have the impact on behavior that was hypothesized. The final section of this chapter suggests that it may have to do with the degree to which the MRFIT information forced the men to reevaluate their lives or to consider the external effects of their actions. But that is just speculation.

COMMUNITY-LEVEL INTERVENTIONS

The successor to individual-level interventions was community-level interventions, designed to change the environment as a whole. These interventions are discussed in two strands. The first strand discusses community-level experiments designed to encourage better health behaviors. The second strand includes public policy interventions such as taxation and regulation that affect what people are allowed to do or the price they pay for doing things.

Community-Level Health Promotion

The implication some people drew from the MRFIT trial was that individual interventions are not enough. People's actions cannot be separated from the environment in which they live. Changing individual behaviors thus requires changing the environment as a whole. The logical implication of this finding is that trials need to be undertaken at the community level, rather than at the individual level.

This conclusion was acted on in the 1980s. Several community interventions were sponsored in that decade. Again, most had the goal of reducing cardiovascular disease risk.[6] The most prominent of these interventions were three related cardiovascular disease risk reduction trials—the Stanford Five City Project (Farquhar et al., 1990), the Minnesota Heart Health Program (Luepker et al., 1994, 1996), and the Pawtucket Heart Health Program (Carleton et al., 1995).

Table 17-2 describes these trials and the individual results. Each trial had one or more treatment cities matched with an equal number of control cities (two treatment and two control cities in the Stanford Five City Project; three treatment and three control cities in the Minnesota Heart Health Program; and one treatment and one control city in the Pawtucket Heart Health Program). The interventions began in the early 1980s and lasted for 5 to 7 years. Data collection began before the intervention and continued for a short time.

Although the goals of the experiments were similar—to reduce coronary heart disease risk—the interventions differed somewhat across sites. The Stanford Five City Project focused on mass media (TV, radio, and newspapers) and direct education (classes, pamphlets and kits, newspapers and letters). Treatment cities received continual exposure to cardiovascular disease education campaigns, along with four to five separate risk factor education campaigns per year. In addition, there were school-based programs for children. The researchers estimated that each adult in the treatment cities was exposed to 527 educational episodes over the 5-year period of the trial, or about 26 hours per adult.

The Minnesota Heart Health Program also used mass media to provide risk factor messages and establish awareness of the program. In addition, health professionals were involved in encouraging healthier behavior. Finally, risk factor screening and individual education were carried out. About 60 percent of adult residents received on-site measurement, education, and counseling; about 30 percent participated in face-to-face intervention programs. The messages stressed self-management and included changes in behaviors, the meaning of those behaviors, and the environmental cues that supported those behaviors. The experiment itself lasted about 5 years.

TABLE 17-2 Results of Community-Level Cardiovascular Disease Intervention Trials

Trial	Years	Intervention	Results
Stanford Five City Project	1980-1987 (6 years of education)	• Two treatment and two control cities • Interventions through media and direct education • General education and four to five risk factor education campaigns per year • Focus on dietary change, physical activity, and medication usage	• Increase in knowledge of Coronary Heart Disease (CHD) risk factors in treatment cities • Positive changes in risk factors for treatment and control cities • Modest differential reduction in blood pressure and obesity in treatment cities in some years • No differential effect on cholesterol, smoking in treatment cities • No differential effect on mortality in treatment cities
Minnesota Heart Health Program	1980-1990 (5 years of education)	• Three treatment and three control cities • Advocated hypertension prevention and control, healthy eating, nonsmoking, and regular exercise • Used community leaders, mass media, and health professionals • Population screening for risk factors	• Significant exposure to program by 3rd year, declining after 5 years • Positive changes in risk factors and health outcomes for treatment and control cities • No differential change in cholesterol, smoking, blood pressure, or Body Mass Index (BMI) • Modest increase in physical activity in treatment cities • No differential effect on cardiovascular disease morbidity or mortality
Pawtucket Heart Health Program	1981-1993 (7 years of intervention)	• One treatment and one control city • Advocated control of cholesterol and blood pressure, reduced smoking and obesity, and increased physical activity • Used community organizations, individual intervention, and community change (e.g., menu labeling) • No mass media	• Positive changes in risk factors and health outcomes for treatment and control cities • No differential change in risk factors across cities with the exception of Body Mass Index (BMI)

SOURCE: Stanford Five City Project: Farquhar et al. (1990); Minnesota Heart Health Program: Luepker, Murray et al. (1994); Luepker et al. (1996); Pawtucket Heart Health Program: Carleton et al. (1995).

The Pawtucket (Rhode Island) Heart Health Program focused on community involvement in behavioral change rather than mass media. Schools, religious and social organizations, large employers, and city government were recruited to encourage behavioral change. The focus of these interventions was to promote awareness and agenda setting, and to train people in skills needed to change behaviors and sustain those changes. Particular emphasis was placed on nutrition, blood pressure, and weight programs. In addition, grocery stores labeled low-fat foods, exercise courses were installed in the community, restaurant menus highlighted heart-healthy foods, and nutrition programs were available in public libraries. It is estimated that the 70,000 people in Pawtucket had more than 110,000 contacts with the program. People particularly liked the nutrition, blood pressure, and weight programs.

In each case, the interventions were more than just the dissemination of knowledge. Although knowledge dissemination was important, each of the studies also stressed messages from social learning theory—people had to learn how to take actions for themselves and what the impact of those actions would be. Furthermore, emphasis was placed on using the medical system appropriately—for example, through screening and treatment of hypertension and high cholesterol. People were not just advised and then left on their own.

In all cases where the data were measured, awareness of cardiovascular disease risk rose in the treatment cities compared to the control cities. In the Stanford Five City Project and the Minnesota Heart Health Program, for example, knowledge of coronary heart disease risk factors rose significantly more in the treatment group than in the intervention group. Thus, the programs achieved their first goal of making people aware of disease risk.

But the other goals were nowhere near as successful. In each of the sites, there were positive changes in risk factors for the treatment cities, but also for the control cities. The differential change in risk factors was small and generally statistically insignificant. There were some successes: blood pressure and obesity declined slightly more in the treatment cities than the control cities in the Stanford site; physical activity increased more in the treatment cities in Minnesota; and Body Mass Index (BMI) increased less in the treatment city in the Pawtucket experiment.

But these successes need to be contrasted with the much greater failures of the interventions. There were no differential changes in smoking in the treatment cities compared to the control cities, cholesterol was generally unaffected, and blood pressure was mostly unaffected. Obesity did not change significantly.

The samples involved in each case were small, because the unit of analysis is the community rather than the individual. But even pooling the data does not suggest large intervention effects. Winkleby, Feldman, and Murray

(1997) estimate that smoking rates fell by an average of –0.3 percent per year in the treatment cities compared to the control cities (p = 0.54), diastolic blood pressure fell by –0.1 mm HG per year (p = 0.68), and cholesterol rose by 0.23 mg/dL per year (p = 0.66).[7] Overall mortality risk was only negligibly affected. This matches the health outcome results. The Minnesota study did not find significantly different trends in outcomes between the treatment and control cities, and the Stanford study found some changes in outcomes, but only for selected people and for a limited period of time.[8]

Thus, the overall conclusion from the cardiovascular intervention studies is that the interventions were largely ineffective in modifying disease risk. This conclusion is particularly important in light of the very substantial cost of running community-level interventions. The Stanford Five City Project, for example, cost $4 per person per year (in 1980 dollars).

Once again, it is important to note that the control cities had changes in behavior as well. The improvement in the risk factor profile in both treatment and control cities was large; only the differential between the two was small.

In addition to these multifaceted interventions, other interventions have focused on particular risk factors. The most important of these was the Community Intervention Trial for Smoking Cessation (COMMIT), conducted between 1988 and 1993 (COMMIT Research Group, 1995). COMMIT randomized 11 communities to receive interventions and matched them with 11 controls. The intervention communities formed task forces for public education, health care providers, work sites, and cessation resources. The idea was to involve volunteers, health professionals, teachers, clergy, and other civic leaders to stress the smoking cessation message. In addition, smoke-free environmental policies were promoted at work sites and other venues.

People in the intervention cities were more likely to recall exposure to smoking control activities than were people in the control cities. But this did not translate into any greater reduction in smoking. About 18 percent of people quit smoking in both the intervention and control cities. There was a small increase in quitting among light to moderate smokers in the intervention sites relative to the control sites (31 percent versus 28 percent), but the difference was not great. The results of the trial as a whole were a major disappointment. The COMMIT trial was one of a series of community-level smoking intervention trials that showed relatively little effect on smoking decisions (Secker-Walker, Gnich, Platt, and Lancaster, 2003).

There is no consensus for why the community-level interventions fared so poorly. The community-level interventions may have failed because they were not carried on long enough to have a significant effect on health behaviors. This seems unlikely, however. In the Stanford Five City Project, the effect on health behaviors was greatest after 2 to 4 years, and then declined toward the end of the trial. In Minnesota, the same pattern was observed in health knowledge and those behaviors that were statistically significantly different in the treatment cities. The time period examined was when the program had its maximal effect; the impact was actually declining by the end.

Furthermore, it is not a case of lack of effort. As best as can be told, the message did get out. Knowledge of cardiovascular disease risk improved when it was measured, and people interacted with the program in the intended ways. Rather, the knowledge did not produce appropriate action.

A third explanation is that the community is not the right level to target. People may take social cues from areas larger than just their local community. In each of the sites, careful attention was directed to this issue. The communities chosen were relatively homogeneous and stable. They were not immediate subsets of a larger metropolitan area, where other messages might conflict. Thus, although the contamination explanation cannot be discounted, it is not likely.

A final explanation is that the programs were not large enough to have the intended effect. Although the interventions cost several million dollars each, they did not fully saturate the communities. The effects of the nutrition and obesity messages may have been drowned out by the enormous volume of food advertising on TV and radio. The national-level data on eating behaviors presented below suggests that larger interventions may have bigger effects than smaller interventions. If so, this argues that only major changes in policy will affect racial and ethnic disparities in health.

Public Policy Interventions

In addition to community-level behavioral interventions, public policy changes have been enacted to influence health behaviors as well. The most important public policy intervention for health is in the area of cigarette smoking.

Public policy affects smoking in several ways. A first mechanism is through taxation. Along with the federal government, most state governments tax cigarettes. These taxes are almost uniformly passed through into prices (Evans, Ringel, and Stech, 1999b) and thus affect the cost of cigarettes for smokers. Governments also spend money on antitobacco advertising, with the goal of counteracting the advertising done by cigarette companies and encouraging people to quit the habit. Finally, the public sector regulates who can smoke and where smoking can occur. Cigarettes are not allowed to be sold to minors (although this is frequently violated), and smoking is now prohibited in many buildings and public spaces.

A vast literature has evaluated the impact of these public policies on smoking behavior. Chaloupka and Warner (2000) and the U.S. Department of Health and Human Services (2000) review this evidence in detail. Most research has focused on the impact of cigarette taxes on utilization. The methodology for measuring the price effects of cigarettes is straightforward. Different states raise tobacco prices at different times. As a result, one can compare cigarette usage before and after the tax increase, differentiating between "treatment" and similar "control" states.

The results of these studies uniformly show large demand responses to price increases. A consensus estimate is that the elasticity of demand for cigarettes is about −0.4; every 10 percent increase in price reduces consumption by 4 percent. Furthermore, the poor seem to be more affected by prices than the rich. Gruber and Kosygi (2002) estimate that the cigarette price elasticity for the poor is greater than −1 in absolute value; the price elasticity for the rich is much smaller. Overall, the finding that cigarette taxes discourage utilization is not in much dispute.

Other public policies also affect cigarette consumption. For example, broadcast advertisements of cigarette ads were effectively banned in 1971. The ban seemed to reduce consumption, but the magnitude that has been estimated is modest.[9] In part, this may be attributable to the many other ways that cigarette companies can advertise their products, including through newspapers, magazines, and direct promotion.

Somewhat more effective is antitobacco advertising. Such advertising was conducted at the federal level in the 1960s, and more recently has been the province of state governments. In each case, evidence suggests relatively sizable impacts of antitobacco messages on consumption. For example, California spent $26 million in the early 1990s on an antitobacco media campaign. Hu et al. (1995) estimate that smoking declined by eight packs per person in response.

Finally, public policies that regulate access to cigarettes and places where smoking is allowed seem to affect consumption as well. In recent years, many governments have adopted smoking bans in many areas, including elevators, public transportation, government buildings, restaurants, shopping malls, and private workplaces. Most of the economic studies of these restrictions find large impacts on consumption, particularly as the regulations become more comprehensive. Workplace smoking bans, for example, are estimated to reduce the share of workers smoking by 5 percent and overall cigarette consumption by 10 percent (Evans, Farrelly, and Montgomery, 1999b).

Restrictions on places where people can smoke may affect cigarette consumption in two ways. First, it increases the effective price of cigarettes. People who must go outside to smoke effectively face a higher cost of cigarette consumption (although not in dollars). Second, it may increase the stigma associated with smoking, or reinforce in people's minds the harms from smoking.

The distinction between price and nonprice effects is important in designing public policy. Although price increases are a good way to discourage smoking, price increases have distributional implications that trouble some people. Because people with lower incomes smoke at much higher rates than those with higher incomes, tax increases would be paid more by those with lower incomes (although the benefits of smoking cessation go to lower income people more than higher income people as well). The very large effect of the workplace smoking bans, combined with the results from limiting tobacco advertising and sponsoring antitobacco advertising, suggests that nonprice policies may be important to combine with price changes.

Summary of Community-Level Interventions

Overall, there is a mixed message about the impact of community-level interventions on health. Experimental programs to change community environments and encourage healthy behavior frequently have been ineffective. That is not to say that all such interventions have failed. Evidence suggests that some workplace health promotion activities and church interventions have been successful (Emmons, 1999). But the record has been more disappointing than encouraging. At the same time, price and nonprice factors undertaken by governments have had a bigger impact on behavior.

It is not clear how to explain the difference between these findings. One hypothesis is that the community-level intervention trials were not large enough to add to the "background" information people were already seeing. The Surgeon General suggests this explanation in a report on smoking cessation (U.S. Department of Health and Human Services, 2000). Alternatively, the public programs may have had more prestige or plausibility than the private interventions. Understanding the difference between these responses has important implications for public policy.

NATIONAL INTERVENTIONS

The third level of intervention is the nation as a whole. Many health interventions are conducted on everyone at the same time. This is valuable because the scale of the intervention is large. But it is more difficult to evaluate the impact of a national intervention than a local one without a control group to determine what would have happened in the absence of the intervention. To present some evidence on the importance of national interventions, the time series evidence is considered as much as possible—looking for sharp breaks around the time of the intervention. To the extent that sharp breaks occurred, it is more plausible to attribute them to the intervention. Still, our understanding of how and why national interventions work is necessarily more limited than for individual or community interventions.

In this section, I review three national interventions: information about the harms of tobacco; the movement against drunk driving; and information about appropriate dietary habits. These interventions were chosen because there is some evidence they were at least partly effective. Choice of these examples does not imply that all national-level interventions were successful; some are not. But the hope is to learn from examples that do work.

Antitobacco Information

The single most successful health intervention of the past half-century has been the movement to reduce smoking. The prevalence of smoking was high and rising in the early 1960s, but it is lower and continuing to fall today.

Figure 17-3 shows the average number of cigarettes consumed per adult over the 20th century.[10] Cigarette smoking rose markedly in the first half of the century, from virtually nothing to more than 4,000 cigarettes per adult. To some extent, the increase in smoking is artificially inflated—hand-rolled cigarettes are missing from the total. But the increase is still impressive. Indeed, public policy encouraged cigarette consumption, for example, by distributing cigarettes to soldiers in the World Wars.

Some information about the harms of smoking was available by mid-century. Cutler and Kadiyala (2002) present results from surveys showing

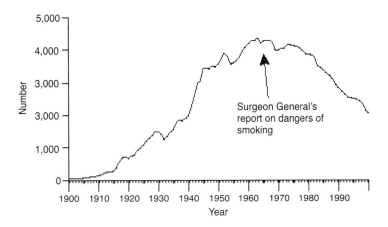

FIGURE 17-3 Average number of cigarettes smoked per adult.
SOURCE: U.S. Department of Health and Human Services (2000).

that about 60 percent of people recognized the harmful effects of cigarettes in the 1950s and 1960s. But people were not greatly attuned to the issue. Many people responded to survey questions by asserting that they did not smoke enough to cause harm to themselves.

That perception ended with the landmark report of the Surgeon General in 1964. The Surgeon General's report showed that smoking caused disease, particularly cancers and likely respiratory disease as well (later strengthened). Furthermore, even moderate amounts of smoking were harmful.

The Surgeon General's report was national news. It was highlighted in the popular press and widely disseminated.[11] The message was clearly heard. By 1970, 90 percent of people reported that they believed smoking was harmful to health. More people recognized the link between smoking and specific ailments such as heart disease and cancer. People recognized that even moderate smoking was harmful to health.

One way to gauge the impact of the Surgeon General's report is to look at smoking changes in the few years just after the report was released. In a relatively short time period, other factors are less likely to change. Using this methodology, the knowledge provision was accompanied by a rapid decline in smoking. Between 1963 and 1970, the share of the population smoking fell by 7 percent.

Over time, the Surgeon General's report was followed by many similar messages, including subsequent reports of the Surgeon General and other organizations such as the American Heart Association and the National Institutes of Health. Smoking continued to decline. By 2000, the number of cigarettes smoked was at roughly half its 1964 level.

This longer term decline has many causes. Price increases played some role in this smoking decline. Cigarette taxes were increased in the 1960s, with the new health information. But taxes were fixed in nominal terms in the 1970s and through the first part of the 1980s. Because inflation was high, the real value of the cigarette tax eroded. In recent years, cigarette taxes have again increased, but this largely makes up for the inflationary erosion of previous decades. Real cigarette taxes today are close to their level in the early 1960s (Gruber, 2001).

Other public policies have affected smoking over this time period, but these too cannot explain all of the trend. Bans on broadcast advertising of cigarettes had a negative effect on consumption, but it was relatively minor. More recent bans on smoking in restaurants, work sites, and public places cannot explain much of the historical trend.

It is clear that much of the response in lower cigarette consumption was individual decisions to quit smoking. What community-level interventions could not do—bring about large changes in smoking rates—the national interventions were able to accomplish.

What is unclear is what factors are most important in this decline. To some extent, smoking reduction is a result of individuals making health decisions in light of new information. This is certainly true about the immediate response to the Surgeon General's report. But social factors or "peer pressure" may also play a role. People may find it more difficult to justify smoking now than they did in the past, even if they would like to smoke. No studies have attempted to differentiate the impact of information from that of social pressure.

In thinking about racial and ethnic disparities in health, it is important to look at the composition of smoking in addition to the level. Figure 17-4 shows racial trends in the share of people who report smoking.[12] Blacks and whites smoke at relatively similar rates, with black rates being slightly higher.[13] Importantly, the trends have tracked each other over time. That is not true about socioeconomic differences, however. Figure 17-5 shows that smoking rates declined by much more for better educated groups than for less educated groups. In 1966, smoking rates were 6 percentage points lower for people with a college degree compared to high school dropouts.[14] By 1995, smoking rates were 19 percentage points lower for college graduates than for high school dropouts. Put another way, smoking declined by 60 percent for college graduates, compared to only 20 percent for high school dropouts. The decline in smoking has raised the socioeconomic disparity in health.

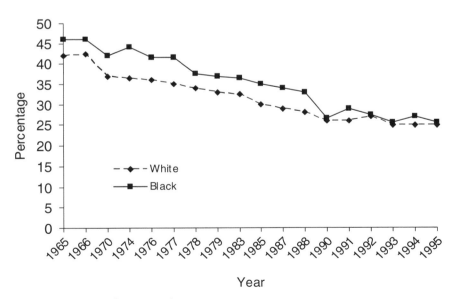

FIGURE 17-4 Smoking rates by race.
SOURCE: U.S. Department of Health and Human Services (1998).

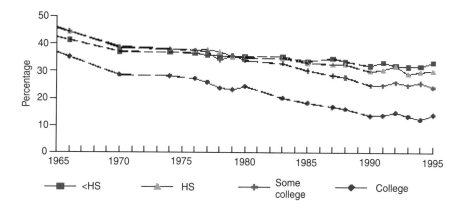

FIGURE 17-5 Smoking rates by education.
SOURCE: U.S. Department of Health and Human Services (1998).

Movement Against Driving

Actions to reduce drunk driving are a second notable chapter in national health interventions. The drunk driving example is so salient because, as with smoking, a national intervention accomplished major behavioral changes that community-level interventions had failed to do.

In the years after World War II, it became increasingly clear that drinking and driving presented a public health challenge. Road mileage increased as rising incomes allowed more people to own a car. People began living farther from work. In addition, alcohol consumption increased. The result was a perceived high rate of drunk driving deaths, although actual data on drunk driving fatalities in this period are sparse.

The prosecution and rehabilitation of drunk drivers is under state control. All states had laws about drunk driving, but police were not trained to stop or test suspected drunk drivers, and the court system was poor at prosecuting them. Rehabilitation efforts were limited. Many drunk drivers got off with a warning or light fine. Thus, through the 1960s, drunk driving became an increasing problem. A sense took hold that something needed to be done, and in particular that a better enforcement and coordination mechanism could substantially reduce the incidence of drunk driving.

Responding to this, the Federal Transportation Department established the Alcohol Safety Action Project (ASAP) in the 1970s (Gusfield, 1996; Voas, 1981). ASAP programs operated in 35 communities.[15] There were numerous specific ASAP interventions, but two themes. The first was to improve the operation of the legal system in dealing with drunk drivers. Arrest procedures were streamlined, improved breath-testing devices were adopted, and mobile vans were deployed to catch drunk drivers. In addition, courts were trained to screen for problem drinkers. The second theme was to encourage rehabilitation of problem drinkers. Identified problem drinkers were provided education and treatment programs to reduce continued drunk driving.

ASAP programs were in place for 2 to 5 years, depending on the community. The project was expensive, costing $88 million between 1970 and 1977 (equivalent to about $275 million today). There is some debate about ASAP's effectiveness, but most analysts believe the programs were not very successful. Some studies find positive effects, others find inconclusive effects, and still others find negative effects. Because the methodology is similar to the community-level cardiovascular disease interventions discussed earlier, details are not presented here. It is sufficient to note that the project was not an enormous success. As of the late 1970s, it was relatively easy for a researcher to conclude that drunk driving was a stubborn social problem, immune to public intervention.

Beginning in the early 1980s, though, drunk driving began a dramatic decline. The initial spur for the decline was the formation of Mothers Against Drunk Driving (MADD) and similar grassroots programs. MADD was organized in 1980 by Candy Lightner, a mother in California whose 13-year-old daughter was killed by a drunk driver. The driver had been arrested a few days before for driving under the influence of alcohol (one of many such arrests for that driver), but had been released. MADD reached national prominence in 1982, when a TV special about the Lightner case was aired. By 1984, there were several hundred MADD chapters around the country.

MADD focused on the passage and enforcement of more severe driving under the influence (DUI) laws. Legally acceptable blood-alcohol levels were lowered, and mandatory penalties for drunk driving were enacted. The legal age for alcohol purchase was increased.

There are no national data on the share of people who drive with blood-alcohol levels above acceptable levels. Thus, it is impossible to know about trends in this area. But data on crash fatality victims are available since 1982. The beginning of the data in 1982 is unfortunate; one would like to measure the trend in drunk driving prior to the MADD experience. But it was only with the increased prominence given to drunk driving by MADD that accurate statistics began to be kept.

The data on the share of fatalities to drunk drivers, presented in Figure 17-6,[16] show a marked decline in the share of fatalities to people who were drunk in the years just after MADD was formed. The share was 30 percent in 1982 and declined to 25 percent by 1987. Although we do not know what the trend was prior to 1982, there does not seem to be a period before an effect is observed.

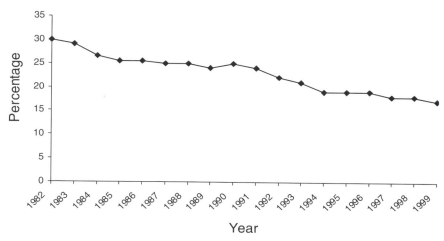

FIGURE 17-6 Share of drivers in fatal crashes with blood alcohol content (BAC) > = 0.10.
SOURCE: U.S. Department of Transportation (2001).

By 1987, drunk driving fatalities seemed to have plateaued. The share was falling only slightly compared to previous years. Around that time, a second campaign was launched, the designated driver campaign (DeJong and Winsten, 1998). The goal here was to have at least one nondrinker available to drive. This program seemed to have worked as well. Shortly after the program was launched, the share of deaths to drunk drivers began another 4-year decline. The share is now 17 percent.

Ironically, the experience of the past two decades, for MADD in particular, violates a central tenet of many public health campaigns. It is frequently stressed in sociology writings that policies should avoid blaming people for their mistakes. The idea is that people respond poorly to being blamed for health problems. Since the early 1980s, however, drunk drivers have been stigmatized in exactly that way. Yet even with this blame, there have been large health improvements.

The contrast between the ASAP programs and the MADD experience is also striking. Both actions focused largely on legal responses to drunk driving. Both targeted police and courts as natural enforcement agents. But one seems to be successful, while the other was not. It is not entirely clear what accounts for the difference. Certainly, the MADD experience drew far more media attention than the ASAP programs. The scale of the intervention may matter a great deal. The deterrent effect of the intervention may also be enhanced by the publicness of the intervention. Laws passed in response to drunk driving concerns were much more noticeable in this era than were the changes brought about by ASAP. Whether these or other aspects account for the difference in response is not known.

Dietary Change

The final intervention to study is perhaps the most complex—changes in diet. Heart disease and many other conditions are affected by the overall amount of caloric intake and the type of calories consumed. Excessive caloric intake leads to obesity, diabetes, and hypertension, all leading risk factors for cardiovascular disease. Excessive fat intake, given the level of calories consumed, leads to high cholesterol and atherosclerosis. For some years, the message to American consumers has been twofold: reduce the overall level of calories and decrease the share of fat in the diet.

The response to these messages has been mixed. Changes in the fat composition of the diet have been exemplary. This response is best seen since the early 1980s. Although it has been known for some time (since at least the 1950s) that high cholesterol leads to heart disease, clinical trials did not show the efficacy of cholesterol intervention programs until 1984. The critical trial, termed the Lipid Research Clinics Coronary Primary Prevention Trial (LRC-CPPT), showed conclusively that cholesterol control significantly reduced mortality risk. The LRC-CPPT was major news. It was covered in newspapers and magazines—often on the cover—and received attention on the evening news.

Time series evidence suggests the message got through. Figure 17-7 shows food issues that are of most concern to consumers.[17] Beginning in the early 1980s, concern about the fat and cholesterol content of food increased from about 10 percent of the population to nearly half. In the

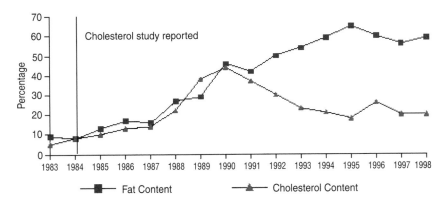

FIGURE 17-7 Nutritional issues that most concern consumers.
SOURCE: U.S. Department of Agriculture (1999).

1990s, public health officials stressed the importance of fat intake over cholesterol intake in explaining high cholesterol. Consumer concern mirrored this changing information.

Food consumption data are shown in Figure 17-8. There are generally not sharp breaks in these series, but the trends are worth noting. The consumption of beef and eggs fell markedly over this period, as consumers shifted into lower fat foods such as chicken and salads (not shown in Figure 17-8). Within these categories, lower fat items were increasingly purchased instead of higher fat items. Coupled with these dietary changes were medical interventions such as increased cholesterol screening and use of anti-cholesterol medication.

Figure 17-9 shows average levels of cholesterol over time. Accurate cholesterol levels require blood samples from a large share of the population, which standard population surveys do not measure. The only viable data are from the National Health and Nutrition Examination Surveys (NHANES). The data presented here are from the early 1970s (1971-1974) and the late 1980s and early 1990s (1988-1994). A more recent NHANES was conducted in the late 1990s, but these data have not yet been publicly released.

Overall, the share of people with high cholesterol fell from 28 percent to 19 percent, a change of about 30 percent. Importantly, the change was common across racial groups. Indeed, high cholesterol rates for blacks declined by more than for whites, while starting from nearly the same base.

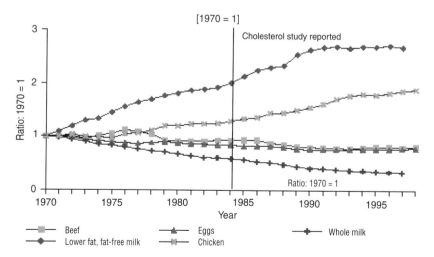

FIGURE 17-8 Trends in food consumption.
SOURCE: U.S. Department of Agriculture (1999).

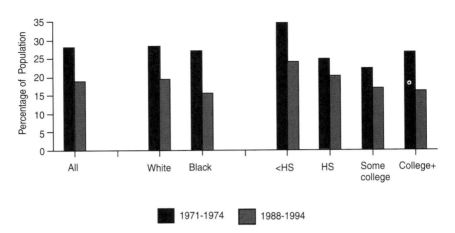

FIGURE 17-9 Share of people with high cholesterol, 1971-1974 and 1988-1994.
SOURCE: Author's calculations form National Health and Nutrition Examination
Surveys (NHANES).

The change was also relatively similar by education groups. People with less
than a high school education and those with a college degree had the largest
declines. There was no substantial change in the socioeconomic status gradient of high cholesterol.

At the same time as cholesterol has been falling, though, the overall
level of caloric intake has increased. Food available for consumption in the
United States increased by 500 calories per person per day between 1970
and 1994. Obesity increased as well, as Figure 17-10 shows.[18] The share of
people who are obese rose by over 10 percentage points between the early
1970s and the late 1980s. Other data show that obesity continued to increase throughout the 1990s. Blacks are more obese than whites. Somewhat
surprisingly, though, obesity increased by more for whites than blacks.
Increases were relatively similar by socioeconomic status. The more educated are less obese than the less educated, but the increase in obesity was
relatively similar across education groups. In this case, the worsening of
health status did not increase the racial or socioeconomic disparities in
health.

Summary of National Interventions

Although the evidence is not crystal clear, many national health interventions seem to have had a large impact on health behaviors. With the
exception of obesity, most health behaviors have improved over time, and
public health interventions are a part of this improvement. In the case of

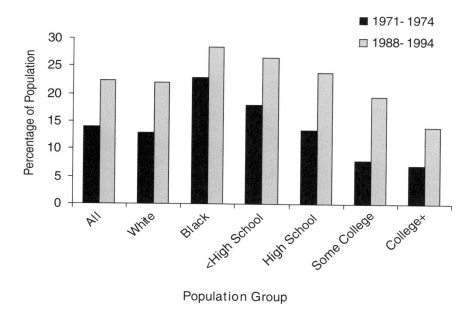

FIGURE 17-10 Obesity rate, 1971-1974 and 1988-1994.
SOURCE: Author's calculations form National Health and Nutrition Examination Surveys (NHANES).

smoking cessation, the health improvement was greater for better educated people. That is not the case with the reduction in high cholesterol or the increase in obesity, however. A lot of changes either narrowed, or left unaffected, the racial, ethnic, and socioeconomic measures of health.

IMPLICATIONS

What makes for a successful behavioral intervention? Making sense of the various facts already presented is not straightforward. There may not be one theory that explains it all. In this section, some empirical regularities are proposed and one possible interpretation is suggested.

Some basics seem to be true. Clearly, the message conveyed to people has to be simple. The harm in each of the national interventions is clear—drunk driving kills children; smoking causes lung cancer. The solution is also clear: don't drive while drunk; stop smoking. People deal with simple messages far better than complex messages.

Beyond that, the situation is murkier. Some theories can be rejected. One theory common in social psychology is that information provision is not enough. People learn new information, the theory goes, but do not act on it readily. One has to change the environment as well. The evidence is not greatly supportive of this theory. Although new information does not always lead to behavioral change, it does sometimes. A good part of the decline in smoking, and certainly the initial decline, is a result of increased public knowledge about the damage from smoking. Changes in fat and cholesterol intake result to a significant extent from the same factors. Information by itself can change behavior.

A second rejected theory is that the form of the message is very important. In particular, negative messages that blame people for their health problems will be less successful than messages that work with people in a positive way. But this theory too is incomplete. The campaign against drunk driving brings this out most prominently. The subtext of this intervention was telling drunk drivers that they were evil people who killed innocent children. They deserved punishment (or possibly reward if they had a nondrinking driver). People responded to this antagonistic message by limiting their drunk driving.

A third theory is that behavioral experiments need to be carried out for a long time to have any effect. Clinical trials of interventions may simply not be long enough. But many of the behavioral experiments that have been conducted lasted for 5 to 7 years. That is a long period of time by the standards of many successful interventions. Within 6 years of the Surgeon General's report on the harms of smoking, for example, cigarette consumption fell by nearly 10 percent. Drunk driving rates changed in that time frame as well, as did food purchasing habits. Behavior can change rapidly when the conditions are right.

While some theories are clearly false, there are other theories that might explain these effects. The first is a theory of *intensity*. One reason why national information interventions may have greater impacts on behavior than community interventions may be the fact that national information permeates more widely and deeply in people's minds. Behavioral change is hard; people always prefer to continue on their current path. In this theory, the key for interventions to succeed is that they force people to take some action. People can continue to do what they were doing, but if the information permeates widely enough, doing nothing becomes a choice that individuals have to rationalize. Once it becomes impossible to continue in the current path without making an explicit decision, people may be more likely to change to new paths.

In this sense, information interventions may be similar to taxes or regulatory interventions. When taxes on cigarettes are raised, people cannot smoke to the extent they formerly could without giving up some other consumption. When smoking is banned in buildings, people have to walk outside to smoke. Similarly, when the information about smoking becomes so clear as to obliterate any doubt about its harms, people cannot continue to smoke without consciously deciding to sacrifice their health.

The national cholesterol intervention seems to fit the same pattern. It was impossible to miss the news about the harms from cholesterol. People had to act on it—for example, by cutting out foods high in fat or cholesterol or visiting the doctor—or consciously recognize that they were not going to do so. As a result, more people changed their behavior.

The focus on the degree to which information permeates is not to deny that the message being conveyed is important. One of the features of all of the successful health information interventions is that their prescriptions are simple: one should not smoke; high cholesterol should be managed; drunk driving is bad. The simplicity of the message is clearly a key to its success.[19] But the simplicity of the message is not enough. It has to impact so deeply that people cannot ignore it.

A second theory has to do with externalities. One of the hallmarks of many interventions is that they stress the harm that people do to others, not just to themselves. Drunk driving was stigmatized because innocent people (frequently children) were killed by it. Cigarette smoking came in for additional scorn when studies linked secondhand smoke to poor health (a subject that is still controversial). People may respond more to the idea that they are hurting others than to the harm they cause themselves. External effects also allow people not engaging in the activity a safer route on which to base negative stigma on those who do.

A third theory is of peer effects. People may decide what is appropriate behavior on the basis of what others are doing, in addition to their own utility from an activity. If more people engage in health-promoting practices, people who would not otherwise engage in those practices might decide to as well. This is often referred to as a "tipping point" phenomenon because it could be that small changes in the behavior of the average person could induce large changes in behavior even among those far away from the average. The tipping point model is similar to the theory of population epidemiology proposed by Rose (1992). It could help explain why national interventions seem to be more effective than community-level or individual interventions, because they result in more changes among the general population.

These theories may or may not be right. Understanding why some health interventions succeed and others fail, though, is essential to making informed decisions about polities directed to health behaviors.

ACKNOWLEDGMENTS

This chapter was prepared for a National Academy of Sciences panel on Ethnic Disparities in Aging Health. I am grateful to Sharon Maccini for research assistance; to Angus Deaton, Sandy Jencks, Jim Smith, Leonard

Syme, and two anonymous reviewers for helpful comments; and the National Institute on Aging for research support.

ENDNOTES

1. Given the limits of this chapter, my discussion is necessarily brief. For a more complete discussion of many interventions, see Sorenson, Emmons, Hunt, and Johnston (1988); Emmons (1999); Syme (2003); and Powell (2001).

2. Note that these are averages over the entire population of men enrolled in the trial, so they are not readily comparable to the goals for men at high risk on any particular dimension.

3. Seven percent of the sample was black—more than 900 men.

4. This is not a result of sample selection; the response rate was about 90 to 95 percent, and was relatively constant after some dropout during the first year.

5. Some evidence shows that women whose husbands were in the MRFIT were more likely to change their risk factors than were women whose husbands were not enrolled (see Sexton et al., 1987).

6. This chapter focuses on trials in the United States. Another trial in Finland was more successful.

7. These results are for men. Changes for women are similar.

8. The Stanford study found evidence of significant health changes using a cohort sample, but not a cross-section sample. Effects were also larger in the 2- to 4-year interval, but not the 6-year interval.

9. Many authors have found that the advertising ban had a small impact on consumption, although others have not. Even the studies finding an effect estimate it to be relatively minor.

10. Cigarette consumption data are tabulated by the Centers for Disease Control and Prevention.

11. Ironically, the Surgeon General's report was not very expensive for the government to produce or disseminate.

12. The data in Figures 17-4 and 17-5 are from periodic years of the National Health Interview Survey, as tabulated by the Surgeon General, U.S. DHHS (2000).

13. These rates are unadjusted for income. Adjusting for income, blacks smoke less than whites.

14. Indeed, the 6 percent differential is probably larger than the difference a few years earlier; when incomes were lower, smoking rates were higher among higher income people than among lower income people.

15. Because the programs were run separately in each community, they are interpreted as community-level interventions, in contrast to information provision for all or a national set of new legislation.

16. The data are from the U.S. Department of Transportation, National Highway Traffic Safety Administration (2001).

17. These data are from surveys conducted by the Food Marketing Institute.

18. Medically, obesity is often defined as having a body mass index (BMI, or weight in kilograms divided by height in meters squared) of 30 or greater.

19. Indeed, it is possible that the lack of a simple prescriptive message is the key to why we have not been able to reduce obesity.

REFERENCES

Carleton, R.A., Lasater, T.M., Assaf, A.R., et al. (1995). The Pawtucket Heart Health Program: Community changes in cardiovascular risk factors and projected disease risk. *American Journal of Public Health*, 85(6), 777-785.

Chaloupka, F.J., and Warner, K.E. (2000). The economics of smoking. In A.J. Culyer and J.P. Newhouse (Eds.), *Handbook of health economics* (Vol. 1b, pp. 1539-1627). Amsterdam: Elsevier.

COMMIT Research Group. (1995). Community Intervention Trial for smoking cessation (COMMIT). Changes in adult cigarette smoking prevalence. *American Journal of Public Health, 85*(2), 193-200.

Connett, J.E., and Stamler, J. (1984). Responses of black and white males to the special intervention program of the Multiple Risk Factor Intervention Trial. *American Heart Journal, 108,* 839-848.

Cutler, D.M., and Kadiyala, S. (2002). The return to biomedical research: Treatment and behavioral effects. In K. Murphy and R. Topel (Eds.), *Evaluating the returns to medical research.* Chicago: University of Chicago Press.

DeJong, W., and Winsten, J.A. (1998). *The media and the message: Lessons learned from past media campaigns.* Washington, DC: National Campaign to Prevent Teen Pregnancy.

Emmons, K.M. (1999). Behavioral and social science contributions to the health of adults in the United States. In B.D. Smedley and S.L. Syme (Eds.), *Promoting health: Intervention strategies from social and behavioral research* (pp. 254-321). Washington, DC: National Academy Press.

Evans, W., Farrelly, M.C., and Montgomery, E. (1999a). Do workplace smoking bans reduce smoking? *American Economic Review, 89*(5), 729-747.

Evans, W., Ringel, J., and Stech, D. (1999b). Tobacco taxes and public policy to discourage smoking. In J. Poterba (Ed.), *Tax policy and the economy* (Vol. 13). Cambridge, MA: MIT Press.

Farquhar, J.W., Fortmann, S.P., Flora, J.A., et al. (1990). Effects of communitywide education on cardiovascular disease risk factors: The Stanford Five City Project. *Journal of the American Medical Association, 264*(3), 359-365.

Gotto, A.M. (1997). The Multiple Risk Factor Intervention Trial (MRFIT): A return to a landmark trial. *Journal of the American Medical Association, 277*(7), 595-597.

Gruber, J. (2001). Tobacco at the crossroads: The past and future of smoking regulation in the U.S. *Journal of Economic Perspectives, 15*(2), 193-212.

Gruber, J., and Koszegi, B. (2002). *A theory of government regulation of addictive bads: Optimal tax levels and tax incidence for cigarette excise taxation.* (NBER Working Paper No. 8777). Cambridge, MA: National Bureau of Economic Research.

Gusfield, J.R. (1996). *Contested meanings: The construction of alcohol problems.* Madison: University of Wisconsin Press.

Hu, T.-W., Sung, H.-Y., and Keeler, T.E. (1995). Reducing cigarette consumption in California: Tobacco taxes versus an anti-smoking media campaign. *American Journal of Public Health, 85*(9), 26-36.

Luepker, R.V., Grimm, R.H., and Taylor, H.L. (1984). The effect of 'usual care' on cardiovascular risk factors in a clinical trial. *Controlled Clinical Trials, 5,* 47-53.

Luepker, R.V., Murray, D.M., Jacobs, D.R., et al. (1994). Community education for cardiovascular disease prevention: Risk factor changes in the Minnesota Heart Health Program. *American Journal of Public Health, 84*(9), 1383-1393.

Luepker, R.V., Rastam, L., Hannan, P.J., et al. (1996). Community education for cardiovascular disease prevention: Morbidity and mortality results from the Minnesota Heart Health Program. *American Journal of Epidemiology, 144*(4), 351-362.

McGinness, J.M., and Foege, W.H. (1993). Actual causes of death in the United States. *Journal of the American Medical Association, 270*(18), 2207-2211.

Multiple Risk Factor Intervention Trial Research Group. (1982). Multiple Risk Factor Intervention Trial: Risk factor changes and mortality results. *Journal of the American Medical Association, 248*(12), 1465-1477.

Multiple Risk Factor Intervention Trial Research Group. (1990). Mortality rates after 10.5 years for participants in the Multiple Risk Factor Intervention Trial. *Journal of the American Medical Association, 263*(13), 1795-1801.

Multiple Risk Factor Intervention Trial Research Group. (1996). Mortality after 16 years for participants randomized to the Multiple Risk Factor Intervention Trial. *Circulation, 94*(5, Supp. 1), 946-951.

Orleans, C.T., Gruman, J., Ulmer, C., Emont, S.L., and Hollendonner, J.K. (1999). Rating our progress in population health promotion: Report card on six behaviors. *American Journal of Health Promotion, 14*(2).

Powell, L.H. (2001). *Behavioral interventions for health promotion and disease management in aging individuals: Issues and future directions.* Unpublished, Rush-Presbyterian-St. Luke's Medical Center.

Rose, G. (1992). *The strategy of preventive medicine.* Oxford, England: Oxford University Press.

Secker-Walker, R.H, Gnich, W., Platt, S., and Lancaster, T. (2003). Community interventions for reducing smoking among adults. *The Cochrane Database of Systematic Reviews, Volume 1.*

Sexton, M., Bross, D., Hebel, J.R., Schumann, B.C., Gerace, T.A., Lasser, N., and Wright, N. (1987). Risk factor changes in wives with husbands at high risk of coronary heart disease (CHD): The spin-off effect. *Journal of Behavioral Medicine, 10*(3), 251-261.

Sherwin, R., Kaelber, C.T., Kezdi, P., Kjelsberg, M.O., and Thomas, H.E., Jr. (1981). The Multiple Risk Factor Intervention Trial (MRFIT) II: The development of the protocol. *Preventive Medicine, 10,* 402-425.

Sorenson, G., Emmons, K.M., Hunt, M.K., and Johnston, D. (1988). Implications of the results of community intervention trials. *Annual Review of Public Health, 19,* 379-416.

Syme, S.L. (2003). *Interventions to reduce health disparities: Should they be specifically targeted or universally applicable?* Unpublished, University of California, Berkeley.

U.S. Department of Agriculture. (1999). *America's eating habits: Changes and consequences* (Agriculture Information Bulletin No. 750). Washington, DC: U.S. Department of Agriculture.

U.S. Department of Health and Human Services. (1998). *Tobacco use among U.S. racial/ethnic minority groups—African Americans, American Indians and Alaska Natives, Asian Americans and Pacific Islanders, and Hispanics: A report of the surgeon general.* Atlanta, GA: U.S. Department of Health and Human Services, Office on Smoking and Health.

U.S. Department of Health and Human Services. (2000). *Reducing tobacco use: A report of the Surgeon General.* Atlanta, GA: U.S. Department of Health and Human Services, Office on Smoking and Health.

U.S. Department of Health and Human Services. (2001). *Health United States, 2001.* Atlanta, GA: U.S. Department of Health and Human Services, National Center for Health Statistics.

U.S. Department of Transportation, National Highway Traffic Safety Administration. (2001). *Alcohol involvement in fatal crashes, 1999.* Washington, DC: Government Printing Office.

Voas, R.B. (1981). Results and implications of the ASAPs. In L. Goldberg (Ed.), *Alcohol, drugs, and traffic safety* (Vol. VIII). Stockholm, Sweden: Almqvist and Wiksell International.

Winkleby, M.A., Feldman, H.A., and Murray, D.M. (1997). Joint analysis of three U.S. community intervention trials for reduction of cardiovascular disease risk. *Journal of Clinical Epidemiology, 50*(6), 645-658.

SECTION V

TWO INTERNATIONAL COMPARISONS

18

Ethnic Disparities in Aging Health: What Can We Learn from the United Kingdom?

James Y. Nazroo

Ethnic inequalities in health have been a major concern in the United Kingdom for several decades. The collection of evidence on the nature, extent, and causes of these has been a focus of numerous studies, both of immigrant mortality (Balarajan and Bulusu, 1990; Harding and Maxwell, 1997; Marmot, Adelstein, Bulusu, and Office of Population Censuses and Surveys, 1984) and difference in morbidity across ethnic groups (Erens, Primatesta, and Prior, 2001; Nazroo, 1997, 2001). Over this time we have seen several paradigm shifts in the focus of studies, with an initial emphasis on genetic and cultural differences, to an emphasis on socioeconomic inequalities, to a more recent emphasis on racism and a revisiting of culture as ethnic identity (Nazroo, 1998; Smaje, 1996). Throughout this work there has been little emphasis on the issues of age and aging, perhaps because of the recency of migration to the United Kingdom for many of the ethnic minority groups studied (and their consequent relatively young age profiles). Nevertheless, given both a concern about the policy implications of ethnic inequalities in health, and the academic interest in using the additional diversity in experience provided by ethnic comparisons to help understand causes, the experiences of older ethnic minority people are very important. Studies of ethnic inequalities in health among older people have the potential to address issues of age, generation, and cohort, which are of fundamental importance to understanding processes and causes. The following specific questions arise in three categories—age, generation, and cohort:

1. Age:
   a. Is the emergence of ethnic inequalities in health intimately linked to the aging process?
   b. If so, how do the factors that lead to ethnic inequalities play out over the life course?
2. Generation:
   a. Are ethnic inequalities in health a consequence of migration experiences? Are they a product of the unique experiences of a migrant generation?
   b. Do they "transmit" to second and subsequent generations and, if so, why?
3. Cohort:
   a. How far are ethnic inequalities in health related to the specific historical context of a new migrant population?
   b. Can we anticipate that the health experiences of younger ethnic minority people will be similar to those of middle-aged and older ethnic minority people?
   c. Or have sufficient shifts occurred in the cultural and economic contexts of their lives to make their experiences of aging different?

The form that migration to the United Kingdom has taken potentially allows us to address these questions, and this chapter sets out to begin to map out elements of the U.K. data on these issues.

MIGRATION OF ETHNIC MINORITY GROUPS TO THE UNITED KINGDOM

Although some black people settled in the United Kingdom prior to World War II (mainly in London and the ports on the west coast of the United Kingdom—Bristol, Cardiff, Liverpool, Glasgow—and primarily related to the slave trade), most of the nonwhite migration to Britain occurred after World War II. This was driven by the postwar economic boom and consequent need for labor, a need that could be filled from British Commonwealth countries—primarily countries in the Caribbean and the Indian subcontinent. This "economic" migration was followed by migration of spouses and children and, sometimes, older relatives, in a climate when the legislation regulating entry into the United Kingdom became increasingly restrictive. Migration from these countries was not evenly spread over time: immigration from the Caribbean and India occurred throughout the 1950s and 1960s, peaking in the early 1960s; from Pakistan, largely in the 1970s; from Bangladesh, mainly in the late 1970s and early 1980s; and from Hong Kong, in the 1980s and 1990s. In addition, there was a notable flow of immigrants from East Africa in the late 1960s and early 1970s, made up of migrants from India to East Africa who were subsequently expelled. Over the past 10 years, migration to the United Kingdom has taken a very different form, including mostly refugees. This pattern of migration means that the vast majority of older, nonwhite ethnic minorities in the United Kingdom are first generation migrants, making the situation different from that in other non-European countries.

However, alongside this "visible" migration, there has been a long history of migration to England from Ireland, which continued during the active recruitment of labor from the Caribbean and the Indian subcontinent. The history of Irish migration to England, as to the United States, holds important lessons on the circumstances of economic migrants and their descendants, and how far skin color is a demarcating factor.

The collection of data on ethnicity in the U.K. Census has happened only twice, for 1991 and 2001. Data from the 2001 Census, which included a fairly comprehensive assessment of ethnicity, have only recently become available. The 1991 Census asked respondents to indicate which ethnic group they belonged to from a range of fixed choices that encompassed both skin color and country of origin, but it did not identify white minority groups. Responses to this question are shown in Table 18-1, along with the percentage in each group who were born in the United Kingdom. The table

TABLE 18-1 Ethnic Composition of United Kingdom Population

Ethnic Group	Number/1,000	Percent	Percent born in United Kingdom
White	51,844	94.5	95.8
All ethnic minorities	3,007	5.5	46.8
All black	885	1.6	55.7
Black-Caribbean	499	0.9	53.7
Black-African	208	0.4	36.4
Black-other[a]	179	0.3	84.4
All South Asian	1,477	2.7	44.1
Indian	841	1.5	42.0
Pakistani	476	0.9	50.5
Bangladeshi	160	0.3	36.7
Chinese and others	644	1.2	40.6
Chinese	158	0.3	28.4
Other-Asian	197	0.4	21.9
Other-other[b]	290	0.5	59.8

[a]The "black-other" group contains people recorded as "black" with no further details, those identifying themselves as "black British," and people with ethnic origins classified as mixed black/white and black/other ethnic group. Most of the "black-other" group members seem to have had Caribbean family origins, but were born in Britain.

[b]The "other-other" group contains North Africans, Arabs, and Iranians, together with people of mixed Asian/white, mixed black/white, and "other" mixed categories.

SOURCE: 1991 Census (Nazroo, 1999).

shows that at the 1991 Census, 5.5 percent of the U.K. population (just over 3 million people) identified themselves as belonging to one of the nonwhite ethnic minority groups.

Table 18-1 also shows that in 1991, just under half of the nonwhite ethnic minority population was born in the United Kingdom, though this varies across specific groups reflecting both period of migration and patterns of fertility. Children formed a third of the ethnic minority population, compared with less than a fifth of the white population. In contrast, while 16 percent of the population as a whole was aged over 65, only just over 3 percent of the ethnic minority population fell within this age group. Differences in age profiles also varied across ethnic minority groups, with the Caribbean, Indian, and Chinese groups having a slightly older profile than the Pakistani and Bangladeshi groups.

SOCIAL AND ECONOMIC CIRCUMSTANCES OF OLDER ETHNIC MINORITIES IN THE UNITED KINGDOM

Ethnic minority and white people live in markedly different areas of the United Kingdom. Analysis of the 1991 Census (Owen, 1992, 1994) has shown that the nonwhite ethnic minority population is largely concentrated in England, mainly in the most populous areas. Key findings are as follows:

- More than half of the ethnic minority population lives in southeast England, where less than a third of the white population lives.
- Greater London contains 44.8 percent of the ethnic minority population and only 10.3 percent of the white population.
- Elsewhere, the West Midlands, West Yorkshire, and Greater Manchester display the highest relative concentrations of ethnic minority people.
- Nearly 70 percent of ethnic minorities live in Greater London, the West Midlands, West Yorkshire, and Greater Manchester, compared with just over 25 percent of whites.
- There are even greater differences when smaller areas, census enumeration districts (equivalent to census tracts in the United States), are considered; more than half of ethnic minorities live in areas where the total ethnic minority population exceeds 44 percent, compared with the 5.5 percent national average.

There are also large differences in household structure among ethnic groups. Analysis of the 1991 Census (Coleman and Salt, 1996) and the Fourth National Survey of Ethnic Minorities (FNS)[1] (Modood et al., 1997) showed that white, Caribbean, Indian, and Chinese families had similar numbers of children, while Pakistani and Bangladeshi families had many more children. South Asian households were also larger because of the number of adults they contained. Half of Pakistani and Bangladeshi households had three or more adults, compared with two-fifths of Indian and Chinese households and less than one-fifth of white and Caribbean households. How this plays out in the household composition of older people has been explored by Evandrou's (2000) analysis of households containing one or more people aged 60 or older using General Household Survey data. This analysis showed that white British, white Irish, and, to a lesser extent, Caribbean people aged 60 or older were more likely to be living alone or as a couple (about 40 percent of the two white groups and 28 percent of the Caribbean group) than Indian (12 percent) or Pakistani and Bangladeshi (6 percent) people. Nearly half of Indians, Pakistanis, and Bangladeshis aged 60 or older were found to be living in large households (three or more adults plus children), compared with about a quarter of white British and white Irish people and 30 percent of Caribbeans.

One consequence of large households is overcrowded accommodation, as shown by analysis of data drawn from a recent Health Survey of England (HSE),[2] which focused on ethnic minority groups, including white minority groups (who have been combined into one group in analyses presented here that encompasses migrants from Ireland, about two-thirds of this group; Scotland; Wales; and mainland Europe). Focusing on respondents aged 50 or older and using an occupancy rate of 1.5 or more people per bedroom as the threshold to define overcrowding, shows the extent of overcrowding in the Bangladeshi and Pakistani groups (63 and 44 percent respectively of those aged 50 or older were in this category), which contrasts with much lower rates in the Caribbean, white minority, and white English groups (all 4 to 5 percent). The Indian group sits in between (20 percent) and, given the similarity in sizes of households among the Indian, Pakistani, and Bangladeshi groups described in the previous paragraph, this suggests that household size is not the only determinant of overcrowding.

Another determinant is, of course, economic position. Tables 18-2 and 18-3, based on HSE data, explore some dimensions of this. The first part of Table 18-2 focuses on men aged 65 or younger (the age of receipt of a state pension for men is 65 in the United Kingdom), showing rates of paid employment for three age groups. Concentrating on the oldest group first, for the white English group just over a third of men aged 50 to 65 were not in paid employment. Figures are higher for all of the ethnic minority groups, except for the Chinese group, with particularly high rates in the Pakistani group (70 percent not in paid employment) and Bangladeshi group (with only one in seven in paid employment). Similar, though smaller, ethnic differences in participation in paid employment can be seen for men aged 30 to 49, with Bangladeshi men again having particularly high rates of not being in paid employment (nearly one in two). Comparing rates for those

TABLE 18-2 Economic Activity and Occupational Class (percent)

	Caribbean	Indian	Pakistani	Bangladeshi	Chinese	White minority	White English
Employed							
Men aged 50-65	42	57	31	16	62	47	63
Men aged 30-49	74	86	78	55	88	84	88
Men aged 16-29	48	49	47	49	39	74	67
Registrar General's class, men aged 50-65							
I/II	12	37	26	9	49	43	39
IIInm	8	9	12	4	1	6	8
IIIm	53	27	29	39	35	30	36
IV/V	27	27	33	48	15	20	17

SOURCE: 1999 HSE (Erens, Primatesta, and Prior, 2001).

aged 50 to 65 with those aged 30 to 49 shows that the fall in participation rates is greater in all but one of the minority groups (Chinese men) compared with the white English group, and is particularly large for Pakistani and Bangladeshi men, for whom rates drop by around two-thirds. Rates of participation in paid employment are low for the youngest group, in part reflecting a large proportion in school, although again rates for white English men are higher than for most other ethnic groups (white minority men are the exception here).

The second part of the table shows occupational class for men aged 50 to 65. The data suggest that the profiles of white English, white minority, and Indian men in this age group are similar, with Chinese men better off and Caribbean, Pakistani, and particularly Bangladeshi men worse off. The striking difference among women in these ethnic groups (not shown in the table) is the level of participation in paid employment. Analysis of the 1999 HSE shows that among women of working age, approximately a quarter of Caribbean, white minority, and white English women are economically inactive, compared with just over a third of Indian and Chinese women and about four-fifths of Pakistani and Bangladeshi women. These figures increase for all groups if women aged 50 to 60 are considered (the age of receipt of a state pension for women is 60 in the United Kingdom), but the broad pattern remains the same. The most stark finding is that only 2 percent of Bangladeshi women in this age group are in paid employment compared with about 10 percent of Pakistani women, just over a third of Indian women, and nearly two-thirds of Caribbean, white minority, and white English women (there were too few Chinese women in this category in the sample to provide an estimate for them).

Table 18-3 shows household income from all sources for households with a respondent aged 50 or older split into tertiles, that is, three bands that reflect the general population income distribution, with a third of the general population (of all ages) in each band. The first part of the table (which is not equivalized to account for variations in household size) suggests that the white groups and the Indian group have similar levels of income, with the Caribbean and Pakistani groups worse off and the Bangladeshi group much worse off—90 percent were in the bottom tertile. The second half of the table is equivalized to account for variations in household size using the McClemens scoring system (Erens et al., 2001). In comparison with the nonequivalized data, the white groups appear to be better off (because older people in these groups live in smaller households) and the Pakistani and Caribbean groups appear a little worse off. The ethnic comparison changes a little for the equivalized data. Again they suggest that the two white groups are equivalent, but with the Indian as well as the Caribbean group worse off, and the Pakistani as well as the Bangladeshi group much worse—three quarters of the Pakistani group and

TABLE 18-3 Household Income: Households with One Person or More Aged 50 or Older (percent)

	Caribbean	Indian	Pakistani	Bangladeshi	Chinese	White minority	White English
Not equivalized							
Bottom tertile	72	53	65	90	—	53	57
Middle tertile	20	29	23	7	—	30	25
Top tertile	8	18	12	2	—	17	18
Equivalized							
Bottom tertile	54	55	77	93	59	36	36
Middle tertile	36	29	19	5	12	35	37
Top tertile	10	17	5	2	29	29	27

SOURCE: 1999 HSE (Erens, Primatesta, and Prior, 2001).

more than 90 percent of the Bangladeshi group were in the bottom tertile. In terms of the top income tertile, the Chinese group is equivalent to the two white groups, but it also has substantially more households in this age group in the bottom tertile.

One of the pervading experiences of ethnic minority people in the United Kingdom (both white and nonwhite) is racial harassment and discrimination. There are no data that allow an adequate exploration of how experiences of racism and discrimination vary by age, but for the adult nonwhite population, this issue was investigated in some depth by the FNS (Modood et al., 1997). This suggested that more than one in eight ethnic minority people had experienced some form of racial harassment in the past year. Although most of these incidents involved racial insults, many of the respondents reported repeated victimization, and a quarter of the ethnic minority respondents reported being fearful of racial harassment. The FNS also showed that among ethnic minority respondents, there was a common belief that employers discriminated against ethnic minority applicants for jobs and widespread experience of such discrimination (Modood et al., 1997). Indeed, when white respondents to the survey were asked about their own racial prejudice, 26 percent admitted to being prejudiced against South Asians, 20 percent to being prejudiced against Caribbeans, and 8 percent to being prejudiced against Chinese. A study by the Commission for Racial Equality has suggested that white minority groups, such as the Irish, also face extensive racial harassment (Hickman and Walters, 1997).

PATTERNING OF ETHNIC INEQUALITIES IN HEALTH IN THE UNITED KINGDOM

The recording of country of birth at the Census and on death certificates has allowed fairly extensive analysis of the patterning of death rates and cause of death by country of birth (Balarajan and Bulusu, 1990; Harding and Maxwell, 1997; Marmot et al., 1984). This is obviously inadequate for understanding the experiences of ethnic minority people born in the United Kingdom and, in the U.K. context, runs the difficulty of conflating migrants returning back to the United Kingdom from British Commonwealth countries and new immigration from those countries. Table 18-4 provides a summary of findings from the most recent analysis of immigrant mortality around the 1991 Census, showing age standardized mortality ratios (SMRs) by country of birth for all causes and four specific causes of death (chosen for illustrative purposes). There are fewer analyses of morbidity, with the key national sources in the United Kingdom being the 1999 HSE (Erens et al., 2001) and the FNS (Nazroo, 1997, 2001). Table 18-5 provides a summary of data on morbidity for the adult population, drawn from the FNS, showing the relative risk for ethnic minority

TABLE 18-4 Standardized Mortality Ratio by Country of Birth for Those Aged 20 to 64, England and Wales, 1991-1993

	All Causes		Coronary Heart Disease		Stroke		Respiratory Disease		Lung Cancer	
	Men	Women	Men	Women	Men	Women	Men	Women	Men	Women
Caribbean	89*	104	60*	100	169*	178*	80*	75	59*	32*
Indian subcontinent	107*	99	150*	175*	163*	132*	90	94	48*	34*
India	106*	—	140*	—	140*	—	93	—	43*	—
Pakistan	102	—	163*	—	148*	—	82	—	45*	—
Bangladesh	137*	—	184*	—	324*	—	104	—	92	—
East Africa	123*	127*	160*	130	113	110	154*	195*	35*	110
West/South Africa	126*	142*	83	69	315*	215*	138	101	71	69
Ireland	135*	115*	121*	129*	130*	118*	162*	134*	157*	143*

*p < 0.05 compared with the total population.
SOURCE: Office for National Statistics (Nazroo, 1999).

TABLE 18-5 Age and Gender Standardized Relative Risk, All Ages, England and Wales, 1993-1994

	Fair or Poor Health	Diagnosed CHD	CHD or Severe Chest Pain	Hyper-tension	Diabetes	Respiratory Symptoms
Caribbeans	1.29*	0.88	0.96	1.47*	3.12*	0.87
All South Asians	1.19*	1.00	1.24*	0.75*	3.65*	0.59*
Indians	1.03	0.79	0.93	0.66*	2.77*	0.55*
Pakistanis/ Bangladeshis	1.48*	1.43*	1.83*	0.91	5.24*	0.67*
Chinese	0.96	0.71	0.56	0.42*	1.77	0.43*

*p < 0.05 compared with white people.
SOURCE: Fourth National Survey (Nazroo, 1999).

people, compared with white people, to report fair or poor health and indicators of four specific conditions (a combination of responses to questions on previously diagnosed conditions and symptoms).

Some general interpretations can be taken from Tables 18-4 and 18-5. First, ethnic minority groups are not uniformly at greater risk of mortality or poor health in the United Kingdom. For example, both data sources suggest that Indians have reasonably good overall health. Second, for some outcomes ethnic minority groups appear to be significantly better off than the ethnic majority (e.g., respiratory symptoms/disease and lung cancer). Third, particular ethnic groups appear to be particularly disadvantaged by different diseases. For example, Caribbeans have high rates of stroke/hypertension and South Asians have high rates of coronary heart disease (CHD)/severe chest pain.

Although there are similarities in the data presented in the two tables, there are also some inconsistencies. For example, people born in the Caribbean have a low all-cause SMR, but a high relative risk of reporting fair or poor general health; men born in India have an elevated SMR for CHD, while the relative risk for a diagnosis or reporting symptoms of CHD is lower for Indians than for whites; men born in the Indian subcontinent have a high SMR from stroke but South Asians have a lower relative risk of reporting hypertension.

These inconsistencies could be a consequence of a number of factors, including the following: the data cover different groups (the mortality data are restricted to those born outside the United Kingdom the morbidity data cover all ethnic minorities); the morbidity data measure prevalence while the mortality data measure a combination of incidence and survival (in the United Kingdom); important cohort effects may be present; or data inaccuracies may exist both in the reporting of symptoms or diagnosis (perhaps because of cultural differences in the experience and reporting of symptoms or differences in opportunities for diagnosis) and in the recording of cause of death, as has been shown to occur for the recording of death by occupational class and gender (Battle et al., 1987; Bloor, Robertson, and Samphier, 1989).

AGE AND ETHNIC INEQUALITIES IN HEALTH

This section will illustrate how the patterning of ethnic inequalities in health varies across age groups. The data to be presented are drawn from the 1999 HSE and so include a white minority group and cover ages 2 and up. The main outcome to be considered is a question asking respondents to rate their current general health (or their child's current general health if she or he is aged less than 12) on a five-point scale: very good, good, fair, bad, and very bad. Throughout the section the scale has been dichotomized into good versus fair or bad.

Figure 18-1 shows how responses to this question vary across ethnic groups for the whole population. It shows the odds ratio for reporting fair or bad health in comparison with the white English group, with 95 percent confidence intervals. The pattern shown is one that is similar to that demonstrated in the 1991 Census and the FNS (Nazroo, 1997), with all non-white minority groups reporting poorer health than the white English group,

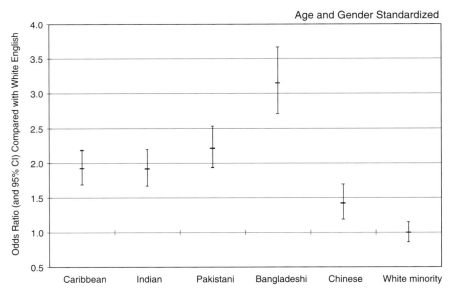

FIGURE 18-1 Reported fair/bad/very bad general health.
SOURCE: 1999 HSE (Erens, Primatesta, and Prior, 2001).

particularly the Bangladeshi group, which has an odds ratio greater than 3. Unlike other morbidity surveys, the 1999 HSE included and identified people in white ethnic minority groups, and Figure 18-1 shows them to have a similar profile to that of the white English group.

Figure 18-2 explores how this pattern varies by age group. It suggests relatively small differences at younger ages, with large differences beginning to emerge in the mid-20s and becoming very large by the mid-30s and remaining large from this age onwards. For the group with the poorest reported health, Bangladeshis, from their mid-40s onwards the rates are about 50 percent higher in absolute terms than those for white English people. Figure 18-3 explores the size of this difference in relative terms, which has the benefit of emphasizing differences at low prevalence of the outcome under consideration. It shows that in relative terms, ethnic inequalities in health are large at young ages and from late 20s onwards, but are more or less absent in teenage years and early 20s, becoming large again at older ages. It is worth noting that the white minority group has a very similar profile to the white English group throughout the age span, and that for the Chinese group is close to these two. The profiles of the Caribbean and Indian groups are similar to each other, and show a worsening in health in comparison with the white English group from the mid-30s to the mid-40s and up, while the Pakistani and Bangladeshi groups have a markedly worse profile than other groups, with differences emerging from the mid-20s and up.

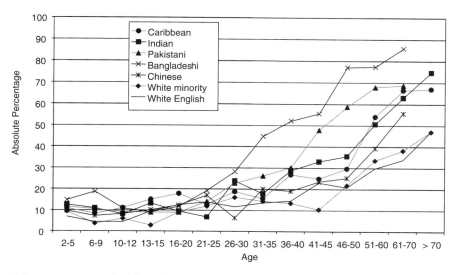

FIGURE 18-2 Fair/bad health by ethnic group and age.
SOURCE: 1999 HSE (Erens, Primatesta, and Prior, 2001).

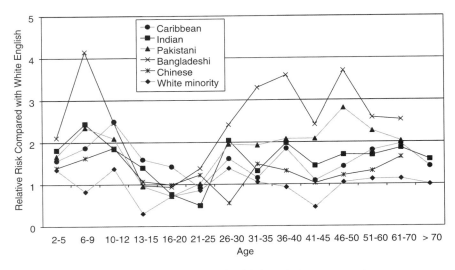

FIGURE 18-3 Relative risk for fair/bad health by ethnic group and age.
SOURCE: 1999 HSE (Erens, Primatesta, and Prior, 2001).

DIFFERENCES IN HEALTH BEHAVIORS

Differences in health behaviors may be important contributors to ethnic differences in health. Table 18-6, which also uses data from the 1999 HSE, shows differences in rates of smoking and alcohol consumption for those aged 50 or older. The first half of the table shows that among women, the two white groups have the highest rates of current and ever smoking, with around three-fifths of white women having smoked at some point in their lives, and one-fifth of white English and a quarter of white minority women currently smoking. All of the nonwhite minority groups had low rates of smoking among women, although rates for Caribbean women were higher than those for other groups of nonwhite minority women. For men the pattern is somewhat different. Similar proportions of white English, white minority, and Caribbean men have never smoked, with few Bangladeshi men having never smoked (only one in five), and more Indian, Pakistani, and Chinese men having never smoked (about three in five for Indian and Pakistani men and half of Chinese men). The pattern for current smoking among men is different again, with the lower rates for Indian and Pakistani men compared with white men disappearing, the rate for Caribbean men becoming higher than that for white men, and the rate for Bangladeshi men becoming higher still—about half of Bangladeshi men reported that they currently smoked. The implication of the difference in the pattern between ever having smoked and currently smoking is that white men have been more successful at giving up smoking.

TABLE 18-6 Smoking and Alcohol Consumption: Aged 50 or Older (percent)

	Caribbean	Indian	Pakistani	Bangladeshi	Chinese	White Minority	White English
Smoking							
Men							
Never	33	57	60	19	52	28	27
Ex-smoker	35	23	15	28	37	48	55
Current smoker	31	20	25	53	11	24	19
Women							
Never	79	95	95	92	87	40	44
Ex-smoker	12	3	0	4	7	36	38
Current smoker	9	1	5	4	6	24	19
Alcohol Consumption							
Men							
Drinks alcohol	83	59	9	3	57	86	91
Drinks over the recommended weekly limit	18	12	0	0	3	24	23
Women							
Drinks alcohol	66	19	0	0	49	81	82
Drinks over the recommended weekly limit	4	0	0	0	0	14	10

SOURCE: 1999 HSE (Erens, Primatesta, and Prior, 2001).

The second half of Table 18-6 shows differences in alcohol consumption. For both men and women, rates of drinking alcohol were highest for the two white groups, with equivalent rates for Caribbean men; slightly lower rates for Caribbean women, Indian men, and Chinese men and women; and low rates for Indian women and for Pakistani and Bangladeshi men and women (who are predominantly Muslim). This pattern is reflected in the measure of drinking more than the recommended weekly limit.

Given the overall pattern shown in Table 18-6, it is unlikely that the poorer health experience of ethnic minorities in the United Kingdom can be explained by differences in health behaviors.

EXPLAINING THE RELATIONSHIP BETWEEN AGE AND ETHNIC INEQUALITIES IN HEALTH

A Migration Effect?

One possible explanation for the patterning of ethnic inequalities in health across age groups that was shown in Figures 18-2 and 18-3 is that this is a consequence of differences between migrants and nonmigrants; that either experiences prior to migration, or factors related to migration, have led to poorer health for migrants, which consequently appears as the emergence of ethnic inequalities in health at older ages. This would also explain the appearance of differences at a younger age for the most recent migrant groups, Bangladeshi and Pakistani. The facts that the period of significant migration for many of these groups was relatively narrow (more or less a decade for most) and that migration generally involved specific age groups (young adults) make the separation of migration and age effects difficult. One possibility is to plot levels of health by age separately for migrant and nonmigrant groups; another is to focus on a group that has had a longer period of migration. Figure 18-4 does both of these, looking at age and reported fair or bad health for migrants and nonmigrants in the white minority group, the only group with a sufficient overlap in age between migrants and nonmigrants to make a graphic representation useful. The figure is striking in that it suggests that the health profile of the two groups is remarkably similar.

Although confounding with age cannot be easily adjusted for when the age profiles of the compared groups do not overlap to any great degree, a regression analysis can begin to unpack separate effects. In this case, regression analysis was used to explore whether age on migration and years since migration contributed to health risk independently of age for each of the migrant groups included in the 1999 HSE (i.e., Caribbean, Indian, Pakistani, Bangladeshi, Chinese, and white minority). No significant, nor large, relationship between age on migration or years since migration and reported fair or bad health was found for four of these groups—Caribbean, Indian, Bangladeshi, and Chinese. For the Irish and Pakistani groups, there

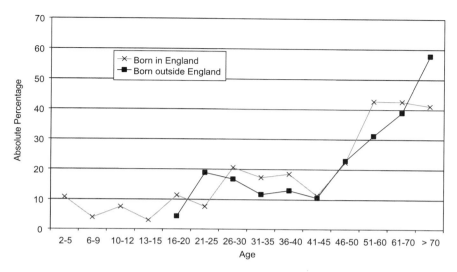

FIGURE 18-4 Fair/bad health by age and migration: White minority.
SOURCE: 1999 HSE (Erens, Primatesta, and Prior, 2001).

was a small but significantly increased risk of fair or bad health with increasing years since migration, which would be consistent with a health selection effect wearing off over time.

Although these findings are clear, their interpretation is not entirely straightforward. Those who migrate are a selected subgroup of the population from which migration occurs, and health may be significant in this selection. Those who are healthier may be more likely to have migrated in certain contexts (long distances and active recruitment into jobs), while those who are less healthy may be more likely to have migrated in other circumstances (short distances). If the latter were the case, we would expect the health of migrants to be poorer than that of nonmigrants. If the former were the case, we would expect the health of migrants to be better than that of nonmigrants. Furthermore, we might expect any health selection effect to wear off over time, with health becoming poorer as time since migration increases. Thus, the evidence of a deterioration in health with time since migration for Irish and Pakistani groups lends some support to the suggestion of positive health selection for them. However, previous evidence has suggested that Irish migrants were not positively health selected (Marmot et al., 1984), and it is not clear why Pakistani migrants would be positively health selected, but not Indian and Bangladeshi migrants. Therefore these findings should be interpreted with care.

An alternative interpretation is that if the process of migration itself, and experiences postmigration, led to a deterioration in health, we might expect the effects of positive health selection to be attenuated, and a pattern similar to that shown graphically in Figure 18-4 to appear; that is, the lack of difference shown in this figure, and in the regression analysis, might be a consequence of the competing drives of positive health selection and the adverse health consequences of migration. Thus the positive health selection effect becomes suppressed. This would then explain why evidence for positive health selection is only present for two of the six migrant groups studied.

Generation Differences

Despite the apparent lack of difference in health between migrants and nonmigrants, the process of migration to the United Kingdom has not been neutral. Ethnic identity is one dimension we might expect to be influenced by the process of migration, the experiences of second generation people, and the globalization of media. Work on ethnic identity, based on the FNS and using factor analysis, identified a number of potential underlying dimensions of ethnic identity, including one reflecting a traditional identity (Karlsen and Nazroo, 2002a). This included dimensions such as:

- wearing traditional clothes;
- speaking traditional languages;
- thinking of oneself as a member of an ethnic minority group;
- not thinking of oneself as British; and
- believing that close relatives should marry a member of the same ethnic group.

This dimension of identity correlated strongly with a number of demographic factors, including age at migration. However, after the inclusion of age, gender, and occupational class in a regression model, it did not correlate with health outcomes (Karlsen and Nazroo, 2002a). The implication is that a change in the strength of traditional ethnic identities is not an explanation for ethnic inequalities in health in general, and does not contribute to the emergence of ethnic inequalities in health at older ages. However, health behaviors appear to be strongly correlated with generation. For example, in the United Kingdom, first generation South Asian migrants have much lower rates of smoking than second generation South Asian migrants (Nazroo, 1998).

There are also economic differences between migrant and nonmigrant ethnic minorities in the United Kingdom. Evidence indicates significant downward social mobility for most postwar migrant groups (Heath and Ridge, 1983; Smith, 1977), and such downward mobility may have impacted on health. There is also evidence of a correction of some of this downward mobility for second generation ethnic minority people. This is illustrated in Table 18-7, which shows the proportion of men who are in a manual rather than nonmanual occupation, focusing on those of working age (16 to 65) and split between migrants and nonmigrants. It shows that

TABLE 18-7 Occupational Class by Country of Birth: Men Aged 16 to 65 (percent)

	In a Manual Occupational Class					
	Caribbean	Indian	Pakistani	Bangladeshi	Chinese	White Minority
Not born in England	73	53	64	77	50	43
Born in England	56	52	43	35	32	53

SOURCE: 1999 HSE (Erens, Primatesta, and Prior, 2001).

although there is no difference for the Indian group, for the white minority group migrants are more likely to be in nonmanual jobs, and for all of the other groups second generation men are less likely to be in a manual job than first generation men. It is worth noting that while the inclusion of men from all ages was necessary because of small samples with more restricted age groups, this leads to underestimation of the relative advantage of second generation men because younger men are more likely to be second generation and at the beginning of an occupational career.

Such differences may be very important. There is an extensive literature on socioeconomic inequalities in health and how these might relate to ethnic inequalities in health (Davey Smith, Wentworth, Neaton, Stamler, and Stamler, 1996; Lillie-Blanton and Laveist, 1996; Navarro, 1990; Nazroo, 1998, 2001; Rogers, 1992). However, most of this work has been applied across the population as a whole. The next section explores socioeconomic effects further.

Socioeconomic Effects

The process of standardizing for socioeconomic position when making comparisons across groups, particularly ethnic groups, is not straightforward. As Kaufman and colleagues (Kaufman, Cooper, and McGee, 1997; Kaufman, Long, Liao, Cooper, and McGee, 1998) point out, the process of standardization is effectively an attempt to deal with the nonrandom nature of samples used in cross-sectional studies—controlling for all relevant "extraneous" explanatory factors introduces the appearance of randomization. But, attempting to introduce randomization into cross-sectional studies by adding "controls" has a number of problems, neatly summarized by Kaufman et al. (1998, p. 147) in the following way:

> When considering socioeconomic exposures and making comparisons between racial/ethnic groups . . . the material, behavioral, and psychological circumstances of diverse socioeconomic and racial/ethnic groups are distinct on so many dimensions that no realistic adjustment can plausibly simulate randomization.

Indeed, an analysis of ethnic differences in income within class groups in the FNS emphasizes this point. Table 6.11 in Nazroo (2001) showed that while total household income adjusted for household size followed the class gradient for each ethnic group, within each class group, ethnic minorities had a smaller income than whites. Indeed, for the poorest groups—Pakistani and Bangladeshi—differences were twofold and equivalent in size to the difference between the top- and bottom-class groups in the white population. A similar pattern existed for other indicators of socioeconomic position.

One way of beginning to deal with this is to enter several indicators of socioeconomic position into the analysis at the same time. Figure 18-5 presents 1999 HSE data where this has been done for the total population. It shows odds ratios of reporting fair or bad health in comparison with the white English group, not adjusted and adjusted for several indicators of socioeconomic position. The natural logarithm of the odds ratio is used, so that the visible size of the difference is more meaningful. Adjustment for socioeconomic indicators produces a reduction in the difference between the ethnic minority group and the white English group for all except the white minority and Indian groups. For the Caribbean, Pakistani, and Bangladeshi groups, the reduction is large. These findings are consistent with other explorations of the contribution of socioeconomic position to ethnic inequalities in health in the United Kingdom, which have suggested that across ethnic groups and across health outcomes, socioeconomic in-

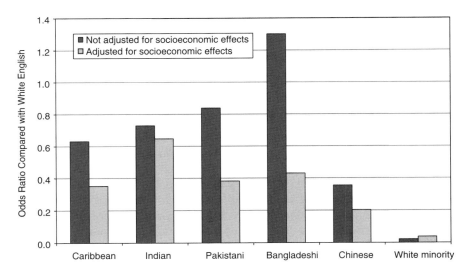

FIGURE 18-5 Odds ratio for reported fair or bad health compared with white English: All ages.
SOURCE: 1999 HSE (Erens, Primatesta, and Prior, 2001).

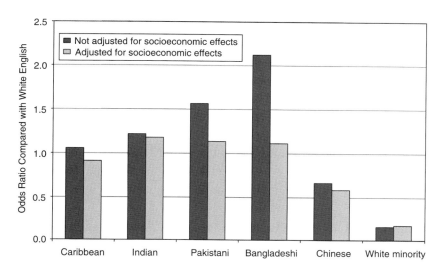

FIGURE 18-6 Odds ratio for reported fair or bad health compared with white English: Aged 50 or older.
SOURCE: 1999 HSE (Erens, Primatesta, and Prior, 2001).

equalities make a major contribution to ethnic inequalities in health, particularly for the poorer groups (Nazroo, 1997, 2001).

Figure 18-6 repeats the analysis shown in Figure 18-5, but for respondents aged 50 or older. Although the overall pattern is similar, the reduction in effects following adjustment is smaller for most groups.

Racial Harassment and Discrimination

Not all of the social disadvantage faced by ethnic minority groups can be summarized with economic variables. As described earlier, experiences of racism and discrimination are commonplace for ethnic minority groups in the United Kingdom. Furthermore, such experiences appear to be related to health in the United Kingdom, as well as the United States (Krieger, Rowley, Herman, Avery, and Phillips, 1993; Krieger and Sidney, 1996). Table 18-8, drawn from analysis of the FNS (Karlsen and Nazroo, 2002b), shows that reporting experiences of racial harassment and perceiving employers to discriminate against ethnic minorities are independently related to likelihood of reporting fair or poor health, and that this relationship is independent of socioeconomic effects. This may represent three dimensions of inequality operating simultaneously: economic disadvantage; a sense of being a member of a devalued, low-status group (British employers dis-

TABLE 18-8 Racial Harassment or Racial Discrimination and Risk of
Fair or Poor Health

	All Ethnic Minority Groups	
	Odds Ratio*	95% Confidence Intervals
Experience of racial harassment		
No attack	1.00	—
Verbal abuse	1.54	1.07-2.21
Physical attack	2.07	1.14-3.76
Perception of discrimination		
Fewer than half of employers discriminate	1.00	—
Most employers discriminate	1.39	1.10-1.76

*Adjusted for gender, age, and occupational class.
SOURCE: Fourth National Survey (Karlsen and Nazroo, 2002b).

criminate); and the personal insult and stress of being a victim of racial
harassment.

Age, Generation, and Cohort

How far the ethnic patterning of health described in previous sections
can be attributed to an aging process, the generation-specific impact of
migration, or contextual effects that vary across age cohorts is not clear,
partly because of the cross-sectional nature of available data. What is clear
is that ethnic inequalities in health in the United Kingdom widen with age,
but are present during early childhood. Such a pattern may be a consequence of an accumulation of risk across the life course, or the playing out
of childhood differences across the life course, with early "exposures" having an impact in early childhood that reappears in adulthood. The fact that
socioeconomic effects appear to be greater when all ages are considered,
rather than just older people, might be a consequence of this—contemporary measures of economic position may have less predictive value for
outcomes that are a consequence of early or accumulated socioeconomic
effects. So it may be that early life experiences are crucial, which in turn
may mean that it will take a few generations of upward social mobility for
ethnic inequalities in health at older ages to diminish.

The evidence presented suggested that the experience of migration,
either in terms of the event itself or longer term consequences, was not an
explanation for the emergence of ethnic inequalities in health at older ages.
However, this may be a premature conclusion to draw, particularly as
effects may have occurred alongside health selection into a migrant group,
with the subsequent suppression of any relationships at a statistical level.

Related to this, it may be that current context is important; that the
contemporary experiences of particular cohorts will determine differences

in health outcomes. Here changes in the economic position of second generation people in comparison with a migrant generation, which occur alongside other shifts, such as those in ethnic identity, may be important. It may be that we cannot predict future health experiences for younger cohorts on the basis of the experiences of older cohorts.

However, one context that does not appear to be changing dramatically in the United Kingdom is experiences of racial harassment and discrimination. The impact of this on health was briefly illustrated earlier, and shown to be a potentially very important determinant of ethnic inequalities in health.

CONCLUSION AND RECOMMENDATIONS

This chapter has raised, but been unable to come to clear conclusions about, a number of issues. How far is the growth of ethnic inequalities in health with age a consequence of aging? The implication of such a consequence is that the inequality is a product of prenatal events or those occurring in childhood (as the observed ethnic inequalities in health in childhood might themselves be), or the product of the accumulation of risk over the life course. In contrast, it might be a consequence of a specific generational effect—the act of migration and its consequences—although the evidence presented suggested this might not be the case. Of course, the experiences of migrants and second generation ethnic minorities are different, with the second generation having less traditional identities and being economically more successful. Such differences between cohorts might suggest different future experiences for younger ethnic minorities compared with the contemporary experiences of middle-aged and older ethnic minorities.

The historical pattern of migration to the United Kingdom means there is a close correlation between age, generation, and period of migration within ethnic minority groups, making it impossible to come to clear conclusions with cross-sectional data such as those reported here, even though we can use them to begin to explore possible explanations. Similar difficulties are likely to exist in other countries, and such difficulties require investment in panel data. While not a panacea, panel data will enable us to begin to sort out age, generation, and cohort effects, and the relevance of these for an understanding of population differences in health is great. The additional diversity in experience offered by studies of ethnicity, and the relationships among age, ethnicity, and health, will greatly strengthen our ability to understand the social mechanisms underlying inequalities in health.

However, it is important to recognize the overriding importance of national and historical context, and how this influences the lives of ethnic minority and migrant populations. Racism can be considered to be fundamentally involved in the structuring of economic, social, and health opportunities for ethnic minorities. At an individual level, experiences and perception of discrimination and harassment appear to be strongly related to health. At an institutional level, discrimination clearly influences the economic opportunities that people have, as well as the quality of health and social services that they receive. In addition, historically racism has fundamentally structured the construction of ethnic minority groups and patterns of migration at both an international level (when, why, and where to) and a national level (which locations, which industries). For example, Fenton (1999), building on the work of Eriksen (1993), has distinguished five types of ethnic-making or migration situations:

1. Urban minorities, who are often migrant worker populations.
2. Proto-nations or ethnonational groups, who are peoples who have and make a claim to be nations and to some form of self-governance.
3. Ethnic groups in plural societies, who are the descendants of populations who have typically migrated as coerced, voluntary, and semivoluntary workers.
4. Indigenous minorities, those dispossessed by colonial settlement.
5. Postslavery minorities: the descendants of (African) people formerly enslaved in the "New World."

Athough this typology might not be comprehensive, it does point to the different contexts within which ethnicity or "race" become mobilized to form distinct groupings. Implicit in the typology is that the differing processes listed will lead to different forms of racialization, of subsequent disadvantage, and to different historical trajectories for the groups involved. Understanding the process and the context within which ethnic groups are "made" should aid in understanding disadvantage and how disadvantage might develop. The value in international studies is that such processes have occurred differently across countries. Understanding how they are related to future trajectories for ethnic minority groups (across generations and cohorts) and individuals (over time) is important to any understanding of ethnic difference, including ethnic inequalities in health.

ACKNOWLEDGMENTS

Work for this chapter was supported by a grant from the U.K. Economic and Social Research Council under the Growing Older Programme, Grant Number: L480254020.

ENDNOTES

1. FNS (Modood et al., 1997) was the fourth in a series of studies on the lives of ethnic minorities in Britain, conducted by the Policy Studies Institute. It was a representative survey of the main ethnic minority groups living in Britain, together with a comparison sample of

whites. Topics covered included economic position, education, housing, health, ethnic identity, and experiences of racial harassment and discrimination.

2. HSE data will be used extensively in this chapter. The HSE is an annual survey conducted jointly by the National Centre for Social Research and University College London on behalf of the Department of Health. Interviews are administered to a nationally representative sample identified using a stratified sampling design. A follow-up biomedical assessment is usually carried out on the sample, which involves measurement of height, weight, blood pressure, etc., and taking a blood sample. The focus of the HSE shifts from year to year. In some years it takes a specific disease focus (e.g., cardiovascular disease), and in other years it focuses on particular population groups (e.g., children). In 1999 the HSE focused on ethnic minorities, providing much of the data shown in this chapter.

REFERENCES

Balarajan, R., and Bulusu, L. (1990). Mortality among immigrants in England and Wales, 1979-83. In M. Britton (Ed.), *Mortality and geography: A review in the mid-1980s, England and Wales* (pp. 104-121). London, England: Her Majesty's Stationery Office.

Battle, R.M., Pathak, D., Humble, C.G., Key, C.R., Vanatta, P.R., Hill, R.B., and Anderson, R.E. (1987). Factors influencing discrepancies between premortem and postmortem diagnoses. *Journal of the American Medical Association, 258*(3), 339-344.

Bloor, M.J., Robertson, C., and Samphier, M.L. (1989). Occupational status variations in disagreements on the diagnosis of cause of death. *Human Pathology, 30*, 144-148.

Coleman, D., and Salt, J. (1996). *Ethnicity in the 1991 Census: Volume 1: Demographic characteristics of the ethnic minority populations.* London, England: Her Majesty's Stationery Office.

Davey Smith, G., Wentworth, D., Neaton, J., Stamler, R., and Stamler, J. (1996). Socioeconomic differentials in mortality risk among men screened for the Multiple Risk Factor Intervention Trial: II. Black men. *American Journal of Public Health, 86*(4), 497-504.

Erens, B., Primatesta, P., and Prior, G. (2001). *Health survey for England 1999: The health of minority ethnic groups.* London, England: Her Majesty's Stationery Office.

Eriksen, T.H. (1993). *Ethnicity and nationalism: Anthropological perspectives.* London, England: Pluto Press.

Evandrou, M. (2000). Social inequalities in later life: The socio-economic position of older people from ethnic minority groups in Britain. *Population Trends, 101*, 11-18.

Fenton, S. (1999). *Ethnicity: Racism, class and culture.* Basingstoke, England: MacMillan Press.

Harding, S., and Maxwell, R. (1997). Differences in the mortality of migrants. In F. Drever and M. Whitehead (Eds.), *Health inequalities: Decennial supplement Series DS no. 15* (pp. 108-121). London, England: Her Majesty's Stationery Office.

Heath, A., and Ridge, J. (1983). Social mobility of ethnic minorities. *Journal of Biosocial Science, 8*(Suppl.), 169-184.

Hickman, M., and Walters, B. (1997). *Disability and the Irish community in Britain: Report of research undertaken for the CRE.* London, England: Commission for Racial Equality.

Karlsen, S., and Nazroo, J.Y. (2002a). Agency and structure: The impact of ethnic identity and racism on the health of ethnic minority people. *Sociology of Health and Illness, 24*(1), 1-20.

Karlsen, S., and Nazroo, J.Y. (2002b). The relationship between racial discrimination, social class and health among ethnic minority groups. *American Journal of Public Health, 92*(4), 624-631.

Kaufman, J.S., Cooper, R.S., and McGee, D.L. (1997). Socioeconomic status and health in blacks and whites: The problem of residual confounding and the resiliency of race. *Epidemiology, 8*, 621-628.

Kaufman, J.S., Long, A.E., Liao, Y., Cooper, R.S., and McGee, D.L. (1998). The relation between income and mortality in U.S. blacks and whites. *Epidemiology, 9*(2), 147-155.

Krieger, N., and Sidney, S. (1996). Racial discrimination and blood pressure: The CARDIA study of young black and white adults. *American Journal of Public Health, 86*(10), 1370-1378.

Krieger, N., Rowley, D.L., Herman, A.A., Avery, B., and Philips, M.T. (1993). Racism, sexism, and social class: Implications for studies of health, disease, and well-being. *American Journal of Preventive Medicine, 9*(Suppl.), 82-122.

Lillie-Blanton, M., and Laveist, T. (1996). Race/ethnicity, the social environment, and health. *Social Science and Medicine, 43*(1), 83-91.

Marmot, M.G., Adelstein, A.M., Bulusu, L., and Office of Population Censuses and Surveys (OPCS). (1984). *Immigrant mortality in England and Wales 1970-78: Causes of death by country of birth*. London, England: Her Majesty's Stationery Office.

Modood, T., Berthoud, R., Lakey, J., Nazroo, J., Smith, P., Virdee, S., and Beishon, S. (1997). *Ethnic minorities in Britain: Diversity and disadvantage*. London, England: Policy Studies Institute.

Navarro, V. (1990, November 17). Race or class versus race and class: Mortality differentials in the United States. *Lancet*, 1238-1240.

Nazroo, J. (1999). Ethnic inequalities in health. In D. Gordon, M. Shaw, D. Dorling, and G. Davey Smith (Eds.), *Inequalities in health: The evidence presented to the Independent Inquiry into Inequalities in Health, chaired by Sir Donald Acheson* (pp. 155-169). Bristol, England: Policy Press.

Nazroo, J.Y. (1997). *The health of Britain's ethnic minorities: Findings from a national survey*. London, England: Policy Studies Institute.

Nazroo, J.Y. (1998). Genetic, cultural or socio-economic vulnerability? Explaining ethnic inequalities in health. *Sociology of Health and Illness, 20*(5), 710-730.

Nazroo, J.Y. (2001). *Ethnicity, class and health*. London, England: Policy Studies Institute.

Owen, D. (1992). *Ethnic minorities in Great Britain: Settlement patterns*. (National Ethnic Minority Data Archive 1991 Census Statistical Paper No. 1). University of Warwick, England: Centre for Research in Ethnic Relations.

Owen, D. (1994). Spatial variations in ethnic minority groups populations in Great Britain. *Population Trends, 78*, 23-33.

Rogers, R.G. (1992). Living and dying in the USA: Socio-demographic determinants of death among blacks and whites. *Demography, 29*, 287-303.

Smaje, C. (1996). The ethnic patterning of health: New directions for theory and research. *Sociology of Health and Illness, 18*(2), 139-171.

Smith, D. (1977). *Racial disadvantage in Britain*. Harmondsworth, England: Penguin.

19

An Exploratory Investigation into Racial Disparities in the Health of Older South Africans

Debbie Bradshaw, Rosana Norman, Ria Laubscher, Michelle Schneider, Nolwazi Mbananga, and Krisela Steyn

South Africa is a middle-income country with a heterogeneous population. The achievements in transforming from its Apartheid past to a nonracial democracy have generated worldwide admiration that almost parallels the notoriety achieved previously for its constitutional racial segregation and exploitation. Structured around a population register of racial classification, the economy, social, and political spheres were mutually reinforcing in building a society steeped in racism and economically favoring the white minority elite. A legacy that South Africa now has to grapple with is an income distribution that is among the most unequal in the world and that more than half of the South African people, mostly black, live in conditions of poverty, with 11.5 percent in conditions of extreme poverty (United Nations Development Programme, 2002).

Currently totaling approximately 46 million, the people of South Africa have diverse origins. Ancestors of the Khoisan flourished in Southern Africa for thousands of years as hunter-gatherers. Around 300 to 500 AD, Bantu-speaking people moved south from West Africa, bringing Iron Age settlements to Southern Africa. Nguni-speaking people settled in the eastern part and Sotho-speaking people settled in the northern part. European explorers reached South Africa many years later and eventually established an outpost at the Cape to provide provisions for the passing sea trade in 1652. An ensuing struggle for land, resources, and political power occurred that involved the British, the Boers, the Xhosa, and the Zulu peoples as well as other smaller groups. The current population profile reflects this diversity, including people of Indian descent who were brought as indentured laborers to work on the sugar plantations or came as "passengers" to trade as merchants. There are 11 official languages, complemented by several other indigenous languages and dialects. The largest organized religion is Christianity; others include Hinduism, Islam, and Judaism. In addition, many people hold a "traditionalist" belief system. The rich heritage of South Africa has resulted in enormous cultural and ethnic diversity.

The complexities of race and ethnicity have been debated extensively by social scientists and are now to a large extent accepted as social and cultural constructs rather than biologically based. These debates have highlighted the fluidity of classifications by race or population group. The current population classification in South Africa is largely based on the practice of the national statistics office, Statistics South Africa, in its collection of demographic and other official statistics. The 1996 Census (Statistics South Africa, 1996) incorporated self-reported population groups: Black/African (77 percent), coloured (9 percent), White (11 percent), Asian/Indian (2.6 percent), and other (0.9 percent). These groupings have evolved from the 1950 Population Registration Act, which racially classified people and formed the basis of Apartheid in conjunction with the Group Areas Act (1950), which defined where people could or could not live and the Bantu Authorities Act (1951), which resulted in forced relocations. This population classification incorporated elements of descent and social standing. While "Black" was defined as "a person who is, or is generally accepted as a member of any aboriginal race or tribe of Africa," the category of "White" incorporated extensive social criteria and the category of "Coloured" was defined in the negative, as a person who is not a white or black. In a critical evaluation of the South African notions of race, West (1988) described these classifications defined by legislation as a "farrago of imprecision" (West, 1988, p. 103) that were far from being based on physical characteristics and concluded that South Africans cannot be categorized easily into the population groups, races, tribes, or cultures. He reiterated that the classification system "existed to divide and control in terms of access to political rights and economic resources and thereby maintain power and privilege" (West, 1988, p. 110).

The profound economic and social impacts of Apartheid and these population group classifications make it important to investigate the resulting inequalities in terms of health and other social dimensions. The 1996 Census reveals that household expenditures differed markedly by population group (Statistics South Africa, 2000). For example, 79 percent of white male-headed households were in the highest expenditure category, compared to only 5.8 percent of African male-headed households (Figure 19-1). Similar trends were observed for female-headed households. Unemployment levels also follow these racial disparities. It is estimated that in 1999, 25 percent of African men were unemployed and 35 percent of African women, compared with 4

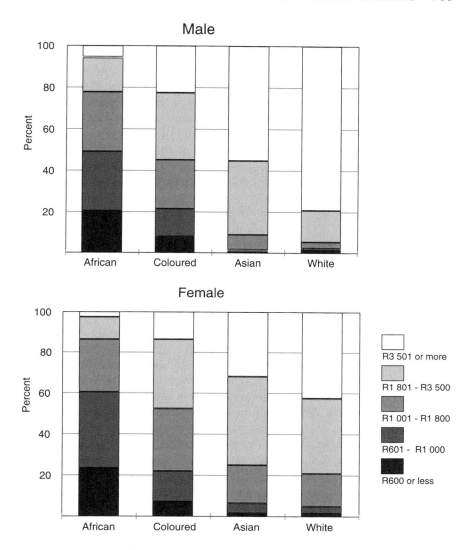

FIGURE 19-1 Monthly household expenditure by population group and gender of
household head.
SOURCE: Statistics South Africa (1996).

percent of white men and 5 percent of white women (Statistics South Africa,
2001b). These figures are based on the more conservative definition of unemployment, which requires that the respondent sought work in the past month
and unemployment can be considered to be higher. The figures hint at the
conflation of race, class, and gender in South African society.

The South African population is undergoing a demographic transition. The total fertility rate has been declining over the past 30 years and has reached a level of 2.9 children (Department of Health, Medical Research Council, and Macro International, 1999). The population is relatively young, with about a third younger than the age of 15, another third between the ages of 15 and 34, and the remaining third aged 35 or older. Just over 5 percent of the population was over the age of 65 at the time of the Census. Although Africans comprise the largest number of elderly, the proportions of whites and Asians who are elderly are larger than that for Africans and coloureds. The Census reveals that a large number of the elderly live in poor conditions. For example, 13 percent live in homes without toilets and 23 percent without running water (Booysen, 2000). South Africa has a social pension that is accessed on the basis of a means test. It is limited (parity purchasing power of approximately \$140 per month in the year 2002), but plays an important role in household income for poor families.

The absolute numbers of elderly can be expected to grow, and their health is of growing social concern. The general disintegration of family care and the lack of institutional care or support poses a threat to the well-being of the elderly. Furthermore, it is not clear how poverty aggravates the ill health of the aged, or how recent retrenchments are likely to affect their health. General unemployment puts added pressure on the old-age pension, with other household expenses, such as school fees competing for the money. There is mounting evidence of the added burden that HIV/AIDS is placing on the elderly, particularly Africans. Not only are they going through the emotional trauma of losing young members of the family and losing the economic support of their children, but they have the added burden of looking after orphaned grandchildren after having nursed a dying child.

This chapter sets out to investigate racial and socioeconomic differentials in aging health in South Africa. Data are examined to describe these differences in health and the prevalence of risk factors. The extent to which such racial differences can be accounted for by socioeconomic factors are then considered, allowing contrasts and comparisons with the situation in the United States.

HEALTH IN SOUTH AFRICA

Efforts to investigate racial disparities in health have been thwarted by the lack of reliable statistics, particularly mortality data. As long ago as 1945, the complete inadequacy of vital statistics for the "native population" (sic) was highlighted (Luke, 1945). For many years, this has been largely ignored. Attempts to extend death registration to Africans living in rural areas during the late 1970s were not successful and analysis of the available statistics showed problems such as underregistration and misclassification of the cause of death (Botha and Bradshaw, 1985). The category "population group" was dropped from the death notification forms in 1991 with the repeal of the Population Registration Act. However, since 1994, the new government has prioritized the development of a national health information system (Department of Health, 1997) and has initiated efforts to improve vital registration and conduct national health surveys. In addition, the importance of monitoring racial disparities has been highlighted and in 1998, a new death notification form was introduced that included population group and other socioeconomic indicators. Because the data have not yet been processed, it is currently impossible to investigate racial disparities in mortality based on vital registrations.

The first comprehensive Census was conducted in 1996 and the first national Demographic and Health Survey (SADHS) was conducted in 1998 (Department of Health, Medical Research Council, and Macro International, 1999). They have revealed clear racial disparities in health status; for example, the infant mortality rate for Africans was found to be 47 per 1,000, compared to 11 per 1,000 for white South Africans.

Although registration of child deaths remains a problem, the registration of adult deaths has improved markedly. Dorrington, Bourne, Bradshaw, Laubscher, and Timaeus (2001) estimate that registration has increased from about 50 percent of adult deaths being registered in 1990 to more than 90 percent in 2000. Although death registration has improved, there is a time lag in the processing of statistics; 1996 is the latest year for which the cause of death statistics are available, but these do not include population group details.

Careful analysis of the available cause of death information suggests that the South African population is undergoing a health transition with the coexistence of both poverty-related diseases, such as tuberculosis (TB) and diarrhea, with the emerging chronic diseases associated with a Western lifestyle. Furthermore, this has been compounded by high rates of injury and more recently by the HIV/AIDS epidemic, which spread rapidly during the 1990s (Bradshaw, Schneider, Dorrington, Bourne, and Laubscher, 2002). The SADHS showed that the previous downward trend in childhood mortality was reversed by the mid-1990s and Dorrington et al. (2001) showed that the age pattern of deaths of adults was shifting toward young adults in the late 1990s. The researchers concluded that the rise in mortality in young adults was largely from AIDS. Statistics South Africa, a government agency, had initially refuted the changing age pattern and then questioned whether the observed change could be attributed to AIDS alone. In a report released in December 2001, on the numbers of deaths for 1997 to 2000 (Statistics South Africa, 2001a), the agency also concludes that there has been a changing age pattern, with an increase in the number of young adult deaths. Statistics South Africa is currently undertaking a project to provide more updated cause of death information. However, it is clear that

South Africa is now experiencing a quadruple burden of disease: poverty-related diseases, chronic diseases, injuries, and AIDS.

The Actuarial Society of South Africa (2001) has developed a demographic model of the impact of the AIDS epidemic. The model incorporates estimates of population group differentials in mortality in 1985 (Bradshaw et al., 1992; Dorrington, Bradshaw, and Wegner, 1999) and the projected trend for the whole population (Dorrington et al., 2001). Assuming no anti-AIDS treatment interventions and calibrated to match the levels of HIV observed among pregnant women attending antenatal services in the public sector during the 1990s, the model is used to project a possible trend in premature adult mortality $(_{45}Q_{15})$ (see Figure 19-2). There is considerable

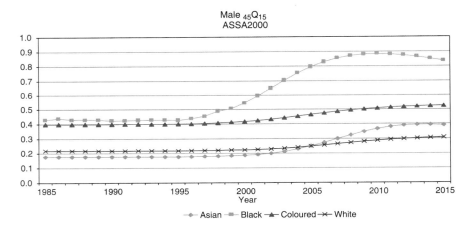

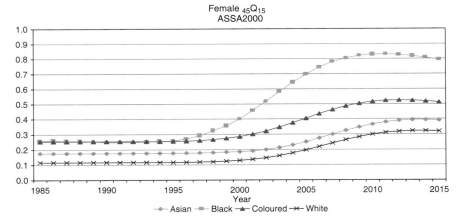

FIGURE 19-2 Projected trends in adult mortality, $_{45}Q_{15}$, based on ASSA2000. SOURCE: Actuarial Society of South Africa (2001).

evidence that the epidemic is having its greatest toll on Africans, but there is less certainty about the extent of the impact on other population groups. The projections are merely a best estimate and should be considered for illustrative purposes only. It should be noted that period estimates exaggerate the effect of AIDS mortality by cumulating the age-specific death rates, all at their highest levels. In reality, an individual is exposed to changing levels of mortality. While cohort estimates would reflect an individual's risk more accurately, it is nonetheless standard to use period estimates of life expectancy and mortality.

INVESTIGATING DISPARITIES IN THE HEALTH OF OLDER SOUTH AFRICANS

Clearly, the South African setting provides extensive scope for investigating racial disparities in the health and health determinants in aging. Data from 1985 show that the mortality for white South Africans 45 years and older was lower than that experienced by African and coloured South Africans (Figure 19-3). The mortality for Asian South Africans was between the groups with high levels of mortality in the oldest ages. The age-specific death rates and the ratios relative to white South Africans are shown for people aged 45 years and older in Table 19-1.

Unfortunately the data limitations severely restrict the opportunities to assess whether these differentials in mortality persist today and whether they can be attributed to differences in socioeconomic conditions. Analysis of the trends in the more recent mortality data suggests that the all-cause mortality in the elderly has not changed (Dorrington et al., 2001), but there is no information on population group differentials. However, making use of two new sources of data, this study aims to investigate population group differences in the cause of death profile among older South Africans and selected adult health indicators for a broader age range. The health indicators are explored for all adults because the sample size is more robust than that for older South Africans and they may reflect trends that extend to the elderly.

Toward the end of 1998, an evaluation of the new death notification form that reintroduced the collection of population group information was conducted by the National Health System of South Africa (NHISS/SA) Technical Committee on Vital Registration and described by Kielkowski et al. (2001). Although the study was designed to provide a nationally representative sample of deaths, the sampling procedures were not followed because of logistical constraints. The realized sample of 16,230 death forms spans the whole country, but because some provinces are overrepresented, the sample cannot be considered nationally representative. Although rates cannot be calculated from these data, by assuming that the bias is independent of the population group of the deceased, the data set can be used as a

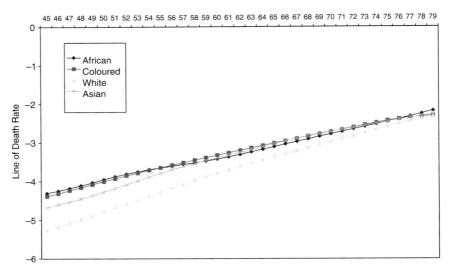

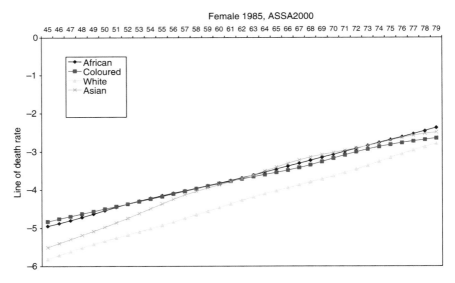

FIGURE 19-3 Death rates for males and females by population group for 1985 from ASSA2000.
SOURCE: Actuarial Society of South Africa (2001).

TABLE 19-1 Death Rates per 100,000 by Population Group and Death Rate Ratios Relative to White South Africans, 1985, Based on ASSA 2000

Panel A: Death Rates Per 100,000

MALE

Age Group	African	Coloured	White	Asian
45-49	7,481	7,076	3,128	5,347
50-54	10,527	10,138	5,112	10,728
55-59	13,357	13,968	8,281	13,556
60-64	17,072	18,772	12,783	17,430
65-69	23,055	24,758	18,719	23,589
70-74	30,622	31,932	26,466	31,331
75-79	40,523	39,040	36,457	41,619

FEMALE

Age group	African	Coloured	White	Asian
45-49	4,095	4,520	1,823	2,507
50-54	6,200	6,217	2,807	6,277
55-59	8,686	8,576	4,318	8,808
60-64	12,027	11,644	6,812	12,329
65-69	17,166	15,534	10,065	17,722
70-74	24,272	22,276	14,985	25,043
75-79	33,927	28,593	23,319	35,734

Panel B: Death Rate Ratios Compared to White South Africans

MALE

Age Group	African	Coloured	White	Asian
45-49	2.39	2.26	1.00	1.71
50-54	2.06	1.98	1.00	2.10
55-59	1.61	1.69	1.00	1.64
60-64	1.34	1.47	1.00	1.36
65-69	1.23	1.32	1.00	1.26
70-74	1.16	1.21	1.00	1.18
75-79	1.11	1.07	1.00	1.14

FEMALE

Age Group	African	Coloured	White	Asian
45-49	2.25	2.48	1.00	1.38
50-54	2.21	2.22	1.00	2.24
55-59	2.01	1.99	1.00	2.04
60-64	1.77	1.71	1.00	1.81
65-69	1.71	1.54	1.00	1.76
70-74	1.62	1.49	1.00	1.67
75-79	1.45	1.23	1.00	1.53

SOURCE: Actuarial Society of South Africa (2001).

case-control study to explore relative differences in the risk of death from a particular cause among people aged 45 and older. This has been done using a logistics regression to estimate the age-adjusted odds ratio and the 95 percent confidence interval for broad categories of cause of death for exploratory purposes. The profile of the causes of death for each population group is presented. Given the hugely different age patterns of the population groups, the proportions of the cause of death for each population group have been weighted to represent the average age distribution of all the deaths in the sample. Thus if the profile of causes differs merely because of the underlying age pattern, the weighted proportions will remove this effect. A fairly large proportion of the sample (77.8 percent) had population group specified, but the remainder (22.2 percent) had no details and could not be included in this analysis.

The second important data source is that of the adult health questionnaire in the South African Demographic and Health Survey conducted in 1998. Selected data will be analyzed in an attempt to sort out the relationships between health and population group, socioeconomic status, urban/rural residence, and education level. The survey did not include a full clinical assessment, but rather had selected indicators that could be measured by lay interviewers after special training. These included the measurement of peak flow, an indicator of respiratory pathology, and hypertension, a risk factor involved in the development of cardiovascular and other chronic diseases. The questionnaire focused, although not exclusively, on chronic respiratory conditions and diseases of lifestyle. For this analysis, the following health outcomes representing the spectrum of conditions in the health transition will be included:

- Peak flow, an objective measure that provides an indicator of respiratory disease (acute and chronic);
- Hypertension, an objective measure of a risk factor for chronic diseases;
- Ever had tuberculosis (TB) (self-reported), a common poverty-related disease;
- Smoking, a risky lifestyle and determinant of future burden in adult health (self-reported); and
- Incidence of injury (self-reported), any type of injury that was treated by a doctor or nurse during the previous 30 days.

An asset index for the sample has been developed using factor analysis based on living conditions and selected household assets (Booysen, 2001). This has been used to rank the households into poverty-related quintiles. In addition, the education level and the urban/rural residence are investigated. Some of these analyses have been presented elsewhere (Norman, Bradshaw, and Steyn, 2001; Steyn, Gaziano, Bradshaw, Laubscher, and Fourie, 2001), but not focusing on population group differences.

Logistic regression analysis was used to calculate adjusted odds ratios (ORs) and 95 percent confidence intervals (95 percent CIs) for males and females separately. The survey set option was used in the STATA statistical package (STATA Corporation, 1999) to take into account the complex sampling design that involved two-stage cluster sampling. A main effects regression model was used to assess the relationship with the mean peak flow, standardized for age, height, and weight (Department of Health, Medical Research Council, and Macro International, 2002). A multinomial logistic regression was used to calculate the relative risk ratios (RRs) and 95 percent CIs for light and heavy smoking compared with no smoking.

In the first instance, a model including only population group and age was fitted to obtain age-adjusted comparison between the population groups (Model I). This was followed by fitting a model that included the asset index quintiles, education, and urban/rural residence in addition to age and population group in order to investigate the independent effects of these factors (Model II). Membership of a medical aid (private health care insurance) was included in the models for self-reported injuries to allow for access to medical care.

CAUSE OF DEATH AMONG PEOPLE AGED 45 YEARS AND OLDER

In the 1998-1999 sample of deaths, there were 8,647 over the age of 45 years. The majority of the deaths in this age range were African (49 percent) while 15 percent were white, 12 percent were coloured, and 1 percent were Asian. Because there were only 109 deaths among Asians (over the age of 45), this group was excluded from the analysis. In this age range, there were more male (54 percent) than female (46 percent) deaths, reflecting the higher male mortality rates.

The profiles of the underlying cause of death for the sample are shown in Figure 19-4 by population group and gender. Although weighted for age to match the overall age distribution of the deaths, it must be reiterated that the sample cannot be considered nationally representative. The age-adjusted ORs of dying from a selected cause, comparing the white and coloured with Africans, are shown in Table 19-2, separately for males and females.

These ORs give an indication of the differences in the profiles, but not the absolute levels of mortality. It can be seen that the ill-defined causes of death have a higher proportion among the Africans than the white and coloured South Africans. (Ill-defined causes of death arise when the death is known to be from natural causes, but information about the conditions resulting in death is insufficient.)

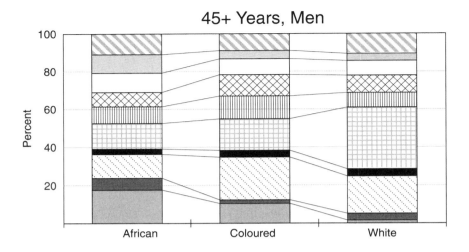

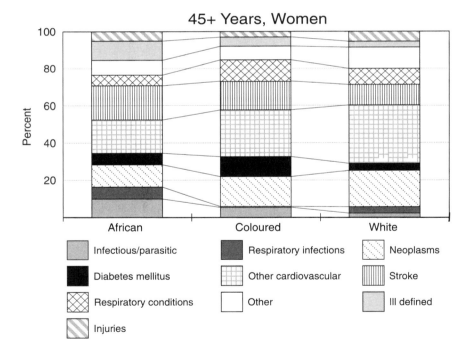

FIGURE 19-4 The age-weighted cause of death profile of the 1998 sample by population group and gender.

TABLE 19-2 Age-Adjusted Odds Ratio* of Death from Specified Causes for 45 Years and Older by Gender, 1998-1999

| | Men | | | Women | | |
Cause of Death	African N=2,290	White N=646	Coloured N=572	African N=1,886	White N=624	Coloured N=507
Natural—ill defined	1.0	0.30 (0.19-0.47)	0.45 (0.30-0.67)	1.0	0.23 (0.15-0.37)	0.44 (0.29-0.67)
Infectious/parasitic	1.0	0.08 (0.04-0.15)	0.58 (0.45-0.77)	1.0	0.24 (0.14-0.42)	0.58 (0.39-0.86)
Respiratory infections	1.0	0.57 (0.37-0.87)	0.29 (0.15-0.54)	1.0	0.56 (0.37-0.86)	0.09 (0.03-0.27)
Neoplasm	1.0	1.71 (1.35-2.17)	1.96 (1.55-2.45)	1.0	2.07 (1.59-2.70)	1.29 (0.97-1.71)
Diabetes	1.0	1.15 (0.71-1.89)	1.18 (0.79-1.97)	1.0	0.68 (0.44-1.08)	1.93 (1.37-2.73)
Ischemic heart disease	1.0	12.8 (9.19-17.76)	4.44 (3.02-6.51)	1.0	6.19 (4.34-8.84)	5.45 (3.75-7.93)
Stroke	1.0	0.82 (0.59-1.12)	1.29 (0.96-1.74)	1.0	0.55 (0.42-0.73)	0.84 (0.63-1.09)
Other cardiovascular	1.0	0.67 (0.49-0.91)	0.54 (0.38-0.78)	1.0	0.94 (0.73-1.21)	0.76 (0.56-1.02)
Respiratory conditions	1.0	1.06 (0.77-1.45)	1.50 (1.11-2.02)	1.0	1.45 (1.01-2.09)	2.19 (1.57-3.06)
Injuries	1.0	1.24 (0.92-1.67)	0.89 (0.65-1.23)	1.0	1.44 (0.95-2.19)	0.59 (0.34-1.03)

*95% confidence intervals shown in parentheses.
SOURCE: Adapted from Kielkowski et al. (2001).

In terms of profiles, it is clear that white South Africans were at much lower risk of dying from infectious diseases, such as diarrhea and TB, and respiratory infectious diseases, such as pneumonia, while they were at higher risk of dying from ischemic heart diseases, cancers, and diabetes than Africans. The risk of dying from stroke was significantly lower among white women than African women. When compared to Africans, the risk profile for coloured South Africans was similar to that of whites. In addition, compared with African women, the coloured women had a much higher risk of respiratory conditions such as asthma and chronic bronchitis. The relative risk of injury death was higher among whites, but this was not statistically significant.

RELATIONSHIP OF POPULATION GROUP AND SELECTED ADULT HEALTH INDICATORS

The 1998 Demographic and Health Survey has been analyzed to investigate the relationship between health and population group, having adjusted for socioeconomic variables. Figure 19-5 shows the mean difference in standardized peak flow for each population group relative to Africans, using Model I, which adjusts for age only, followed by Model II, which adjusts for the other socioeconomic variables as well as age. The approximate 95 percent CIs for the mean effect shown on the graph and the differences that are statistically significant are indicated with an asterisk. The standardized peak flow is in the form of a Z-score of the relative difference from the expected value for a given age, height, weight, and sex.

Figure 19-5 shows that the mean peak flow for white men is significantly higher than that for African men even after socioeconomic factors are taken into account. The peak flow for white women is significantly higher than that for African women, but this is not significant once the socioeconomic factors are taken into account. Figure 19-5 also shows that the mean peak flow for Asian women is significantly lower than that for African women, even after socioeconomic factors are taken into account. In the SADHS report (Department of Health, Medical Research Council, and Macro International, 2002), it is noted that there is a bias in the data, affecting the low peak flow readings. Measuring peak flow requires that the respondent be coached to blow with full effort. In an attempt to obtain accurate readings, the highest of three attempts is used. The fieldwork instructions required that respondents with a peak flow of less than 200ml be referred to the nearest clinic for examination. Analysis of the data revealed an unexpected concentration of observations just above 200ml. This could have arisen through misreporting of values by fieldworkers to avoid having to write a referral letter for the respondent concerned. Alternatively, this could have arisen through the fieldworker giving more encouragement

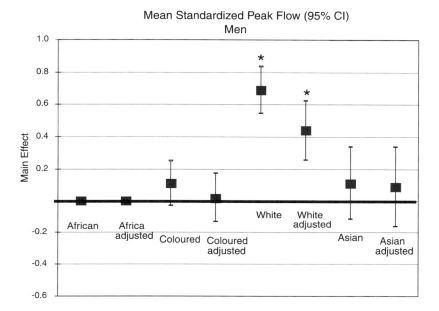

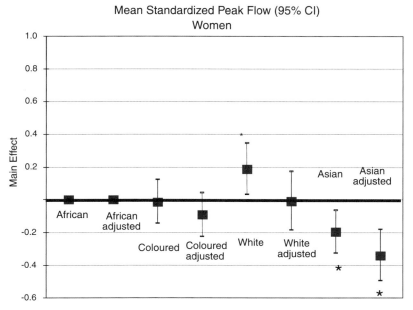

FIGURE 19-5 Comparison of standardized peak flow, adjusted for age only (Model I) and adjusted for other socioeconomic factors and age (Model II). SOURCE: Norman et al. (2001).

to the respondent when the readings were low compared to higher readings. Because women generally have a smaller physique than men and consequently have lower peak flow, the impact of this bias has a greater effect on the data for women.

Figures 19-6 through 19-9 show the adjusted odds ratios of the outcome for each population group relative to the African group using Model I and Model II. The first odds ratio is adjusted for age only, while the second odds ratio is adjusted for the other socioeconomic factors as well. The confidence intervals for the odds ratios are displayed on the figures and those that are statistically significantly different are indicated with an asterisk. Full details of the analyses are shown in Tables 19-3a through 19-5.

Hypertension is significantly higher among white and Asian men compared with African men using Model I, but the differences are not significant when adjusted for socioeconomic factors using Model II (Figure 19-6). The prevalence of hypertension is significantly higher among coloured and white women, but remains significant, even after adjusting for socioeconomic factors, only for the coloured women.

The results based on the self-reported information about ever having had TB diagnosed by a doctor or a nurse are shown in Figure 19-7. These suggest that white and Asian South Africans have been protected from having this disease, but when the other socioeconomic factors are taken into account, they are not significantly different. Coloured men and women had significantly higher prevalence of TB once the socioeconomic factors had been taken into account. Figure 19-8 shows that for heavy smoking, African men smoke significantly less than coloured, white, or Asian men, regardless of socioeconomic variables. African women smoke significantly less than women in the white and coloured population groups, and this population group difference is particularly marked with heavy smoking. For light smoking, no significant differences were observed between white men and African men after adjusting for socioeconomic status, but coloured and Asian men had significantly higher levels of light smoking than African men in the fully adjusted model. As Figure 19-9 indicates, self-reported incidence of injury in the previous month was significantly higher among white men and women once socioeconomic factors were considered.

DISCUSSION

This study is based on secondary analysis of data sets that were not specifically designed to answer questions regarding the health of the elderly, and the analyses have several limitations. The mortality data have the problem that the underlying cause of death was not known in a proportion of the deaths, and this varied according to population group (highest proportion among Africans). Furthermore, the lack of current mortality rates

TABLE 19-3a Racial Disparities in Mean Peak Flow Among Men, SADHS 1998

Demographic Variables	P-Value Model	Estimate	Standard Error	P-Value Estimate	Design Effect
Model I (R-square = 0.0339)					
Intercept	0.0018	−0.0110	0.0357	0.7588	1.75
Population group	<0.0001				
African		0.0000			
Coloured		0.1079	0.0718	0.1331	2.26
White		0.6896	0.0735	<0.0001	2.10
Asian		0.1095	0.1156	0.3448	1.91
Age	0.0018				
15-24		0.0000			
25-34		−0.0725	0.0498	0.1458	1.36
35-44		−0.1845	0.0553	0.0009	1.56
45-54		−0.1492	0.0691	0.0310	1.87
55-64		−0.2257	0.0810	0.0054	2.05
65+		−0.1993	0.0722	0.0059	1.56
Model II (R-square = 0.0484)					
Intercept	0.9292	−0.0468	0.1053	0.6566	1.80
Population group	<0.0001				
African		0.0000			
Coloured		0.0176	0.0775	0.8208	2.18
White		0.4385	0.0928	<0.0001	1.96
Asian		0.0868	0.1279	0.4974	1.99
Age	0.0404				
15-24		0.0000			
25-34		−0.0909	0.0501	0.0701	1.37
35-44		−0.1731	0.0545	0.0016	1.49
45-54		−0.1040	0.0702	0.1385	1.81
55-64		−0.1577	0.0855	0.0655	2.07
65+		−0.1085	0.0814	0.1827	1.68
Asset index (quintiles)	0.4220				
Poorest group		0.0000			
Second poorest		−0.0419	0.0643	0.5149	1.32
Middle group		0.0491	0.0692	0.4787	1.47
Fourth poorest		0.0491	0.0849	0.5627	1.83
Richest group		0.1250	0.0916	0.1728	1.57
Education	<0.0001				
None		0.0000			
1-7 years		−0.0551	0.0741	0.4570	1.61
8-12 years		0.1018	0.0764	0.1835	1.62
>12 years		0.3075	0.1006	0.0023	1.49
Geographic setting	0.0342				
Urban		0.0000			
Rural		−0.1207	0.0567	0.0342	2.13

SOURCE: Norman et al. (2001).

TABLE 19-3b Racial Disparities in Mean Peak Flow Among Women,
SADHS 1998

Demographic Variables	P-Value Model	Estimate	Standard Error	P-Value Estimate	Design Effect
Model I (R-square = 0.0044)					
Intercept	0.0236	−0.0030	0.0326	0.9275	1.59
Population group	0.0018				
African		0.0000			
Coloured		−0.0127	0.0679	0.8511	2.37
White		0.1885	0.0792	0.0176	2.92
Asian		−0.1952	0.0668	0.0035	0.89
Age	0.0018				
15-24		0.0000			
25-34		−0.0231	0.0448	0.6062	1.36
35-44		−0.0566	0.0481	0.2399	1.42
45-54		−0.1185	0.0557	0.0337	1.61
55-64		−0.1038	0.0557	0.0624	1.41
65+		−0.0697	0.0556	0.2871	1.83
Model II (R-square = 0.0162)					
Intercept	<0.0001	−0.0858	0.0830	0.3017	1.66
Population group	0.0002				
African		0.0000			
Coloured		−0.0908	0.0671	0.1764	1.92
White		−0.0062	0.0910	0.9460	2.29
Asian		−0.3378	0.0799	<0.0001	1.05
Age	0.8073				
15-24		0.0000			
25-34		−0.0187	0.0450	0.6779	1.35
35-44		−0.0191	0.0498	0.7007	1.44
45-54		−0.0533	0.0588	0.3651	1.61
55-64		−0.0030	0.0626	0.9619	1.54
65+		0.0591	0.0740	0.4250	1.92
Asset index (quintiles)	0.8556				
Poorest group		0.0000			
Second poorest		−0.0063	0.0480	0.8957	1.06
Middle group		0.0188	0.0535	0.7258	1.23
Fourth poorest		−0.0356	0.0785	0.6507	2.06
Richest group		0.0261	0.0842	0.7564	1.75
Education	0.011				
None		0.0000			
1-7 years		0.0700	0.0552	0.2055	1.54
8-12 years		0.2012	0.0663	0.0025	1.98
>12 years		0.3058	0.0914	0.0009	1.57
Geographic setting	0.0021				
Urban		0.0000			
Rural		−0.1821	0.0589	0.0021	2.82

SOURCE: Norman et al. (2001).

TABLE 19-3c Racial Disparities in Hypertension (BP≥160/95 mmHg ± antihypertensive medication), SADHS 1998

Sociodemographic Characteristics	Men: Hypertensives = 704 Normatensives = 5,049		Women: Hypertensives = 1,280 Normatensives = 6,793	
	Odds Ratio	95% CI	Odds Ratio	95% CI
Model I				
Population group				
African	1.00	—	1.00	—
Coloured	1.18	0.87-1.61	1.75	1.33- 2.30
White	1.98	1.50-2.62	1.33	1.04- 1.70
Asian	1.60	1.04-2.46	1.40	0.99- 1.99
Age				
15-24	1.00	—	1.00	—
25-34	2.76	1.67- 4.56	3.29	2.10- 5.14
35-44	7.53	4.65-12.18	8.20	5.34-12.60
45-54	18.09	11.35-28.87	21.20	13.89-32.35
55-64	20.08	12.54-32.17	35.80	23.48-54.60
65+	29.90	18.45-48.45	43.00	28.58-64.70
Model II				
Population group				
African	1.00	—	1.00	—
Coloured	0.87	0.61- 1.25	1.40	1.04- 1.89
White	1.28	0.84- 1.96	1.23	0.87- 1.76
Asian	1.02	0.62- 1.70	1.08	0.71- 1.65
Age				
15-24	1.00	—	1.00	—
25-34	2.79	1.69- 4.61	3.41	2.16- 5.38
35-44	7.98	4.94-12.87	8.26	5.31-12.83
45-54	19.21	12.00-30.75	22.26	14.31-34.62
55-64	21.10	13.08-34.02	39.62	25.12-62.51
65+	32.74	19.91-53.86	48.27	30.72-75.85
Asset index (quintiles)				
Poorest group	1.00	—	1.00	—
Second poorest	1.14	0.78- 1.68	1.00	0.74- 1.35
Middle group	1.11	0.75- 1.67	1.00	0.73- 1.36
Fourth poorest	1.77	1.15- 2.73	1.33	0.94- 1.87
Richest group	2.20	1.35- 3.59	1.13	0.75- 1.72
Education				
None	1.00	—	1.00	—
1-7 years	0.99	0.70- 1.39	1.19	0.94- 1.50
8-12 years	1.19	0.84- 1.68	1.11	0.84- 1.46
> 12 years	0.75	0.43- 1.31	0.58	0.36- 0.92
Geographic setting				
Urban	1.00	—	1.00	—
Rural	1.06	0.82- 1.37	0.63	0.50- 0.80

SOURCE: Norman et al. (2001).

TABLE 19-3d Racial Disparities in "Ever Had TB," SADHS 1998

Sociodemographic Characteristics	Men: Ever Had TB = 188 Not Had TB = 5,539		Women: Ever Had TB = 196 Not Had TB = 7,848	
	Odds Ratio	95% CI	Odds Ratio	95% CI
Model I				
Population group				
African	1.00	—	1.00	—
Coloured	1.37	0.80- 2.34	1.69	1.05-2.70
White	0.19	0.05- 0.74	0.61	0.25-1.47
Asian	0.67	0.18- 2.40	0.17	0.02-1.19
Age				
15-24	1.00	—	1.00	—
25-34	3.10	1.54- 6.26	1.40	0.77-2.55
35-44	5.40	2.72-10.72	1.64	0.91-2.92
45-54	7.48	3.72-15.02	2.12	1.18-3.80
55-64	5.61	2.62-12.00	1.84	1.02-3.31
65+ years	7.02	3.48-14.18	2.59	1.43-4.65
Model II				
Population group				
African	1.00	—	1.00	—
Coloured	1.89	1.13- 3.18	3.05	1.80-5.17
White	0.50	0.13- 1.99	2.36	0.88-6.36
Asian	1.25	3.42- 4.56	0.51	0.07-3.67
Age				
15-24	1.00	—	1.00	—
25-34	3.12	1.54- 6.30	1.45	0.79-2.67
35-44	5.14	2.52-10.49	1.67	0.92-3.04
45-54	6.57	3.12-13.83	2.11	1.15-3.86
55-64	4.27	1.89- 9.40	1.74	0.94-3.24
65+	5.59	2.56-12.21	2.36	1.19-4.66
Asset index (quintiles)				
Poorest group	1.00	—	1.00	—
Second poorest	0.82	0.43- 1.56	0.53	0.33-0.83
Middle group	0.50	0.30- 0.84	0.43	0.26-0.71
Fourth poorest	056	0.28- 1.12	0.39	0.20-0.74
Richest group	0.38	0.17- 0.83	0.16	0.07-0.36
Education				
None	1.00	—	1.00	—
1-7 years	0.96	0.62- 1.49	1.35	0.85-2.15
8-12 years	0.70	0.40- 1.22	1.03	0.60-1.78
> 12 years	0.14	0.03- 0.64	0.59	0.15-2.30
Geographic setting				
Urban	1.00	—	1.00	—
Rural	0.80	0.47- 1.39	1.07	0.68-1.68

SOURCE: Norman et al. (2001).

TABLE 19-4a Racial Disparities in Light Smoking (1-14 tobacco equivalents*/day), SADHS 1998

Sociodemographic Characteristics	Men: Light Smokers = 2,051 Nonsmokers = 2,678		Women: Light Smokers = 780 Nonsmokers = 6,276	
	Odds Ratio	95% CI	Odds Ratio	95% CI
Model I				
Population group				
African	1.00	—	1.00	—
Coloured	1.80	1.46-2.22	11.77	9.08-14.26
White	0.41	0.46-0.67	3.50	2.33- 5.25
Asian	1.30	0.88-1.93	1.52	0.88- 2.61
Age				
15-24	1.00	—	1.00	—
25-34	3.70	3.01-4.55	1.66	1.15- 2.37
35-44	4.92	3.94-6.14	3.31	2.30- 4.76
45-54	3.14	2.41-4.10	3.63	2.50- 5.27
55-64	3.68	2.78-4.85	1.97	1.29- 3.00
65+	3.30	2.50-4.34	1.72	1.11- 2.64
Model II				
Population group				
African	1.00	—	1.00	—
Coloured	2.28	1.75-2.97	18.34	13.34-25.23
White	0.84	0.48-1.45	12.96	7.55-22.24
Asian	2.19	1.38-3.49	3.20	1.68- 6.11
Age				
15-24	1.00	—	1.00	—
25-34	3.84	3.11-4.75	1.47	1.01- 2.13
35-44	4.94	3.92-6.21	2.61	1.79- 3.80
45-54	2.91	2.19-3.87	2.54	1.71- 3.78
55-64	3.16	2.36-4.24	1.22	0.77- 1.95
65+	2.76	2.04-3.73	0.96	0.59- 1.56
Asset index (quintiles)				
Poorest group	1.00	—	1.00	—
Second poorest	0.77	0.60-0.98	0.88	0.59- 1.32
Middle group	0.57	0.44-0.73	0.99	0.65- 1.50
Fourth poorest	0.61	0.46-0.82	0.72	0.44- 1.17
Richest group	0.37	0.25-0.54	0.39	0.22- 0.71
Education				
None	1.00	—	1.00	—
1-7 years	0.88	0.68-1.13	0.65	0.48- 0.89
8-12 years	0.73	0.56-0.95	0.26	0.17- 0.38
> 12 years	0.35	0.23-0.54	0.16	0.09- 0.31
Geographic setting				
Urban	1.00	—	1.00	—
Rural	0.72	0.59-0.87	0.53	0.36- 0.77

SOURCE: Norman et al. (2001).

TABLE 19-4b Racial Disparities in Heavy Smoking (≥ 15 tobacco equivalents*/day), SADHS 1998

Sociodemographic Characteristics	Men: Heavy Smokers = 477 Normatensives = 2,678		Women: Heavy Smokers = 153 Normatensives = 6,276	
	Odds Ratio	95% CI	Odds Ratio	95% CI
Model I				
Population group				
African	1.00	—	1.00	—
Coloured	3.84	2.71- 5.43	49.67	25.02- 98.61
White	7.68	5.57-10.58	86.17	41.54-178.78
Asian	5.93	3.79- 9.28	2.73	0.76- 9.79
Age				
15-24	1.00	—	1.00	—
25-34	5.44	3.64- 8.12	2.70	1.23- 5.91
35-44	6.89	4.57-10.39	4.78	2.34- 9.78
45-54	6.42	4.14- 9.94	3.39	1.53- 7.50
55-64	4.77	2.94- 7.75	3.27	1.52- 7.05
65+	4.48	2.68- 7.50	0.93	0.26- 3.31
Model II				
Population group				
African	1.00	—	1.00	—
Coloured	3.81	2.57- 5.61	49.32	21.59-112.67
White	10.04	5.95-16.93	161.46	62.82-414.97
Asian	6.17	3.64-10.48	3.09	0.81- 11.79
Age				
15-24	1.00	—	1.00	—
25-34	5.80	3.85- 8.76	2.71	1.22- 6.05
35-44	7.21	4.78-10.87	4.66	2.19- 9.92
45-54	6.33	4.07- 9.85	2.95	1.36- 6.41
55-64	4.57	2.71- 7.69	2.57	1.15- 5.75
65+	4.29	2.45- 7.54	0.68	0.19- 2.53
Asset index (quintiles)				
Poorest group	1.00	—	1.00	—
Second poorest	1.11	0.60- 2.06	0.48	0.11- 2.13
Middle group	0.64	0.33- 1.21	0.73	0.18- 3.01
Fourth poorest	0.86	0.45- 1.66	1.07	0.25- 4.54
Richest group	0.79	0.38- 1.64	0.79	0.18- 3.55
Education				
None	1.00	—	1.00	—
1-7 years	0.99	0.62- 1.59	0.51	0.21- 1.27
8-12 years	0.82	0.49- 1.36	0.26	0.10- 0.66
> 12 years	0.42	0.20- 0.85	0.09	0.03- 0.27
Geographic setting				
Urban	1.00	—	1.00	—
Rural	0.62	0.42- 0.93	0.68	0.18- 2.55

SOURCE: Norman et al. (2001).

TABLE 19-5 Racial Disparities in Self-Report Injury in Past Month, SADHS 1998

Sociodemographic Characteristics	Men: Injured = 80 Not Injured = 5,673		Women: Injured = 95 Not Injured = 7,978	
	Odds Ratio	95% CI	Odds Ratio	95% CI
Model I				
Population group				
African	1.00	—	1.00	—
Coloured	0.69	0.28- 1.66	1.67	0.76- 3.67
White	1.58	0.54- 4.63	2.49	0.85- 7.33
Asian	0.53	0.11- 2.48	0.79	0.11- 5.82
Age				
15-24	1.00	—	1.00	—
25-34	1.55	0.51- 4.71	0.76	0.33- 1.76
35-44	2.10	0.88- 5.02	0.90	0.51- 1.57
45-54	2.22	0.87- 5.66	1.07	0.58- 1.98
55-64	1.81	0.65- 5.03	0.79	0.30- 2.08
65+	0.97	0.24- 3.89	1.04	0.50- 2.17
Medical Aid				
Yes	1.00		1.00	
No	0.91	0.42- 2.00	0.96	0.43- 2.15
Model II				
Population group				
African	1.00	—	1.00	—
Coloured	0.92	0.37- 2.29	1.97	0.85- 4.58
White	3.24	1.08- 9.78	5.17	1.71-15.64
Asian	0.84	0.18- 3.96	1.33	0.18- 9.54
Age				
15-24	1.00	—	1.00	—
25-34	1.56	0.53- 4.60	0.73	0.31- 1.70
35-44	2.31	0.96- 5.54	0.83	0.46- 1.51
45-54	2.71	0.99- 7.40	1.00	0.49- 2.05
55-64	2.36	0.73- 7.67	0.79	0.32- 1.98
65+	1.49	0.31- 7.02	1.02	0.43- 2.41
Medical aid				
Yes	1.00		1.00	
No	0.74	0.31- 1.76	0.82	0.35- 1.94
Asset index (quintiles)				
Poorest group	1.00	—	1.00	—
Second poorest	1.12	0.35- 3.57	2.63	0.85- 8.13
Middle group	0.69	0.20- 2.37	2.09	0.59- 7.44
Fourth poorest	0.55	0.18- 1.64	1.62	0.44- 5.93
Richest group	0.22	0.06- 0.81	0.63	0.16- 2.45
Education				
None	1.00	—	1.00	—
1-7 years	2.89	0.86- 9.69	1.31	0.54- 3.16
8-12 years	3.65	1.04-12.88	0.90	0.31- 2.63
> 12 years	1.20	0.20- 7.07	0.75	0.16- 3.40
Geographic setting				
Urban	1.00	—	1.00	—
Rural	0.40	0.18- 0.88	0.37	0.14- 0.99

SOURCE: Norman et al. (2001).

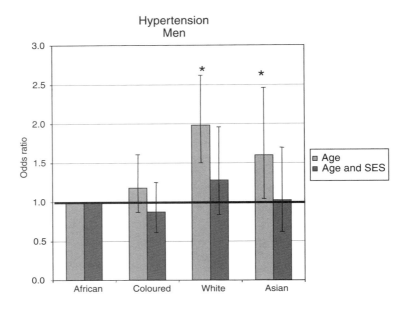

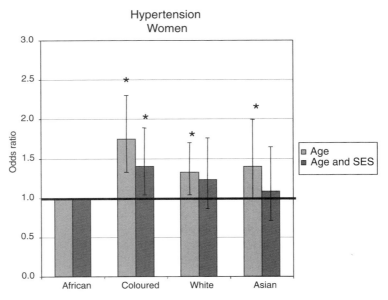

FIGURE 19-6 Comparison of odds ratio for hypertension, adjusted for age only (Model I) and other socioeconomic factors and age (Model II).
SOURCE: Norman et al. (2001).

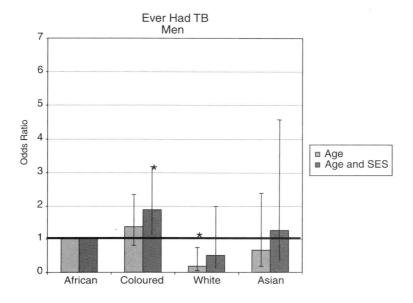

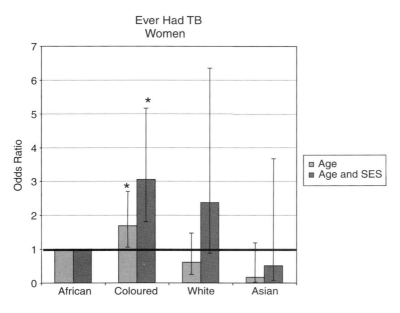

FIGURE 19-7 Comparison of odds ratio for "ever had TB" adjusted for age only (Model I) and other socioeconomic factors and age (Model II).
SOURCE: Norman et al. (2001).

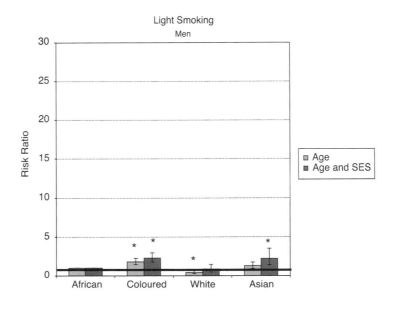

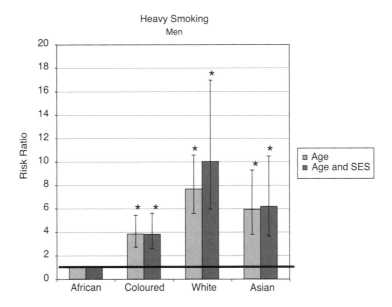

FIGURE 19-8 Comparison of odds ratio for light and heavy smoking, adjusted for age only (Model I) and other socioeconomic factors and age (Model II).
SOURCE: Norman et al. (2001).

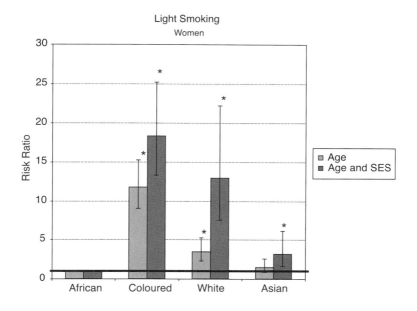

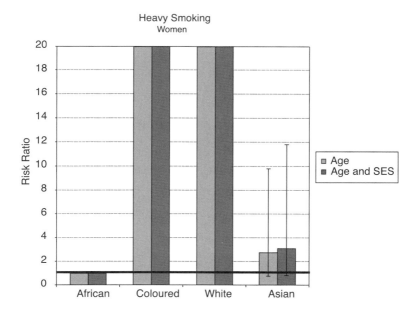

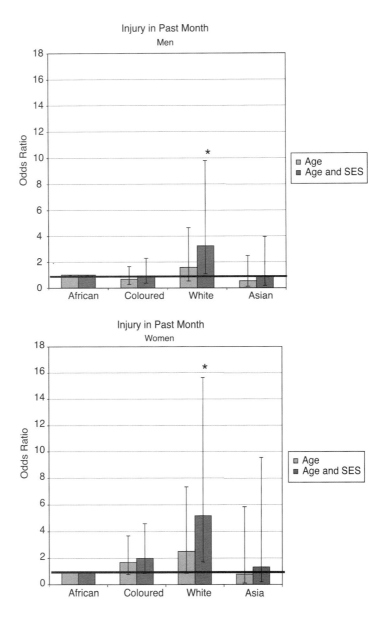

FIGURE 19-9 Comparison of odds ratio for self-reported injury in the past month, adjusted for age only (Model I) and other socioeconomic factors and age (Model II). SOURCE: Norman et al. (2001).

limits the analysis to a comparison of the cause of death patterns experienced by the population groups. The Demographic and Health Survey is a cross-sectional study with consequent limits on analyses. Nevertheless, the discussion attempts to consolidate the findings that have been observed through these exploratory analyses.

Whether the higher mortality of Africans and coloureds has persisted over the past 15 years is unclear. However, the current cause of death profile suggests that the population groups remain at different stages of the health transition with Africans affected more by the infectious diseases and coloured and white South Africans affected more by noncommunicable diseases. This pattern would tend to suggest that the differences in mortality rates have persisted.

The mean standardized peak flow for white men and women was significantly higher than for African men and women. This would be consistent with a lower mortality experienced by whites. The peak flow of the other population groups was not significantly different, with the exception of Asian women, who had a lower peak flow. This may result from the higher prevalence of underweight among this group of women, but also could be related to the upward bias observed in the lower peak flow values that occurred as a result of the fieldwork requirements. Although this upward bias did not affect large numbers of observations, it affected the results for women more than for men due to the smaller body size of women.

For peak flow, the difference between white and African men remained significant even after the socioeconomic factors were considered. However, for women, the difference between whites and Africans was no longer significant, while the difference with Asians was even greater. Without additional information from other studies, drawing conclusions is difficult.

The hypertension patterns are particularly interesting. Although the prevalence was lower among Africans, in general, this effect was removed when socioeconomic factors were taken into account. The exception is for coloured women, who had significantly higher prevalence than African women. This is likely to be associated with other determinants of hypertension; in particular, the somewhat higher use of alcohol among coloured women could play a role.

Cooper, Rotimi, and Ward (1999) note that although 25 percent of all Americans are hypertensive, 35 percent of black Americans have hypertension. Furthermore, the disease is particularly virulent for black Americans, accounting for 20 percent of their deaths—double the figure for whites in the United States. These authors suggest that in order to understand this phenomenon, conventional hypotheses concerning race should be abandoned. Instead, it should be acknowledged that hypertension arises through different pathways and involves complex interactions among external factors and internal physiology. The external factors include diet and/or stress. Many Americans have known behavioral risk factors for hypertension, such as obesity, high salt intake, long-term psychological stress, alcohol abuse, and a sedentary lifestyle. The internal physiology includes biological systems that regulate blood pressure as well as the genes involved in controlling blood pressure. Genetic factors have been determined to account for 25 to 40 percent of the variability in blood pressure among people, and as many as 10 to 15 genes can play a role in this variation. In addition, the environmental influences necessary to result in the expression of these hypertension-causing traits are essential. An individual with a given mix of alleles may be susceptible to high blood pressure, but hypertension will only develop for these people when exposed to a specific setting.

Studying the African diaspora is invaluable for evaluating changing environmental and social effects on the expression of the disease in the African population. In Cooper, Rotimi, and Ward's study (1999), the American and Jamaican blacks shared on average of 75 percent of their genetic heritage with the Nigerians, the other participating group. The investigators found that the incidence of hypertension drops dramatically from America across the Atlantic to Africa. The greatest difference was between urban African Americans (33 percent) and rural Nigerians (7 percent), and Jamaicans were in between at 26 percent.

Cooper et al. (1999) suggest that race does not explain why hypertension is so high in African Americans. Race is not the underlying cause. Instead, racial designation is but a proxy measure for other variables such as socioeconomic status. The findings in our study would tend to confirm their observations that race is not a determinant of hypertension. However, in South Africa, hypertension is associated with increasing socioeconomic status, while in the United States, hypertension appears to be associated with disadvantage. This can be explained by the fact that socioeconomic status has been used on a relative scale within each country. The average gross domestic product, an indicator of economic wealth, in the United States is somewhat higher than the average in South Africa. In 2000 it was PPP $34,142 in the United States compared with PPP $9,401 in South Africa (United Nations Development Programme, 2002). Furthermore, the range and distribution of socioeconomic conditions differ enormously between these countries.

Popkin (2001) has developed a model of the nutrition transition of societies in different stages of development. Starting with a pattern based on hunting and gathering (collecting food) and moving into a deficient diet (famine), passing through an adequate diet (receding famine) and moving into a stage of overnutrition (nutrition-related noncommunicable disease), the final stage is one of a "healthy alternative" (behavioral change). The determinants of this transition also affect other lifestyles that would be related to hypertension, such as physical activity and alcohol use. The contrasting relationships between hypertension and socioeconomic status seen in South Africa and the United States can be explained in terms of the Popkin model that South Africa is in an earlier stage of development than the United States.

The differences in tobacco smoking in South Africa persist even after socioeconomic factors have been taken into account, suggesting that cultural factors also play a role in determining smoking patterns in South Africa. This highlights the complexities of an investigation into racial disparities in health where race is not only a proxy measure of socioeconomic status, but includes a cultural/ethnic dimension.

The findings regarding injuries are difficult to interpret. The higher incidence of self-reported injury observed among the white South Africans in the Demographic and Health Survey could be an artifact of the subjective nature of the question and better access to medical care (despite the statistical adjustment for having medical aid/private insurance) because the definition of injury in this study is based on it being "severe enough to seek medical attention." The cause of death data from the 1998-1999 sample of deaths shows that the proportion of injury deaths was higher among whites compared to Africans (for people older than age 45). However, this does not necessarily confirm the observation from the Demographic and Health Survey because it provides no information about the injury death rate, and it may be possible that the rate for white South Africans is lower than it is for Africans. On the other hand, the pattern of self-reported injury observed in the survey correlates with reported alcohol use, a known risk factor for injury. Alcohol use was highest among the white South Africans (71 percent of men and 51 percent of women), followed by coloured South Africans (45 percent of men and 23 percent of women), Africans (41 percent of men and 12 percent of women), and Asians (37 percent of men and 9 percent of women), and would tend to suggest that cultural and lifestyle factors may play a role in the determination of injury patterns. Clearly, this needs further investigation.

CONCLUSIONS

This exploratory attempt to investigate racial differentials has highlighted both the complexities of the issues and the lack of longitudinal data. It does suggest that population group differences are likely to be confounded by socioeconomic factors as well as cultural factors that influence health outcomes through health-related behaviors. In the case of hypertension, interesting anomalous findings between South Africa and the United States can be explained by the fact that South Africa is not as wealthy as the United States. However, observations from both countries suggest that race is a proxy measure for other variables such as socioeconomic status and is not a determinant of hypertension per se.

Compared to many developing countries, South Africa can be considered data rich. However, this investigation reveals that there is a need for improved data to compile a more complete description of the differentials in health, in this case, for the older segment of the population. Once the death statistics, post-1998, containing the population group of the deceased become available, there will be more scope to describe the differentials and examine the relationships among population group, socioeconomic factors, and mortality. However, the mortality data will have limitations, making it timely to reflect on the issues that need to be investigated with a view to conducting more directed data collection for investigating racial disparities in health.

In terms of the well-being of older South Africans, we clearly face many challenges, and it is imperative to obtain more coherent information to monitor inequalities arising from the legacy of Apartheid and also new trends in health. Investigating the differential impact of AIDS on the older population will be particularly important.

REFERENCES

Actuarial Society of South Africa. (2001). *The AIDS and demographic model*. Available: http://www.assa.org.za/aidsmodelo.asp [accessed May 30, 2002].

Booysen, D. (2000). *Profiling those South African 65 years and older*. Pretoria, South Africa: Statistics South Africa.

Booysen, F. (2001). The measurement of poverty. In D. Bradshaw and K. Steyn (Eds.), *Poverty and chronic diseases in South Africa* (Medical Research Council Technical Report; pp. 5-38). Parowvallei, South Africa: Medical Research Council.

Botha, J.L., and Bradshaw, D. (1985). African vital statistics—a black hole? *South African Medical Journal, 67*, 977-981.

Bradshaw, D., Schneider, M., Dorrington, R., Bourne, D., and Laubscher, R. (2002). South African cause of death profile in transition: 1996 and future trends. *South African Medical Journal, 92*, 624-628.

Cooper, R.S., Rotimi, C.N., and Ward, R. (1999, February). The puzzle of hypertension in African-Americans. *Scientific American*, 56-63.

Department of Health. (1997). *White paper for the transformation of the health system in South Africa* (*Government Gazette*, 17910, Notice 667 of 1997). Pretoria, South Africa: Author.

Department of Health, Medical Research Council, and Macro International. (1999). *South African Demographic and Health Survey 1998* (Preliminary Report). Pretoria, South Africa: Department of Health.

Department of Health, Medical Research Council, and Macro International. (2002). *South African Demographic and Health Survey 1998*. (Full Report). Pretoria, South Africa: Department of Health.

Dorrington, R., Bourne, D., Bradshaw, D., Laubscher, R., and Timaeus, I.M. (2001). *The impact of HIV/AIDS on adult mortality in South Africa*. (MRC Technical Report). Cape Town, South Africa: Medical Research Council.

Dorrington, R.E., Bradshaw D., and Wegner, T. (1999). *Estimates of the level and shape of mortality rates in South Africa around 1985 and 1990 derived by applying indirect demographic techniques to reported deaths.* (MRC Technical Report). Cape Town, South Africa: Medical Research Council.

Kielkowski, D., Bah, S., Bradshaw, D., Cassim, M., Esterhuizen, E., Khotu, S., Mavimbela, N., Sitas, F., and Urban, M. (2001). *Evaluation of the New Death Notification Form (BI 1663)* (Final Report). NHISS/SA Technical Committee of Vital Registration. Pretoria Department of Health, Medical Research Council, and Statistics South Africa.

Luke, F.R. (1945). The National Health Service (Presidential Address). *South African Medical Journal, 19,* 18-21.

Norman, R., Bradshaw, D., and Steyn, K. (2001). Chronic diseases, risk factors and lifestyles based on the South Africa Adult Demographic and Health Survey. In D. Bradshaw and K. Steyn (Eds.), *Poverty and chronic diseases in South Africa* (Medical Research Council Technical Report; pp. 53-103). Parrowvallei, South Africa: Medical Research Council.

Popkin, B.M. (2001). An overview on the nutrition transition and its health implications: The Bellagio meeting. *Public Health Nutrition, 5*(1A), 93-103.

STATA Corporation. (1999). *Statistical software: Release 7.0.* College Station, TX: STATA Corporation.

Statistics South Africa. (1996). *The People of South Africa Population Census, 1996. Census in Brief.* (Report No. 03-01-11). Pretoria, South Africa: Statistics South Africa.

Statistics South Africa. (2000). *Measuring poverty in South Africa.* Pretoria, South Africa: Statistics South Africa.

Statistics South Africa. (2001a). *Advanced release of recorded deaths, 1997-2000.* (Statistical Release P0309.1). Pretoria, South Africa: Statistics South Africa.

Statistics South Africa. (2001b). *South Africa in transition: Selected findings from the October Household Survey of 1999 and changes that have occurred between 1995 and 1999.* Pretoria, South Africa: Statistics South Africa.

Steyn, K., Gaziano, T., Bradshaw, D., Laubscher, J.A., and Fourie, J.M. (2001). Hypertension in South African adults: Results from the Demographic Health Survey, 1998. *Journal of Hypertension, 19*(9), 1717-1725.

United Nations Development Programme. (2002). *Deepening democracy in a fragmented world: Human Development Report 2002.* New York: Oxford University Press.

West, M. (1988). Confusing categories: Population groups, national state and citizenship. In E. Boonzaier and J. Sharp (Eds.), *The uses and abuses of political concepts* (pp. 78-99). Cape Town and Johannesburg, South Africa: David Phillip.